Handbook of Sports Medicine:

A Symptom-Oriented Approach

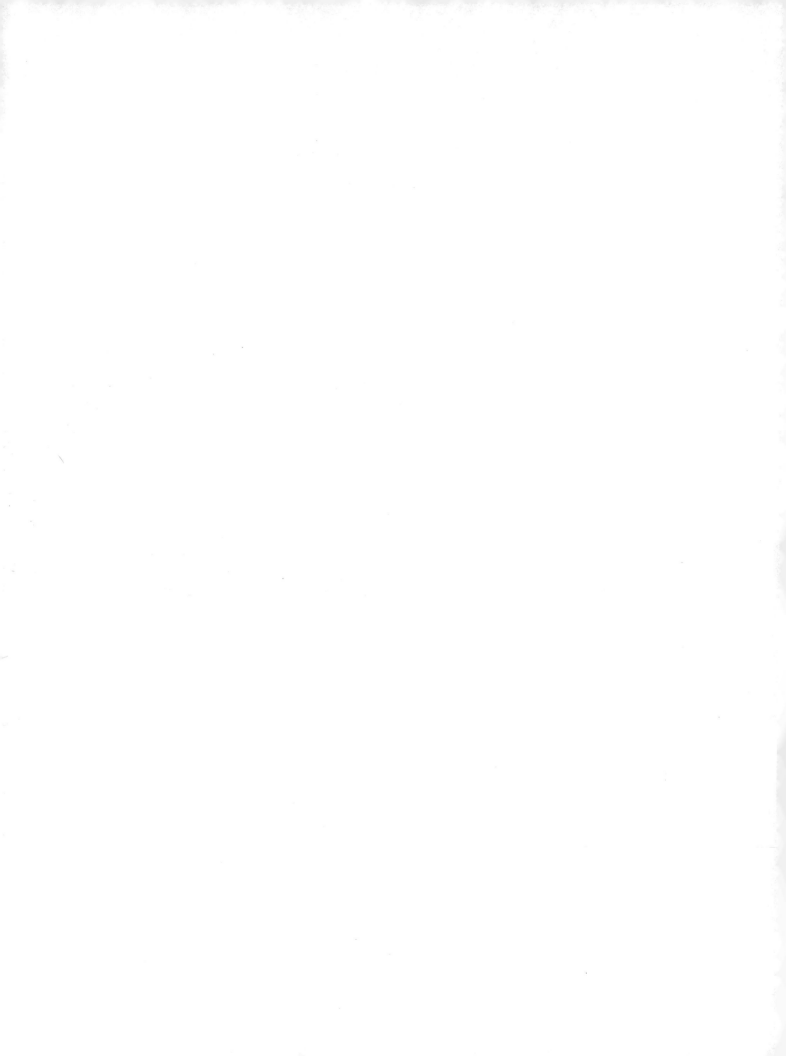

Handbook of Sports Medicine:
A Symptom-Oriented Approach

SECOND EDITION

WADE A. LILLEGARD, M.D.

Co-Director, Sports Medicine, Department of Orthopedics,
St. Mary's/Duluth Clinic, Duluth, Minnesota; Assistant Professor of
Family Practice, University of Minnesota—Duluth School of Medicine

JANUS D. BUTCHER, M.D.

Staff Physician, Sports Medicine, Department of
Orthopedics, St. Mary's/Duluth Clinic, Duluth, Minnesota;
Associate Clinical Professor of Family Practice, University
of Minnesota—Duluth School of Medicine

KAREN S. RUCKER, M.D.

Chairman and Herman J. Flax, M.D., Professor, Department of
Physical Medicine and Rehabilitation, Virginia Commonwealth
University School of Medicine and Hospitals, Richmond; Executive
Medical Director, The HealthSouth Rehabilitation
Hospital of Virginia, Richmond

Foreword by
KARL B. FIELDS, M.D.

Professor and Associate Chairman of Family Medicine, University of North Carolina
at Chapel Hill School of Medicine; Program Director and Sports Medicine Fellowship
Director, Department of Family Practice Residency, The Moses H. Cone Memorial
Hospital, Greensboro, North Carolina

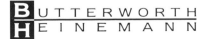
BUTTERWORTH
HEINEMANN

Boston • Oxford • Johannesburg • Melbourne • New Delhi • Singapore

Copyright © 1999 by Butterworth–Heinemann

ⓡ A member of the Reed Elsevier group

Every effort has been made to ensure that the drug dosage schedules within this text are accurate and conform to standards accepted at time of publication. However, as treatment recommendations vary in the light of continuing research and clinical experience, the reader is advised to verify drug dosage schedules herein with information found on product information sheets. This is especially true in cases of new or infrequently used drugs.

∞ Recognizing the importance of preserving what has been written, Butterworth–Heinemann prints its books on acid-free paper whenever possible.

Library of Congress Cataloging-in-Publication Data
Handbook of sports medicine : a symptom-oriented approach / [edited
by] Wade A. Lillegard, Janus D. Butcher, Karen S. Rucker. -- 2nd ed.
    p.   cm.
    Includes bibliographical references and index.
    ISBN 0-05-064041-0 (alk. paper)
    1. Sports medicine--Handbooks, manuals, etc. I. Lillegard, Wade
A. II. Butcher, Janus D. III. Rucker, Karen S.
    [DNLM: 1. Sports Medicine handbooks. 2. Athletic Injuries
handbooks. QT 29H236 1999]
RC1211.H36 1999
617.1'027—dc21
DNLM/DLC
for Library of Congress   98-26931
                                                            CIP

British Library Cataloguing-in-Publication Data
A catalogue record for this book is available from the British Library.

The publisher offers special discounts on bulk orders of this book.
For information, please contact:
Manager of Special Sales
Butterworth–Heinemann
225 Wildwood Avenue
Woburn, MA 01801-2041
Tel: 781-904-2500
Fax: 781-904-2620

For information on all Butterworth–Heinemann publications available,
contact our World Wide Web home page at: http://www.bh.com

10 9 8 7 6 5 4 3 2 1

Printed in the United States of America

Contents

Contributing Authors

Paul W. Baumert, Jr., M.D.
Clinical Associate Professor, Department of Community and Family Medicine, University of Missouri–Kansas City School of Medicine; Staff Physician, College Park Family Care Center, P.A., Overland Park, Kansas

B. Wayne Blount, M.D., M.P.H.
Vice Chair of Family and Preventive Medicine, Emory University School of Medicine, Atlanta; Chair of Family Practice, Crawford Long Hospital, Atlanta

Janus D. Butcher, M.D.
Staff Physician, Sports Medicine, Department of Orthopedics, St. Mary's/Duluth Clinic, Duluth, Minnesota; Associate Clinical Professor of Family Practice, University of Minnesota—Duluth School of Medicine

John W. Cassels, Jr., M.D.
Assistant Professor of Clinical Obstetrics and Gynecology, University of Missouri–Columbia School of Medicine

Mark A. Crowe, M.D.
Assistant Chief, Dermatology Service, Madigan Army Medical Center, Tacoma, Washington; Clinical Instructor of Medicine, University of Washington School of Medicine, Seattle

Stephen M. Davis, M.D.
Assistant Clinical Professor of Plastic Surgery, Vanderbilt University School of Medicine, Nashville, Tennessee; Plastic Surgeon, Centennial Medical Center/HCA, Nashville

John W. Dietz, Jr., M.D.
Orthopedics and Spine Surgeon, Orthopedics Indianapolis, Inc.

Ted Epperly, M.D.
Chairman, Department of Family and Community Medicine, Eisenhower Army Medical Center, Fort Gordon, Georgia; Associate Clinical Professor of Family Medicine, Uniformed Services University of the Health Sciences, F. Edward Hébert School of Medicine, Bethesda, Maryland

Timothy W. Flynn, Ph.D., P.T., O.C.S.
Assistant Professor, U.S. Army Baylor University Graduate Program in Physical Therapy, Fort Sam Houston, Texas

Robert C. Gambrell, M.D.
Assistant Professor, Department of Family Medicine and Department of Surgery, Center for Sports Medicine, Medical College of Georgia School of Medicine, Augusta

Arlon H. Jahnke, Jr., M.D.
Director, Orthopaedic Surgery Residency, and Chief, Sports Medicine Service, Eisenhower Army Medical Center, Fort Gordon, Georgia

Robert E. Jones, M.D., F.A.C.P., F.A.C.E.
Associate Professor of Medicine, Division of Endocrinology, Metabolism, and Diabetes, University of Utah School of Medicine, Salt Lake City

Daniel R. Kraeger, D.O., A.T.C.
Director, Primary Care Sports Medicine, The Sports Medicine Center, Stevens Point, Wisconsin; Affiliate Staff, Department of Family Practice, Saint Michael's Hospital, Stevens Point

Richard W. Kruse, D.O., F.A.A.O.S.
Clinical Associate Professor in Surgery, Uniformed Services University of the Health Sciences, F. Edward Hébert School of Medicine, Bethesda, Maryland; Clinical Associate Professor, Department of Orthopedic Surgery, Jefferson Medical College of Thomas Jefferson University, Philadelphia; Pediatric Orthopaedic Surgeon, Alfred I. duPont Institute, Wilmington, Delaware

John P. Kugler, M.D., M.P.H.
Assistant Clinical Professor of Family Practice, Uniformed Services University of the Health Sciences, F. Edward Hébert School of Medicine, Bethesda, Maryland; Deputy Commander for Primary/Managed Care and Chief of Family Practice, DeWitt Army Community Hospital, Fort Belvoir, Virginia

Wade A. Lillegard, M.D.
Co-Director, Sports Medicine, Department of Orthopedics, St. Mary's/Duluth Clinic, Duluth, Minnesota; Assistant Professor of Family Practice, University of Minnesota—Duluth School of Medicine

Thomas H. Mader, M.D.
Chief of Ophthalmology, Department of Surgery, Madigan Army Medical Center, Tacoma, Washington; Clinical Professor of Surgery, Uniformed Services University of the Health Sciences, F. Edward Hébert School of Medicine, Bethesda, Maryland

David J. Magelssen, M.D.
Clinical Associate Professor of Obstetrics and Gynecology, University of Washington School of Medicine, Seattle; Obstetrician/Gynecologist, St. Clare Hospital, Lakewood, Washington

Christopher A. McGrew, M.D.
Associate Professor of Orthopaedics and Sports Medicine and Family and Community Medicine, University of New Mexico School of Medicine and Health Sciences Center, Albuquerque

Mark Thomas Messenger, D.P.M.
Podiatrist, McDuffie County Hospital, Thomson, Georgia; Consultant, Orthopaedic Surgery Residency Training Program, Eisenhower Army Medical Center, Fort Gordon, Georgia

William F. Miser, M.D., M.A., A.A.F.P.
Clinical Associate Professor of Family Medicine, University of Washington School of Medicine, Seattle; Staff Family Physician, Primary Care Providers, Renton, Washington

Joseph C. Mulrean, D.M.D.
Private Practice, South Sound Oral Surgery, Olympia, Washington; Consultant, Oral and Maxillofacial Surgery Residency Program, Madigan Army Medical Center, Tacoma, Washington

Robert P. Nirschl, M.D., M.S.
Founding Director, Nirschl Orthopedic Clinic, Arlington, Virginia; Director of Orthopedic and Family Practice Sports Medicine Fellowship Programs in association with Columbia Arlington Hospital, Arlington; Associate Clinical Professor of Orthopedic Surgery, Georgetown University School of Medicine, Washington, D.C.

Francis G. O'Connor, M.D., F.A.C.S.M.
Assistant Professor of Family Medicine and Director, Primary Care Sports Medicine Fellowship Program, Uniformed Services University of the Health Sciences, F. Edward Hébert School of Medicine, Bethesda, Maryland

Carl O. Ollivierre, M.D., F.A.C.S.
Lake Centre for Orthopaedics and Sports Medicine, Leesburg, Florida

Jeffrey D. Patterson, M.D.
Orthopedic Surgeon, St. Clare Hospital, Lakewood, Washington

J. David Pitcher, M.D.
Assistant Chief of Orthopaedic Surgery Service and Orthopaedic Oncologic Surgeon, Madigan Army Medical Center, Tacoma, Washington

William O. Roberts, M.D., M.S., F.A.C.S.M.
Associate Clinical Professor of Family Practice and Community Medicine, University of Minnesota Medical School—Minneapolis; Private Practice, MinnHealth Family Physicians, White Bear Lake, Minnesota

Karen S. Rucker, M.D.
Chairman and Herman J. Flax, M.D., Professor, Department of Physical Medicine and Rehabilitation, Virginia Commonwealth University School of Medicine and Hospitals, Richmond; Executive Medical Director, The HealthSouth Rehabilitation Hospital of Virginia, Richmond

Wayne A. Schirner, D.O., M.P.H.
Deputy Commander for Clinical Services, Irwin Army Community Hospital, Fort Riley, Kansas

Gregory W. Sorensen, M.D.
Chief, Dermatology Service, Madigan Army Medical Center, Tacoma, Washington; Assistant Clinical Professor of Medicine, University of Washington School of Medicine, Seattle

Seth John Stankus, D.O.
Staff, Departments of Neurology and Family Practice, Dwight David Eisenhower Army Medical Center, Augusta, Georgia

Patrick St. Pierre, M.D.
Chief of Sports Medicine and Shoulder Service, Madigan Army Medical Center, Tacoma, Washington; Clinical Assistant Professor of Surgery, Uniformed Services University of the Health Sciences School of Medicine, F. Edward Hébert School of Medicine, Bethesda, Maryland

Gregg W. Taylor, M.D.
Chief of Orthopaedic Surgery, Tripler Army Medical Center, Honolulu

Richard Tenglin, M.D.
Staff Hematologist and Medical Oncologist, Womack Army Medical Center, Fort Bragg, North Carolina

Laura Jean Trombino, M.D.
Clinical Instructor of Orthopaedics, University of Minnesota—Duluth School of Medicine; Attending Orthopaedic Surgeon, St. Mary's Medical Center, Duluth, Minnesota

Monte C. Uyemura, M.D.
Site Coordinator, Wray Family Practice Residency, Rural Training Tract, Wray, Colorado; Staff Family Physician, Wray Community District Hospital, Wray, Colorado

William C. Walker, M.D.
Assistant Professor of Physical Medicine and Rehabilitation, Virginia Commonwealth University School of Medicine, Richmond

David R. Webb, M.D.
Co-Director, Sports Medicine, Department of Orthopedics, St. Mary's/Duluth Clinic, Duluth, Minnesota; Clinical Assistant Professor of Family Medicine, University of Minnesota—Duluth School of Medicine

Joseph F. Yetter III, M.D., M.P.H.
Director, Faculty Development Fellowship, Department of Family Practice, Madigan Army Medical Center, Tacoma, Washington

Foreword

Handbook of Sports Medicine: A Symptom-Oriented Approach, Second Edition, serves as a guide not only for team physicians and sports medicine specialists but for most primary care doctors. This book fills a special role as sports medicine increasingly has become part of mainstream medicine. Studies show that even for elderly patients, most dysfunction in aging relates to deconditioning rather than to the process of growing older. In 1989, a landmark study by Blair and colleagues pointed out the strong association of fitness level with longevity. Numerous studies have linked better physical fitness with improvement in conditions as diverse as hypertension, osteoporosis, and depression. As primary care physicians, our challenge to our patients is to awaken the athlete within them and to return to the precept advised in the seventeenth century by John Dryden:

> Better to search the fields for health unbought
> Than to fee the physician for a nauseous drought
> The wise for a cure on exercise depend
> God never made his work for man to mend

For children, soccer leagues, gymnastic classes, ice skating, and other sports often begin before entry into school. As patients become more athletic, however, they also increase certain risks. Foremost of these is musculoskeletal injury. This text provides a ready reference for appropriate differential diagnostic entities, the latest treatment advice, and a general guide to rehabilitation and return to sport.

Sport sometimes worsens existing medical conditions and occasionally triggers conditions, such as exercise-induced asthma, that relate closely to activity level. A general review of the major medical conditions and treatment modalities in the athletic population is provided as a guide. Treatment that not only expedites return to sport but also improves overall health care is the focus of these chapters.

Changes in the organization of sport have led to increasing numbers of participants involved in mass competitions. Whether for youth soccer tournaments, cross-country ski races, swimming carnivals, or road races, physicians have increasingly become the coordinators and planners for events that require medical supervision to ensure the safety of participants. Practical guidelines for performing these roles and handling exercise in environmental extremes are necessary for standard medical practice. Having up-to-date information about organizing medical care for major events allows the physician to become a resource for his or her community.

The editors and authors of *Handbook of Sports Medicine: A Symptom-Oriented Approach*, Second Edition, should be congratulated on assembling practical, timely information on injury, illness, and supervision of sport into one valuable text. The timing of this second edition coincides with efforts by the U.S. Public Health Service, the American College of Sports Medicine, the American Heart Association, and other organizations to encourage greater physical activity among Americans. The primary care physician will find this text an excellent resource in guiding care for the increasing numbers of participants in organized sports and for emerging athletes.

Karl B. Fields, M.D.

Preface

Physicians, athletic trainers, and physical therapists are confronted daily with a wide variety of injuries and medical problems in the athletes they treat. In a training room environment, approximately 60% of these problems are musculoskeletal and 40% nonmusculoskeletal in nature. The medical training of each of these varied health care providers differs significantly and is inherently deficient in some areas. Most athletic trainers and physical therapists have not been trained in medical management of asthma or cardiovascular problems, and many primary care physicians or nonorthopedic specialists have not had extensive training in injury evaluation and treatment, yet all of these providers are occasionally called on to address problems they have not been trained to handle in counseling or treating the athlete. As primary care providers to athletes, we appreciate the difficulty in keeping abreast of the numerous medical illnesses and injuries with which the athlete can present. The purpose of this book is to provide a reference that addresses both injuries and medical problems in a systemic manner, including initial assessment, evaluation, and treatment.

The book is divided into three sections: general considerations, injuries, and medical problems. The preparticipation physical examination chapter includes the most recent recommendations for performing the examination and practical guidelines on qualification for participation. The chapters on anti-inflammatory medicines and modalities succinctly review the appropriate use of these in the management of acute and chronic injuries. Because the athlete generally presents with a specific symptom, the sections of this book devoted to injuries and medical problems are based on these symptoms wherever possible. Algorithms are used in most of these chapters to help the practitioner form a quick differential diagnosis. For example, when evaluating an athlete reporting chronic posterior elbow pain, the reader can refer to the section on elbow pain, look under *chronic posterior*, and know immediately to evaluate for triceps tendinitis, olecranon impingement, olecranon bursitis, and olecranon apophysitis. Each of these entities is then discussed in terms of pertinent anatomy, pathophysiology, clinical findings, radiographic assessment, and treatment. If the athlete reports a rash in the groin area, the chapter on dermatologic problems will lead the clinician to categorize it as *papular/nodular* (molluscum contagiosum, scabies, venereal warts), *vesicular* (herpes), or *papulosquamous* (tinea cruris), and determine the diagnosis and treatment of each.

The symptom-oriented approach was thought by readers of the first edition to be quite useful in managing patients in a busy practice or training room. This format is maintained in the second edition, but a number of improvements have been made based on suggestions from these same readers. A chapter on mass-participation event coverage has been added, as many physicians are asked to cover these events with little background training or education. The author of that chapter is one of the nation's experts in this area, and he thoroughly addresses environmental considerations, personnel requirements, logistics, and necessary supplies. As the approach to back pain differs in children compared with adults, a separate chapter has been dedicated to this. Special considerations in the pediatric athlete have also been included in the other musculoskeletal chapters. The shoulder and ankle injury chapters have been greatly expanded as they tend to be common—yet frequently difficult—problems to evaluate. Finally, we have added more radiographs, figures, and tables to reinforce the text.

The contributors have again been selected based on their interest in athletes and expertise in their field, and they have continued to emphasize the primary care approach. We appreciate their efforts and think they have done a remarkable job in synthesizing a massive amount of information in a clinically useful format for the "front-line" health care provider.

W.A.L.
J.D.B.
K.S.R.

I

General Considerations

1

Preparticipation Athletic Examinations for the High School and College Athlete

CHRISTOPHER A. McGREW

The preparticipation athletic examination (PPAE) is the foundation for the health care system of competitive high school and college athletes. Millions of examinations are performed annually, requiring millions of health care provider hours.[1] Because of this large demand, the PPAE must be a rational and efficient exercise. Since the writing of this chapter for the first edition, a consensus document has been produced (the *Preparticipation Physical Evaluation* monograph, now in its second edition) that has helped to set a standard for these examinations.[2] This consensus monograph and the recent guidelines issued by the American Heart Association (AHA) concerning the cardiovascular examination[3] are the source of most of the updates for this chapter.

OBJECTIVES

The major question asked in the PPAE is "Will this athlete be at any *greater* risk of injury or illness than would normally be expected from participation in this sport?" Many other questions can be raised during the PPAE; these are discussed by various authors[4-8] and have been summarized in the consensus monograph (Table 1-1).

The PPAE is not a substitute for routine health care of the child or adolescent. Certainly, the PPAE could be incorporated into the routine health care maintenance examinations recommended by various health care groups; however, athletes and parents should be informed that the PPAE alone does not substitute for this routine preventive care. One study revealed that 78% of athletes examined in a PPAE believed that it fulfilled all of their health care needs for the year.[9]

TIMING OF THE PREPARTICIPATION ATHLETIC EXAMINATION

Scheduling the PPAE 4–6 weeks before the start of preseason practice sessions allows time for correction of any problems that are discovered, but the examination is close enough to the first practice session that many additional problems are not likely to occur. However, this ideal situation may be impractical for many school systems with limited resources and personnel. Additionally, it may be difficult to schedule examinations for athletes during the middle of the summer. PPAEs are usually scheduled sometime between the end of the school year in May or June and right before the fall sports season, regardless of whether the sport starts in the fall. For sports that begin later, the history since the last examination should briefly be reviewed by the trainer or coach before practice sessions begin. This is a useful way to help detect problems that have occurred since the last PPAE. Positive findings on this review should be referred to a physician for further evaluation.

FREQUENCY OF THE PREPARTICIPATION ATHLETIC EXAMINATION

At the high school level, state requirements vary greatly, although most states still require yearly examinations.[10] At the collegiate level, the *NCAA Sports Medicine Handbook*[11] recommends that an initial full evaluation be done on an athlete's entrance into the institution's intercollegiate athletics program. (This handbook is used not only by National Collegiate Athletic Association [NCAA] insti-

TABLE 1-1
Objectives of the Preparticipation Physical Evaluation

Primary objectives
  Detect conditions that may predispose to injury
  Detect conditions that may be life threatening or disabling
  Meet legal and insurance requirements
Secondary objectives
  Determine general health
  Counsel on health-related issues
  Assess fitness level for specific sports

tutions but is often adopted by non-NCAA institutions.) In subsequent years, a limited, focused history and appropriate physical examination based on positive findings should be done. It seems reasonable that this system would work equally well in the high school—that is, after the initial, entry-level physical examination is done, subsequent examinations should be focused, with a screening history and pertinent physical examination for the positive findings. These subsequent examinations should also include vital signs and visual testing. A specific cardiovascular assessment is recommended each year in the recent guidelines put forth by the AHA.[3] This specific recommendation was not incorporated into the *Preparticipation Physical Evaluation* monograph.[2]

A system of entry-level complete examinations followed by interim examinations in successive years will be successful only if medical records are available from year to year and are clearly understandable by the examining physicians. If these criteria are not met, it is probably best to do a complete physical examination and history every year.

TYPES OF EXAMINATIONS

The two most common methods of examination are (1) the individual office physical examination conducted by the athlete's personal physician and (2) the station examination, in which large numbers of athletes are screened during a single session using a well-planned and organized team approach. The athlete moves through an assembly line of "stations," in which multiple personnel (e.g., nurses, trainers, coaches, physical therapists, physicians) act as a unit to evaluate the athletes in a systematic fashion. There are pros and cons to both examinations.

The advantages of the individual office examinations are (1) the physician's knowledge of the athlete's past medical history; (2) an established doctor-patient relationship, ideally with good rapport for greater ease of

communication about sensitive subjects such as drug use and developmental concerns; and (3) greater continuity and follow-up if further evaluation is needed after initial screening.

Disadvantages of individual office examinations include (1) lack of interest or skill in the preparticipation physical examination on the part of some health care providers, (2) lack of consistency among individual examiners, (3) increased cost per athlete, (4) lack of interaction between the physician and school athletic staff, and (5) an athlete's lack of a personal physician.

The advantages of the station examination method are (1) lower cost for the athlete, (2) potentially higher rate of problem detection, and (3) greater consistency and efficiency of examinations.

Disadvantages of the station examination method include (1) loss of continuity of care and rapport with the athlete's personal physician (if the athlete has one), (2) less knowledge of past medical and injury history, and (3) difficulty in discussing adolescent health maintenance issues and giving preventive counseling.

Some features could be added to the standard station examination to make it more comprehensive. This could include a list of community health resources to which the athlete lacking access to regular health care could be referred (this problem is less frequent in the college student athlete population). A nurse or other health care provider could be made available to answer more sensitive questions privately and to hand out pamphlets on adolescent health care topics. The examination process should be tailored to local needs and resources and should result from group planning among all the personnel involved.

CONTENT OF THE PREPARTICIPATION ATHLETIC EXAMINATION

At the high school level, there are currently no national standards for PPAEs.[10] It is wise to discuss the local rules and regulations concerning the PPAE with local school officials, including principals, athletic directors, and school health personnel.

At the collegiate level, the *NCAA Sports Medicine Handbook* does list some guidelines.[11] There is a wide variation between NCAA schools as to how extensive the PPAE is. Additionally, one must look at the collegiate level as somewhat different from the traditional community high school. In many cases, college-level athletes are in a "boarding school" situation in which they are away from home and their primary care physicians. The sports medicine team may be providing primary care throughout the 4–5 years of athletic competition for these athletes. In these cases, more extensive evaluation and counseling with the PPAE may be necessary.

In general, the PPAE is composed of a focused history that can be covered in 10–15 questions. It also includes a focused physical examination that includes a comprehensive orthopedic examination and cardiovascular evaluation. It may include other areas, both within the history and the physical examination, as dictated by the needs of the individual athlete. The form should be relatively short and easy to fill out (Figures 1-1 and 1-2).

Health History

The health history is the cornerstone of any medical examination. It is particularly important in the PPAE, because approximately two-thirds of the findings in the PPAE are identified by the history. The health history should cover cardiovascular risk, previous musculoskeletal injury, previous neurologic injury, missing organs, allergies, chronic diseases, medication use, symptoms of exercise-induced asthma, special equipment needs, immunization record, and in females, the menstrual history. An example of a preparticipation history form is shown in Figure 1-1.

All athletes, especially minors, should be helped by parents or guardians to complete the health history form. The athlete and parents or guardians of minors should sign the form. After the form has been reviewed, it should be signed by the health care provider performing the examination. The importance of having both the athlete and the parents or guardians complete the form cannot be overemphasized; one study[12] showed that when separate history forms were completed by parents or guardians and athletes, only 39% of the forms matched. Additionally, the form should be reasonably brief and in language that is easy to understand (sixth-grade reading level). Finally, the history is not foolproof. In one group of athletes studied by Risser and colleagues,[13] one-third were referred for orthopedic problems. None of these problems had been mentioned on the history form despite the athlete's awareness of the problem.

Cardiovascular History

The most common causes of sudden cardiovascular death in young athletes younger than 35 years of age are hypertrophic cardiomyopathy, congenital coronary artery anomalies, and, less commonly, aortic rupture associated with Marfan syndrome and atherosclerotic coronary artery disease. It has been estimated that the frequency of sudden death in young athletes is approximately 1 in 100,000.[14] Because of this relative rarity, it is difficult to determine

the value of screening questions in detecting and preventing sudden cardiovascular death. However, a review of the histories of many athletes who died suddenly suggests that there is value in asking questions that might identify at least some of those at risk.[14] Such questions concern sudden nontraumatic death of a family member at an early age (younger than 50 years old), a history of syncope with exercise, and a family history of Marfan syndrome. Other questions about dizziness, chest pain, and easy fatigue with exercise are useful. It is also important to ask if there has been a history of high blood pressure or if the patient has ever had a heart murmur or irregular heartbeats (see the history form in Figure 1-1 and reference 3 for further detail). There is no foolproof system of identifying all athletes at risk, even with the use of extensive—and expensive—testing, such as echocardiograms and treadmill stress testing. Such testing is not recommended.[3, 15]

Musculoskeletal History

The history of musculoskeletal injury covers the most common problem area in the PPAE. A history of previous injury puts the athlete in a higher-risk group for an injury to that site, especially if rehabilitation has not been complete.[16]

Neurologic History

Neurologic history should include questions about previous concussion, loss of consciousness, seizures, and stingers or burners. A positive response to any of these questions should mandate a thorough neurologic history and examination. A return to play should be based on absolute lack of symptoms, full function, full range of motion, lack of sensory deficits, and full muscle strength. Liberal use of consultants is encouraged in difficult situations. A history of craniotomy is an absolute contraindication to a return to contact sports.

Physical Examination

Physical examination should focus on the cardiovascular and musculoskeletal systems. The examination should be guided by a sport-specific frame of reference as well as areas of concern in the history. An example of a PPAE form is shown in Figure 1-2.

Vital signs should be obtained: height, weight, blood pressure, and pulse. Vision problems should be screened for by the use of Snellen's chart.

The cardiovascular examination should be performed in a quiet area. The simple presence of a murmur is common, so the focus of the examination is to identify the murmurs likely to indicate disease process. Hypertrophic

Preparticipation Physical Evaluation

HISTORY

DATE OF EXAM _____

Name _____ Sex _____ Age _____ Date of birth _____

Grade ____ School _____ Sport(s) _____

Address _____ Phone _____

Personal physician _____

In case of emergency, contact

Name _____ Relationship _____ Phone (H) _____ (W) _____

Explain "Yes" answers below.
Circle questions you don't know the answers to.

	Yes	No
1. Have you had a medical illness or injury since your last check up or sports physical?	☐	☐
Do you have an ongoing or chronic illness?	☐	☐
2. Have you ever been hospitalized overnight?	☐	☐
Have you ever had surgery?	☐	☐
3. Are you currently taking any prescription or nonprescription (over-the-counter) medications or pills or using an inhaler?	☐	☐
Have you ever taken any supplements or vitamins to help you gain or lose weight or improve your performance?	☐	☐
4. Do you have any allergies (for example, to pollen, medicine, food, or stinging insects)?	☐	☐
Have you ever had a rash or hives develop during or after exercise?	☐	☐
5. Have you ever passed out during or after exercise?	☐	☐
Have you ever been dizzy during or after exercise?	☐	☐
Have you ever had chest pain during or after exercise?	☐	☐
Do you get tired more quickly than your friends do during exercise?	☐	☐
Have you ever had racing of your heart or skipped heartbeats?	☐	☐
Have you had high blood pressure or high cholesterol?	☐	☐
Have you ever been told you have a heart murmur?	☐	☐
Has any family member or relative died of heart problems or of sudden death before age 50?	☐	☐
Have you had a severe viral infection (for example, myocarditis or mononucleosis) within the last month?	☐	☐
Has a physician ever denied or restricted your participation in sports for any heart problems?	☐	☐
6. Do you have any current skin problems (for example, itching, rashes, acne, warts, fungus, or blisters)?	☐	☐
7. Have you ever had a head injury or concussion?	☐	☐
Have you ever been knocked out, become unconscious, or lost your memory?	☐	☐
Have you ever had a seizure?	☐	☐
Do you have frequent or severe headaches?	☐	☐
Have you ever had numbness or tingling in your arms, hands, legs, or feet?	☐	☐
Have you ever had a stinger, burner, or pinched nerve?	☐	☐
8. Have you ever become ill from exercising in the heat?	☐	☐
9. Do you cough, wheeze, or have trouble breathing during or after activity?	☐	☐
Do you have asthma?	☐	☐
Do you have seasonal allergies that require medical treatment?	☐	☐

	Yes	No
10. Do you use any special protective or corrective equipment or devices that aren't usually used for your sport or position (for example, knee brace, special neck roll, foot orthotics, retainer on your teeth, hearing aid)?	☐	☐
11. Have you had any problems with your eyes or vision?	☐	☐
Do you wear glasses, contacts, or protective eyewear?	☐	☐
12. Have you ever had a sprain, strain, or swelling after injury?	☐	☐
Have you broken or fractured any bones or dislocated any joints?	☐	☐
Have you had any other problems with pain or swelling in muscles, tendons, bones, or joints?	☐	☐

If yes, check appropriate box and explain below.

☐ Head ☐ Elbow ☐ Hip
☐ Neck ☐ Forearm ☐ Thigh
☐ Back ☐ Wrist ☐ Knee
☐ Chest ☐ Hand ☐ Shin/calf
☐ Shoulder ☐ Finger ☐ Ankle
☐ Upper arm ☐ Foot

	Yes	No
13. Do you want to weigh more or less than you do now?	☐	☐
Do you lose weight regularly to meet weight requirements for your sport?	☐	☐
14. Do you feel stressed out?	☐	☐

15. Record the dates of your most recent immunizations (shots) for:

Tetanus _____ Measles _____

Hepatitis B _____ Chickenpox _____

FEMALES ONLY

16. When was your first menstrual period? _____

When was your most recent menstrual period? _____

How much time do you usually have from the start of one period to the start of another? _____

How many periods have you had in the last year? _____

What was the longest time between periods in the last year? _____

Explain "Yes" answers here: _____

_____

_____

_____

_____

_____

_____

_____

_____

I hereby state that, to the best of my knowledge, my answers to the above questions are complete and correct.

Signature of athlete _____ Signature of parent/guardian _____ Date _____

FIGURE 1-1

The preparticipation medical history. (Reprinted with permission from American Academy of Family Physicians, American Academy of Pediatrics, American Medical Society for Sports Medicine, American Orthopaedic Society for Sports Medicine, American Osteopathic Academy of Sports Medicine. Preparticipation Physical Evaluation [2nd ed]. Minneapolis: The Physician and Sportsmedicine [McGraw-Hill], 1997.)

Preparticipation Physical Evaluation

Name _____ Date of birth _____

Height _____ Weight _____ % Body fat (optional) _____ Pulse _____ BP___/____ (___/___ , ___/___)

Vision R 20/ _____ L 20/ _____   Corrected: Y N   Pupils: Equal _____   Unequal _____

	NORMAL	ABNORMAL FINDINGS	INITIALS*
MEDICAL			
Appearance			
Eyes/Ears/Nose/Throat			
Lymph Nodes			
Heart			
Pulses			
Lungs			
Abdomen			
Genitalia (males only)			
Skin			
MUSCULOSKELETAL			
Neck			
Back			
Shoulder/arm			
Elbow/forearm			
Wrist/hand			
Hip/thigh			
Knee			
Leg/ankle			
Foot			

* Station-based examination only

CLEARANCE

❏ **Cleared**

❏ **Cleared after completing evaluation/rehabilitation for:** _____

_____

_____

_____

❏ **Not cleared for:** _____ **Reason:** _____ _____

Recommendations: _____

_____

_____

_____

Name of physician (print/type) _____ **Date** _____

Address _____ **Phone**_____

Signature of physician _____ , **MD or DO**

FIGURE 1-2

Sample sports preparticipation medical evaluation. (Reprinted with permission from American Academy of Family Physicians, American Academy of Pediatrics, American Medical Society for Sports Medicine, American Orthopaedic Society for Sports Medicine, American Osteopathic Academy of Sports Medicine. Preparticipation Physical Evaluation [2nd ed]. Minneapolis: The Physician and Sportsmedicine [McGraw-Hill], 1997.)

TABLE 1-2
Two-Minute Musculoskeletal Examination

Athletic Activity (instructions)	Observations
1. Stand facing examiner	Acromioclavicular joints; general habitus
2. Look at ceiling, floor, over both shoulders; touch ears to shoulder	Cervical spine motion
3. Shrug shoulders (examiner resists)	Trapezius strength
4. Abduct shoulders 90 degrees (examiner resists at 90 degrees)	Deltoid strength
5. Full external rotation of arms	Shoulder motion
6. Flex and extend elbows	Elbow motion
7. Arms at sides, elbows at 90 degrees flexed; pronate and supinate wrists	Elbow and wrist motion
8. Spread fingers; make fist	Hand and finger motion and deformities
9. Tighten (contract) quadriceps; relax quadriceps	Symmetry and knee effusion; ankle effusion
10. "Duck walk" four steps (away from examiner)	Hip, knee, and ankle motion
11. Back to examiner	Shoulder symmetry; scoliosis
12. Knees straight, touch toes	Scoliosis; hip motion; hamstring tightness
13. Raise up on toes, heels	Calf symmetry; leg strength

Source: Reprinted with permission from D McKeag. Pre-participation screening of the potential athlete. Clin Sports Med 1989;8:391.

cardiomyopathy (HCM) is a leading cause of sudden death in young athletes, and physicians should be aware of the characteristics of the murmur found with this condition. The murmur of HCM typically is best heard at the left sternal border and begins shortly after the first heart sound. It is accentuated by maneuvers that reduce the volume of blood flow returning to the left side of the heart. The maneuver that the AHA specifically recommends is to auscultate the precordium first in the supine position and then while the athlete is standing (the murmur of HCM will increase with standing). For further review of the cardiovascular examination of the young athlete, see Strong and Steed[17] or Chapter 24 (Cardiovascular Problems).

It has been noted[3, 17] that the history and physical examinations have a limited sensitivity in detecting potential causes of sudden cardiac death; however, they remain the most cost-effective method of detecting some of the problems that athletes develop. Routine electrocardiograms and other expensive cardiovascular diagnostic processes are not indicated because of the limited prevalence of cardiac disease in this age group. (If indicated by the history or physical examination, then they should be done.)

The musculoskeletal examination identifies approximately two-thirds of the identifiable risk factors for participation in sports. Three areas should be considered: (1) a total screening examination, which can be accomplished in approximately 2 minutes (Table 1-2); (2) sports-specific areas, which should receive special attention (Table 1-3); and (3) areas of old injuries, which should be examined specifically and thoroughly. Ligamentous laxity, muscle tendon inflexibility, and biomechanical problems are worth observing and noting; it is believed

that these might contribute to injury, although there is no conclusive proof that they are reliable predictors of injury.[18, 19]

Maturity Classification

Maturity classification is an aspect of the physical examination that remains controversial and not widely used. An excellent review of this topic is found in the article by Caine and Broekhoff.[20] The preparticipation monograph[2] does not recommend maturity staging as a routine part of the preparticipation examination.

Other Areas of Concern

Other parts of the examination may be those tied to a particular sport or suggested by a particular item found

TABLE 1-3
Examples of Sport-Specific Emphasis in Physical Examination

Sport	Emphasis
Football	Neck, knee, ankle
Basketball	Ankle, knee
Baseball	Shoulder, elbow
Swimming	Shoulder (ears)
Wrestling	Shoulder, elbow, back, neck (skin)
Gymnastics	Wrist, shoulder, back, ankle
Soccer	Ankle, knee, foot, hip
Running	Lower-extremity alignment
Volleyball	Shoulder, knee, ankle

Source: Reprinted with permission from C McGrew. Pre-participation athletic examinations for the junior and senior high school athlete. J Back Musculoskel Rehabil 1991;1:16.

TABLE 1-4
Miscellaneous Physical Examination Items

Skin: important for wrestlers for detection of conditions such as herpes, impetigo, or scabies
Ears: important in swimmers and divers in whom infections of the external canal and injuries to the tympanic membrane would limit participation
Nose and throat: examine if indicated by history
Eyes: should be examined for pupil size and inequality
Neck: indicated by history
Lungs: indicated by history
Abdomen: should be checked for organomegaly, especially in contact and collision sports

in the history. A sampling of these items is presented in Table 1-4.

Laboratory Testing

No laboratory tests are routinely recommended.[2, 21] Because of the high incidence of anemia in young females, a screening hematocrit could be justified in female athletes.[22] Urine testing (by dipstick) produces a high false-positive rate for proteinuria and is not recommended.[23, 24] Other laboratory testing should be guided by the history and physical examination. Testing for bloodborne pathogens, in particular hepatitis and human immunodeficiency virus (HIV), should not be considered routine. Mandatory testing for these entities is not recommended, but voluntary testing should be encouraged for athletes with special risk factors.[25]

Special Testing

Endurance, muscle strength, muscle power, speed, flexibility, and agility testing may be useful in monitoring training progress and can serve as a baseline if the athlete is injured.[26] No specific testing is routine, however, and none has been shown to help consistently predict or prevent injury.

Drug Testing

There are several instances of local high school districts incorporating drug testing into their criteria for allowing students to play interscholastic sports, but they are not considered part of the examination per se. Drug testing should not be considered a standard part of the PPAE for the high school athlete at this time. An American Academy of Pediatrics policy statement states that "student athletes should not be singled out for involuntary screening for drugs of abuse. Except for health related purposes, such testing should not be a condition for participation in sports or any school function."[27]

At the collegiate level, many institutions test for drugs routinely at the preparticipation examination and throughout the year. The NCAA has drug testing at championship events and year-round for certain sports, such as football and track and field, but it makes no specific recommendation for preparticipation testing. If such testing is considered, it should be accompanied by appropriate counseling and rehabilitation opportunities. To be most effective as a deterrent to use, drug testing should be unannounced and random throughout the year, both in season and out of season; preparticipation drug screening would not seem to fit into these criteria.

ASSESSMENT AND CLASSIFICATION FOR PARTICIPATION

Based on the results of the physical examination, the physician may approve an athlete's participation in sports. This clearance may be divided into four categories: (1) clearance without limitations for the indicated sports, (2) clearance deferred pending further evaluation, (3) clearance for certain sports but not the one originally evaluated for, and (4) disqualification for all participation. Category 4 is rarely used. The goal of the classification process is to find the appropriate participation level for all students. The athlete should be informed that alternative activities that are deemed permissible are healthier than no activity at all.

The American Academy of Pediatrics has proposed workable and specific guidelines for competitive sports and recommendations for qualification and disqualification for these sports (Tables 1-5 through 1-7).[28] However, these are recommended only as guidelines. Therefore, each athlete should be evaluated individually to determine the proper level of participation. For the junior high and senior high school athlete, parents or guardians should be involved in decisions that determine qualification for various sports. Even at the college level, it is important to try to involve parents or guardians; however, this will vary according to the different ages of legal adulthood among states.

FORMS

One copy of the PPAE form should be available for all practices and games, especially when the athlete is traveling.

TABLE 1-5

Classification of Sports by Contact

Contact or Collision	Limited Contact	Noncontact
Basketball	Baseball	Archery
Boxing*	Bicycling	Badminton
Diving	Cheerleading	Body building
Field hockey	Canoeing and kayaking (white water)	Bowling
Football	Fencing	Canoeing and kayaking (flat water)
Flag	Field	Crew or rowing
Tackle	High jump	Curling
Ice hockey	Pole vault	Dancing
Lacrosse	Floor hockey	Field
Martial arts	Gymnastics	Discus
Rodeo	Handball	Javelin
Rugby	Horseback riding	Shot put
Ski jumping	Racquetball	Golf
Soccer	Skating	Orienteering
Team handball	Ice	Power lifting
Water polo	In-line	Race walking
Wrestling	Roller	Riflery
	Skiing	Rope jumping
	Cross-country	Running
	Downhill	Sailing
	Water	Scuba diving
	Softball	Strength training
	Squash	Swimming
	Ultimate Frisbee	Table tennis
	Volleyball	Tennis
	Windsurfing and surfing	Track
		Weight lifting

*Participation not recommended.

TABLE 1-6

Classification of Sports by Strenuousness

	High to Moderate Intensity			
Dynamic and Static Demands	Dynamic and Low Static Demands	Static and Low Dynamic Demands	Low Intensity Dynamic and Static Demands
---	---	---	---
Boxing*	Badminton	Archery	Bowling
Crew/rowing	Baseball	Auto racing	Cricket
Cross-country skiing	Basketball	Diving	Curling
Cycling	Field hockey	Equestrian	Golf
Downhill skiing	Lacrosse	Field events (jumping)	Riflery
Fencing	Orienteering	Field events (throwing)	
Football	Ping-pong	Gymnastics	
Ice hockey	Race walking	Karate or judo	
Rugby	Racquetball	Motorcycling	
Running (sprint)	Soccer	Rodeoing	
Speed skating	Squash	Sailing	
Water polo	Swimming	Ski jumping	
Wrestling	Tennis	Waterskiing	
	Volleyball	Weight lifting	

*Participation not recommended.
Source: Reprinted with permission from American Academy of Pediatrics Committee on Sports Medicine and Fitness. Medical conditions affecting sports participation. Pediatrics 1994;94:391.

TABLE 1-7
Medical Conditions and Sports Participation*

Condition	May Participate?
Atlantoaxial instability (instability of the joint between cervical vertebrae 1 and 2)	Qualified yes
Explanation: Athlete needs evaluation to assess risk of spinal cord injury during sports participation.	
Bleeding disorder	Qualified yes
Explanation: Athlete needs evaluation.	
Cardiovascular diseases	
Carditis (inflammation of the heart)	No
Explanation: Carditis may result in sudden death with exertion.	
Hypertension (high blood pressure)	Qualified yes
Explanation: Those with significant essential (unexplained) hypertension should avoid weight and power lifting, body building, and strength training. Those with secondary hypertension (hypertension caused by a previously identified disease) or severe essential hypertension need evaluation.	
Congenital heart disease (structural heart defects present at birth)	Qualified yes
Explanation: Those with mild forms may participate fully; those with moderate or severe forms, or who have undergone surgery, need evaluation.	
Dysrhythmia (irregular heart rhythm)	Qualified yes
Explanation: Athlete needs evaluation because some types require therapy or make certain sports dangerous, or both.	
Mitral valve prolapse (abnormal heart valve)	Qualified yes
Explanation: Those with symptoms (chest pain, symptoms of possible dysrhythmia, or evidence of mitral regurgitation [leaking]) on physical examination need evaluation. All others may participate fully.	
Heart murmur	Qualified yes
Explanation: If the murmur is innocent (does not indicate heart disease), full participation is permitted. Otherwise the athlete needs evaluation (see Congenital heart disease and Mitral valve prolapse above).	
Cerebral palsy	Qualified yes
Explanation: Athlete needs evaluation.	
Diabetes mellitus	Yes
Explanation: All sports can be played with proper attention to diet, hydration, and insulin therapy. Particular attention is needed for activities that last 30 minutes or more.	
Diarrhea	Qualified no
Explanation: Unless disease is mild, no participation is permitted, because diarrhea may increase the risk of dehydration and heat illness. See Fever below.	
Eating disorders	Qualified yes
Anorexia nervosa	
Bulimia nervosa	
Explanation: These patients need both medical and psychiatric assessment before participation.	
Eyes	Qualified yes
Functionally one-eyed athlete	
Loss of an eye	
Detached retina	
Previous eye surgery or serious eye injury	
Explanation: A functionally one-eyed athlete has a best-corrected visual acuity of less than 20/40 in the worst eye. These athletes would experience significant disability if the better eye was seriously injured as would those with loss of an eye. Some athletes who have previously undergone eye surgery or had a serious eye injury may have an increased risk of injury because of weakened eye tissue. Availability of eyeguards approved by the American Society for Testing Materials and other protective equipment may allow participation in most sports, but this must be judged on an individual basis.	
Fever	No
Explanation: Fever can increase cardiopulmonary effort, reduce maximum exercise capacity, make heat illness more likely, and increase orthostatic hypotension during exercise. Fever may rarely accompany myocarditis or other infections that may make exercise dangerous.	
Heat illness, history of	Qualified yes
Explanation: Because of the increased likelihood of recurrence, the athlete needs individual assessment to determine the presence of predisposing conditions and to arrange a prevention strategy.	
Human immunodeficiency virus infection	Yes
Explanation: Because of the apparent minimal risk to others, all sports may be played that the state of health allows. In all athletes, skin lesions should be properly covered, and athletic personnel should use universal precautions when handling blood or body fluids with visible blood.	
Kidney, absence of one	Qualified yes
Explanation: Athlete needs individual assessment for contact or collision and limited contact sports.	

Continued

TABLE 1-7
(continued)

Condition	May Participate?
Liver, enlarged	Qualified yes
Explanation: If the liver is acutely enlarged, participation should be avoided because of risk of rupture. If the liver is chronically enlarged, individual assessment is needed before collision or contact or limited contact sports are played.	
Malignancy	Qualified yes
Explanation: Athlete needs individual assessment.	
Musculoskeletal disorders	Qualified yes
Explanation: Athlete needs individual assessment.	
Neurologic disorders	
History of serious head or spine trauma, severe or repeated concussions, or craniotomy	Qualified yes
Explanation: Athlete needs individual assessment for collision or contact or limited contact sports, and also for noncontact sports if there are deficits in judgment or cognition. Research supports a conservative approach to management of concussion.	
Convulsive disorder, well controlled	Yes
Explanation: Risk of convulsion during participation is minimal.	
Convulsive disorder, poorly controlled	Qualified yes
Explanation: Athlete needs individual assessment for collision or contact or limited contact sports. Avoid the following noncontact sports: archery, riflery, swimming, weight or power lifting, strength training, or sports involving heights. In these sports, occurrence of a convulsion may be a risk to self or others.	
Obesity	Qualified yes
Explanation: Because of the risk of heat illness, obese persons need careful acclimatization and hydration.	
Organ transplant recipient	Qualified yes
Explanation: Athlete needs individual assessment.	
Ovary, absence of one	Yes
Explanation: Risk of severe injury to the remaining ovary is minimal.	
Respiratory disorders	
Pulmonary compromise, including cystic fibrosis	Qualified yes
Explanation: Athlete needs individual assessment, but generally all sports may be played if oxygenation remains satisfactory during a graded exercise test. Patients with cystic fibrosis need acclimatization and good hydration to reduce the risk of heat illness.	
Asthma	Yes
Explanation: With proper medication and education, only athletes with the most severe asthma will have to modify their participation.	
Acute upper respiratory infection	Qualified yes
Explanation: Upper respiratory obstruction may affect pulmonary function. Athlete needs individual assessment for all but mild disease. See Fever above.	
Sickle-cell disease	Qualified yes
Explanation: Athlete needs individual assessment. In general, if the status of the illness permits, all but high exertion, collision or contact sports may be played. Overheating, dehydration, and chilling must be avoided.	
Sickle cell trait	Yes
Explanation: It is unlikely that individuals with sickle cell trait have an increased risk of sudden death or other medical problems during athletic participation except under the most extreme conditions of heat, humidity, and possibly increased altitude. These individuals, as all athletes, should be carefully conditioned, acclimatized, and hydrated to reduce any possible risk.	
Skin: boils, herpes simplex, impetigo, scabies, molluscum contagiosum	Qualified yes
Explanation: While the patient is contagious, participation in gymnastics with mats, martial arts, wrestling, or other collision or contact or limited contact sports is not allowed. Herpes simplex virus probably is not transmitted via mats.	
Spleen, enlarged	Qualified yes
Explanation: Patients with acutely enlarged spleens should avoid all sports because of risk of rupture. Those with chronically enlarged spleens need individual assessment before playing collision or contact or limited contact sports.	
Testicle, absent or undescended	Yes
Explanation: Certain sports may require a protective cup.	

*This table is designed to be understood by medical and nonmedical personnel. In the Explanation sections, "needs evaluation" means that a physician with appropriate knowledge and experience should assess the safety of a given sport for an athlete with the listed medical condition. Unless otherwise noted, this is because of the variability of the severity of the disease or of the risk of injury among the specific sports in Table 1-5, or both.
Source: Reprinted with permission from American Academy of Pediatrics Committee on Sports Medicine and Fitness. Medical conditions affecting sports participation. Pediatrics 1994;94:16.

SUMMARY

Even though the PPAE has not been completely justified in the sports medicine literature, it seems to be a worthwhile preventive exercise. However, its usefulness demands a systematic and focused approach.

REFERENCES

1. Ryan A. Qualifying examinations: a continuing dilemma. Phys Sports Med 1980;8:10.
2. American Academy of Family Physicians, American Academy of Pediatrics, American Medical Society for Sports Medicine, American Orthopaedic Society for Sports Medicine, American Osteopathic Academy of Sports Medicine. Preparticipation Physical Evaluation (2nd ed). Minneapolis: The Physician and Sportsmedicine (McGraw-Hill), 1996.
3. American Heart Association. American Heart Association scientific statement: cardiovascular preparticipation screening of competitive athletes. Circulation 1996;94:850–856.
4. McKeag D. Pre-participation screening of the potential athlete. Clin Sports Med 1989;8:373–397.
5. Lombardo J. The pre-participation physical exam. Prim Care 1984;11:3–21.
6. Linder C, Durant R, Seckleckl D, et al. Pre-participation health screening of young athletes: results of 1268 exams. Am J Sports Med 1981;9:187–193.
7. Alman J. Prevention and emergency care of sports injuries. Fam Pract Recert 1983;5:141–163.
8. McGrew C. Pre-participation athletic examinations for the junior and senior high school athlete. J Back Musculoskeletal Rehab 1991;1:19–20.
9. Goldberg B, Saraniti A, Witman P, et al. Pre-participation sports assessment: an objective evaluation. Pediatrics 1980;66:736–744.
10. Feinstein R, Soileau E, Daniel W. A national survey of pre-participation examination requirements. Phys Sports Med 1988;16:51–59.
11. National Collegiate Athletic Association. Policy 1B: Medical Evaluations, Immunizations and Records. In 1996–1997 NCAA Sports Medicine Handbook (9th ed). Overland Park, Kansas: National Collegiate Athletic Association, 1996;8.
12. Risser W, Hoffman H, Bellah G. Frequency of pre-participation sports examinations in secondary school athletes: are the university intra-scholastic lead guidelines appropriate? Tex Med 1985;61:35–39.
13. Risser W, Hoffman HM, Bellah GG, et al. A cost benefit analysis of pre-participation sports examinations of adolescent athletes. J Sch Health 1985;55:270–273.
14. Amsterdam E, Laslet L, Holly R. Exercise and sudden death. Cardiol Clin 1987;2:341.
15. Braden D, Strong W. Pre-participation screening for sudden death in high school and college athletes. Phys Sports Med 1988;16:126–140.
16. Roby J, Blyghe C, Mueller F. Athletic injuries: application of epidemiologic methods. JAMA 1971;27:184–189.
17. Strong WB, Steed D. Cardiovascular examination of the young athlete. Prim Care 1984;11:61–75.
18. Lysens B. The predictability of sports injuries. Sports Med 1984;1:6–10.
19. Jackson D. Injury prediction in the young athlete. Am J Sports Med 1978;6:6–10.
20. Caine D, Broekhoff J. Maturity assessment: a viable preventive measure against physical and psychological insult to the young athlete? Phys Sports Med 1987;15:67–80.
21. American Academy of Pediatrics Committee on Sports Medicine. Sports Medicine: Health Care for Young Athletes. Evanston, IL: American Academy of Pediatrics, 1983.
22. Taylor W, Lombardo J. Pre-participation screening of college athletes: value of the complete blood count. Phys Sports Med 1990;18:106–118.
23. Goldberg B, Sarantini A, Witman P, et al. Pre-participation sports assessment: an objective evaluation. Pediatrics 1980;66:736–744.
24. Peggs J, Reinhart RW, O'Brien JM. Proteinuria in adolescent sports physical examinations. J Fam Pract 1986;22:80–81.
25. American Medical Society for Sports Medicine and the American Orthopedic Society for Sports Medicine. Human immunodeficiency virus and other blood-borne pathogens in sports. Clin J Sport Med 1995;5:199–204.
26. Bar-Or O, Lombardo J, Rowland T. The pre-participation sports exam. Patient Care 1988;Oct 30:75–102.
27. American Academy of Pediatrics Committee on Adolescence, Committee on Bio-Ethics, and Provisional Committee on Substance Abuse. Screening for drugs of abuse. Pediatrics 1989;84:396–398.
28. American Academy of Pediatrics Committee on Sports Medicine. Recommendations for participation in competitive sports. Pediatrics 1994;94:757–760.

2

Inflammation and the Role of Anti-inflammatory Medications

Seth John Stankus

Today's sports physician is challenged by a wide variety of clinical entities, the majority of which result from some traumatic or overuse injury and the resultant inflammation. Therefore, it is imperative that the sports physician have a working knowledge of the inflammatory process as well as the safe use of nonsteroidal anti-inflammatory drugs (NSAIDs) and injectable corticosteroids. The nonmedicinal modalities used to reduce inflammation and restore function are described elsewhere in this book (see Chapter 3).

INFLAMMATION

Acute Inflammation

Acute inflammation is the normal response in tissue to any traumatic or noxious insult. The purpose of the inflammatory response is to contain the injury, remove the offending agent or irreparable tissue, and restore function by reestablishing structural integrity. Through a series of complex biochemical and cellular processes, acute inflammation results in (1) increased vascular flow to injured tissues, (2) increased vascular permeability, and (3) leukocyte exudation and emigration to the inflammatory site. These physiologic changes produce the classic signs of inflammation that were described by Virchow.[1] These include (1) rubor (redness), (2) tumor (swelling), (3) calor (heat), and (4) dolor (pain).

The acute inflammatory response predominates during the first 48 hours after injury. Initially, inflammation is mediated by the local vasoactive compounds histamine, bradykinin, and serotonin, which are released from mast cells and result in increased vascular flow and permeability. Their effects are generally limited to the first 60 minutes after injury.

The inflammatory response is maintained, in part, by a powerful class of mediators known as the *eicosanoids*, which are the products of arachidonic acid metabolism (Figure 2-1). There are two pathways that arachidonic acid may follow: the cyclooxygenase enzyme system, which leads to the formation of the prostaglandins, and the lipoxygenase enzyme system, which leads to the formation of the leukotrienes. The prostaglandins can best be viewed as locally acting hormones, their end result being increased vascular permeability and vasodilation.

A variety of other mediators maintain and enhance the inflammatory process, including the complement system, bradykinin, and fibrinopeptides. Many mediators, such as cytokines, also serve as chemoattractants during cellular response. It is beyond the scope of this chapter to detail each of the mediators or include all aspects of the inflammatory process instead, the major mediators and most common aspects are detailed.

After the initial 24–48 hours, the cellular response begins to play a more active role and functions to "clean up" the inflammatory site. This marks the beginning of the reparative phase. The spent products of inflammation are phagocytized and digested. The cells most involved in acute inflammation are the neutrophils and tissue macrophages. In the process of phagocytosis and digestion, some of the enzymatic compounds in the lysosomes will "spill out" and come in contact with healthy tissues. This can lead to injury of healthy tissues and further injury to areas already affected by the inflammatory process. As the spent products of inflammation are removed, reestablishment of structural integrity by fibroblasts can take place.

15

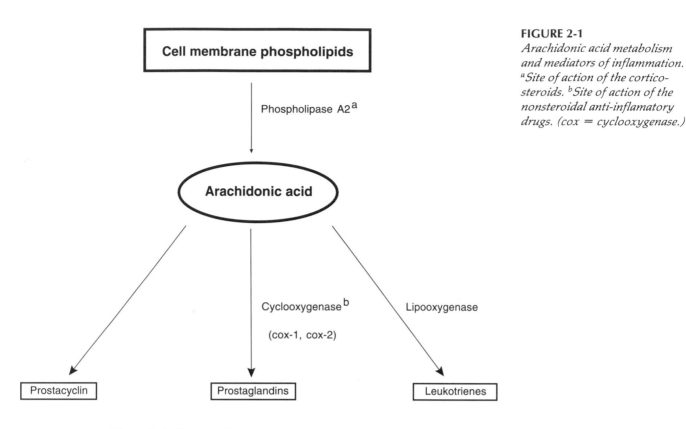

FIGURE 2-1
Arachidonic acid metabolism and mediators of inflammation. [a]*Site of action of the cortico-steroids.* [b]*Site of action of the nonsteroidal anti-inflamatory drugs. (cox = cyclooxygenase.)*

Chronic Inflammation

The transition from acute to chronic inflammation is vague and best viewed as a continuum with overlapping features. Chronic inflammatory changes tend to develop with (1) repeated microtrauma, as with overuse injuries, and (2) increased or continued tissue damage as a result of the acute inflammatory response. The presence of a continued acute inflammatory process may result in inhibition of the normal evolution or resolution of inflammation and thereby trigger the abnormal cellular and chemical processes that form the basis of chronic inflammation. An autoimmune component in acute sports injuries has been suggested by some authors as a mechanism for the development of chronic inflammation.[2] Chronic inflammation leads to the formation of granulation tissue and fibrosis. Clinically, this may result in pain and impaired function of muscles, ligaments, tendons, and joints.

NONSTEROIDAL ANTI-INFLAMMATORY DRUGS

NSAIDs have been in use, in one form or another, since the eighteenth century.[3] In 1963, however, indomethacin was introduced, thus marking the beginning of active research and development of modern NSAIDs. Hopefully, as more specific details of the inflammatory response are described, newer NSAIDs that target inflammatory sites while sparing healthy tissues will be developed, resulting in greater efficacy and fewer adverse effects.

Mechanisms of Action

Although the NSAIDs have been used for more than two centuries, there is an incomplete picture of how they work. The inhibition of cyclooxygenase and the resultant decreased production of prostaglandins is the best-described (but far from only) mechanism of action.[4-6] Two isoforms of cyclooxygenase have been found. Cyclooxygenase-1 is found in the stomach, kidneys, and platelets. It appears to be involved in the maintenance of normal function in these organs and cells. Cyclooxygenase-2 is thought to be more involved in the inflammatory response.[7] Most NSAIDs have little or no effect on the production of the other inflammatory mediators such as prostacyclin and the thromboxanes. The NSAIDs also act by altering intracellular communication and the normal inflammatory response of neutrophils.[3]

Selection

The selection of which NSAID to use for a particular condition remains more an art than a science. There is no consistent clinical evidence to support the use of one NSAID over another in any given inflammatory condition.[8, 9] Additionally, the literature gives little guidance about how to change from one NSAID to another. However, some general principles will enhance the safe and efficacious use of NSAIDs.

As is true of many other medications, NSAIDs reach steady-state serum concentrations after three to five half-lives. Therefore, as half-life increases, more time is needed to judge clinical response. It is generally believed that at least 2–3 weeks of an adequate dose is needed to define an adequate trial. It is advisable to increase the dose of a particular NSAID to the maximum recommended before deciding the medication is not effective. There is no evidence to support the need to change NSAID classes when switching medications. The use of multiple NSAIDs has not been shown to be more effective than monotherapy and increases the likelihood of complications; therefore, this practice should be avoided. However, the simultaneous use of acetaminophen and an NSAID is safe and results in better pain relief. NSAIDs should be considered adjunctive therapy to proper rest and rehabilitation. The NSAIDs have been used safely in children; however, dosage calculation corresponding to weight is recommended. The use of NSAIDs during pregnancy is not recommended.[10] Tables 2-1 and 2-2 compare dosages of frequently used prescription and over-the-counter NSAIDs, respectively. Ketorolac tromethamine (Toradol) is not indicated for use as an anti-inflammatory agent in sports injuries. It should be used only as a short-term analgesic agent.

TABLE 2-1
Dosage Comparison of Commonly Used Prescription Nonsteroidal Anti-inflammatory Drugs

Generic Name	Proprietary Name	Recommended Doses per Day	Recommended Total Daily Dosage (mg)
Acetylsalicylic acid (aspirin)	Ecotrin	4–6	325–6,000
Diclofenac	Voltaren, Cataflam	2–3	75–225
Diflunisal	Dolobid	2–3	500–1,500
Etodolac	Lodine	3–4	600–1,200
Fenoprofen	Nalfon	3–6	800–3,200
Ibuprofen	Motrin, Advil	2–4	1,200–3,200
Indomethacin	Indocin	2–4	50–200
Ketoprofen	Orudis	3–4	150–300
Meclofenamate	Meclomen	4	200–400
Mefenamic acid	Ponstel	4	500–1,000
Nabumetone	Relafen	1–2	1,000–2,000
Naproxen	Naprosyn, Anaprox	2–3	250–1,500
Oxaprozin	Daypro	1	600–1,200
Phenylbutazone	Azolid, Butazolidin	2–3	300–600
Piroxicam	Feldene	1	10–20
Salsalate	Disalcid	2–4	1,500–3,000
Sulindac	Clinoril	2	300–400
Tolmetin	Tolectin	4–6	800–1,600

TABLE 2-2
Dosage Comparison of Over-the-Counter Nonsteroidal Anti-inflammatory Drugs

Generic Name	Proprietary Name	Formulation (mg)	Recommended Doses per Day	Recommended Total Daily Dosage (mg)
Acetylsalicylic acid (aspirin)	Ascriptin Ecotrin	325	4–6	325–6,000
Ibuprofen	Advil Motrin IB Nuprin	200	4–6	800–2,400
Ketoprofen	Actron Orudis KT	12.5	4–6	50–75
Naproxen sodium	Aleve	220	2–3	440–660

Complications

The complications seen with NSAID use primarily result from the inhibition of prostaglandin synthesis. In order of decreasing relative frequency, the major NSAID-induced complications include gastrointestinal (GI) (gastritis, GI bleeding), renal (interstitial nephritis), dermatologic (rash), and central nervous system changes.[4]

NSAID-induced gastropathy is possibly the most common side effect of any currently used prescription medication. This ranges from simple dyspepsia to fatal GI hemorrhage. Although bothersome, dyspepsia does not correlate with more serious complications. The populations at highest risk of developing GI complications are the elderly; smokers; and people with current or recent systemic corticosteroid use, prior GI disease, prior NSAID intolerance, or NSAID use for longer than 3 months.

The stomach is the most common site of injury. The prophylaxis and treatment of gastric erosions and ulcerations is controversial. Misoprostol (Cytotec), a synthetic prostaglandin E_1 analog, has been shown to decrease gastric injury.[11, 12] It should be reserved for those patients at high risk, and it is dosed at 200 μg four times daily. Some authors suggest beginning misoprostol at 100 μg twice daily and increasing slowly based on tolerance.[13] The primary side effects responsible for discontinuation are nausea, diarrhea, and abdominal cramping. There is little evidence to support prophylaxis with H_2-blockers. Short-term studies of omeprazole (Prilosec), 40 mg per day, however, have shown promising results in preventing NSAID-induced gastric ulcerations. The H_2-blockers are effective in the treatment of NSAID-induced gastric lesions if NSAIDs are concurrently discontinued. Contrary to popular practice, sucralfate (Carafate) has no role in the prophylaxis or treatment of NSAID-induced gastropathy. Nabumetone (Relafen), a new NSAID that preferentially inhibits cyclooxygenase-2, appears to decrease prostaglandins at the inflammatory site while preserving prostaglandin levels in the stomach. Etodolac (Lodine) may have a similar gastric protective effect; however, long-term studies are needed to confirm this.

Prostaglandins play an integral role in autoregulation of renal blood flow. Acute renal failure has been reported in as few as 7–11 days after initiation of NSAID therapy. Patients at highest risk of renal complications are the elderly, those with pre-existing renal disease, hypertension, hypovolemia, hypoalbuminemia, or congestive heart failure. In patients at high risk, it is reasonable to obtain a urinalysis and monitor blood urea nitrogen (BUN), creatinine, and serum electrolytes every 1–2 weeks for the first month. For additional screening recommendations, see Surveillance.

Urticaria is the most common dermatologic reaction to NSAIDs. This is most often seen with acetylsalicylic acid and usually resolves when the medication is discontinued. Erythema multiforme and Stevens-Johnson syndrome have been reported. It is always important to be aware of hypersensitivity reactions. The triad of nasal polyposis, asthma, and rhinitis may be an indication of increased risk of NSAID-induced hypersensitivity reaction.

Central nervous system changes are relatively uncommon. Indomethacin has been the most frequently implicated NSAID in central nervous system complications. Most commonly, this is manifested as headache. However, tinnitus, depression, aseptic meningitis, mental status changes, and coma have been reported.

All of the NSAIDs impair the normal function of platelets. Acetylsalicylic acid decreases platelet aggregation for the life of the platelet. Therefore, prolongation of bleeding time may persist for 10–12 days after the last dose. The remainder of the NSAIDs generally affect platelet function for no longer than 24–48 hours after discontinuation.

The NSAIDs may alter blood pressure control and potentially decrease the effectiveness of antihypertensive medications. The medications most commonly affected are hydrochlorothiazide, furosemide, beta-blockers, and angiotensin-converting enzyme inhibitors.

Surveillance

Patients should be screened routinely for possible side effects of NSAIDs. This is most advisable for those taking NSAIDs on a chronic basis, for example, longer than 3 months. A reasonable plan would be to monitor the complete blood count, urinalysis, liver function tests, BUN, creatinine, and serum electrolytes at 1 month after initiation of NSAID therapy and then every 3–6 months. Patients should be informed of potential side effects, reasons to discontinue NSAID use, and when to contact their physician. Some of these include the following:

1. Rash or itching of skin
2. Unusual weight gain
3. Swelling of legs or feet
4. Shortness of breath or difficulty breathing
5. Blood in urine or stool; black or "tarry" stools
6. Nausea, vomiting, abdominal pain, or diarrhea

Additionally, patients should be instructed to avoid concomitant use of other NSAIDs, both prescription and over-the-counter.

TABLE 2-3
Recommended Corticosteroid and Lidocaine Dosages for Injection

Site of Injection	Dose of 1% Lidocaine (cc)	Dose of Triamcinolone (mg)	Dose of Betamethasone (mg)
Abductor tendon of thumb	2–3	40	6
Carpal tunnel	0	40	6
Flexor tendon sheath (trigger finger)	1	20	3
Lateral or medial epicondyle	5	40	6
Biceps tendon	5	40	6
Subacromial space	9	40–60	6–9
Glenohumeral joint	9	40–60	6–9
Acromioclavicular joint	2–3	40	6
Sacroiliac joint	2–3	40	6
Symphysis pubis	5	40	6
Trochanteric bursa	10	40–60	6–9
Anserine bursa	5	40	6
Intraarticular knee	10–15	40–60	6–9
Plantar fascia	5	40	6
Metatarsophalangeal capsule	1–2	20	3

CORTICOSTEROIDS

The most common use of corticosteroids is to reduce inflammation. In athletes, these are given almost exclusively in the injectable form. Local corticosteroid treatment results in high drug concentrations at the inflammatory site with few systemic side effects. Table 2-3 lists recommended doses of corticosteroid and local anesthetic for various sites.

Mechanism of Action

Corticosteroids act by a variety of mechanisms. They inhibit the synthesis of prostaglandins and leukotrienes by inhibiting the formation of arachidonic acid from cell membrane phospholipids. Corticosteroids are more potent inhibitors of the inflammatory process than NSAIDs because they act at a more proximal site in the inflammatory cascade. Additionally, they decrease the migration of leukocytes and stabilize lysosomes. When used in the setting of chronic inflammation, they decrease fibroblast proliferation and deposition of collagen fibers.[14] Although they decrease inflammation, they do not treat the underlying condition.

Selection

Corticosteroids may be divided by potency and duration of action (Table 2-4). Generally, as the potency increases, so does the duration of action. It is often helpful to combine a short- and long-acting preparation so as to hasten the onset of relief while providing adequate duration of treatment. An anesthetic may be added for rapid pain relief, assurance of correct placement of corticosteroid, and treatment of posttraumatic neuropathic conditions.

Complications

If administered correctly, injectable corticosteroids can be safer than NSAIDs. However, they are not without potential complications. Skin pigment changes, subcutaneous fat atrophy, and tendon rupture have been observed after corticosteroid injections. It is thought that the corticosteroid transiently decreases the tendon strength; therefore, it is recommended that strenuous activity be avoided for approximately 2–3 weeks after an injection. In fewer than 10% of patients treated with combined corticosteroid and local anesthetic, a painful flare will develop at the injection site. This is caused by crystalline precipitation of the local anesthetic and is treated with rest and ice.

TABLE 2-4
Potency Comparisons of Commonly Used Corticosteroids

Generic Name	Proprietary Name	Relative Potency	Relative Duration
Cortisone	Cortone	0.8	Short
Hydrocortisone	Hydrocortone	1.0	Short
Prednisolone	Hydeltrasol	4.0	Intermediate
Triamcinolone	Aristocort	5.0	Intermediate
Dexamethasone	Decadron	25.0	Long
Betamethasone	Celestone	25.0	Long

Some evidence suggests that repeated joint space injections lead to early articular cartilage degeneration. Septic arthritis is rare.

Systemic side effects are unusual but possible. They are more often encountered with large doses of high-potency preparations or with too frequent use. Some of the systemic side effects are glucose intolerance, peptic ulcer disease, hypertension, osteoporosis, and mental status changes.

Diabetic patients should be counseled that their blood sugars may be markedly elevated for a few days to a few weeks after a steroid injection.

The use of NSAIDs and injectable corticosteroids have greatly enhanced the ability to treat acute and chronic athletic injuries. When used as recommended in low-risk patients, they are also safe.

REFERENCES

1. May SA, Lees P, Higgins AJ, Sedgwick AD. Inflammation: a clinical perspective. Vet Rec 1987;120:514–517.
2. Friedlander GE, Jokl P, Horowitz MC. The auto-immune nature of sports-induced injury: a hypothesis. In WB Leadbetter, JB Buckwalter, SL Gordon (eds), Sports-Induced Inflammation. Park Ridge, IL: American Academy of Orthopaedic Surgeons, 1990;619–627.
3. Weissman G. Aspirin. Sci Am 1991;264:84–90.
4. Mortensen ME, Rennebohm RM. Clinical pharmacology and use of nonsteroidal anti-inflammatory drugs. Pediatr Clin North Am 1989;36:1113–1139.
5. Vane J. The evolution of non-steroidal anti-inflammatory drugs and their mechanisms of action. Drugs 1987;33 (suppl 1):18–27.
6. Vane J, Botting R. Inflammation and the mechanism of action of anti-inflammatory drugs. FASEB J 1987;1:89–96.
7. DeWitt DL, Meade EA, Smith WL. PGH synthase isoenzyme selectivity: the potential for safer nonsteroidal anti-inflammatory drugs. Am J Med 1993;95(suppl 2A):40–44.
8. Pincus T, Callahan L. Clinical use of multiple non-steroidal antiinflammatory drug preparations within individual rheumatology private practices. J Rheumatol 1989;16:1253–1258.
9. Day RO, Brooks PM. Variations in response to non-steroidal anti-inflammatory drugs. Br J Clin Pharmacol 1987;23:655–658.
10. O'Brien WM, Bagby GF. Rare adverse reactions to nonsteroidal antiinflammatory drugs. J Rheumatol 1984;12:785–790.
11. Jiranek GC, Kimmey MB, Saunders DR, et al. Misoprostol reduces gastroduodenal injury from one week of aspirin: an endoscopic study. Gastroenterology 1989;96:656–661.
12. Graham DY, Agrawal NM, Roth SH. Prevention of NSAID-induced gastric ulcer with misoprostol: multicentre, double-blind, placebo-controlled trial. Lancet 1988;2:1277–1280.
13. Ament PW, Childers RS. Prophylaxis and treatment of NSAID-induced gastropathy. Am Fam Physician 1997;55:1323–1332.
14. Kerlan RK, Glousman RE. Injections and techniques in athletic medicine. Clin Sports Med 1989;8:541–560.

3

Modalities in Rehabilitation

PAUL W. BAUMERT, JR.

Therapeutic modalities modify the body's response to injury so that it can manage the associated inflammatory condition and achieve rapid, optimal healing. Pain, edema, loss of motion, muscle atrophy, and joint dysfunction are all possible results of the series of vascular and cellular reactions referred to as *inflammation*. The traditional modalities of cold and heat, as well as ultrasound and electrical stimulation, can be combined with therapeutic exercises to create a healing environment and facilitate the athlete's return to competition in a minimal amount of time.

CRYOTHERAPY

The use of ice as a therapeutic modality is one of the oldest known means to reduce swelling and pain. Ice can be easily applied, is readily accessible at most athletic events, and has relatively few contraindications. Ice packs, ice massage, cold whirlpools, cooling sprays, and cold compression units are some of the common methods of cryotherapy. Ice massage is generally the most effective method of cryotherapy. Ice packs tend to provide more cooling than the gel packs available. Vapocoolant sprays are used in the "spray and stretch" technique to increase muscle response to stretching.

Physiologic Effects

When cold is applied to the skin immediately after injury, the first response is vasoconstriction of cutaneous blood vessels, resulting in reduced blood flow. In acute injuries, the restriction of blood flow to the area reduces swelling and minimizes extravasation of blood into the skin and surrounding tissues; this, in turn, limits the extent of inflammation.

Application of cold during the initial 24–72 hours after injury elicits a number of other beneficial physiologic responses.[1] It reduces cellular metabolism and oxygen demand, which may prevent some of the tissue damage that results from oxygen deprivation. It also reduces the release of vasodilators, such as histamine, which would otherwise increase the swelling. Muscle spasm can also be relieved by an application of cold. This may be brought about by a reduction of muscle spindle firing or by a reflex response of sensory nerves overlying the muscles.[2] The nerve conduction velocities of gamma motor neurons and sensory neurons carrying pain impulses have been shown to decrease with the therapeutic application of cold.[3] Despite its widespread use, cryotherapy remains a subject of scientific discussion because of difficulties in explaining the physiologic mechanisms behind every observed clinical effect.[4]

Indications and Contraindications

Therapeutic applications of cold are indicated in the following acute conditions found in sports medicine: sprains, strains, contusions, fractures, and the acute phases of inflammatory bursitis, tendinitis, and tenosynovitis (Table 3-1). The benefits of ice or cold treatment extend beyond the acute phase of injury management. Cryotherapy can also be used in the later stages of rehabilitation to help minimize swelling after therapeutic exercise. Contraindications for the use of cryotherapy include Raynaud's phenomenon, cold hypersensitivity, cryoglobulinemia, and compromised local circulation. Cold packs should not be applied directly over a superficial motor nerve such as the peroneal nerve at the fibular head or the ulnar nerve at the medial humeral epicondyle. Also, cryotherapy should not involve continuous application to the skin for more than 30 minutes. Athletes should be advised against returning to participation in a sport immediately after a therapeu-

TABLE 3-1
Indications and Contraindications for Cryotherapy

Indications	Contraindications
Acute painful injuries	Cold hypersensitivity
Acute inflammation	Raynaud's phenomenon
Muscle spasm	Cryoglobulinemia
Chronic inflammation (tendinitis, bursitis)	Compromised circulation

tic cold application to an injured area, because it can compromise the body's protective pain mechanism.

Application Techniques

The most inexpensive, efficient, and convenient method of cold application is the placement of a plastic bag or towel filled with chipped, flaked, cubed, or crushed ice directly on the skin. The size of the pack can be varied according to the area treated. McMaster et al. reported that ice consistently produced the greatest decrease in tissue temperature over a 60-minute period, compared with other cryotherapy modalities.[5] Treatment time varies, but 15–30 minutes should be sufficient to lower tissue temperature to desired levels. During the first 24–72 hours after an acute injury, cryotherapy should be performed several times a day as often as every other hour, depending on the amount of initial pain and swelling.

Commercially available gel packs can also be used in the application of cryotherapy. These reusable packs consist of a silica gel mixture in a heavy vinyl case and are usually kept in a freezer until ready for use. Gel packs should be applied over a wet towel for up to 20 minutes. There have been some reports of cold injury or "burn" when these packs are applied directly to the skin. An economic, reusable ice pack can be made by filling a self-sealing plastic bag with ice, water, and isopropyl alcohol in a 2 to 1 to 1 ratio. The bag will not freeze solid if kept in a freezer, and it can be used many times.

Massage of the affected area with ice in a foam cup or frozen on a stick is an effective method of cold application. Water is frozen in a foam cup, then the top portion of the cup is peeled away to expose the ice. The cup can be held while the ice is massaged over the injured area in small, overlapping circles. The athlete should be instructed that he or she may experience several distinct sensations—intense cold, burning, aching, and finally, analgesia. When analgesia is reached, the massage should be discontinued because of the risk of cold injury.

Immersion of an extremity in an ice bucket ensures circumferential cold application to the extremity, but it is usually uncomfortable for the athlete and can be tolerated for only a few minutes. Cold whirlpools at 12.8°–18.3°C (55°–65°F) are more commonly used for immersion of larger body parts.

Ethyl chloride has been used to reduce muscle spasm. The affected area is sprayed at an acute angle in parallel sweeps 1.5–2.0 cm apart from a distance of 12–18 in. (30–45 cm). The rate of spraying is approximately 10 cm per sec and should be continued until the entire muscle has been covered. Repeated applications may lower skin temperature enough to cause tissue damage, so caution should be used.

Cold compression units—such as the Cryotemp (Jobst Institute, Inc., Toledo, OH) and the CryoCuff (Aircast, Summit, NJ), which circulate cooled water through a sleeve applied over an elevated extremity—are another type of cold modality. Intermittent pressure and cold provide a pumping action to reduce edema from the extremity.

THERMOTHERAPY

Thermotherapy, or the application of heat, has been used as an analgesic, an antispasmodic, and a sedative. In the subacute or chronic stage of injury, heating agents are used to relieve pain, increase blood flow, facilitate tissue healing, and prepare stiff joints and tight muscles for exercise. Consequently, thermotherapy is one of the most common modalities used in the treatment of athletic injuries. Moist hot packs, warm whirlpools, and contrast baths are a few of the application methods used in thermotherapy. Ultrasound is also considered a heating modality and is discussed later in the chapter.

Physiologic Effects

An increase in tissue temperature is associated with vasodilation and an increase in blood flow to the tissues. For a physiologic response to occur, heat must be absorbed into the tissue and the temperature of the tissue must be elevated to between 40° and 45°C (104°–113°F).[6] It is important to understand that the chemical activity and metabolic rate in cells increase two- to threefold for each 10°C that the temperature rises.[7] If the temperature rises past 45°C, however, the tissues burn because the metabolic activity required to repair the tissue is not capable of keeping up with thermally induced protein denaturation.

Indications and Contraindications

Therapeutic heat is primarily indicated for the treatment of musculoskeletal pain, muscle spasm, and joint stiffness

(Table 3-2). After the acute phase of injury, heat is useful in treating contusions, strains, bursitis, tendinitis, tenosynovitis, and capsulitis. Contraindications to thermotherapy include the use of heat in the first 48–72 hours after injury, continued swelling, loss of sensation in the injured area, decreased arterial circulation, and use directly over the eyes, genitals, or abdomen in pregnancy. Generalized superficial heat application, such as warm whirlpools, should be avoided after exercise unless the body is allowed to cool down for a period of at least 20–30 minutes. For increasing muscle flexibility, moist heat tends to be more effective than dry heat. Stretching of tight muscles can be maximized if done immediately after 20 minutes of moist heat.

Application Techniques

Superficial heat can be easily and inexpensively applied using warm, moist towels. However, the heat is retained more effectively by commercially available hydrocolator packs. These packs are heated by conduction and should remain immersed in thermostatically controlled hot water at a temperature of 71°–79°C (160°–174°F) until they are ready to be used. The pack should be covered with six layers of dry towels or a commercial cover before it is directly applied to an injured area. Treatment time is usually 15–20 minutes. The towels should be removed one layer at a time as the pack cools to maintain continuous heat next to the skin.

The water temperature of warm whirlpool baths must vary according to each patient's tolerance and the stage of injury. Temperatures of 33.9°–36.7°C (93°–98°F) are used initially after an acute injury has stabilized. Later in the healing process, water temperatures of 36.7°–40°C (98°–104°F) can be used for 20–30 minutes. For chronic injuries, 37.8°–43.3°C (100°–110°F) water may be used for 20 minutes at a time. The agitator must always be properly positioned so that flow is not aimed directly at an acute lesion.

Some athletes have found contrast baths, in which 2 minutes in hot water at 40.6°–43.3°C (105°–110°F) is

TABLE 3-2
Indications and Contraindications for Thermotherapy

Indications	Contraindications
Chronic painful injuries	Compromised circulation
Chronic inflammation	Over area of sensory loss
Muscle spasm, trigger points	Over the eyes or genitals
Joint stiffness	Over pregnant abdomen
	Inflammatory connective tissue disease, such as acute episode of rheumatoid arthritis

alternated with 2 minutes in cold water at 12.8°–18.3°C (55°–65°F) for a period of 20 minutes (five cycles), to be helpful in the rehabilitative phase of the injury. Active range-of-motion exercises should be encouraged, especially in the heat phase of the contrast. The hot to cold ratio may progress from 2 to 2, to 3 to 2, to 4 to 2 as the injury matures. The final minutes are usually cold to minimize any reactive swelling after the rehabilitative exercises. The appropriate use of cold and heat in the treatment of athletic injury is summarized in Table 3-3.

ULTRASOUND

Since the 1940s, high-frequency acoustic energy has been used to produce beneficial thermal and mechanical effects in tissues. An electrical generator is used to deliver an appropriate voltage via a coaxial cable to a transducer or "sound head." The crystal in the transducer experiences elastic deformation at a resonant frequency from the applied current, creating the therapeutic sound waves. Clinical ultrasound has a frequency of 1–3 MHz. Attenuation of ultrasonic energy increases as frequency increases, so a 1-MHz signal penetrates deeper than a 3-MHz signal. Adequate transmission of the energy to the tissues requires a

TABLE 3-3
Comparison of the Use of Cold and Heat in Athletic Injury

	Cold	Heat
When to use	Immediately after injury Initial 72 hrs postinjury or until swelling stops	72 hrs postinjury, if swelling has stopped Chronic conditions without significant swelling
Treatment time	15–20 mins	15–20 mins
Number of treatments	3–5 per day	3–5 per day
Blood flow	Decreased to injury site	Increased to injury site
Forms	Ice bag or cup Gel pack Cool whirlpool	Warm, moist towel Hydrocollator heat pack Warm whirlpool

conductive medium such as a commercial gel, water, lotion, mineral oil, or glycerol.

Physiologic Effects

Sound waves are absorbed well by homogeneous tissues, especially those with a high protein content, such as muscle and connective tissue. The acoustic transmission properties of skin, fat, muscle, and bone are similar but not identical. At the irregular muscle-bone interface, sound waves are absorbed and reflected. Any periosteal disruption, such as an early stress fracture, may be quickly irritated by the absorption and reflection of the ultrasound.[8] Another mechanical effect of ultrasound is micromassage, the result of the alternating positive and negative pressures of the sound waves.

Indications and Contraindications

Ultrasound is used to relieve pain and muscle spasms, promote tissue healing, and increase range of motion (Table 3-4). It is frequently used to treat tendinitis, bursitis, joint sprains, and muscle strains as well as calcific tendinitis, calcaneal exostoses, and plantar warts. It should not be used in areas of acute thrombus or hemorrhage, tumor, or active infection; around the eyes; over the open epiphyses of young children; or on pregnant women.

Topical medications, usually anti-inflammatory or analgesic, can be driven into targeted superficial tissues with ultrasound energy. This noninvasive method of introducing medication into the skin is called *phonophoresis* (discussed in a following section).

Application Techniques

Therapeutic ultrasound is applied by two treatment methods: (1) stationary transducer and (2) moving transducer.

With the stationary technique, lower intensities are necessary to prevent tissue damage. With the moving technique, the transducer is slowly moved over the tissue surface using firm, partially overlapping linear or circular strokes. Burns may occur if there is insufficient coupling agent on the skin, if the intensity is too great, if the transducer is applied directly over a bony prominence, or if the transducer head is moved too slowly. However, the transducer should not be moved faster than 1–2 in. per second to deliver adequate energy to the tissues.

Two modes of output are available with modern clinical ultrasound: continuous and pulsed. Continuous ultrasound provides an uninterrupted flow of energy and generates both thermal and nonthermal responses. In the pulsed mode, bursts of energy result primarily in nonthermal effects. These effects are primarily mechanical, the result of alternating positive and negative pressures of the sound waves passing through the tissues. The pulsed mode is most appropriate in the acute phase of injury, when additional heating may have detrimental effects on the injured tissue. The continuous mode is preferred for most athletic applications.

Intensity of the acoustic energy is determined by dividing the total wattage by the radiating area of the crystal. Acoustic energy of 10 W delivered over a 10-cm^2 crystal provides 1.0 W/cm^2 average intensity. Intensities of 0.5–2.0 W/cm^2 are considered the effective range of therapeutic ultrasound. Recommended duration of treatment is 5 minutes over an area three times that of the transducer head.

Phonophoresis

Molecules of a topical anti-inflammatory or analgesic medication can be transferred to superficial tissues via the thermal effect and the acoustic streaming of the ultrasound. Medications of a higher concentration, such as

TABLE 3-4
Indications and Contraindications for Other Modalities

Modality	Indications	Contraindications
Ultrasound	Chronic inflammation Promotion of tissue healing Increased range of motion of soft tissue Soft tissue calcification	Overacute thrombus or hemorrhage; can be used to help resolve 72-hr-old hematomas in muscle of patient with no blood disorder Tumor or active infections Over the eyes Over open physes
Phonophoresis	Use of topical medication with ultrasound	Same as above Drug hypersensitivity
Iontophoresis	Use of topical medication with electrical stimulation	Over abraded skin or scars Drug hypersensitivity

10% hydrocortisone cream, have been shown to produce the best results.[9] The cream is rubbed into the skin, and a layer of coupling gel is spread over the area, or it can be premixed by a pharmacist (12.5 g hydrocortisone powder and 8.45 fl oz of coupling gel).[10] Normal ultrasound procedures are used to deliver the medication throughout the treatment time. This technique should only be used when the target area is very superficial, such as biceps tendon and in thin individuals. It should not be used for piriformis syndrome when the muscle is too deep for phonophoresis to reach.

ELECTRICAL STIMULATION

Many types of electrical stimulation units are available for use during the care and rehabilitation of athletes. These units can be categorized by the physical characteristics of the stimulation they provide (e.g., alternating current vs. direct current, high voltage vs. low voltage). The reported effects of the various forms of electrical stimulation are often similar. Muscle relaxation, acceleration of healing, increased strength, pain reduction, diminished edema, and retardation of muscle atrophy are all effects commonly attributed to electrical stimulation. A complete description of the various types of electrical stimulation and their uses is beyond the scope of this discussion. However, several of the types of stimulators commonly used in the rehabilitation of athletes are briefly discussed.

Transcutaneous Electrical Nerve Stimulation

Transcutaneous electrical nerve stimulation is the introduction of low-voltage electrical stimulation across the skin with the purpose of relieving pain. It is frequently used for postoperative pain control, pain from fractures, and any pain that is appropriate to mask.

Microcurrent Electrical Neuromuscular Stimulation

Microcurrent electrical neuromuscular stimulation is treatment with low-voltage, long-pulse duration current used for point stimulation. Microcurrent has two primary uses: promotion of wound healing and, more recently, pain relief.

Interferential Current

Interferential current refers to the application of two slightly different medium-frequency currents (approximately 4,000 Hz) to the body simultaneously that are allowed to cross.

A new frequency is created when these currents cross that can stimulate both sensory and motor nerves. Thus, pain relief and muscle relaxation are the two most common indications for using interferential current.

Neuromuscular (Russian) Stimulation

Neuromuscular stimulation uses alternating current delivered in bursts to facilitate muscle contraction and is used primarily for muscle strengthening.

High-Voltage Pulsed Current

High-voltage pulsed current (HVPC), formerly termed *galvanic stimulation*, uses direct current delivered in very short pulses (less than 200 ms) making higher voltages (up to 500 V) safe and comfortable, unlike uninterrupted direct current. Decreased edema, decreased pain, wound healing, reduction of muscle spasm, and neuromuscular stimulation are all reported with HVPC.

Iontophoresis

Iontophoresis is the technique of introducing ions into the tissues by means of continuous, low-voltage direct current. The manner in which a specific compound ionizes must be known, as well as whether the compound is to be driven into the skin by the positive or negative electrode. Ions of medication that have the same charge as the source electrode are repelled from it and driven into the skin.

Indications and Contraindications

Iontophoresis has several advantages over local injection of anti-inflammatory medication. It is noninvasive, delivers a low systemic dose of medication, is less painful, and does not cause the tissue damage that may be seen with injection (see Table 3-4). Entities that are treated with this modality include tendinitis, bursitis, epicondylitis, fasciitis, myofascial trigger points, and arthritic conditions. Contraindications include drug hypersensitivity and placement of electrodes over abraded skin or scars.

Application Techniques

Two models of iontophoretic devices currently on the market have widespread sports applications. Most of these devices have built-in sensors for determining the level of skin resistance. There are a number of different drug combinations used for specific situations.[11] The one most often used for sports-related injury is a combination of 4% lidocaine hydrochloride noninjectable solution and dexamethasone sodium phosphate (4 mg/ml) in a 2 to 1 ratio in the electrode.[10] The treatment surface must first be cleaned with alcohol or povidone-iodine (Betadine). Then, the active electrode (the positive electrode in the case of lidocaine and dexamethasone) is placed directly over the painful area and the dispersive pad is placed approximately 2 in. away (usually proximally). The electrodes are filled, and the current is turned on slowly. The current is usually increased by 1 mA per minute up to 4–5 mA per minute with the patient's comfort level always a guideline. Treatment time using these continuous, direct current devices is usually limited to 10–15 minutes because of the possibility of electrochemical burns with longer treatment times. Advances, such as the buffering of medications and the use of modulated current, may allow longer treatment times without risk of electrochemical injury.[12] A therapeutic trial of three treatments per week for 2 weeks will usually determine if a significant clinical response will occur with this method. Protocols for iontophoresis may vary.

REFERENCES

1. Silver HL, Poole RM. Therapeutic Modalities in Sports Rehabilitation. In CL Baker Jr (ed), The Hughston Clinic Sports Medicine Book. Philadelphia: Williams & Wilkins, 1995; 627–635.

2. Loane SR. Cryotherapy—Using Cold to Treat Injuries. In O Appenzeller (ed), Sports Medicine: Fitness, Training, Injuries. Baltimore: Urban & Schwarzenberg, 1988;447–452.

3. Kowal MA. Review of physiologic effects of cryotherapy. J Orthop Sports Phys Ther 1983;5:66–73.

4. Swenson C, Sward L, Karlsson J. Cryotherapy in sports medicine. Scand J Med Sci Sports 1996;6:193–200.

5. McMaster WC, Liddle S, Waugh TR. Laboratory evaluation of various cold therapy modalities. Am J Sports Med 1978;6:291–294.

6. Lehmann JF, deLateur BJ. Therapeutic Heat. In JF Lehmann (ed), Therapeutic Heat and Cold (3rd ed). Baltimore: Williams & Wilkins, 1982.

7. Hardy JD, Bard P. Body Temperature Regulation. In VD Mount Castel (ed), Medical Physiology 2 (13th ed). St. Louis: Mosby, 1974.

8. Gieck JH, Saliba EN. Application of modalities in overuse syndromes. Clin Sports Med 1987;6:427–466.

9. Kleinkort JA, Wood F. Phonophoresis with 1 percent versus 10 percent hydrocortisone. Phys Ther 1975;55:1320–1324.

10. Gray D, Gamino B. Physical Modalities in Rehabilitation. In B Reider (ed), Sports Medicine: The School-Age Athlete. Philadelphia: Saunders, 1996;75–93.

11. Costello CT, Jeske AH. Iontophoresis: applications in transdermal medication delivery. Phys Ther 1995;75:554–563.

12. Howard JP, Drake TR, Kellogg DL Jr. Effects of alternating current iontophoresis on drug delivery. Arch Phys Med Rehabil 1995;76:463–466.

4

Mass-Participation Events

WILLIAM O. ROBERTS

The medical administration and care of athletes in mass-participation events requires advance planning to ensure the safety of the competitors. Whenever large numbers of athletes gather to pursue the pleasure of sport and competition, the shear mass of athletes will guarantee an active medical event based on the intrinsic risk of physical activity. A well-planned event with input from the medical staff in the early stages of development will give the athletes the best opportunity for a peak performance in a safe environment. The functions of the medical operations team are two-fold: The primary purpose is to ensure competitor safety, and the secondary purpose is to prevent unnecessary use of the local emergency medical facilities. Event planning can be divided into three phases: pre-event or pre-race planning, event or race-day medical operations, and event or race review and modification. Acknowledging the inherent risk for medical and trauma casualties in sport, a mass-participation event should be approached as a planned disaster.

PRE-EVENT PLANNING FOR SPECTATOR AND ATHLETE CARE

Spectator Care

In many circumstances, spectator care will not be handled by the same medical team as athlete care. At some mass-participation events, the spectator care will, by default, fall into the hands of the athlete medical team. It is important to establish early in the planning process if the event medical team will have primary responsibility for spectators and athletes. The general problems of spectators will be exacerbations of chronic disease and acute events related to cardiovascular compromise, anaphylaxis, or trauma. The general event care plan will remain unchanged, but the addition of spectator care requires a change in staffing ratios and supply requisitions. Spectator care will be radically influenced by high heat and humidity, extreme cold, and waiting times in transportation and venue access lines.

Athlete Care

Athlete care at events is the most public of the sports medicine roles. The general considerations for athlete care outlined in Table 4-1 are the same for road races and large team gatherings. A well-organized medical plan will improve the image of the sports medicine team and ensure prompt medical attention for injured athletes.

The number of participants will influence every part of the medical plan, and an early estimate is crucial. Larger numbers increase the number of common medical casualties and increase the risk of rare or uncommon medical problems. Therefore, more medical support will be needed, from personnel to supplies.

The injury rates in a given activity will also influence medical planning. The predicted incidence of injury during an event will be used to project the needs for staff, supplies, and equipment and can be estimated by this equation: (anticipated number of participants) × (casualty incidence). After 2–3 years of experience, an event-specific injury rate can be calculated. This will provide a more accurate estimate of casualty occurrence and improve the accuracy of staffing and supply requests. For new events, estimates will be based on literature ranges as outlined in Tables 4-2 and 4-3.[1, 2]

The risk of sudden cardiac death in road racing is in the range of 1 in 50,000 to 1 in 100,000 entrants.[3] Preparations for cardiac arrest will be necessary, but the protocols will not be used very often in mass-participation events. Injury types and distributions are also critical to

TABLE 4-1
Medical Care for Mass-Participation Events

Event Planning for Athlete Care	Race-Day Medical Operations	Event Review and Modification
Number of participants	Personnel and staffing	What went right
Injury rates	Equipment and supplies	What went wrong
Selection of event day(s)	Communications	Proposed changes
Starting time	Transportation	
Event modification parameters	Treatment protocols	
Shelter		
Medical records		
Preparticipation screening		
Competitor and volunteer education		
Expected problems		
Emergency services notification		
Hazardous waste precautions		

TABLE 4-2
Literature-Based Injury Rates for Endurance Activities

Activity	Injury Rate
Running (41 km)	1–20%
Running (<21 km)	1–5%
Triathlon (225 km)	15–30%
Nordic skiing (55 km)	5%
Triathlon (51 km)	2–5%
Cycling (variable)	5%

Source: Adapted from BH Jones, WO Roberts. Medical Management of Endurance Events. In RC Cantu, LJ Micheli (eds), ACSM: Guidelines for the Team Physician. Philadelphia: Lea and Febiger, 1991; 266–286.

TABLE 4-3
National Collegiate Athletic Association Injury Studies

Sport	Injury Rate*
Football	35.9
Wrestling	30.6
Women's gymnastics	22.0
Men's soccer	19.7
Women's soccer	16.4
Men's ice hockey	16.4
Men's basketball	9.7
Women's basketball	8.9
Baseball	6.1
Women's volleyball	5.2

*Game injury rate per 1,000 athlete exposures.
Source: Adapted from National Collegiate Athletic Association. NCAA Ice Hockey Surveillance System Report 1994–95 (NCAA 10157-11/94). Overland Park, KS: Sports Sciences National Collegiate Athletic Association, 1995.

the medical plan. Trauma increases the need for specialized equipment and will require the team to be prepared for transport as well as on-site care. The injury classification from the Twin Cities Marathon is listed in Table 4-4.

Selection of Event Days

Placing an event on the annual calendar may be the single most important administrative decision with regard to competitor safety in continuous and prolonged outdoor events or indoor events without air-conditioned facilities. When scheduling a new event, choose a time of the year that avoids the extremes of temperature, especially high ambient temperatures combined with high humidity. Existing events should consider moving to a safer part of the calendar if there has been a history of excessive heat- or cold-related problems. The historical average high and low temperatures and relative humidities for a proposed race day will suggest the likely risk of environmental injury. If a wet bulb globe temperature (WBGT) greater than 82°F (28°C) is anticipated in the coolest part

of the suggested day, consider scheduling the race for a cooler time of the year. If the weather data is not in acceptable risk ranges for the proposed start and finish times, regional and national sanctions should be withheld from the event. In urban areas, it is important to consider the stored heat energy that will accumulate in the streets and buildings during a hot, sunny day.

Starting Time for an Endurance Event

Schedule the start and finish during the coolest part of the day for spring, summer, and fall months and during the warmer parts of the day during winter in the temperate latitudes. Starting in the early morning for historically "hot" days will allow a finish in reasonable conditions for the slower competitors. When advising an existing race, make every effort to move starting times to the early morn-

TABLE 4-4
Injury Classification

Medical
  Exercise-associated collapse
    Hyperthermia
    Hypothermia
    Normal body temperature
  Leg cramps
  Cardiac arrest
  Anaphylaxis
  Insulin shock
  Other
Trauma
  Microtrauma
    Tendinitis
    Fasciitis
    Blister
    Bursitis
  Macrotrauma
    Closed head injury
    Concussion
    Neck
    Chest
    Abdominal
    Vascular
    Muscle
    Skeletal
    Skin

ing hours to give the elite competitors the coolest hours for optimum performance and the citizen runners a chance to finish before the temperatures start to drop if the race day is unexpectedly cool.

Armstrong and Maresh stated in their review of acclimatization for heat that the risk of heat injury rises above 21°C (70°F) and 50% relative humidity.[4] Data from Grandma's Marathon in Duluth, Minnesota, showed the odds ratio for medical illness rises in both the half- and full-marathon distance if the starting temperature is higher than 15°C (60°F).[5] The Twin Cities Marathon experience is similar, with the highest percentage of injury (26–30 per 1,000 entrants) when the starting temperatures have been higher than 15°C, compared with fewer than 18 per 1,000 entrants when the starting temperatures have been lower than 15°C.[6] In comparison, the Boston Marathon often has injury rates in the 5–10% range with a noon start and the start temperature higher than 15°C.[1] The average daily high and low temperatures are nearly identical for the Twin Cities and the Boston Marathons, but the injury rates are considerably lower with the early-morning start at the Twin Cities Marathon.

Performance in distance races at the college level generally decreases as WBGT increases.[7] The Minnesota State High School League State Track Meet held in mid-June often has midafternoon high temperatures in the 80°–100°F (26°–39°C) range. Moving the start of the 3,200-m race from 4 P.M. to 11 A.M. has resulted in a dramatic drop in postrace collapse with the virtual elimination of intravenous fluid administration to collapsed athletes. Precooling the body increases exercise endurance in hot, humid conditions, implying that starting with a "cooler" body in the early morning may afford racers some protection from heat stress.[8] Races longer than 5 k with anticipated high humidity and an ambient temperature higher than 80°F during the race should have a start near sunrise or sunset.

Event Cancellation or Modification Parameters and Hazardous Conditions

Normal, prudent behavioral adaptations used by athletes in training are abandoned for competition, and in athletic contests the decisions regarding adverse conditions are "transferred" by the athletes to the event administration or officials. Hazardous conditions can be defined as any situation that threatens the health or safety of the athlete beyond the "normal" risk of that activity. Examples include lightning, heat and humidity, cold, wet or icy surfaces that interfere with traction, wind, obstructions, and air pollution. Lightning is a deadly force and postponement or cancellation is an accepted response. Athletes should be moved to buildings or cars when lightning is in the vicinity. Heat with high humidity and cold conditions deserve similar consideration for the athlete's safety. The options to consider when the conditions pose a risk to the competitors are to alter, postpone, or cancel the event. The protocol for modifying events in high-risk situations should be established and published in advance. A reasonable safety plan should announce environmental risks at the start of competition, evacuate the area when appropriate and before danger is imminent, and provide adequate shelter or protection for the athletes and spectators. Volunteer safety must also be considered in the decision to continue or alter an event.

It is difficult to imagine canceling a major mass-participation event, especially when television and sponsors are involved. The responsibility of the event administration lies not only with the competitors but with the volunteers who are exposed and may be at risk when hazardous conditions are present. It is difficult to convince many race officials that lightning, extreme heat, and severe cold are equally hazardous to the health of the entrants and that event modification, including cancellation, may need to be considered. The event administration should be especially cautious of an extremely

TABLE 4-5
Wet Bulb Globe Temperature (WBGT) Heat Safety Cascade and Flag System

The WBGT and color-coded flags to indicate the risk of thermal stress are:

Black flag (extreme risk). WBGT is above 28°C (82°F). Races should be canceled, postponed, or modified if conditions exceed this level at starting time. If unable to cancel the event, it may be prudent to advise the participants of the risks and advise no competition.

Red flag (high risk). WBGT is 23°–28°C (73°–82°F). This signal indicates that all runners should be aware that heat injury is possible and any person particularly sensitive to heat or humidity should probably not run. Advise participants to slow pace and stress hydration.

Yellow flag (moderate risk). WBGT is 18°–23°C (65°–73°F). It should be remembered that the air temperature and radiant heat load will increase during the course of the race if conducted in the morning or early afternoon.

Green flag (low risk). WBGT is below 18°C (65°F). This does not guarantee that heat injury will not occur, only that the risk is low. Both hyperthermia and hypothermia are likely to occur in this temperature range.

White flag (lower risk for hyperthermia, but increasing risk for hypothermia). WBGT is below 10°C (50°F). Hypothermia may occur, especially in slow runners during long races and in wet and windy conditions.

Blue flag (increasing risk for frostbite and hypothermia). Ambient temperature less than 0°C (32°F).

Black flag. Cancel Nordic ski races for ambient temperatures less than –4°F (–20°C) because of generated windchill in the severe risk range.

Source: Adapted from American College of Sports Medicine. Position statement on heat and cold illnesses during distance running. Med Sci Sports Exerc 1996;28:i–vii.

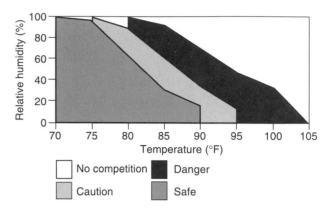

FIGURE 4-1
Event modification temperature and relative humidity graph (does not include radiant or black globe contribution to heat stress). (Adapted from National Weather Service tables.)

hot race day that is preceded by one or more extremely hot days, or in multiday competitions in which there is no opportunity for respite from the heat. The risk of heat stroke rises dramatically in these situations as heat gradually accumulates in the competitors. A warm day after several days of cool weather can also increase the risk to competitors who may not be acclimatized to the heat.

The risk of heat illness increases above 70°F (21°C) and 50% relative humidity, and suspicion for heat illness should be high in warm, humid conditions.[4] The American College of Sports Medicine has suggested a temperature cascade for risk modification in endurance running events using the WBGT, which measures the combined thermal stress from the wet bulb thermometer (WBT), dry bulb thermometer (DBT), and radiant energy or black globe thermometer (BGT) (WBGT = 0.7 WBT + 0.2 BGT + 0.1 DBT).[9] A corresponding colored-flag system can be used to visually signal the thermal injury risk of current weather conditions to competitors (Table 4-5).

The dewpoint temperatures may be used as a guide when the WBGT is not available. Dewpoints in the 60s are stressful, 70s are oppressive, and 80s are extremely dangerous for athletes competing at high levels of exertion. Another simple guideline for judging the level of heat stress is to add the ambient temperature in degrees Fahrenheit to the relative humidity. A sum greater than 150 implies that very high-risk conditions for heat illness exist, and postponement, modification, or cancellation should be considered. A temperature-humidity competition recommendation is illustrated in Figure 4-1, but it should be recognized that this cascade does not include the radiant heat load of the sun. Liability for allowing practice or competition in higher-risk conditions will increase with the current data regarding heat illness and prevention.

Cold temperatures less than 32°F (0°C), especially with wind chill, require clothing precautions for hypothermia and frostbite. Eye protection should be required for fast-moving sports in cold temperatures to prevent frostbite of the cornea. Tight-fitting alpine ski race boots markedly increase the risk of frostbite of the toes, and alpine events should use extreme caution at subzero temperatures. At temperatures less than –4°F (–20°C), Nordic ski races should be postponed, and at temperatures less than –20°F (–40°C), practices should be canceled. Windchill increases heat loss and risk of hypothermia and frostbite injury and should be considered in the decision to continue or postpone an event in cold environments. Windchill can even have an effect at moderate temperatures. A simple rule is the following: At 50°F with a 20-mph wind speed, the windchill factor or cooling rate is equal to 32°F.

Shelter should be provided for both well and ill or injured competitors along the race course or at the event venue to prevent the progression of environmentally induced problems.

Medical records should be kept to document care, calculate incidence of casualties, project future needs for staffing and supplies, research injury rates and trends, and document environmental conditions. An example from the Twin Cities Marathon is shown in Figure 4-2. Similar forms can be developed for any event or tournament geared toward the most common problems of the specific activity. Race records of entrants, finishers, casualties, and weather conditions should be kept to allow comparison from year to year and event to event. In longer events, the historic data become critical to ensure adequate medical staffing at peak injury-risk times.

Body fluid and hazardous waste precautions are necessary in the care of athletes who potentially carry blood-borne diseases. A blood-borne pathogens policy should be implemented using modified universal precautions as a minimum standard. Sharp instruments and contaminated waste disposal should be provided in convenient locations throughout the medical area.

Preparticipation screening is costly in mass-participation settings and may not be cost-effective in reducing injury or illness. In wrestling tournaments, a precompetition skin examination should be done to eliminate competitors with active viral (herpes), bacterial, and fungal skin infections. Education programs for competitors and volunteers will be helpful for injury prevention and intervention. Written and oral presentations should outline the expected problems and prevention strategies and should be included with race registration materials and in the race home page if one is available on the Internet. The medical problems outlined in Table 4-4 fall into two simple groups: common and rare-random. The injury profile will be unique for each event type but will generally be the same for similar event types. Medical protocols include simple first aid, cardiopulmonary resuscitation (CPR), advanced cardiac life support (ACLS), advanced trauma life support (ATLS), and exercise-associated collapse (EAC) protocols.

DEVELOPING MEDICAL OPERATIONS FOR MASS-PARTICIPATION RACES AND TOURNAMENTS

Mass-participation events include road races on foot, bicycles, or in-line skates; Nordic ski races; and open-water distance swims with courses spanning many miles. Large tournaments involving individual and team competitions in swimming, wrestling, soccer, rugby, volleyball, or basketball usually have a more geographically defined competition area, but will share many of the logistic problems of mass-participation events. The potential for trauma will influence the staffing and equipment needs for all events. The safety considerations for mass races and large tournaments should be included in the early phases of event development.

Road Races

A representative of the medical team should be present for course development and review to protect the safety of the competitors. The start should be located away from steep downhill areas, especially if wheelchairs will be involved in running races. Some variations that may decrease the risk of injury that is due to crowding at the start include wave (sequential) and split starts. The wave start has been very effective in decreasing start problems in Nordic ski races and also allows a better chance for an accurate course time for the competitor. The course should be assessed for hills, turns, immovable objects, altitude changes, and open water, which may increase the risk to athletes. A procedure for traffic control is essential in races that use roads normally reserved for motorized vehicles.

A scheme of aid stations should be developed for the course. Medical aid stations are usually stationary and located at regular intervals along the course. Courses that have adequate space for vehicles can deploy mobile medical aid teams in buses or vans supplied with medical equipment to respond rapidly to medical problems on the course. Fluid stations can be combined with stationary medical aid stations. The type and location of course aid stations should be established well in advance of the race so competitors know the locations in advance. Medical aid station options include major aid stations, which provide full medical care, and minor aid stations, which provide comfort care, fluids, and first aid. Major aid stations are generally located at the finish area and at high-injury locations along the course. Stationary aid stations should be located every 15–20 minutes at the average race pace along the course. The interval may need to be shortened for very large fields to improve access to aid and fluids for the competitors. First-response teams on motorcycles or bicycles equipped with an automatic defibrillator can decrease the time to defibrillation in a cardiac arrest.

Some form of shelter for dropped participants will be necessary for inclement weather. Along the race course, school buses can be used for well dropouts and a stationary ambulance or a tent can provide shelter for ill dropouts. At the Twin Cities Marathon, these shelter vehicles are parked at the medical aid stations on the course.

The finish area should be equipped and staffed with a major medical station or field hospital located 50–200 yd

Marathon Medical Record—Confidential   19_____

Race #: _____   Location: Finish/Aid station mile: _____   Arrival time: _____

Name: _____   Discharge time: _____

Age: _____   Gender: M / F   Finish time: _____

Previous marathons: # Entered: _____   # Finished: _____   Best previous time: _____

Weekly mileage: _____   Pre-race injury/illness: Y / N

                   Describe: _____

Skin, Bones, and Joints

Complaint:	Pain	Blister	Abrasion	Bleeding	Cramps	Swelling

                  Other: _____

Tissue:	Skin	Muscle	Tendon	Ligament	Bone

                  Other: _____

Location:

Toe	R / L		Knee	R / L
Foot	R / L		Thigh	R / L
Ankle	R / L		Hip	R / L
Calf	R / L		Back	R / L

                  Other: _____

Diagnosis:

Blister		Tendinitis
Sprain		Abrasion
Strain		Cramps
Bursitis		Stress fracture (suspected)
Fasciitis		

                  Other: _____

Notes:

Medical Problems   Arrival time: _____

Race #: _____   Discharge time: _____

Symptoms and signs

Exhaustion	Lightheaded	Stomach cramps
Fatigue	Confused	Leg cramps
Hot or fever	Headache	Rapid heart rate
Vomiting	Nausea	Palpitations
Unconscious	CNS changes	Muscle spasms

                  Other: _____

Mental status: Alert   or   Responds to: Voice / Touch / Pain

Orientation: Person / Place / Time

Walking status: Alone / With assistance / Unable

Other: _____

Time	Temperature	BP	Pulse	IV fluids	Meds/Rx
_____	_____	_____	_____	_____	_____
_____	_____	_____	_____	_____	_____
_____	_____	_____	_____	_____	_____
_____	_____	_____	_____	_____	_____

Notes:

Diagnosis

EAC		Other _____	IV fluid	Y / N
Hyperthermic:	mild / mod / severe	_____	$D_{50}W$	Y / N
Normothermic:	mild / mod / severe	_____	ER transfer	Y / N
Hypothermic:	mild / mod / severe	_____	Discharge home	Y / N

FIGURE 4-2

Sample road race medical form tailored to common problems in the marathon finish area. (BP = blood pressure; CNS = central nervous system; $D_{50}W$ = 50% dextrose in water; EAC = exercise-associated collapse; ER = emergency room; IV = intravenous; Meds = medications; mod = moderate; Rx = treatment.)

beyond the finish line. At the Twin Cities Marathon, where the injury rate is about 18 per 1,000 entrants, the medical tent is between 1,500 and 2,400 sq. ft in area. Because the conditions are usually cool, the tent is heated with a propane furnace. The medical tent or building should have the space to accommodate the peak flow of injuries and the average length of stay of the casualties. The injury peak at the Twin Cities Marathon is at 3.5 hours after the start, and the average length of stay is 30–60 minutes.

The medical area can be subdivided into triage, intensive medical, intensive trauma, minor medical, minor trauma, and skin areas (or tents). A medical records coordinator and crew will improve the collection of medical data. The medical team will also be responsible for triage in the finish line chutes, the postchute finish areas, and the family meeting area. Sweep teams can be used to patrol the areas away from the finish line for casualties. For true emergencies, such as cardiac arrest, an advanced life support ambulance should be available for immediate transport to the nearest hospital emergency facility. Shelter should be available for well finishers in inclement weather. In hot conditions, fanning out the finishers will increase the ability to remove heat. Individual detection chips are now available and used in many races. The chip is attached to the shoe and can be detected electronically to record finish times. With the advent of chip-detection computerized timing systems, the need for chutes and the artificial slowing of runners after the finish will be removed, and the rate and severity of collapse may decrease in many races. The area of most frequent collapse may move farther downstream from the finish line with the use of the chip. Race medical teams will need to adjust their triage strategies as more races implement this technology.

The public permit for a race course on city streets will often limit the amount of time available to complete the event. Course time limits and scheduled closure should be published in advance to ensure appropriate competitor entry into the field. Traffic control with barricades and traffic control personnel at all intersections should be maintained until the course is closed. It is not uncommon for slow competitors to continue along the route after the course is closed, but the medical team and race administration should make it known if race services will continue after course closure. The Twin Cities Marathon does not leave unattended fluids along the course after it has been closed for fear of willful contamination of the fluids. A common time limit for the marathon is 6 hours. An "end of race vehicle" traveling at the race closure pace can serve to notify participants of course closure and mark the "official" end of race services for competitors and volunteers.

Communication among the medical team members will help ensure adequate care and rapid response to emergency situations and dropped-out runners. Communications systems should be developed for the medical team to discuss information with spotters and medical personnel on the course and at the aid stations. Portable or hardwire phones and handheld radios can be used along the course. A communications coordinator at a central dispatch station located in the medical area at the finish line can ensure course coverage and response. In urban areas, the race communications system can be augmented by telephone access to the 911 emergency system. The role of the 911 system should be clarified with the volunteers, because activation of the 911 system will set the protocols in motion that may remove an ill competitor from the care of the race medical team. A separate communications network should be developed for the finish area to assist the medical team in triage and transport of runners who have problems away from the immediate finish-line medical team.

Transportation should be provided for competitors who cannot finish the event. Well dropout competitors will need some form of transportation to the finish area. The Twin Cities Marathon uses small vans that sweep the course in 2-mile segments until the closing vehicle passes. The dropout runners are let off at the next aid station to enter the shelter bus, which moves to the finish line when it is full. The New York City Marathon uses the subway system, which can be accessed for free with a race entry number. As many as 40% of entrants may drop out of a marathon in hot conditions. Ill or injured competitors should be transported to prevent the progression of illness or injury. Ambulance transport is probably the most prudent transportation for ill competitors. In the finish area, wheelchairs, litters, and stretchers are used to transport casualties who are unable to walk with assistance to the medical evaluation area.

Fluids and foods should be available at the start, finish, and transition areas and at every aid station along the course. Fluid stations should be located on the outside (farthest from the tangent line) of the course every 15–20 minutes at the average pace and every 10 minutes for very large fields (more than 15,000 participants). At each fluid station there should be 6–12 oz of each fluid type for every competitor. Maintaining adequate hydration will decrease the risk of exertional hyperthermia and heat stroke.[10, 11] The amount of fluid should be doubled for the start, finish, and transition areas. Water is an adequate fluid for shorter races.[12] Carbohydrate-electrolyte solutions can improve performance for events more than 50 minutes in duration.[10, 12] An electrolyte solution will decrease the risk of water overload and hyponatremia and may be safer for ultramarathon and long triathlon distances.[13-15] Estimate the number of cups at three per entrant per aid station along the course and six per entrant at the start, finish, and transition areas. High-carbohydrate foods and fruits should be selected based on competitor preferences and made available at the finish and along the course for longer events. The fluid and food types and the fluid station course locations should be published in advance of the event so competitors can use the same fluids and foods in training. Volunteers will also need fluid and food, especially in events of long duration.

An impaired competitor policy should be developed and published before the event to allow the medical staff to intervene in cases of suspected life-threatening medical emergency, such as heat stroke, hypothermia, or cardiovascular compromise. Medical personnel at the Twin Cities Marathon use the following triage criteria for an athlete to proceed in the race:

- Oriented to person, place, and time
- Progressing with straight line movement toward the finish
- Maintaining a good competitive posture
- Appearing "clinically fit"

Competitors should not be disqualified for a medical evaluation during the event and should be allowed to return to competition if criteria for safe return are met. The criteria for returning a competitor to the event after trauma and injury or illness should be determined by the medical team in advance of the event.

When the start and finish areas are separated, a shuttle should be provided to move dry clothes from the start to the finish area to ensure warm, dry clothing is available to the competitors at the finish. Volunteers should be assigned to retrieve the dry clothes for the runners in the medical tent. In cold conditions, a portable clothes dryer will allow casualties to dry sweaty clothing so that they do not leave the medical area in wet clothing. This is especially important at medical aid stations away from the finish area.

Part of the purpose of the medical team is to relieve the local emergency facilities from minor race casualties. Emergency medical services should be notified of the event date, location, start and finish times, and the anticipated casualty types and numbers. Ambulance services should be enlisted and emergency medical service protocols integrated into the race medical protocols to ease the transfer of care to emergency rooms and hospitals.

Special considerations are necessary for some specific competitions. Wheelchair racers should be given an earlier start than runners to minimize the risk of collision between slower runners and wheelchair competitors who can reach high speeds on the downhill segments of the course. In biking events, the injury rates have been in the range of 5%, but the risk for major trauma is increased.[16] The course should be swept clear of loose gravel and sand, especially at the corners, where good traction is imperative for the safety of the racers. Swimming events require the ability to perform water rescue and the presence of spotters in or on the water. Cold-water races below 65°F (19°C) should require wet suits for hypothermia protection. Nordic ski races at the 55-km distance also have an injury rate of 5%.[17, 18] Congestion at the starts, severe cold conditions, and evacuations from remote course sites pose the greatest concern for the medical team. Combination sports, such as the triathlon, have injury rates at the 51-km distance in the 2–5% range; in the long-course triathlon, injury rates can range as high as 35%.[13, 19] All of the problems of individual sport events can be compounded in the multisport events.

Team Sports

Team and individual sport tournaments present the same general medical considerations for the care of large numbers of athletes, but the competitions often last for several days. The site selection should consider the proximity to medical care and on-site facilities for medical care.

Sports with collision potential should prepare both for trauma and for the athlete who collapses from prolonged or repeated exercise bouts. Some representative game injury rates from the National Collegiate Athletic Association injury registry are listed in Table 4-3.[2] Data from boys youth ice hockey (ages 11–19 years) showed an average injury rate of 117 per 1,000 player hours (PH) and 26 per 1,000 athlete exposures.[20] Since 1986, the USA Cup Soccer Tournament has had an all-injury rate for boys and girls of 15–20 per 1,000 PH (S. Elias, personal communication, June 9, 1998).

For large tournaments, such as the USA Soccer Cup (with more than 10,000 athletes competing on 54 pitches for a span of 6 days), communication and transportation systems are essential for adequate medical care. In the summer months, a plan for hot weather should be in place before the opening of the tournament to respond quickly to increases in heat-related collapse, as youth athletes are at even greater risk than adults.[21] For unexpectedly hot conditions, it is helpful to encourage athletes to spend as much of their day as possible in a cool, air-conditioned environment. When trauma is expected, it may be useful to arrange for a portable radiography unit to be on site for the duration of the tournament. All of the other considerations for medical planning of mass-participation events also apply to tournaments.

RACE DAY AND EVENT MEDICAL OPERATIONS

Personnel and Staffing

The medical team for an athletic event is usually staffed by physicians, acute care nurses, paramedics, emergency medical technicians (EMTs), certified athletic trainers (ATCs), physical therapists, first aid–trained persons, and nonmedical assistants. Common sources of medical volunteers beyond the local hospital and clinic rosters include the community ambulance services, the state Athletic Trainers Association, the National Ski Patrol, the Civil Bicycle Patrol, the Civil Defense, the American Red Cross, the Explorer Scouts, and the National Guard or Armed Services Reserves. A physician should be the medical director and should be in direct dialog with event administration. The medical director should be involved in pre-event planning and represent the medical team. The Twin Cities Marathon, with 6,000–7,000 entrants, has 250–300 medical volunteers. Within this group there are 25–30 physicians, 30–40 nurses, 100–120 EMTs, and 20–30 ATCs. Most of the physicians are trained in family practice, emergency medicine, or critical care medicine. The nurses are generally recruited from the area hospital critical care units or emergency rooms. It is important for the competitors, coaches, other volunteers, and spectators that medical personnel be readily identified. Distinctive shirts, hats, jackets, and vests have been used with success at many events. Both the Twin Cities Marathon and the USA Soccer Cup use red shirts for easy visibility and recognition.

Staff Placement and Responsibilities

The finish line at a road race and the main medical area of a tournament will usually be staffed by physicians, nurses, and physical therapists. Course and sideline first aid can be handled by EMTs and ATCs. Course and secondary event aid stations should have a physician present. The medical team at a road race finish should divide into chute- and finish-area triage teams and a medical tent team. One or two physicians should act as tent supervisors to assist the smaller treatment teams with difficult case-management issues. An arrest team should be appointed and specific roles assigned so the team can function quickly and efficiently in the event of a cardiac arrest. Triage teams are located in the chutes and finish area to assess competitors and direct those in need of care to the medical tent. Protocol at the Twin Cities Marathon is formulated to keep on-course injuries away from the finish area, and all on-course injuries are transported to local

emergency rooms. Aid station physicians assume care of the injured athlete until the advanced life support ambulance can take over management of the athlete. Paramedics from the local emergency network should be enlisted for transport of critically injured or ill athletes to an emergency facility. Nonmedical volunteers are used in medical records and as runners to fetch dry clothing and food for injured athletes.

Equipment and Supplies

Equipment and medical supplies for a major aid station are listed in Tables 4-6 through 4-8; equipment and supplies for minor aid stations are listed in Table 4-9. The following intravenous solutions are recommended for fluid replacement in athletes who collapse during prolonged events and who are unable to take oral fluids: For events less than 4 hours in duration, use dextrose $(D)_{5\%}$ ½ normal saline (NS) or $D_{5\%}$ NS; for events greater than 4 hours, use $D_{5\%}$ NS for first liter of replacement fluid.[13] Consider changing to ½ NS or NS beyond the first liter of intravenous fluid to prevent hyperglycemia.[13] It is prudent to avoid fluids containing K^+ until a serum K^+ has been measured. If there is a high potential for hyponatremia during an event, such as in a long-distance triathlon or an ultramarathon, arrangements should be made to measure the serum sodium and potassium on site.[13, 15] Lactate solutions should not be used if there is a risk for hypothermia, because the cold liver will not metabolize lactate.[22] Medications that have proved useful at the Twin Cities Marathon and other races are listed in Table 4-10.

Triage and Treatment Protocols

Medical protocols should be agreed on in advance to speed the diagnosis and treatment of multiple casualties. Some standard intervention protocols include CPR, ACLS, and ATLS. CPR and ACLS are begun if cardiac arrest or unexplained syncope occurs. The chances of surviving a cardiac arrest are low in the marathon, especially in the last 15 km of the race, but successful resuscitation is possible. Cardioversion should be attempted as soon as the cardiac rhythm is determined. An automatic defibrillator can be used by first responders to speed access to defibrillation. Consider the following modifications to the ACLS protocol early in the resuscitation effort: substrate repletion with 50% D in water, high-dose intravenous epinephrine (5–10 mg), and sodium bicarbonate. ATLS protocol should be used for collision events and suspected trauma casualties in road races. For closed head injury and concussion in sports that use helmets, casualties should be

TABLE 4-6
Medical Equipment and Supplies for an Event*

Equipment	Trauma	Skin and Wound Care	Airway and ACLS	IV Fluid	Medications	Cooling
Bandage scissors	Aluminum padded splint	1% lidocaine	Bulb suction or turkey baster	Butterfly catheter (18-, 22-, and 25-gauge)	Acetaminophen	Ice
Batteries	Backboard	Alcohol swabs	Cricothyrotomy kit	$D_{5\%}$ ½ NS	Albuterol nebulizers	Tubs or wading pools
Blue light	Blankets	Bacitracin ointment	Defibrillator and monitor	$D_{5\%}$ NS	Albuterol MDI	Fans
Coins	Cast padding (3-in., 4-in., 6-in. rolls)	Band-Aids	Endotracheal tube (3 mm, 5 mm, 7 mm)	½ NS	Atropine cardiac	—
Cotton-tip applicators	Cervical collar (hard)	Benzoin adherent	Laryngoscope (plastic adult and pediatric size)	NS (500- or 1,000-ml bags)	$D_{50\%}$ W (50 ml)	—
Cups	Cervical collar (soft)	Elastic bandage (4 in. and 6 in.)	Mouth-to-mouth mask	IV administration sets	Demerol	—
Emesis bags (airline type)	Crutches	Forceps	Nasal pharyngeal airway (three sizes)	Tourniquet	Diazepam	—
Emesis basin	Elastic bandage (2-in., 3-in., 4-in., 6-in. rolls)	Irrigation syringe or bag	Oral airway (three sizes)	Vein catheters (16-, 18-, and 22-gauge)	Diphenhydramine	—
Examination gloves	Garbage bags	Kling gauze	Oxygen tank and administration set	—	Epinephrine 1:10,000	
Eye patch pads	Ice	Nasal packing	Ventilation bag, mask, and reservoir with CO_2 whipple	—	Epinephrine 1:1,000	
Flashlight	Ice chest	Needle holder	—	—	Lidocaine 1% local	—
Fluorescence stain strips	Knee immobilizer	Needles (30-, 25-, 22-, and 18-gauge)	—	—	Magnesium sulfate	—
Measuring tape	Plastic bags	Normal saline for irrigation (250–1,000 ml)	—	—	Morphine	—
Moist towelettes (individual)	Sand bags	Petroleum jelly	—	—	Na bicarbonate	—
Oto-ophthalmoscope	Screwdriver	Povidone-iodine	—	—	Naloxone	—
Paper	Splints: cardboard, inflatable	Scalpel (Nos. 10, 15, 11)	—	—	Nitroglycerin SL	—
Paper bags (lunch size)	Stretcher	Scissors	—	—	Ophthaine	—
Pen	Turkey baster (suction bulb)	Silvadene cream	—	—	Propranolol	—
Plastic zippered bags	—	Soap (small can of shaving cream)	—	—	—	—
Red bag	—	Sterile strips	—	—	—	—

TABLE 4-6
(continued)

Equipment	Trauma	Skin and Wound Care	Airway and ACLS	IV Fluid	Medications	Cooling
Reflex hammer	—	Sterile gloves	—	—	—	—
Safety pins	—	Sterile barrier (full and fenestrated)	—	—	—	—
Sharps box	—	Sterile dressing (2 in. × 2 in., 4 in. × 4 in., 8 in. × 7½ in.)	—	—	—	—
Slings	—	Sterile basin	—	—	—	—
Sphygmoma-nometer	—	Suture (3-0, 4-0, and 5-0 nylon)	—	—	—	—
Stethoscope	—	Suture kits	—	—	—	—
Suction machine	—	Syringes (10 cc, 5 cc, and 3 cc)	—	—	—	—
Telephone	—	Tape: Adhesive (½ in., 1 in., 2 in.), paper (½-in., 1-in. rolls)	—	—	—	—
Thermometer (rectal): clinical, high temperature, low temperature	—	—	—	—	—	—
Tin snips	—	—	—	—	—	—
Tongue blades	—	—	—	—	—	—
Urinals	—	—	—	—	—	—
Water jug	—	—	—	—	—	—

*Equipment may vary from event to event.
ACLS = advanced cardiac life support; $D_{50\%}W$ = 50% dextrose in water; IV = intravenous; MDI = metered dose inhaler; Na= sodium; NS = normal saline; SL = sublingual.

transported with the helmet on if the airway is open and breathing is adequate. This issue is most often encountered in football and ice hockey when the shoulder pads elevate the trunk and make safe removal of the helmet more difficult on the field of play. In bicycle racing, the helmet may be easily removed.

Syncope and near-syncope are common after endurance events. An EAC protocol can be used to standardize and speed the care of collapsed athletes.[23] Collapse before the finish line is often associated with more serious medical problems than collapse after the finish line.[24] Symptoms of EAC include exhaustion, fatigue, hot, cold, nausea, stomach cramps, light-headedness, headache, leg cramps, and palpitations. Signs of EAC include abnormal rectal temperature, unconsciousness, altered mental status, central nervous system changes, inability to walk unassisted,

leg muscle spasms, tachycardia, vomiting, and diarrhea. The classification scheme is outlined in Table 4-11.

The management protocol includes diagnosis and initiating documentation, fluid redistribution and replacement, temperature correction and maintenance, fuel (energy) replacement, and transfer to a medical facility or release from the race medical tent. In mild casualties, fluid redistribution is promoted with ambulation to keep the muscle pump active. In athletes who are unable to walk, fluid redistribution is promoted by placing them in the supine position with the legs and buttocks elevated to restore pooled blood to the circulation.[24, 25] Oral fluid replacement is the preferred method of rehydration in all mild and moderate EAC cases who can tolerate it.[23-25] Intravenous fluids are administered when an athlete is unable to tolerate oral fluids or if severe volume deficits

TABLE 4-7

Equipment for Mass-Participation Endurance Events at Major Aid Stations[a]

Air conditioner
Ambulance: advanced cardiac life support (one)[b]
Blankets, wool or synthetic (100)
Chairs (12)
Clothes dryer, portable
Cots (50)
Extension cords (three)
Fans
Flashlights (six)
Heater (one propane gas with fuel for 8 hours)
Ice (six 40-pound bags)
Lights (trouble or clamp) (12)
Massage towels (100)
Mylar-aluminum or plastic blankets (6,000)
Plug strips (three)
Portable toilet (one at finish tent)
Portable electric generator (one)
Portable telephone (one)
Respiratory humidifier (two)
Security fencing (400 ft)
Shelter:
    Tent (30 ft × 50 ft in finish area)[c]
    Vehicles
    Buildings
Stretchers
Tables (six)
Tubs for immersion cooling
Wash stand (one at finish tent)
Wheelchairs (10)

[a]See also Table 4-6.
[b]Twin Cities Marathon numbers for 6,500 participants and an injury rate of 18 per 1,000 entrants.
[c]Larger size required for higher injury rates.

TABLE 4-8

Medical Supplies for Mass-Participation Endurance Events at Major Aid Stations[a]

No. 11 scalpel blades (100)[b]
⅛-in. cord (100 ft)[c]
Advance cardiac life support kits (three)
Automatic finger stick apparatus (one)
Blood glucose sticks (one box)
Clipboards (50)
Contaminated waste container bag (four)
$D_{50\%}$W—50 ml preloads (50)
Defibrillator-monitor pack (one)
Automatic defibrillator
Diaper pins (three dozen)
Examination gloves (three boxes)
Facial tissue (six boxes)
Home glucose monitor (one)
Intravenous setups (one)
Intravenous fluids: 500- or 1,000-ml bags
    $D_{5\%}$ NS for events >4 hrs
    $D_{5\%}$ ½ NS for events <4 hrs (50)
    ½ NS or NS for second bag
Medical record forms (200)
Oxygen tanks with regulators and masks (two)
Pens (50)
Physician's kit (see Table 4-6)
Sharp instrument disposal container (four)
Thermometer covers (200)
Thermometers (rectal)
    High temperature range—110°F (49°C) (one)
    Clinical (100)
    Low temperature range—70°F (21°C) (10)
Wet wipes (six boxes)

$D_{50\%}$W = 50% dextrose in water; NS = normal saline.
[a]Estimate numbers for expected casualties.
[b]Twin Cities Marathon numbers for 6,500 participants and an injury rate of 1.8 per 1,000 entrants.
[c]For hanging intravenous bags.

exist.[23–25] Temperature correction is important for rapid recovery in hyperthermic and hypothermic EAC, and temperature maintenance is essential for normothermic EAC. Athletes running shorter, faster-paced races are at greater risk for heat stroke in hot, humid conditions because of the rapid production of metabolic heat that cannot be effectively removed from the body.[26] Body temperature should be measured by the rectal route, which is the most accurate estimate of core temperature for sideline and event medicine.[27–30] Ice-water immersion has been shown to be the most rapid form of body cooling in the field.[31–35] Hypothermic athletes who cannot be warmed with simple external or endogenous warming methods should be transferred to an emergency facility. Body energy stores should be replaced with oral glucose solutions, high-carbohydrate foods, intravenous glucose solutions with 5% D, or D 50% in water ($D_{50\%}$W) 50 ml by intravenous push. Severe hyperglycemia will slow the

recovery process. Blood glucose should be measured from the great toe or ear lobe with a home glucose monitor to detect hypoglycemia and to monitor blood glucose levels when more than a liter of 5% D or more than 50 ml of $D_{50\%}$W is administered to avoid hyperglycemia. An athlete who does not respond to the usual treatment protocol should be transferred to an emergency facility. The athlete who responds to the management protocol, is clinically stable, and is normothermic can be discharged from the race medical facility with instructions to continue fluid and energy replacement, and criteria for re-evaluation.

Hyponatremia has been shown to occur in marathon and longer races, and hyponatremia may be a reason for poor response to treatment in EAC.[13, 15, 36] There are two types of symptomatic hyponatremia in events of long duration.[13–15] One type is associated with dehydration, high Na⁺ losses through sweat, and fluid replacement with "unsalted" fluids. This type usually responds well to intra-

TABLE 4-9
Minor Aid Station Supplies

No. 11 scalpel blades
4 in. × 4 in. gauze pads
Albuterol metered dose inhaler
Alcohol or povidone-iodine (Betadine) preparations
Automatic defibrillator
Bacitracin ointment
Adhesive strip bandages
Chairs
Clinical rectal thermometer
Clipboard
Cots
Elastic wrap
Emesis bags
Facial tissue
Garbage bags*
Disposable wipes
Ice
Medical record forms
Moleskin
Mylar or plastic "blankets"
Nonsterile tongue blades
Paper towels
Pen
Penlight
Pocket mouth-to-mouth mask
Adhesive tape: ½ in. and 1 in.
Petroleum jelly—1-lb jars (three to six)
Wool blankets

*Cut head and arm holes for windbreaker.

TABLE 4-10
Commonly Used Medications at Endurance Events

Advanced cardiac life support drugs
    Epinephrine
    Atropine
    Lidocaine
    Procainamide
    Bretylium
    Verapamil
    Sodium bicarbonate
    Morphine
50% Dextrose in water
Albuterol metered dose inhaler and nebulizer
Epinephrine (EpiPen)
Diphenhydramine (antihistamine)
Diazepam
Magnesium sulfate
Acetaminophen

venous fluid replacement with normal saline.[13, 15] The second type is associated with slower competitors who overhydrate with large amounts of salt-free fluids and collapse with dilutional hyponatremia, which can result in seizures and other life-threatening events.[14] This group of casualties may have a temporary inability to regulate body fluid and will require hospitalization with slow removal of excess free water and replacement of Na⁺.[15, 36] Noakes and Hiller have observed this type of hyponatremia at a rate of 1 per 1,000 entrants in the Comrades Marathon and the Hawaii Ironman competitions (personal communication, May 1996).

Leg muscle cramps are common after prolonged exercise. Exercise muscle cramping has been considered a result of dehydration or heat exposure, but evidence suggests at least a partial neural etiology for postexercise muscle cramping. Muscle cramping is also seen with hyponatremia and can be quite severe. Fluid and fuel replacement, assisted walking, massage, and neuromuscular inhibition techniques all seem to help relieve the cramps. Neuromuscular inhibition techniques often relieve cramps when other interventions have failed. Occasionally, medications are necessary to relieve the painful muscle spasms, and both diazepam in 1–5 mg intravenous push aliquots and magnesium sulfate in 1–5 g intravenous aliquots have been used successfully.[13, 15] Dantrolene sodium may be another alternative, especially in the presence of exertional heat stroke.[37, 38]

TABLE 4-11
Exercise-Associated Collapse Classification Matrix

	Mild	*Moderate*	*Severe*
Hyperthermic	T ≥ 103°F (39.5°C)	T ≥ 105°F (40.5°C)	T ≥ 106°F (41°C)
Normothermic	97°F ≤ T ≤ 103°F	97°F ≤ T ≤ 103°F	97°F ≤ T ≤ 103°F
Hypothermic	T ≤ 97°F (36°C)	T ≤ 95°F (35°C)	T ≤ 90°F (32°C)
Key symptoms and signs	Any symptom or sign	No oral intake	CNS changes
	Walk with or without assistance	Extra fluid loss	Unconsciousness
		Unable to walk	
		Severe muscle spasm	

CNS = central nervous system; T = temperature.
Source: Adapted from WO Robert. Exercise associated collapse in endurance events: a classification system. Phys Sportsmed 1989;17:49–55.

Other common medical intervention protocols include allergic or exercise anaphylaxis treated with subcutaneous epinephrine and intramuscular diphenhydramine (50 mg); insulin shock or hypoglycemia treated with concentrated oral glucose solutions, $D_{50\%}W$ 50 ml by intravenous push, or subcutaneous glucagon; and status asthmaticus treated with nebulized albuterol or subcutaneous epinephrine.

In cold-weather competitions there is a risk for frostbite. The digits, face, ears, and genitals are most commonly affected in athletes. The affected area should be insulated to avoid further cold damage and the athletes returned to a sheltered environment. Once there is no danger of second freeze damage to the tissue, immersion of the affected tissue in warm water (104°–106°F [40°–41°C]) should be done for rapid thawing of the tissue.[39, 40] If hypothermia is also present, rewarming should be done in a controlled setting and not on the field.[41] Initial first aid should include removing wet clothing and insulating the body to prevent continued decrease in core temperature.

Transfer protocols for severe medical problems should be determined in advance to avoid delays when problems present to the medical area. Participants with suspected cardiac chest pain should be transported to a hospital emergency facility rather than delay with an evaluation in the race medical facility. "Automatic transfers" at the Twin Cities Marathon include suspected cardiac chest pain, cardiac arrest, respiratory arrest, hyperthermia with seizure, rectal temperature less than 94°F (34°C), and shock. All protocols should be integrated into the emergency medical services system.

EVENT REVIEW AND MODIFICATION

Take the opportunity during and immediately after the event to improve the quality of the medical care and the safety of the athletes. Ask three basic questions: What went right and could it be better? What went wrong and how should it be modified? What can be done to improve the event safety and medical operations? Proposed changes for the next event should be integrated into pre-event planning. Develop a time line for changes and continued practices, review and update the medical database, and begin the pre-event planning process again.

SUMMARY

Competitor safety is the primary goal of the medical team. Mass-participation events are "planned disasters." The duties of the medical team include implementing injury prevention strategies before the event begins, pre-

venting injury progression once the event is under way, and relieving local emergency facilities of the burden of minor and moderate injury generated by the event. The medical team should agree on treatment protocols in advance of the event and work with the event administration to develop a rational and prudent response to hazardous environmental conditions that may arise during the course of the event, increasing the risk to competitors and volunteers above the inherent risk of the sport. Emergency medical and hazardous condition protocols for the event should be easy to comprehend and execute. For collision and contact events, be prepared to evaluate and treat trauma with emergency backup for evacuation. Return to competition criteria should be included in the medical plan. It is acceptable to challenge traditions and suggest alternatives for the safety of the athlete.

REFERENCES

 1. Jones BH, Roberts WO. Medical Management of Endurance Events. In RC Cantu, LJ Micheli (eds), ACSM: Guidelines for the Team Physician. Philadelphia: Lea and Febiger, 1991;266–286.
 2. National Collegiate Athletic Association. NCAA Ice Hockey Surveillance System Report 1994–95 (NCAA 10157-11/94). Overland Park, KS: Sports Sciences National Collegiate Athletic Association, 1995.
 3. Maron B, Poliac LC, Roberts WO. Risk for sudden death associated with marathon running. J Am Coll Cardiol 1996; 28:428–431.
 4. Armstrong LE, Maresh CM. The induction and decay of heat acclimatisation in trained athletes. Sports Med 1991;12: 302–312.
 5. Crouse B, Beattie K. Marathon medical services: strategies to reduce runner morbidity. Med Sci Sports Exerc 1996; 28:1093–1096.
 6. Roberts WO. The 1982 to 1994 Summary of Twin Cities marathon medical injury rates (submitted for publication).
 7. McCann DJ, Adams WC. Wet bulb globe temperature index and performance in competitive distance runners. Med Sci Sports Exerc 1997;29:955–961.
 8. Booth J, Marino F, Ward JJ. Improved running performance in hot humid conditions following whole body precooling. Med Sci Sports Exerc 1997;29:943–949.
 9. American College of Sports Medicine. Position statement on heat and cold illnesses during distance running. Med Sci Sports Exerc 1996;28:i–vii.
10. Coyle EF, Montain SJ. Benefits of fluid replacement with carbohydrate during exercise. Med Sci Sports Exerc 1992;24(suppl):S324–S330.
11. Sawka MN, Young AJ, Latzka WA, et al. Human tolerance to heat strain during exercise: influence of hydration. J Appl Physiol 1992;73:368–375.

12. American College of Sports Medicine. Position statement on exercise and fluid replacement. Med Sci Sports Exerc 1996;28:i–vii.
13. Laird RH. Medical care at ultra endurance triathlons. Med Sci Sports Exerc 1989;21(suppl):S222–S225.
14. Noakes TD. Dehydration during exercise: what are the real dangers? Clin J Sport Med 1995;5:123–128.
15. O'Toole ML, Douglas PS, Laird RH, Hiller WDB. Fluid and electrolyte status in athletes receiving medical care at an ultradistance triathlon. Clin J Sport Med 1995;5:116–122.
16. McLennan JG, McLennan JC, Ungersma J. Accident prevention in competitive cycling. Am J Sports Med 1988;16:266–268.
17. Gannon DM, Derse AR, Bronkema PJ, Primley DM. Emergency care network of a ski marathon. Am J Sports Med 1985;13:316–320.
18. Murphey P. Treating the wounded and the weary at a large cross-country ski marathon. Phys Sportsmed 1987;15:170–183.
19. Weinberg S. The Chicago Bud Light Triathlon. In RH Laird (ed), Report of the Ross Symposium on Medical Coverage of Endurance Athletic Events. Columbus, OH: Ross Laboratories, 1988;74–78.
20. Roberts WO, Brust JD, Leonard BJ. Youth ice hockey injury: tournament injury rates and patterns (submitted for publication).
21. Elias S, Roberts WO, Thorson DC. Team sports in hot weather: guidelines for modifying youth soccer. Phys Sportsmed 1991;19:67–80.
22. Mills WJ. Field care of the hypothermic patient. Int J Sports Med 1992;13(suppl 1):199–202.
23. Roberts WO. Exercise associated collapse in endurance events: a classification system. Phys Sportsmed 1989;17:49–55.
24. Holtzhausen LM, Noakes TD, Kroning B, et al. Clinical and biochemical characteristics of collapsed ultramarathon runners. Med Sci Sports Exerc 1994;26:1095–1101.
25. Noakes TD, Berlinski N, Solomon E, Weight L. Collapsed runners: blood biochemical changes after IV fluid therapy. Phys Sportsmed 1991;19:70–82.
26. Noakes TD, Myburgh KH, du Pliessis J, et al. Metabolic rate, not percent dehydration, predicts rectal temperature in marathon runners. Med Sci Sports Exerc 1991;23:443–449.
27. Armstrong LE, Maresh CM, Crago AE, et al. Interpretation of aural temperatures during exercise, hyperthermia, and cooling therapy. Med Exerc Nut Health 1994;3:9–16.
28. Brengelman GL. The Dilemma of Body Temperature Measurement. In K Shiraki, MK Yousef (eds), Man in Stressful Environments: Thermal and Work Physiology. Springfield, IL: Thomas, 1987.
29. Deschamps A, Levy RD, Cosio MG, et al. Tympanic temperature should not be used to assess exercise induced hyperthermia. Clin J Sport Med 1992;2:27–32.
30. Roberts WO. Assessing core temperature in collapsed athletes. Phys Sportsmed 1994;22:49–55.
31. Armstrong LE, Crago AE, Adams R, et al. Whole-body cooling of hyperthermic runners: comparison of two field therapies. Am J Emerg Med 1996;14:355–358.
32. Brodeur VB, Dennett SR, Griffin LS. Exertional hyperthermia, ice baths, and emergency care at the Falmouth Road Race. J Emerg Nurs 1989;15:304–312.
33. Costrini AM. Emergency treatment of exertional heat stroke and comparison of whole body cooling techniques. Med Sci Sports Exerc 1990;22:15–18.
34. Hayward JS, Collis M, Eckerson JD. Thermographic evaluation of relative heat loss areas of man during cold water immersion. Aerospace Med 1973;44:708–711.
35. Roberts WO. Managing heatstroke: on-site cooling. Phys Sportsmed 1992;20:17–28.
36. Surgenor S, Uphold RE. Acute hyponatremia in ultraendurance athletes. Am J Emerg Med 1994;12:441–444.
37. Bouchama A, Cafege A, Devol EB, et al. Ineffectiveness of dantrolene sodium in the treatment of heatstroke. Crit Care Med 1991;19:176–180.
38. Channa AB, Seraj MA, Saddique AA, et al. Is dantrolene effective in heat stroke patients? Crit Care Med 1990;18:290–292.
39. Heggers JP, Robson MC, Manavalen K, et al. Experimental and clinical observations on frostbite. Ann Emerg Med 1987;16:1056–1062.
40. McCauley RL, Heggers JP, Robson MC. Frostbite: methods to minimize tissue loss. Postgrad Med 1990;88:67–77.
41. Weinberg AD. Hypothermia. Ann Emerg Med 1993;22:370–377.

II

Injuries

5

Ocular Sports Injuries

Thomas H. Mader

Although constituting less than 0.25% of the body surface, the eye is uniquely vulnerable to injury. Even minor trauma to the eye or ocular adnexa can result in severely debilitating injury with the potential for vision loss. This chapter provides a quick reference for the evaluation and management of common ocular injuries that may occur as a result of sporting events. The extent of the examination depends on the available equipment, but even in a remote area a meaningful examination can be performed—one that directly affects the patient's eventual outcome.

HISTORY

In cases of ocular trauma, the mechanism of injury may help to determine the extent of the examination and treatment. It is important to obtain specific answers to questions about the injury. For example, the statement "I hurt my eye during a soccer game" is not as informative as "I was poked in the eye with a finger" or "Somebody kicked dust in my eye."

PHYSICAL EXAMINATION

The basic anatomy of the eye and lid is illustrated in Figures 5-1 and 5-2. For simplicity, the lids and eyes are always examined from front to back, and abnormalities are recorded as they are found. One must mentally check several parameters of each anatomic structure as the examination proceeds (Table 5-1).

A stepwise approach to the examination allows specific injuries to be identified and either treated or properly referred. The injury pictured in Figure 5-3 occurred when a young man ran into a stick protruding from a tree. An examination was conducted at the site of the injury, and a lid laceration and probable intraocular foreign body were noted. A shield was placed to protect the eye from further trauma. This was the only treatment necessary before triage. A brief explanation of each part of the ocular examination follows.

Lids

The lids and periocular area are examined first. The basic anatomy is illustrated in Figures 5-1 and 5-2. The tarsus is the thick, tough layer of connective tissue that maintains the lid contour. The puncta are the openings positioned medially into which tear fluid is drained (Figure 5-4). The fluid drains further into the canaliculi and finally into the nose.

A lacerated or avulsed lid can lead to corneal exposure, which can cause corneal damage. A lid laceration can also communicate with the globe. Although thorough exploration of wounds is not appropriate in the field, such an examination in the emergency room is imperative. A wound can gently be probed with an applicator tip or other instrument. If a wound tract or foreign body is directed toward the eye, it should be assumed that an ocular laceration exists. For example, in Figure 5-3, the dark wood foreign body appears very near the globe. Therefore, the eye was assumed to be open and was triaged as such.

The lid margin should be examined thoroughly for its normal smooth contour and lash position. The puncta should be identified in their normal medial position. The orbicularis oculi muscle tends to pull a lid wound apart such that normal anatomic position may be greatly distorted if a canalicular laceration exists (see Figure 5-4). Such a lid laceration requires repair by an ophthalmologist. Because this type of lid laceration may be accompa-

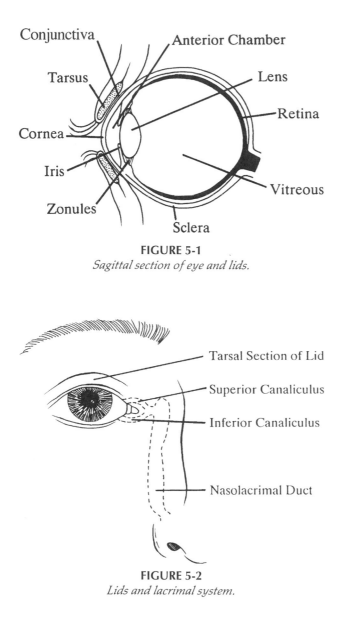

FIGURE 5-1
Sagittal section of eye and lids.

FIGURE 5-2
Lids and lacrimal system.

TABLE 5-1
Examination Checklist

Lids
　Lid margin
　Puncta
Visual acuity
Intraocular pressure
Extraocular motility
Cornea
　Epithelium
　Stroma*
　Endothelium*
Conjunctiva
　Normal translucence
　Smooth contour
Anterior chamber
　Depth
　Cells*
Pupil
　Afferent defect
　Shape
Lens
　Proper position
　Clarity
Vitreous
　Clarity
Fundi
　Disk
　Vessels
　Macula
　Background

*Slit-lamp needed.

nied by ocular injury, a thorough ocular examination is mandatory.

Visual Acuity

The measurement of visual acuity is the single most important part of the examination. An eye chart is not necessary, but some form of best-corrected visual acuity must always be obtained. This helps to establish the degree of incapacitation and a baseline level of vision. This measurement can be obtained in the field by reading newspaper print, a distant sign, or a license plate. If visual acuity is not 20/20, a measurement of pinhole visual acuity should also be obtained, as this largely eliminates the effect of a refractive error. The purpose of the pinhole is to block out peripheral light rays entering the eye such that only central parallel rays enter the anatomic pupil and focus clearly on the macula. If visual acuity is severely impaired, the patient may only be able to count fingers, see hand motion, or detect light. Whatever the extent of vision loss, an accurate documentation of acuity is always necessary.

Intraocular Pressure

In any trauma patient, the intraocular pressure should be evaluated. In the field, the eye can be gently palpated through the closed lid for a rough assessment of intraocular pressure. Comparison with the normal eye is helpful. In an office setting, an applanation tonometer or Tono-Pen can work well. A Schiötz tonometer should be avoided, because this instrument puts pressure on the eye and can cause corneal epithelial damage.

Knowledge of the precise intraocular pressure is not necessary, but obtaining the pressure relative to the other eye is essential. A low intraocular pressure is very suggestive of a lacerated globe. A high intraocular pressure

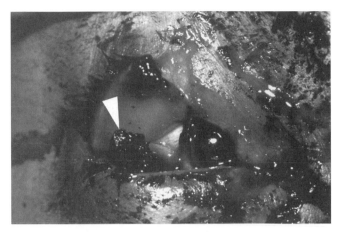

FIGURE 5-3
Severe ocular trauma. Arrow shows wood foreign body.

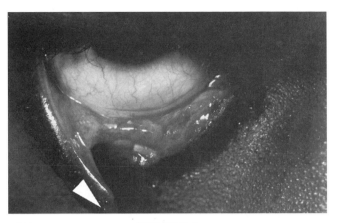

FIGURE 5-4
Lower right lid and canalicular laceration. Arrow shows position of inferior puncta.

may be associated with retrobulbar bleeding, intraocular bleeding, or inflammation.

Extraocular Motility

The assessment of extraocular motility is necessary after blunt trauma to the eye or periocular area. This is best accomplished simply by having the patient follow the tip of the examiner's finger up, down, left, and right. The patient with adequate visual acuity should also be instructed to report any symptoms of double vision (diplopia). The report of diplopia in a particular field of gaze may point out a subtle muscle imbalance.

Cornea

The cornea is the tough, transparent anterior shell of the eye. It is well innervated such that a patient with even the slightest corneal abrasion will call attention to the injury. Nearly all corneal injuries are accompanied by intense photosensitivity, which may sometimes appear out of proportion to the injury. Therefore, examination in a dark place is usually more comfortable for the patient. The use of topical anesthetic drops, such as proparacaine 0.5%, is also extremely helpful. In an eye with blepharospasm, a drop may be instilled by leaning the head back and pulling down the lower lid to expose the lower conjunctival cul-de-sac into which a drop is placed. This drop quickly anesthetizes the entire corneal and conjunctival surface.

The corneal epithelium is examined first. A sterile fluorescein strip is useful in demonstrating corneal epithelial defects. Wet the tip of the fluorescein strip with a drop of sterile saline or proparacaine, and touch the wet tip to the inferior conjunctival cul-de-sac while the eye is look-ing up. Do not apply directly to the cornea as it may abrade the corneal epithelium and lead to diagnostic confusion. The abrasion will fluoresce a bright green under a Woods' lamp or penlight equipped with a cobalt blue filter. Once topical anesthetic drops are applied, the patient should not be allowed to participate in sports until the effect of the drops has worn off to avoid inadvertent damage to an anesthetized cornea.

With a slit-lamp, the corneal stroma is also examined for clarity. The stroma is completely clear in its normal state, and any opacification is abnormal. The corneal endothelium should also be studied. It is normally a barely discernible corneal cell layer, composing the deepest layer of the cornea.

Anterior Chamber

The anterior chamber should be assessed for depth. Directing the beam of a penlight from the temporal side across the iris plane demonstrates anterior chamber depth, because the iris may protrude anteriorly and cast a shadow over the nasal side. It is important to compare eyes. Aqueous leakage from a corneal wound produces a very shallow anterior chamber, whereas vitreous loss from a ruptured sclera leads to a very deep chamber. A detailed examination of the anterior chamber can be made only with a slit-lamp. When a slit-lamp is available, the anterior chamber should be examined for cells and flare, which result from traumatized iris vasculature.

Pupil

Although frequently neglected, the examination of the pupil can be highly informative. The pupil should be checked for reaction to light. In the case of recent trauma, the pupil may be nonreactive or minimally reactive as a result of iris trauma. Such a lack of reaction may be differentiated from a true afferent defect by the swinging flashlight test. In this test, the flashlight is slowly swung from one eye to the other. Normally, both pupils will promptly constrict. In an eye with an afferent lesion, that eye will paradoxically dilate. The roundness of the pupil should always be evaluated, because this may provide extremely valuable information.

Lens

The clear lens is held in place by hundreds of zonules that suspend it behind the pupil. The lens is best examined with the use of a slit-lamp, but a meaningful examination of lens clarity can be accomplished with a direct ophthalmoscope. The scope is held approximately 18 in. in front of the eye, and the pupil is examined from this distance with the direct ophthalmoscope setting on infinity. Using this method, lenticular opacities present as dark spots through the viewing hole.

Vitreous

The vitreous is the gel-like portion of the eye, lying between the posterior lens capsule and the retina. The vitreous is normally clear, and any variation from this clarity represents some form of ocular pathology. Ideally, the vitreous is examined with a slit-lamp. Only approximately the anterior one-third of the vitreous is in focus with a slit-lamp alone.

Retina

The retina is a complex neurosensory layer that requires careful examination. Ideally, the examination is performed with the aid of a dilated pupil using one drop of 1% tropicamide, but dilation in the field is rarely indicated. Once pupillary reactivity and shape are recorded, however, the use of a mydriatic in the office or emergency room is appropriate. Once dilated, the retina is examined in a systematic fashion. First, the disk is examined. This is best done with a 90 diopter (D) lens using a slit-lamp, but a direct ophthalmoscope is adequate. The advantage of the 90 D lens is that it gives the examiner a detailed stereoscopic view of the disk. Second, the major retinal vessels are followed out from the disk to the periphery. The macula is then examined. Finally, a general sweep of the retinal periphery is performed. This peripheral examination is again ideally accomplished with an indirect ophthalmoscope, but a standard direct ophthalmoscope may be more

practical. Making a specific diagnosis is not the objective of the examination; rather it is to identify an abnormality that can then be specifically diagnosed and treated by an ophthalmologist.

SPECIFIC DIAGNOSES

This section discusses specific diagnoses that are commonly encountered in sports medicine. It is by no means all-encompassing. The treatment of common ocular injuries is summarized in Table 5-2.

Extraocular Motility

Poor extraocular motility may be indicative of a blowout fracture with muscle entrapment or may result from temporary periocular edema. Poor extraocular motility is not in itself an emergency, but further study may be necessary to define the etiology. Because associated ocular injuries are common, all motility abnormalities should be referred to an ophthalmologist.

Cornea

Abrasion

Corneal epithelial defects heal by proliferation and migration of the cells at the margin of the abrasion over the denuded area. The treatment of an abrasion varies according to the patient and the extent of injury. In the case of a minor abrasion, an antibiotic drop (for example, sulfacetamide) used four times per day until the epithelium is healed is adequate treatment. Patching of minor abrasions is normally not necessary and should be avoided if possible. Patching the eye results in a natural culture medium and could theoretically predispose a corneal defect to bacterial infection. In addition, once an eye is patched, antibiotic drops can no longer be easily instilled. Thus, antibiotic levels necessary to prevent corneal infection may not be achieved.

It may be prudent to apply antibiotic ointment and a tight patch with corneal abrasions larger than 10 mm². Although patching large abrasions does not necessarily lessen pain, photophobia, tearing, or foreign body sensation, healing may occur faster compared with unpatched eyes.[1] If a patch is used, it should always be applied tightly with tape. A loose-fitting patch is both uncomfortable and useless. Antibiotic ointment (e.g., erythromycin) is usually applied before taping on the patch. The patient should always be seen the following day for a thorough examination, preferably with a slit-lamp. During this follow-up examination, the patient is frequently more comfortable, and a more thorough eye examination may be performed.

Corneal Laceration

A corneal laceration may be either partial- or full-thickness. Either type should prompt examination by an ophthalmologist as soon as possible to rule out serious ocular damage. Diagnosis by slit-lamp examination is usually straightforward. A corneal laceration appears as a slit-like opacification. Fluorescein highlights the edges of the laceration. If a slit-lamp is available, a wet, sterile fluorescein strip may be touched to the wound. An area of fluorescein dilution or frank aqueous leakage indicates a full-thickness wound (positive Schirmer's test). Once the diagnosis of a corneal laceration is made or strongly suspected, a shield should be placed over the eye to prevent pressure on the globe. A piece of cardboard or a paper cup is perfectly adequate if taped securely over the eye so that no pressure is exerted on the globe.

Corneal Foreign Body

The presence of a corneal foreign body is suggested by persistent ocular discomfort and foreign body sensation.

Topical proparacaine should be applied for ease of examination. Larger corneal foreign bodies may be seen with the naked eye, but frequently a slit-lamp or other magnification device may be necessary to identify a small foreign body. The best way to make this diagnosis without a slit-lamp is by shining a penlight in the eye from the temporal side to broadly illuminate the iris surface. This retro-illuminates the cornea, and the foreign body shows up as a dark spot on the bright background of the iris. Any time a foreign body is suspected, the conjunctivae of the upper and lower lids should be examined. The lower conjunctiva is examined simply by pulling down on the lower lid (everting it) and exposing the lower conjunctival cul-de-sac for examination. The upper lid should also be everted and examined.

If a superficial corneal foreign body is noted, it is best removed with the tip of a 25- to 27-gauge sterile needle. This is usually done with the aid of a slit-lamp but can be accomplished with loupes or even—in the case of a large foreign body—with the naked eye. The tip of the needle is placed under the foreign body, which is gently lifted from the cornea. Although a sharp needle near the eye may seem intimidating to some practitioners, it is a

TABLE 5-2

Ocular Sports Injuries

Diagnosis	Symptoms	Signs	Treatment
Extraocular motility (limited movement)	Pain or diplopia	Limited eye movement	Ice and referral within 24 hrs
Corneal abrasion	± Decreased vision Photosensitivity Foreign-body sensation	Epithelial defects with fluorescein stain	Antibiotic drops Patching prn—with abrasions >10 mm²
Corneal laceration	± Decreased vision Photosensitivity Foreign-body sensation	Corneal laceration Shallow anterior chamber (if full-thickness)	Immediate referral
Corneal foreign body	± Decreased vision Photosensitivity Foreign-body sensation	Corneal foreign body	Removal Antibiotics and patching Referral prn
Conjunctiva (subconjunctival blood)	Foreign-body sensation ± Pain	Blood beneath conjunctiva	Antibiotics Referral prn
Traumatic iritis	Eye pain Photosensitivity	Cells in anterior chamber	Homatropine Referral within 24 hrs
Hyphema	Decreased vision Pain	Blood in anterior chamber	Bed rest Immediate referral
Irregular pupil	Decreased vision ± Pain	Irregularly shaped pupil	Immediate referral
Lens damage	Decreased vision ± Pain	Cloudy lens Dislocated lens	Immediate referral
Vitreous opacities	Decreased vision ± Pain	Vitreous opacities	Immediate referral
Retinal damage	Decreased vision	Distorted retinal anatomy and blood	Immediate referral

± = with or without; prn = as needed.

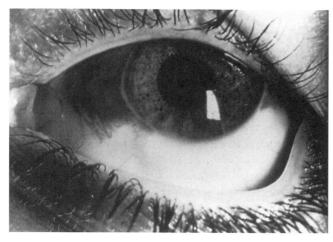

FIGURE 5-5
Subconjunctival hemorrhage extending medial and lateral to cornea. (Reprinted with permission from FG Bergson. Basic Ophthalmology for Medical Students and Primary Care Residents. San Francisco: American Academy of Ophthalmology, 1993;85.)

very precise instrument and only rarely causes iatrogenic injury. The cornea is extremely tough tissue, and complete penetration from the needle would require considerable force. Using a cotton swab for foreign body removal is not recommended because it rarely dislodges the foreign body and may cause epithelial damage to surrounding tissue. Deep corneal foreign bodies should be removed by an ophthalmologist. Multiple corneal foreign bodies that appear superficial may be removed by irrigation.

After removal of a metallic foreign body, a residual rust ring is commonly present. If this is prominent or near the visual axis, it may be removed with a dental burr by a physician skilled in its use. As for patients with corneal abrasions, antibiotics should be used four times per day after removal. These patients should always be examined daily until the epithelium is healed to assess for a corneal ulcer or other pathology.

Conjunctiva

Damage to the conjunctiva is common after ocular trauma because of its considerable exposure. Because of extensive vascularity, even a minor insult to the conjunctiva can cause a laceration. This leads to extensive subconjunctival hemorrhage, which may appear out of proportion to the actual damage. Such a hemorrhage is composed of extravasated blood from the conjunctiva, which dissects between the conjunctiva and the sclera. It usually appears as a flat, homogeneous, bright red area,

which may cover a large portion of the bulbar conjunctiva (Figure 5-5).

Despite the striking appearance, most conjunctival lacerations do not require surgical intervention and can simply be treated with antibiotic drops four times per day until the defect heals. Some subconjunctival hemorrhages, however, may be associated with underlying scleral lacerations and intraocular injury. Such serious injuries usually present with a prominent conjunctival elevation in the area of the hemorrhage. This elevation may be caused by displaced vitreous, retinal tissue, or even a lens that has been expulsed from the eye and become entrapped under the conjunctiva. After such extensive injuries, the eye may appear soft and distorted in shape. If any question exists regarding the extent of the injury that may be associated with a subconjunctival hemorrhage, the patient should be referred immediately to an ophthalmologist.

Anterior Chamber

Traumatic Iritis
A history of blunt trauma with persistent photosensitivity, a red eye, and droning eye pain is suggestive of iritis. A small to midsized pupil sluggishly reactive to light is common. Cells may be readily apparent on slit-lamp examination. Even with significant pain, surprisingly few cells may be seen. The initial treatment is homatropine for cycloplegia. Further treatment and follow-up should be provided by an ophthalmologist, because this condition may be associated with other ocular pathology.

Hyphema
A hyphema is the presence of visible blood in the anterior chamber of a traumatized eye (Figure 5-6). Regardless of the precise origin of the blood, a hyphema is a serious injury, and the patient should always be evaluated by an ophthalmologist to rule out associated injury. This should be done promptly, if possible. If a patient cannot be sent to an ophthalmologist immediately, the patient should be kept at bed rest with the head of the bed elevated 10–20 degrees. This encourages blood to layer in the inferior angle instead of along the entire circumference of the anterior chamber angle. The eye need not be patched. There is no harm in watching television or reading, but other than bathroom privileges, the patient should remain at bed rest for at least several days. The main purpose of bed rest is to prevent rebleeding, as this is associated with a higher complication rate. Although oral steroids or aminocaproic acid are usually indicated for treatment, they are best used in consultation with an ophthalmologist.

Pupil

An irregularly shaped pupil may be indicative of significant ocular trauma. Specifically, a teardrop pupil (Figure 5-7) is an ominous sign and nearly always represents a ruptured globe or other serious injury. Such pupillary distortion may be caused by iris tissue being entrapped within a hole in the cornea. Although this usually requires surgical correction, plugging of a corneal laceration may be temporarily beneficial as it may prevent further loss of intraocular contents. It should be noted that such a plug of iris may actually protrude from the corneal surface and should not be confused with a dark-colored corneal foreign body. Any irregular pupil requires immediate referral to an ophthalmologist.

Lens

Two major injuries may affect the lens: traumatic cataract or lens dislocation. A traumatic cataract may form after either blunt or penetrating injury and cause an opacified lens. This may require eventual surgical removal and replacement. If the lens capsule is violated, cortical lens material may escape from the lens and cause a significant inflammatory reaction, greatly elevating the intraocular pressure. Such an occurrence requires surgical intervention.

The lens can also become traumatically dislocated as a result of broken zonules. Such a dislocation can occur in any direction, and a grossly dislocated lens is usually readily identified. When only a few zonules are broken, the lens may maintain a roughly normal position, but it will quiver during blinking or eye movements. Any lens injury requires evaluation by an ophthalmologist.

Vitreous

Red blood cells, pigment, or other debris present in the vitreous is strongly suggestive of retinal trauma and should prompt a referral to an ophthalmologist. The specific diagnosis is not significant, but any vitreous opacity may be associated with major intraocular damage. Prompt examination by an ophthalmologist is indicated.

Retina

Commotio-retinae is probably the most common manifestation of retinal trauma. It represents retinal edema and is usually seen as a result of a contrecoup injury. It is manifested by a pale, flat retina. This is self-limiting and does not require treatment. Such an injury may be associated with more significant damage, and examination by an ophthalmologist is indicated.

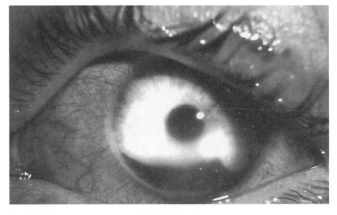

FIGURE 5-6
Hyphema.

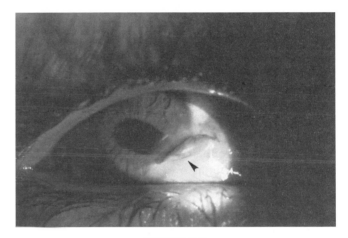

FIGURE 5-7
Teardrop pupil after corneal laceration. Arrow points to prolapsed iris tissue.

Retinal damage is common in blunt or penetrating trauma. This can take the form of choroidal rupture, retinal tear, or subretinal hemorrhage. In all cases, the patient has significantly decreased visual acuity, and the normal anatomy is bloody and disrupted. The specific diagnosis in cases of retinal trauma is not important. However, it is important to identify that an abnormality exists and to promptly refer any patient with suspected retinal damage directly to an ophthalmologist.

OCULAR PROTECTIVE DEVICES

Approximately 90% of all recreation-related ocular trauma is preventable if ocular protective devices are used.[2-4] Baseball, ice hockey, and racquet sports are

TABLE 5-3
Eye Protectors*

Type	Uses
Polycarbonate lenses (2-mm center thickness)	In streetwear frames; usually give adequate, cosmetically acceptable protection in day-to-day use for active people; constant wear suggested for the functionally one-eyed
Polycarbonate lenses (3-mm center thickness)	In sports frames for sports that use a ball or have contact potential
Polycarbonate sports eye protectors	With no prescription; for use by contact lens wearers or those who usually do not wear glasses; protectors should pass the racket sport protector standards
Industrial safety glasses with polycarbonate lenses and side shields	For use around machinery, storage batteries, and flying particles
Industrial safety goggles with polycarbonate lenses	Provide better protection than safety glasses; may be worn over regular streetwear spectacles
Face mask-helmet combinations	For collision sports (e.g., hockey, football, lacrosse); functionally one-eyed people should wear sports eye protectors under the face mask for added protection

*Note: Glass lenses, ordinary plastic lenses, open (lensless) eyeguards, and contact lenses do not provide adequate protection for active people.
Source: Reprinted with permission from B Shingleton, P Hersh, K Kenyon. Eye Trauma. St. Louis: Mosby–Year Book, 1991;399.

responsible for the greatest number of injuries.[5] Impact-resistant polycarbonate lenses and frames provide excellent protection for nearly all sports, and they are readily available. Such devices are described in Table 5-3. For maximum protection, all polycarbonate lenses should be at least 3-mm thick at the thinnest point and supported by frames that meet impact-resistance standards. Prescription polycarbonate lenses are available from –25 D to +12 D with up to 4 D of cylinder.[5]

Spectacle correction lenses, standard sunglasses, contact lenses, and lensless goggles do not provide adequate protection. In fact, standard spectacles or sunglasses may shatter on impact and cause further injury, such as a corneal abrasion or globe perforation. Although contact lenses alone afford no eye protection, adequate ocular protection can be achieved with wraparound plano polycarbonate lenses used in conjunction with contact lenses. Individuals who have had globe weakening surgical procedures, such as cataract surgery, corneal transplantation, or radial keratotomy, are predisposed to ocular rupture with trauma. Therefore, eye protection should always be used by these individuals and any athlete with only a single functioning eye.

The specific device used for optimal ocular protection varies from sport to sport. Standards currently exist for eye and face protective wear for racket sports, hockey,

baseball, football, skiing, and motorcycling.[6] In ice hockey, football, and motorcycling, the ocular protection is usually incorporated into a helmet or face mask. In some sports, such as baseball, it may be necessary to change ocular protection depending on the position played. A player may need a helmet with a face shield while at the plate but only polycarbonate lenses while catching a fly ball in center field. The risk of injury in some sports, such as karate and boxing, is very high because adequate eye protection is not practical.

REFERENCES

1. Kaiser PK. A comparison of pressure patching versus no pressure patching for corneal abrasions due to trauma or foreign body removal. Ophthalmology 1995;102:1936–1942.
2. Jones NP. Eye injury in sport. Sports Med 1989;7:163–181.
3. National Society to Prevent Blindness: 1993 Eye Injuries Associated with Sports and Recreational Products (FS09). Schaumberg, IL: National Society to Prevent Blindness, July 1993.
4. Pashby T. Eye injuries in sports. J Ophthalmic Nurs Tech 1989;8:99–101.
5. Napier SM, Baker RS, Sanford DG, et al. Eye injuries in athletics and recreation. Surv Ophthalmol 1996;41:229–244.
6. Pine D. Preventing sports related eye injuries. Physician Sports Med 1991;19:129–134.

6

Maxillofacial Injuries

JOSEPH C. MULREAN AND STEPHEN M. DAVIS

Maxillofacial injuries occur frequently in sporting activities. Although seldom life-threatening, these injuries can be extremely debilitating and disfiguring if not properly managed. This chapter outlines the most common injuries and provides a systematic method of evaluation and treatment of this most critical area. The discussion centers on initial management and on soft tissue, bony, and dentoalveolar injuries.

INITIAL MANAGEMENT OF FACIAL TRAUMA

History

An attempt should be made to obtain information regarding the mechanism of injury, loss of consciousness, treatment rendered, past medical history, past injuries, present medications, and allergies.

Airway Assessment

All patients sustaining maxillofacial trauma must be evaluated for airway obstruction. Airway embarrassment may be acute or insidious in its onset, and it may vary with the level of consciousness, thus mandating continuous evaluation. Injuries that are particularly prone to causing airway obstruction are a "flail" mandible; maxillary fractures; lacerations of the tongue; hematomas of sublingual, nasopharyngeal, lateral pharyngeal, or retropharyngeal areas; and a fractured larynx.[1] The tongue is the most common cause of upper airway obstruction in the obtunded patient.

Diagnosis

Diagnosis of upper airway obstruction is done primarily by clinical examination with good light and suction. If the patient is conscious and can talk, the airway is patent. Partial obstruction is evident by stridor, use of accessory muscles of respiration, and tachypnea.

Sublingual, lateral pharyngeal, and retropharyngeal hematomas are suggested by swelling, ecchymosis, and elevation of the tongue or deviation of the soft palate. A severe open bite with only the posterior teeth occluding may indicate a posteriorly and inferiorly displaced maxilla or bilateral fractures of the mandible. The former can result in obstruction of the airway secondary to the soft palate, and the latter can result in airway obstruction by the tongue. Palpation of the anterior neck is done to assess the position and contour of the thyroid cartilage and to note crepitus, edema, and subcutaneous emphysema.

Treatment

In the unconscious patient, the examiner must look, listen, and feel for respiration. If the airway is obstructed, it is examined for foreign material, which is removed. An attempt should be made to open the airway with the chin lift without hyperextending the neck, in case cervical spine injuries exist. An oral or nasopharyngeal airway is placed to maintain patency.

If the patient is conscious, but obtunded, a nasopharyngeal airway is more tolerable, but it must be continuously suctioned and checked for patency. If the patient is alert and able to maintain his or her airway, no adjuncts are necessary.

Endotracheal intubation is indicated if the airway is considerably compromised or if its integrity is deteriorating as a result of progressive swelling. If the patient is suspected of having a cervical spine injury, oroendotracheal intubation is contraindicated (even with in-line traction, it has been shown to cause significant displacement of the cervical spine).[2] If time permits, a blind nasoendotracheal intubation should be performed. In the setting of

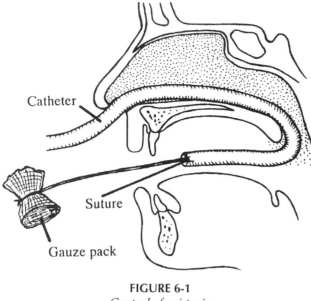

FIGURE 6-1
Control of epistaxis.

severe maxillofacial injuries, however, nasoendotracheal intubation may result in intubation of the cranial cavity.

Alternatives to oroendotracheal intubation and blind nasoendotracheal intubation, besides surgical intervention, include percutaneous transtracheal ventilation, intubation over a flexible fiberoptic endoscope, intubation using a lighted stylet, and translaryngeal guided intubation.[3]

Translaryngeal guided intubation is particularly useful when trying to secure an airway in the combative patient who refuses to lie down because of continuous bleeding into the pharynx.[4] It involves placement of a guidewire into the trachea through the cricothyroid membrane, which is then passed cephalad into the oral cavity. The endotracheal tube is then passed over the wire. The patient's oxygenation can be maintained during this procedure; therefore, it can be a lifesaving technique. In the hands of trained personnel, these techniques may provide alternatives to cricothyroidotomy and tracheostomy. If the preceding fails, cricothyroidotomy is the emergent surgical technique of choice, whereas tracheostomy is done electively.

Lower Airway Obstruction

Although it may present early, lower airway obstruction typically produces delayed respiratory obstruction. This usually presents with postural dyspnea, dysphonia, and pain on swallowing. Examination of the anterior neck may reveal loss of prominence of the thyroid cartilage, subcutaneous emphysema, and ecchymosis.

The presence of air within the prevertebral tissue of the neck is pathognomonic for cervical perforation of the esophagus.[5]

Bronchoscopy must be done to rule out a disruption of the larynx or trachea.[6] Intubation may cause a total separation of the trachea and is contraindicated. Tracheostomy is indicated when subcutaneous emphysema in the neck and retropharyngeal space is progressive. Once an airway is obtained, ventilation must be assured.

Control of Hemorrhage

Bleeding from maxillofacial injuries is seldom so severe as to lead to shock, but it can happen, particularly in scalp lacerations or from severe nasopharyngeal bleeding secondary to maxillary fractures.

Treatment
Control of hemorrhage can usually be accomplished most effectively by direct pressure, which is normally successful as a temporary measure. A partially severed vessel (e.g., superficial temporal or facial) eventually should be ligated, but this should not be blindly attempted with hemostats by inexperienced personnel, as it can damage neurovascular structures.

Maxillary Fractures
Profuse bleeding associated with maxillary fractures in the nasopharyngeal area can be frequently controlled with digital pressure on the hard palate to superiorly reposition the maxilla and tamponade the sphenopalatine or greater palatine arteries.[7]

Nasal Epistaxis
Usually, nasal epistaxis can be controlled with pressure on the alar bases and head elevation. If these are ineffective, the origin of the bleeding should be determined, which requires good light, suction, anesthesia (4% cocaine soaked in cotton), and a nasal speculum. Posterior bleeding may require posterior nasal packs, which are placed by insertion of a Foley catheter (16 French [F]–18F) with inflation of the balloon (30 cc). Alternatively, a red Robinson or Foley catheter can be passed through the nasal cavity, visualized in the posterior pharynx, grasped, and pulled through the oral cavity, where it is tied to 4-in. by 4-in. gauze packs with O silk suture and pulled back through the nose. Meanwhile, a finger, posteriorly positioned, pushes the pack superiorly and anteriorly into the posterior nasal cavity (Figure 6-1).

An anterior pack is then placed to control bleeding anteriorly. If this fails, the patient should be referred for an arteriogram to localize the bleeding site, followed by either ligation or embolization of the offending vessel[8] with an absorbable gelatin sponge (Gelfoam [Pharmacia and Upjohn, Inc., Bridgewater, NJ]).

Circulation must be restored with infusion of intravenous fluids. Monitoring of vital signs, urinary output, and level of consciousness is done to assess adequacy of resuscitation.

SOFT TISSUE INJURIES

Before discussing specific areas, the following terms are defined:

- *Abrasion*: the denuding of skin, partial- or full-thickness
- *Contusion*: a bruise; a soft tissue injury with no disruption in the skin
- *Laceration*: a tear, cut, or a disruption of skin
- *Avulsion*: the complete removal of a part from the body
- *Hematoma*: a collection of blood, usually under the skin, which can be seen with all of the preceding

Physical Examination

The face is a structure that is readily accessible for physical examination. The examination should begin at the top and move downward. The patient is observed while speaking to note appropriate and symmetric movement of the lips, eyes, and eyebrows or some evidence of paralysis secondary to nerve injury or muscle damage. The forehead, cheeks, and mandible are lightly stroked to check for intact sensation.

Scalp
Scalp is evaluated by inspection and palpation. The face and especially the scalp are densely vascular structures, and their injury can cause a patient to lose a large volume of blood very quickly. Direct pressure is of great benefit. It is essential to remember that underlying skull fractures may exist, exposing the brain. It is critical that this type of wound be diagnosed immediately and that it be managed by a neurosurgeon. In some cases, the patient's hair can be tied to approximate the wound temporarily and reduce bleeding.

Face
Most structures on the face are bilateral, which allows comparison of the two sides. The integrity of the skin and disruption of major structures, such as eyebrows, eyelids, and lips, are observed. If any tissue has been avulsed and it is obtainable, it should be wrapped in a moist saline gauze and kept with the patient. Major lacerations with hematomas should not be wiped away to assess the deeper structures, as this may exacerbate the bleeding. Areas that are active in bleeding can usually be controlled with direct pressure; if this does not control the bleeding, specialized medical care is needed immediately. The mechanism of injury directs the examination for foreign bodies (such as rocks, glass, and dirt). Superficial debris can easily be removed, whereas deeper objects may require more specialized care.

Wound Care

The patient's tetanus status must be determined and immunization administered as appropriate. As a general rule, antibiotics are not necessary with isolated soft tissue injuries; cleansing the wound is far more important. If soft tissues are the only structures involved, then they can be addressed immediately. If underlying fractures exist, repair is delayed until fractures are evaluated.

Superficial Wounds
Superficial wounds can be treated with gentle cleansing, usually using normal saline-soaked gauzes, followed by the application of a sterile topical ointment and dressing. If these wounds have ground-in dirt, tar, or any foreign bodies, then more extensive cleansing is indicated. Technically, one can use saline-soaked gauze, or for wounds that are more severely tattooed, a surgical scrub brush. To carry out such a debridement usually requires the administration of local anesthesia. It is essential to remember to check for facial animation and sensation before injection. If these wounds involve some separation of the epidermis, cuticular suturing or Steri-Strips (Medical Surgical Division 3M, St. Paul, MN) may be used for approximation. Closer alignment of the skin produces a higher-quality result.

Lacerations
Lacerations of the face should be treated with irrigation ("the solution to pollution is dilution"), minimal debridement, and control of bleeding. If the bleeding is minimal, then the use of a small, battery-operated, handheld cautery unit works well. The proper suturing of the wounds is extremely important. The wound is closed in layers to eliminate dead space and reapproximate the tissues. The deeper structures are closed using absorbable material (4-0 or 5-0 Vicryl, Ethicon, Inc., Johnson & Johnson, Somerville, NJ); the skin is closed with nylon (6-0). These wounds must be sutured together like a puzzle, placing each individual piece into its original position. This technique helps to naturally break up the line of the scar and make it some-

what less obvious. Dressings usually are light gauze and a topical antibiotic ointment.

Scalp

Injuries in this area may vary from simple lacerations to avulsions. Injuries around the skull may involve fractures and frontal sinus injuries. These must be ruled out radiographically and, if present, referred for definitive treatment. Simple lacerations are repaired with 3-0 Prolene (Ethicon, Inc., Johnson & Johnson).

Eyebrows

Injuries in this area should always include a careful ophthalmologic evaluation (see Chapter 5). After this is completed, the wounds should be carefully cleansed and minimally debrided. The brow should not be shaved, because the hair may not regrow in the same pattern. The hair follicles are used to guide suture placement. It is essential to place cutaneous alignment sutures first, before repairing the deeper layers. Prolene suture (6-0) is suitable because its blue color makes it easy to find in dark hair.

Eyelids

An ophthalmologic evaluation is mandatory before any attempted therapy, for the patient's sake and for the medicolegal ramifications. Once this is accomplished, simple abrasions can be treated as described in the preceding paragraphs; however, complete lid lacerations, avulsions, and any orbital trauma require specialized care. Rarely is eyelid skin truly avulsed; it is usually retracted secondary to disruption of the orbicularis oculi muscle. If skin is avulsed and retrieved, however, it should be gently cleansed and wrapped in a normal saline-soaked gauze for potential grafting. If care is not available for some period, it is preferable to close the skin with cuticular sutures (6-0 nylon) and to protect the eye with moist dressings until the patient can be seen by the appropriate specialist.

Nose

The nose has three components: (1) mucosa as lining, (2) cartilage and bone as support, and (3) skin as cover. Therefore, when repairing injuries in this area, all three tissues should be evaluated and repaired as necessary. As with eyebrows and lids, key sutures should be placed first to allow for the alignment of cosmetic units. Notching, step deformities, and contour irregularities are far more readily noticed than scarring, so these key sutures are crucial. Damage to the nasal septum must not be overlooked. A hematoma here can be devastating by leading to septal necrosis. It is easily treated by needle aspiration or a small incision in a dependent portion of the hematoma.

This is followed by anterior nasal packs for a period of several days to appose the mucoperichondrium and prevent recurrence.

Cheeks

Deep wounds may involve the facial nerve, parotid gland, and Stensen's duct. Nerve function is assessed, and the parotid duct catheterized to rule out injury to these critical structures. If the catheter appears in the wound, the duct is severed. The proximal end is found by compressing the parotid gland to express saliva. Superficial lacerations are treated as discussed; complicated wounds should be handled by specialized personnel. If there will be a long interval before definitive treatment can be rendered, the wound can be gently cleansed and lightly closed with sutures. In large avulsions, skin should be sutured directly to mucosa (4-0 or 5-0 nylon).

Ears

Trauma to the ears can be simple (skin laceration, hematoma) or complex (crushed tissue, exposed cartilage, or avulsion). Treatment of superficial abrasions is similar to treatment of abrasions elsewhere on the face. A simple laceration with exposed but undamaged cartilage can be sutured with fine cuticular sutures (5-0 or 6-0 nylon). If cartilage is traumatically disrupted, it should be debrided as minimally as possible and the skin closed over it (the cartilage itself should not be sutured). Traumatic hematomas are drained in a dependent position using an 18-gauge needle. A standard otoplasty dressing is fashioned, using wet saline gauze to contour to the ear, followed by a head wrap for 5 days. Injuries that involve volume and cartilage loss should be sent for specialized care. If the avulsed parts (especially cartilage) are obtainable, they should be wrapped in saline-soaked gauze and sent with the patient.

Lips

The lips are prominent structures of the face and are easily injured. As in the eyelid, disruption of the circular orbicularis oris muscle leads to great distraction of the wound and an apparent tissue loss. Even when avulsions are present, however, up to one-third of the upper and lower lips can be lost without significant aesthetic effect. After thorough inspection and palpation to rule out foreign bodies (frequently teeth), the wound is prepared in standard fashion. If underlying bony fractures exist, definitive closure of the wound should be delayed until the bony fractures are evaluated. The vermilion border is identified and reapproximated with a positional suture, then it is closed in three layers, from inside out: mucosa, muscle, and skin.

Tongue

The tongue is a vascular organ that can bleed profusely when damaged. The first priority of treatment is to control hemorrhage. Direct pressure with gauze temporarily brings it under control. The wound is then anesthetized and inspected, and large vessels are ligated. Once the bleeding is controlled, the tongue is extended by the patient to observe deviation and rule out hypoglossal nerve damage (the tongue will deviate to the affected side). The tongue is repaired in two layers (muscle and mucosa) with 3-0 chromic. Extensive lacerations or hematomas from blunt trauma, particularly those in the posterior region, may develop significant swelling and obstruct the airway. Admission for observation should be considered and intubation performed before the airway is in critical condition. If not admitted, the patient should be instructed to return at the first signs of respiratory distress or inability to handle oral secretions. Even if asymptomatic, he or she should return for reevaluation in 48 hours and then in 7 days for suture removal.

BONY INJURIES

Physical Examination

Examination of the patient with maxillofacial injuries should consist of inspection, palpation, manipulation, and functional evaluation. A history of the injury should be obtained if possible, because knowing the mechanism of injury will guide the examiner and frequently assist in diagnosis. The examination must be thorough and systematic. One method is to start at the top and work downward.

Scalp and Skull

The scalp is inspected for lacerations, contusions, and bleeding, and it is palpated bimanually for hematomas, swelling, asymmetry, and foreign bodies. Open wounds must not be deeply probed, because bony fragments can be pushed into the brain or venous sinuses and cause significant hemorrhage.

Ears

The ears are inspected for laceration, subperichondrial hematomas, perforation of external auditory canal (indicative of condylar fracture of mandible), and drainage of blood or cerebrospinal fluid (otorrhea).

The tympanic membrane is examined for perforation and hemotympanum. The skin behind the ears and along the sternocleidomastoid muscle is examined for presence of ecchymosis (Battle's sign), which is indicative of basal skull fracture of the middle cranial fossa. Blood from the ear is removed, and if the patient is conscious, hearing is grossly assessed.

Orbits

The orbits are inspected for periorbital ecchymosis, lacerations, and contusions. The eyes are examined for subconjunctival hemorrhage (if present without posterior limit, it is pathognomonic of orbital wall fracture), blood in anterior chamber of eye (hyphema), and pupillary level. Funduscopic examination should be done, if possible, to assess retinal damage and papilledema (see Chapter 5).

Bony orbits are palpated bimanually and bilaterally to detect asymmetry, step-offs, tenderness, and soft tissue emphysema. Visual acuity, extraocular muscle function, and diplopia are assessed if the patient is conscious. If the patient is unconscious, optic and oculomotor nerves can be evaluated by consensual light reflex and muscle entrapment by a forced duction test.

Supratrochlear and infraorbital nerve function is assessed by light touch to the forehead, cheeks, and upper lip. Anesthesia of the cheek suggests a zygomaticomaxillary complex fracture or blow-out fracture of the orbital floor.

Naso-Orbital Area

The medial canthal angle, the inclination of the palpebral fissure, and the nasal bridge are inspected. Presence of an obtuse medial canthal angle, mongoloid inclination of the palpebral fissure, and a flat nasal bridge indicate displacement of frontal process of the maxilla or avulsion of medial canthal ligament.

The intercanthal distance should be approximately 32–33 mm and equal to the width of the palpebral fissure. Telecanthus indicates a fracture or disruption of the medial canthal ligament.

Additionally, lateral traction can be applied to the eyelids while the medial canthal tendon is palpated. If it is displaced, no resistance to lateral displacement will be felt.[9]

Nose

The nasal bridge and tip are inspected for asymmetry, deviation, and swelling. Periorbital ecchymosis, most severe in medial areas, is indicative of nasal fracture. Medial subconjunctival hemorrhage indicates involvement of the medial wall or roof of the orbit. Intranasal bleeding is evaluated (unilateral bleeding from the nose may indicate zygomaticomaxillary complex fracture). One should look for septal hematoma, exposed cartilage, and displacement. The nose is palpated bimanually for tenderness, crepitus, and instability (swelling may make it difficult to palpate deformities).

Anosmia will be difficult to assess acutely because of blood and swelling, but it should be assessed. Persistent anosmia is indicative of anterior cranial fossa fracture.

Cerebrospinal fluid rhinorrhea can be detected with filter paper. Presence of a bull's-eye or halo indicates cerebrospinal fluid. Alternatively, a glucose determination can be done. Glucose levels above 30 mg/100 cc are suggestive of a cerebrospinal fluid leak.[10] The concentration of glucose in cerebrospinal fluid should be at least 50% of serum glucose. A glucose dipstick may give a false-positive result, but if negative, it rules out cerebrospinal fluid as the tested fluid.[11]

Maxilla

The cheeks are inspected for gross bilateral edema, periorbital ecchymosis, and lengthening of the face, the presence of which is pathognomonic for maxillary fractures.

The soft tissues are palpated for subcutaneous emphysema and hematomas. The maxilla is manipulated bimanually by palpating the nasofrontal suture while attempting to move the maxilla by grasping the maxillary teeth to diagnose Le Fort II and III fractures (see Maxillary Fractures). If this is stable, the superior hand is moved intraorally to the malar buttress area, and another attempt is made to move the maxillary teeth to diagnose a Le Fort I fracture. Lack of mobility does not rule out a fracture, because it may be severely impacted. If movement is questionable, maxillary teeth can be percussed. The presence of the sound of a cracked cup indicates a maxillary fracture.

Intraorally, the dentition is inspected for unstable dentoalveolar segments and fractured, missing, or avulsed teeth. The occlusion is then evaluated. A maxillary fracture causes an open bite that is due to the posterior and inferior displacement of the maxilla. The buccal maxillary fold is palpated for crepitus, emphysema, and tenderness and is examined for ecchymosis. Presence of these signs indicates maxillary or zygomaticomaxillary complex fractures.

Mandible

The mandible is inspected for swelling, ecchymosis, and asymmetry in preauricular, submandibular, and submental areas. Intraorally, step-offs in the occlusion, loose or missing teeth, and ecchymosis of mucosa are noted. Ecchymosis in the floor of the mouth is pathognomonic of mandibular fracture.

The inferior border, angle, and preauricular areas of the mandible are palpated while step deformities and tenderness are noted. Instability, crepitus, and pain with manipulation indicate a fracture. The patient is instructed to open his or her mouth while the condyles are palpated in the preauricular areas. Failure of the condyles to move with mandibular movement is indicative of condylar fracture.

The mandible should be observed when the patient opens his or her mouth for deviation, which will occur to the side of the injury. A limited opening (trismus) may indicate a mandibular fracture or possibly a depressed

zygomatic arch fracture with impingement on the coronoid process of the mandible.

The mental nerve is assessed for anesthesia by light touch to the lower lip. Anesthesia indicates either direct injury to mental nerve or more probably a fracture of the mandible. The dental occlusion is assessed by first asking if the patient perceives a change. Patients are very sensitive to even minimal changes. An anterior open bite may indicate a Le Fort fracture, a bilateral condylar fracture of the mandible, a dislocation, or a pre-existing malocclusion.

Radiographic Evaluation

A routine facial series should be obtained when a facial fracture is suspected. The suspected fracture should be viewed in at least two planes, preferably three. Cervical spine x-ray studies in three views (odontoid, posteroanterior, and lateral) should also be obtained to rule out cervical spine injury when indicated.

Panoramic radiography is an excellent method of evaluating mandibular injuries. Panoramic zonography has been developed for superior visualization of orbital, zygomatic, and maxillary areas. Panoramic zonography offers convenience (patient is examined in the recumbent position with minimal repositioning) and minimal radiation exposure.[12] Computed tomography should be obtained for complex facial fractures in axial and coronal planes.

Treatment

Maxillofacial bony fractures may consist of any combination of orbital, zygomaticomaxillary, naso-orbital, ethmoidal, nasal, maxillary, and mandibular fractures. They may be associated with skull fractures, basal skull fractures, cervical spine injuries, and head injuries, all of which are serious and warrant evaluation but are beyond the scope of this discussion.

Initial Management

Orbital Fractures

Orbital fractures include orbital rim fractures, blow-out fractures of orbital floor or walls, and zygomaticomaxillary complex fractures. Generally, urgent care is not indicated, unless there is a sudden deterioration in vision or sudden onset of proptosis or pain suggesting a retrobulbar hemorrhage; this requires immediate consultation with an ophthalmologist and is an ophthalmologic emergency.

Maxillary Fractures

Maxillary fractures are classically described by René Le Fort and fall into one of three categories (Le Fort I, II,

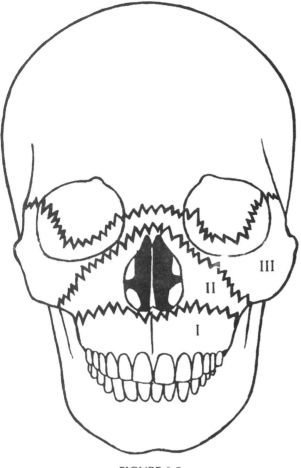

FIGURE 6-2
Le Fort fractures (I, II, III) of the midface.

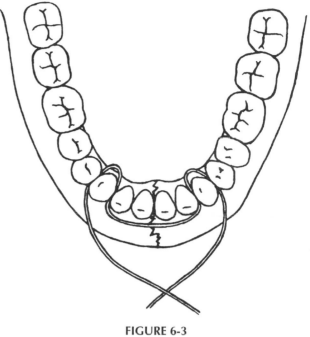

FIGURE 6-3
Temporary stabilization of mandibular fractures.

III) depending on the level of the fracture (Figure 6-2). Urgent care consists of controlling the airway and bleeding. If the patient is conscious and other injuries permit, he or she should be allowed to assume the position in which breathing is most comfortable. If the cervical spine is cleared and there is a danger of becoming unconscious, the patient should be placed in a semiprone position to allow drainage of secretions. The patient must be referred for definitive treatment.

Mandibular Fractures

Urgent care consists of securing the airway and controlling the bleeding. Progressive swelling may lead to insidious onset of upper airway obstruction.

If the fracture exists within the dental arch, it may be temporarily reduced and stabilized with circumdental 24-gauge stainless steel wire passed two teeth distal to the fracture on both sides and tightened. This will require infiltration of local anesthesia. Temporary immobi-

lization will decrease pain, bleeding, and swelling (Figure 6-3).

Lacerations are not repaired around the lips if facial fractures exist, because manipulation of bony tissue will disrupt the repair. Tacking sutures can be placed to temporarily stabilize soft tissue to decrease bleeding. The patient should be referred for definitive treatment.

Nasal Fractures

Nasal fractures are the most common of facial fractures. Because of rapid swelling, acute assessment and treatment are difficult to accomplish. It is advisable to wait 3–4 days to allow the swelling to resolve before reevaluation. If swelling is still present, it is preferable to wait an additional 3–4 days before treatment. Definitive treatment should be done within the first 10–14 days; beyond this time, healing has begun, complicating treatment. The only acute care indicated is to control bleeding, close open wounds, and drain septal hematomas.[13]

The patient should be advised to keep his or her head elevated and place ice packs for the first 24–48 hours to control swelling. The patient should also be placed on oral antibiotics.

When the swelling has sufficiently resolved, a closed reduction may be accomplished with the use of a Boies or Sayre elevator. These are blunt, single-bladed instruments that allow more control in the reduction of the fractured segments. This should not be attempted by inexperienced personnel unfamiliar with the anatomy.

After proper reduction, internal support is provided by nasal packs coated with antibiotic ointment. This should remain in place 3–4 days with the patient taking oral antibiotics while the nose is packed. External support is provided by a splint molded to the nose.

DENTOALVEOLAR INJURIES

Dentoalveolar injuries may vary in complexity from a partially avulsed tooth to comminution of large dentoalveolar segments. Evaluation consists of counting the teeth, assessing mobility, and radiographic examination. All teeth must be accounted for; if this is not possible, chest and abdominal x-ray films must be obtained to rule out aspiration or swallowing.

Treatment

Partial Avulsion
The area is anesthetized with 2% lidocaine hydrochloride (Xylocaine) (if available), and an attempt is made to digitally reposition the tooth into its socket. The patient is asked to close his or her mouth to ensure that the tooth does not occlude prematurely.

If the patient has a mouth guard, this can be inserted to temporarily stabilize the tooth or teeth. If unstable, the tooth should be stabilized with a semirigid splint. This can be done by acid-etching resin and 26-gauge wire to stable teeth on both sides. The wire should be fixed first to the stable teeth. The patient then bites on a bite block to intrude the tooth into the socket, and it is then fixed to the wire. The patient should be placed on oral antibiotics, given

pain medication, and told to report to a dentist within 24 hours.

Complete Avulsion
When complete avulsion occurs, the tooth should be replanted as soon as possible. The most important factor in the success of replantation is the speed in which the tooth is replanted. Dirt should be removed from the root with milk, saline, or water; however, the tooth should be handled only by the crown and not be brushed, particularly the root. If the tooth cannot be replanted immediately, it should be transported immediately to a dentist or emergency room in the best medium available. Storage media in order of preference are a physiologic solution, such as Hank balanced salt solution (commercially available as Save-A-Tooth, Biologic Rescue Products, Conshohocken, PA), milk, normal saline, and saliva (the buccal vestibule).[14]

If the tooth can not be replanted within 15 minutes, it should be soaked in Hank balanced salt solution for 30 minutes before replantation (Table 6-1). This restores the vitality of the cells of the periodontal ligament and markedly decreases the probability of external resorption of the tooth.[15]

If the avulsed tooth has an immature apex, revascularization of the pulp is possible and enhanced by soaking the tooth in a solution of 1 mg doxycycline in 20 cc of normal saline for 5 minutes. If the tooth has a mature apex, root canal therapy will be necessary and should be done in 7 days.

If the tooth is not replanted within 2 hours and has been allowed to dry, the periodontal cells can not be restored and should be removed before replantation by soaking the tooth in bleach for 30 minutes to dissolve the organic debris on the root surface. This is followed by 5-minute soaks

TABLE 6-1
Treatment of the Avulsed Tooth

Storage Medium	Extraoral Time	Treatment: Periodontal	Treatment: Pulpal Immature Apex	Mature Apex	Replant	Stabilize	Analgesic Antibiotic
Dry	<15 mins	Rinse HBSS	AB soak 5 mins*	RCT 1 wk	Yes	Yes	Yes
	15–120 mins	Soak HBSS 30 mins	AB soak 5 mins	RCT 1 wk	Yes	Yes	Yes
	>120 mins	Refer	RCT immediately	RCT immediately	No	No	Yes
HBSS	<15 mins	—	AB soak 5 mins	RCT 1 wk	Yes	Yes	Yes
	15 mins–24 hrs	—	AB soak 5 mins	RCT 1 wk	Yes	Yes	Yes
Milk, water, saliva	<15 mins	Rinse HBSS	AB soak 5 mins	RCT 1 wk	Yes	Yes	Yes
	15–360 mins	Soak 30 mins HBSS	AB soak 5 mins	RCT 1 wk	Yes	Yes	Yes
	>360 mins	Refer	RCT immediately	RCT immediately	No	No	Yes

AB = antibiotic; HBSS = Hank balanced salt solution; RCT = root canal therapy.
*AB soak = 1 mg doxycycline in 20 cc of normal saline.

in citric acid, 2% stannous fluoride, and 5% doxycycline solutions. Because these solutions are unlikely to be available outside a dentist's office, it will probably be necessary to refer the patient for this treatment. Root canal therapy can also be done at this time with the tooth out of the patient's mouth.

After replantation, the tooth will need stabilization for 2 weeks. If alveolar fractures are present, 6–8 weeks are required. The patient is placed on 500 mg pen v k qid × 7 days and analgesics and is advised to see an endodontist as soon as possible.

Fractured Teeth

Fractures of the teeth may involve the enamel, dentin, or pulpal tissues. Fractures of only the enamel are the least serious, asymptomatic, and do not require immediate attention. Fractures involving the dentin are sensitive to air and thermal changes, but pose no immediate risk to the vitality of the tooth. If the fractured segment can be retrieved, it should be brought to a dentist who may be able to lute it to the tooth. If the pulp is minimally exposed, the vitality of the tooth may be preserved, particularly if the tooth is immature, but it must be sealed from the oral cavity. If the pulp is grossly exposed, it should be removed, and the canal protected with a temporary filling. Fractures of the root are detected by clinical and radiographic examination. Usually, these teeth are very mobile. The prognosis of root fractured teeth is poor, and they should be extracted and replaced with an implant at a later date.

Mouth Guards

Mouth guards are well-known protective devices that help prevent injuries to the teeth, gingiva, tongue, lips, and temporomandibular joints. To be effective, they must be comfortable, resilient, cover all the teeth, and not interfere with breathing. Although available in stock form, the best-fitting models are custom made by the dentist. If a strap attachment is made, it must be of a breakaway type to prevent dislocation and whiplash injuries.[16]

Field Emergency Kit

For the purposes of treating dentoalveolar injuries, a basic kit can be assembled. It should include examination gloves, a mouth mirror, a penlight, topical anesthesia, tongue depressors, sterile gauze, the emergency tooth preserving system Save-A-Tooth, instant cold ice packs, and an irrigating solution such as normal saline.

REFERENCES

1. Teichgraeber JF, Rappaport NH, Harris JH. The radiology of upper airway obstruction in maxillofacial trauma. Ann Plast Surg 1991;27:103–109.
2. Bivins HG, Ford S, Bezmalinovic Z, et al. The effect of axial traction during orotracheal intubation of the trauma victim with an unstable cervical spine. Ann Emerg Med 1988;17:25–29.
3. Kellman R. The cervical spine in maxillofacial trauma: assessment and airway management. Otolaryngol Clin North Am 1991;24:1–13.
4. Hwa-Kou K. Airway managements of patients with maxillofacial trauma. Acta Anesthesiol Sin 1996;34:213–220.
5. Henry CH, Hill EC. Traumatic emphysema of the head, neck, and mediastinum associated with maxillofacial trauma: case report and review. J Oral Maxillofac Surg 1989;47:876–882.
6. Leigh J, Garfield J, Rowe NL, Williams J. Primary Care. In Rowe W (ed), Maxillofacial Injuries. Edinburgh, Scotland: Churchill Livingstone, 1985.
7. Pollock R, Dingman RO. Management and Reconstruction of Athletic Injuries to the Face, Anterior Neck and Upper Respiratory Tract. In RC Schneider, JC Kennedy, ML Plant (eds), Sports Injuries: Mechanisms, Prevention, and Treatment. Baltimore: Williams & Wilkins, 1985.
8. Murakami WT, Davidson TM, Marshall LF. Fatal epistaxis in craniofacial trauma. J Trauma 1983;23:57–61.
9. London PS, Rowe NL, Williams JL. Definitive Clinical Exam. In W Rowe (ed), Maxillofacial Injuries. Edinburgh, Scotland: Churchill Livingstone, 1985.
10. Ommaya AK. Spinal fluid fistulae. Clin Neurosurg 1975;23:363–392.
11. Marentette LJ, Valentino J. Traumatic anterior fossa cerebrospinal fluid fistulae and craniofacial considerations. Otolaryngol Clin North Am 1991;24:151–163.
12. Hartman LC, Wolfgang L, Hall RE. The application of panoramic zonography to the diagnosis of maxillofacial fractures. Oral Surg Oral Med Oral Pathol Oral Radiol Endod 1989;67:214–219.
13. Renner GJ. Management of nasal fractures. Otolaryngol Clin North Am 1991;24:195–213.
14. Trope M. Clinical management of the avulsed tooth. Dent Clin North Am 1995;39:93–112.
15. Krasner P, Rankow HJ. New philosophy for the treatment of avulsed teeth. Oral Surg Oral Med Oral Pathol Oral Radiol Endod 1995;79:616–623.
16. Padilla R, Balikov S. Sports dentistry: coming of age in the '90s. CDA J 1993;21:27–37.

7

Cervical Spine Injuries

John W. Dietz, Jr., and Wade A. Lillegard

Catastrophic injury to the cervical spine in athletes is, thankfully, uncommon. However, most athletes and health care providers alike can name several outstanding performers whose careers or lives have been cut short by untimely spinal cord injury in sports. All agree that athletes' cervical spines should be protected by both the best equipment and rules of participation to minimize the chances of permanent spine injury. The purpose of this chapter is to detail the various types of cervical spine injuries, their prevention, immediate treatment, and guidelines for return to activity (Figure 7-1).

INITIAL ASSESSMENT

To the injured athlete, the most important person is the first examiner. Prompt recognition of serious neck injuries and the proper immobilization of a potentially unstable spine can protect the athlete from further harm. Most injuries to the neck are minor, but the initial evaluation must both rule out serious injury and protect the injured structures. When there is doubt about the seriousness of the injury, the athlete should be removed from competition until further evaluation is performed.

The Unconscious Athlete

If the athlete is unconscious after a fall or a blow to the head, the examiner must always consider the diagnosis of cervical spine injury along with head injury. The association between head and face trauma and cervical spine injuries is well known based on the evidence of motor vehicle and motorcycle accident victims. The initial assessment should include checking the airway and breathing and checking the circulation. If the patient is to be moved, one examiner should stabilize the head to the shoulders

while two attendants logroll the shoulders and hips into the supine position for examination. The athlete relies on the examiner to protect the spinal cord anytime the athlete is unable to do so. The examiner should always treat an unconscious athlete as if an unstable cervical spine injury is present and should continue to protect the cervical spine when the athlete regains consciousness.

Basic life support, if necessary, should begin immediately. If a helmet is in place, it should not be removed, but rather the face mask should be cut away with bolt cutters, leaving the rest of the helmet until after the initial radiographic examination. Some of the newer helmet designs have removable face masks. The procedure for removal of the face mask should be rehearsed by the examiner and staff early in the athletic season. An athlete who remains unconscious should be treated as if a cervical spine injury is present until such an injury is radiographically and clinically ruled out. Care should be taken to protect the airway from obstruction as a result of emesis or the patient's tongue. The unconscious athlete should be constantly monitored.

Neck Injury in the Conscious Athlete

After determining that the patient is awake and breathing, the first examiner at the scene should control the head while two assistants logroll the patient into the supine position. From this position, a brief assessment of cervical spine tenderness and location of pain can be performed, as well as a neurologic screening examination (Table 7-1). The level of consciousness, pupillary response, response to pain, abnormal posturing, and flaccidity or rigidity should be noted. Next, a brief motor examination should be performed of the upper- and lower-extremity muscle groups and reflexes, and a Babinski test should be done. Obviously, it is not possible to do every assessment listed in Table 7-1 on the field, but the neurologic examination should

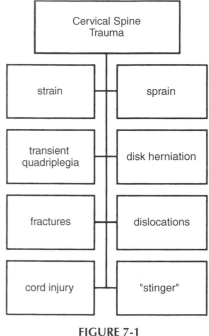

FIGURE 7-1
Cervical spine injuries.

progress and be repeated often if deficits exist. Again, the helmet should be left in place during the initial assessment.

If there is significant neck pain or if any neurologic deficit is appreciated, the patient should be transported to the nearest medical facility, using proper cervical spine immobilization techniques. If there is only mild neck discomfort and spasm and the neurologic screen is normal, the athlete can be taken to the sideline for further examination. Range of motion should then be assessed. The athlete can remove the helmet and then gently move his or her own neck. The

TABLE 7-1

Assessment of Upper- and Lower-Extremity Muscle Groups by Nerve Level

Nerve Level	Motor	Sensory
C5	Deltoid	Lateral shoulder
C6	Wrist extension	Thumb and index fingers
C7	Wrist flexion	Long finger
C8	Finger flexion	Ring and small fingers
T1	Hand intrinsics	Axilla
T2–T12	None	Trunk sensation
L1–L2	Hip flexion	Anterior upper thigh, groin
L3–L4	Quadriceps	Anterior and medial thigh
L4	Ankle dorsiflexion	Medial calf
L5	Great toe dorsiflexion	Lateral calf, dorsum of foot
S1	Ankle plantar flexion	Lateral and plantar foot
S2–S4	Rectal tone	Perianal

examiner should not attempt to push the athlete beyond the range of comfortable motion. Detailed palpation should also be done. If there is point tenderness over the spinous processes or if there is any decreased range of active motion of the cervical spine, the athlete should be removed from the sport until radiographic examination is done or range of motion improves. Likewise, if there is any paresthesia, numbness, tingling, or muscle weakness, the athlete should not return to competition. Although most high-level athletes are careful to follow directions from the physician or trainer, occasionally an athlete attempts to return to the game despite warning. The most effective way to ensure compliance with the order to stay on the sidelines is to take the athlete's helmet and hold it.

Transportation

If a cervical spine injury is considered, the athlete should be transported using proper immobilization of the cervical spine. The most experienced member of the health care team should take control of all movements, and no action should be taken without direction from this person. The "captain" should control the head at all times and not be responsible for any lifting. Two to three assistants should evenly divide the body weight. The first movement is to the supine position, where the brief assessment of neurologic function can begin. The second movement is onto a backboard, where the cervical spine is immobilized with sandbags and tape, and the body is held to the board with straps. In an athlete with altered consciousness or profound neurologic deficit, the face mask should be cut off during transport to avoid problems that might occur from emesis or if basic life support is necessary. Once on the backboard, the athlete can be transferred to an ambulance. Again, one person is in charge, and all movements are at that individual's direction. The head and shoulders should move as a unit without any rotation, twisting, or pulling.

Although the situation of possible cervical spine injury is rare, it is a good idea to rehearse the entire procedure at least once at the beginning of the season. The rehearsal is simple and quick, and the penalty for confusion in a critical situation may be disaster. One principle to remember is "First, do no harm."

SOFT TISSUE INJURIES TO THE CERVICAL SPINE

Cervical Strain

The diagnosis of cervical strain connotes an injury to the cervical musculature. This diagnosis is one of exclusion after a careful physical examination and imaging studies have ruled out underlying fracture or instability. There are numerous muscle groups that may be injured, including the paraspinals, trapezia, and sternocleidomastoids. In practice, it is not possible to assess whether the apparent strain injury involves only muscular elements or also includes the muscular insertions, facet joints, and other structures. Garrett[1] has shown that muscular injuries probably occur at the musculotendinous junction, rather than within the body of the muscle. Hemorrhage from a tear at the musculotendinous junction then results in inflammatory response, muscle spasm, pain, and decreased range of motion. It is known that muscle heals with fibrous bridging of the defect, rather than regeneration of the muscle fibers, and that fibrous tissue achieves 90% of its tensile strength in 6 weeks. Nevertheless, experience has shown that athletes can resume activity much earlier. It is considered safe for the athlete to return to competition when spasm has significantly resolved and active range of motion has returned to normal and when strength lost during convalescence has been regained. The health care consultant should avoid letting an athlete return to a contact sport before the athlete has acquired adequate strength and range of motion to protect the cervical spine from further injury. The cervical musculature and flexibility are key elements in dissipating energy in a high-energy injury, as is discussed in the section on cervical spine fractures and dislocations.

Treatment of cervical strains is symptom directed. Emphasis should be placed on decreasing the inflammatory response to muscle injury. Nonsteroidal anti-inflammatory medication in therapeutic doses given on a regular schedule is recommended. Many nonsteroidal anti-inflammatory agents are available (see Chapter 2). In practice, there is no significant difference among brands, and the practitioner should use one that is inexpensive and familiar. The anti-inflammatory effect usually requires faithful adherence to the recommended dose regimen and often takes several days to become effective. Additional pain relief may be safely obtained with acetaminophen in therapeutic doses as needed.

Ice massage is a convenient method of relieving spasm and pain. Direct ice massage should be done for 8–10 minutes at regular intervals during the acute phase of inflammation. This treatment can be self-directed. Although its mechanism of action is unclear, ice massage remains a practical and inexpensive treatment for both the spasm and pain associated with muscle injury (see Chapter 3).

Active range-of-motion exercises may be started as soon as they are tolerated. Motion should be limited to the painless arc and gradually increased. Resisted strengthening exercises should be postponed until the painless range of motion returns to normal. Isometric exercises should be started first, followed by resisted motion.

In general, treatment with costly modalities such as whirlpool, electrical stimulation, ultrasound, or specialized exercise equipment does not speed healing or return to activity, although they may enhance patient comfort to some degree. The key principles are gentle, active range-of-motion exercises followed by isometric and elastic-band, progressive-resistance exercises before returning to activity. There is no place for manipulative treatment of acute cervical spine injuries because of the risk of damage to healing structures or neurologic elements.

Further evaluation should be considered if (1) the muscle pain does not improve in the expected 2–3 weeks, (2) painless range of motion does not promptly improve to normal, or (3) neck pain with normal motion persists longer than 6 weeks. Any persistent neurologic deficit or paresthesia should be evaluated earlier. An advancing neurologic deficit or any evidence of developing spasticity should prompt immediate referral.

Cervical Sprains and Instability

The term *cervical sprain* connotes injury to the restraining ligaments of the cervical spine. A sprain can be categorized as follows: mild (grade I), meaning that the ligaments have been damaged but are not lengthened; moderate (grade II), meaning some laxity remains after the injury, but the ligament is not totally disrupted; or severe (grade III), meaning that the ligament is completely disrupted. This classification is applicable to cervical spine strains and serves to emphasize that sprains represent a spectrum of injuries from the mild, stable injury to the severe, mechanically unstable injury.

In practice, cervical sprains rarely occur alone; the symptoms of muscle spasm and pain may lead to a diagnosis of cervical strain. The unstable spine must not be misdiagnosed. If severe spasm and pain persist more than a few minutes after the injury, then radiographs should be obtained. In a more mild injury, radiographs should be obtained if range of motion and spasm do not normalize in a matter of hours to days. If no fracture is identified on a routine cervical spine series, lateral flexion and extension views should be done to assess for instability. In the normal spine, horizontal movement of one vertebral body on another should not exceed 3.5 mm, and the angular displacement of one vertebral body on the next is less than 11 degrees[2] (Figures 7-2 through 7-4). Displacement or angulation equal to or greater than these numbers indicates frank instability, which may warrant operative intervention. Younger individuals may normally have ligamentous laxity that may be confused with instability. If there is any question, the injured patient should be treated

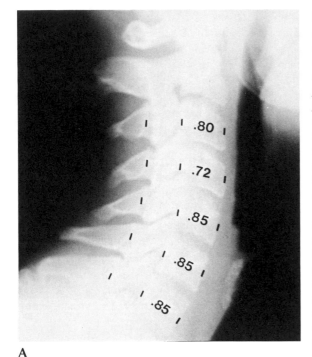

A

FIGURE 7-2

A 26-year-old athlete who sustained three episodes of transient quadriplegia in sports. The initial injury occurred when he struck his head on the wall of a racquetball court while diving for the ball. The second and third episodes were from blows to the head while playing football. After each injury, he was quadriplegic for 15–20 minutes, followed by gradual recovery of motor function. After the third episode, he developed clonus at both ankles, a positive Hoffmann sign for spasticity of the upper extremities, and left-arm weakness. On flexion or extension of the neck, he experienced paresthesia in both upper and lower extremities (Lhermitte sign). This case illustrates spinal cord injury resulting from both developmental stenosis and cervical instability. A. A lateral radiograph demonstrates the Torg ratio for developmental cervical spinal stenosis measured at each level. The ratio is calculated by dividing the sagittal diameter of each vertebral body by the distance from the spinolaminar line to the posterior aspect of the vertebral body. The ratio should be greater than 1.0. If it is less than 0.80, developmental stenosis is considered to be present, such as at C3 and C4 in this case. B. A lateral radiograph in extension of the same patient also demonstrates 4.0 mm of posterior displacement of C3 on C4, indicating cervical instability. C. A partial vertebrectomy of C4 with a two-level fusion was performed to decompress the spinal cord and stabilize the unstable segment. A cervical plate was used for fixation.

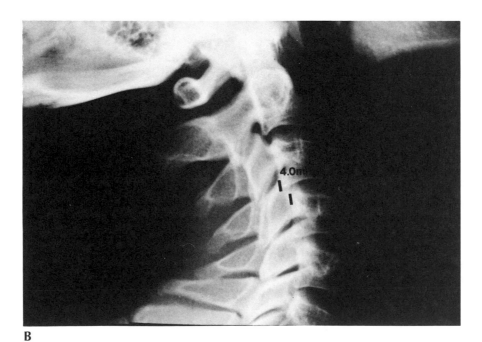

B

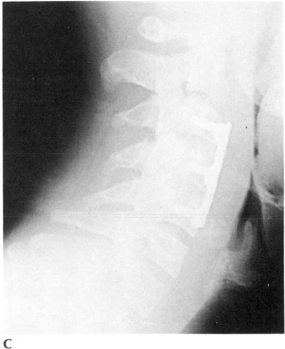

C

FIGURE 7-3

Evaluation of the lateral cervical spine radiograph may include an assessment of translation, or step-off, between vertebral bodies and a measurement of developmental or congenital spinal stenosis.

Sagittal translation is measured as follows: A mark is made on the posterosuperior corner of the lower vertebral body (1) and on the posteroinferior corner of the upper vertebral body (5). Next, a line is drawn along the superior border of the lower vertebral body (2). Two lines are drawn perpendicular to 2 and passing through 1 and 5. These are shown as 3 and 4 on the diagram. The translation A is measured as the distance between 3 and 4 and should be less than 3.5 mm or 20% of the sagittal diameter of the vertebral body. B is the sagittal diameter of the vertebral body.

Developmental cervical stenosis may be recognized on the lateral radiograph by measuring the ratio as follows: Measure the distance from the center of the spinolaminar line to the midpoint of the posterior aspect of the vertebral body (c). Next, measure the sagittal diameter of the vertebral body at its midpoint (d). The ratio of c to d should be 1.0. If it is less than 0.80, then it is abnormal. (Adapted from AA White, MM Panjabi [eds]. Clinical Biomechanics of the Spine. Philadelphia: Lippincott, 1990.)

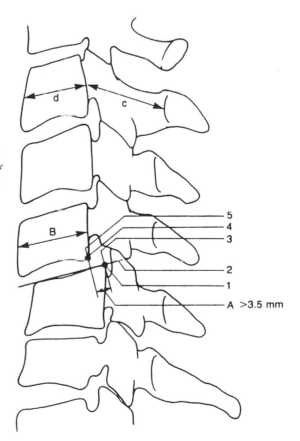

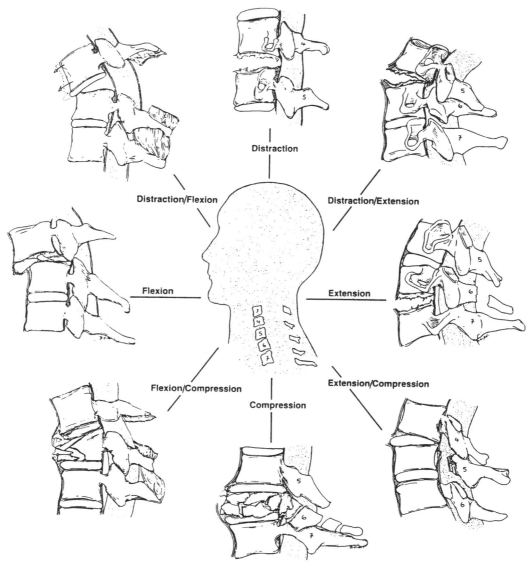

FIGURE 7-4

Lower cervical spine injuries involve C3 through C7 and follow patterns based on the mechanism of injury maximum injury vector. In this "clock" diagram, the points on the clock represent the injury vectors: 12 o'clock is pure distraction, 3 o'clock is pure exten-sion, 6 o'clock is pure compression, 9 o'clock is pure flexion, and all other points are combinations of these vectors.

At 12 o'clock, pure distraction causes disruption of a disk. Pure distraction, however, usually causes upper cervical spine injuries. At 1 o'clock, distraction with extension produces a common cervical instability pattern with posterior displacement of the cephalad verte-bra on the caudal vertebra. The injuries depicted at the 3 and 4 o'clock positions result from extension and are mostly ligamentous. These injuries are most common in the elderly population with some degree of degenerative disk changes and low-energy injury, such as a fall.

The fractures at 7 and 8 o'clock are often severe, high-energy injuries. In pure compression (6 o'clock) the vertebra may be crushed, and this is often called a burst fracture. Tension in the ligaments may pull most of the fragments back into reasonable alignment, making diagnosis more difficult. At the time of fracture, there is a more dramatic displacement. This fracture is common in athletic injuries in which the player strikes an opponent with the top of his or her head, causing compression on a straightened cervical spine. At 8 o'clock, flexion and compression combine to produce fracture of the anterior vertebral body with tearing of the poste-rior ligaments. Often, the anterior fracture will take the form of a teardrop broken off of the upper corner of the vertebral body. The small size of the teardrop fragment hides the fact that significant ligamentous damage has led to severe instability.

The injuries at 9 o'clock and 11 o'clock demonstrate pure flexion or flexion and distraction, producing dislocation of the cervical facets with anterior displacement of one vertebra on another. Facet dislocations may be unilateral with significant rotation on the anteropos-terior radiograph or bilateral with significant anterior displacement and angulation. (Adapted from PC McAfee. Cervical Spine Trauma. In JW Frymoyer, TB Ducker, NM, Hadler et al. [eds], The Adult Spine. New York: Raven, 1991;1080–1081.)

with a hard cervical collar, and flexion and extension radiographs should be repeated in 2–4 weeks. If these films are normal or show no evidence of progression, it is unlikely that a significant injury has occurred, and the injury may be treated as a sprain.[3]

Cervical instability without fracture may exist even in the presence of normal flexion and extension radiographs after the injury if muscle spasm acutely masks abnormal motion. In this case, the athlete should be protected until muscle spasm has subsided, and flexion and extension radiographs should be repeated in 7–10 days (but before the return to activity). No amount of muscular strengthening can safely overcome excessive ligamentous laxity in the cervical spine. If instability is noted radiographically, immediate referral is indicated, and the athlete should be protected in a hard cervical collar or other adequate immobilization. The athlete depends on the examiner to protect the spinal cord when the athlete cannot do so him- or herself. If radiographic instability is present, the athlete may need 6–12 weeks of immobilization in a rigid orthosis, and surgery may be required. Increased angulation or displacement greater than normal but less than 11 degrees or 3.5 mm, respectively, may represent a relative contraindication to contact sports.

If the initial radiographs were normal, then treatment may progress for the cervical strain, with care taken not to force motion beyond the painful limit. If spasm and pain continue, further studies with flexion and extension tomograms or computed tomography (CT) are warranted. Even a mild cervical sprain takes longer to become asymptomatic than a strain, and athletes require protection from activity for at least 6 weeks to allow for adequate strength of the healing ligaments. No athlete should return to competition until painless range of motion—with and without axial compression—is restored. Cervical strains and sprains are the most commonly encountered injuries. Constant vigilance is required to avoid missing the occult unstable injury.

NEUROLOGIC INJURIES WITHOUT FRACTURE

Stingers and Burners

"Stingers" and "burners" refer to a transient shooting or burning pain or paresthesia in one arm related to shoulder or neck trauma. There are two proposed mechanisms: traction on the brachial plexus or nerve root impingement within the cervical neural foramen from compression.[4] Most injuries at the high school level are the traction type, whereas the compressive type predominate in collegiate and professional players. Affected individuals report a shocklike sensation and numbness in a C5–C6 distribution. Weakness is unusual and generally transient. If symptoms are bilateral or involve the lower extremities, it is not a stinger, and spinal cord injury must be considered.

The athlete may safely return to competition if all symptoms resolve in minutes and there is full, painless neck range of motion. If symptoms persist longer than 15 minutes, a full workup to include plain radiographs and magnetic resonance imaging (MRI) should be considered to evaluate for instability, herniated disk, or other compressive pathology.[4] Persistent weakness beyond 3 weeks should be evaluated with electromyography. Preventive strategies include the use of high shoulder pads with a soft cervical roll, neck strengthening exercises, and review of blocking and tackling technique.

Transient Quadriplegia and Cervical Cord Neurapraxia

Immediate complete quadriplegia after a blow to the head or neck is the most feared injury in sports. Two sets of athletes present in this fashion: those with spinal cord injury from cervical fracture or dislocation and those with transient spinal cord shock. The latter recover function in 10–20 minutes, and they usually regain normal neurologic function without any residual effects. The initial treatment for both groups, however, should be identical until the diagnosis is firmly established. The medical team should first evaluate the athlete's ability to breathe and move the limbs. If the spinal cord injury extends above C2 to C4, the phrenic nerves may be paralyzed and diaphragm function compromised. The cervical spine should be protected while lifesaving measures are taken, and the athlete should be transported on a backboard to the nearest medical facility.

The syndrome of transient quadriplegia has been well described[5-15] and is also known as *cervical cord neurapraxia* (CCN). *Transient quadriplegia* and *CCN* refer to an athlete who experiences an acute transient neurologic episode originating from the traumatized cervical spinal cord. This is caused by spinal cord compression secondary to a blow to the head or a flexion/extension-type injury to the neck. Symptoms involve both legs, both arms, or an ipsilateral arm and leg. They may be sensory or sensory and motor. Sensory changes include burning pain, numbness, or tingling; motor changes range from mild weakness to complete paralysis. Symptoms generally last less than 15 minutes but can persist for 24 hours or longer.[16]

Affected athletes should be initially treated like any spinal cord injury patient, with spine board immobilization and emergency transport. When symptoms resolve, attention should be directed toward assessing

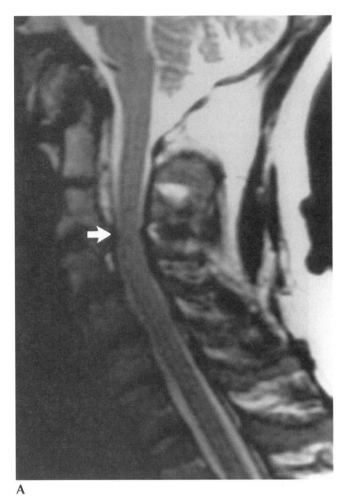

A

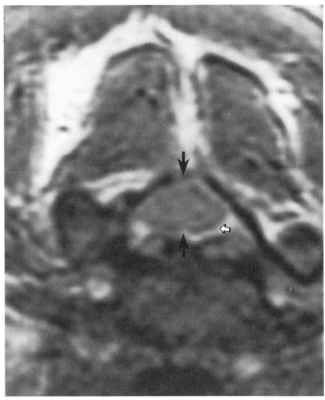

B

FIGURE 7-5

Magnetic resonance image of cervical spinal stenosis. A. Sagittal view. This athlete has congenital fusion of C2 and C3 with degenerative changes and a posterior bulge between C3 and C4. There is considerable narrowing of the spinal canal at the C3–C4 level (white arrow) with virtually no cerebrospinal fluid (white density) surrounding the cord at this level. This decrease in functional reserve potentially places the spinal cord at increased risk as hyperextension may narrow the canal another 30% from infolding of the interlaminar ligaments. B. This axial image demonstrates the decreased space available for the cord at the C3–C4 level. Note the scant amount of cerebrospinal fluid (open arrow) surrounding the cord (between black arrows).

anatomic factors that predispose to spinal cord insult. Initial evaluation should include routine cervical spine radiographs and possibly tomograms or CT scans to evaluate for subtle fractures. If these are normal, lateral flexion and extension views should be done to assess for ligamentous instability (see Figures 7-2 through 7-4). If no bony or ligamentous injury is identified, an MRI should be done to look for intrinsic or extrinsic cord abnormalities and nerve root compression (Figure 7-5). Torg et al.[16] performed a detailed analysis of 110 athletes who experienced a witnessed episode of CCN. Abnormalities were identified on plain radiographs in 93% and on MRI in 92%. Plain radiograph abnormalities included spinal stenosis (86%), osteophytic ridges (50%), degenerative disk disease (28%), lordotic reversal (21%), congenital vertebral fusion (7%), compression fracture (6%), limbus vertebrae (5%), atlantodens interval greater than 5 mm (2%), and teardrop fracture (1%). MRI abnormalities included degenerative disk disease (81%), osteophytic ridges (55%), neuroforaminal compromise (47%), disk protrusion (36%), spinal cord compression (34%), thecal sac effacement (25%), disk herniation (13%), lordotic reversal (8%), abnormal cord signal (8%), and posterior stenosis (4%).

Once the symptoms of CCN have resolved, two critical radiographic determinations must be made: assessment of instability and the presence or absence of cervical spinal stenosis. Lateral flexion and extension views should be done to assess instability. In the normal spine, horizontal movement of one vertebral body on another should not exceed 3.5 mm (see Figures 7-2 through 7-4), and the angular displacement of one vertebral body on the next is less than 11 degrees.[2] Measurements equal to or greater than these indicate instability is present, and patients should be referred.

Determination of spinal stenosis is somewhat more difficult on plain radiographs. The lateral radiograph is used most often to determine spinal stenosis (see Figure 7-3). Direct measurement of the spinal canal from the posterior vertebral body to the anterior interlaminar line should be more than 13 mm. Differences in projection and magnification make this measurement less reliable than Torg and Pavlov's method, which uses the ratio of the sagittal measurement of the spinal canal to the sagittal diameter of the vertebral body.[13] The normal ratio is thought to be 1.0, and ratios of less than 0.80 are suggestive of spinal stenosis. The Torg and Pavlov method, however, has a low predictive value. Herzog et al.[17] reported a ratio of less than 0.80 in 49% of 80 asymptomatic professional football players, and they calculated the Torg ratio to have a positive predictive value of only 12%. As the narrowing of the spinal canal cannot be determined by bone measurements alone, MRI is used to assess both the diameter of the cord and canal narrowing that is due to ligamentous hypertrophy or disk protrusion. The amount of protective cerebrospinal fluid (CSF) surrounding the spinal cord is called the *functional reserve*, and its absence on MRI is considered functional spinal stenosis[18] (see Figure 7-5). This lack of functional reserve may place the cord at risk, because hyperextension of the neck may narrow the canal another 30% from infolding of the interlaminar ligaments.[3]

RETURN-TO-PLAY CRITERIA

If there is no radiographic evidence of spinal instability or spinal stenosis, then return to collision sports is considered safe.[4, 16] If there is evidence of cervical instability after an episode of transient quadriplegia, the athlete should be precluded from collision sports. With no instability, but underlying congenital or acquired spinal stenosis, the decision is much more difficult. Cantu[18] believed that athletes who have had spinal cord–related symptoms and have true functional spinal stenosis should not be allowed to participate in contact sports. As evidence, he cited the work of Matsuura et al.,[19] who found the sagittal diameters of 42 spinal cord injury patients to be sig-

nificantly smaller than that of 100 noninjured controls. Additionally, MRI has documented functional spinal stenosis in 6 of 11 patients rendered quadriplegic.[20] Finally, Cantu noted that a small cervical spinal canal predisposes to a poor outcome when spinal injury does occur. Interpreting data from the National Center for Catastrophic Sports Injury between 1987 and 1996, he noted that no quadriplegic patients who had fracture dislocation with underlying stenosis completely recovered. Conversely, 20% of initially quadriplegic patients who had fracture dislocation with normal size canals went on to complete recovery.[18]

Torg et al.[16] have suggested that CCN is a transient phenomenon that does not pose an increased risk of catastrophic injury. They analyzed 110 patients with witnessed CCN; 86% had spinal stenosis defined as a spinal canal (SC) to vertebral body (VB) ratio of less than 0.80. Thirty-four percent had MRI evidence of spinal cord compression. Sixty-three patients (57%) with CCN returned to contact sports after the initial occurrence, and 32 of these had a recurrent episode. Of those with a recurrence, 17 retired after the second episode, and the remaining 15 continued with an average recurrence of 3.1 ± 4.0 episodes. There were no permanent neurologic injuries among the 45 patients who continued to play, with follow-up ranging from 15 to 43 months. The authors concluded that CCN is a transient phenomenon that is due to cord compression caused by trauma in a patient with developmental or spondylolytic narrowing of the sagittal diameter of the cervical canal. They suggested that patients without spinal instability can return to contact sports without risk of permanent neurologic injury. The risk of recurrence, however, was 56% overall and is strongly related to the degree of stenosis as assessed by the SC/VB ratio (plain radiographs) or disk-level canal measurement on MRI. Clearly, the decision to return athletes with CCN and underlying spinal stenosis to play is controversial. If such an athlete insists on continuing in contact or collision sports, it is advisable to obtain the opinions of multiple consultants.

SPINAL CORD INJURIES IN ATHLETES

Three sports have accounted for the majority of cervical spinal cord injuries in recent history: football, trampoline (gymnastics), and diving. Of these, organized football and gymnastics are most amenable to preventive changes, because they are generally well controlled. Diving accidents are often recreational and not part of an organized sport; therefore, high-risk behavior is more difficult to change.

TABLE 7-2
Incidence of Football (FB) Injuries[a]

Year	Intracranial Hemorrhages	Cranial Deaths	Cervical Spine Fractures	Permanent Quadriplegia	Source
1959–1963	3.39	1.58	1.36	0.73	Schneider[b]
1971–1975	1.15	0.92	4.14	1.58	FB registry[c]
1976 (year of rule changes)	1.07	1.07	7.72 high school 30.66 college	2.24 high school 10.66 college	FB registry
1984	2.12	0.91	3.65 high school 6.66 college	0.40 high school 0.00 college	FB registry
1987	1.78	0.10	2.31 high school 10.66 college	0.73 high school 0.00 college	FB registry

[a]Number of injuries per 100,000 participants.
[b]RC Schneider. Head and Neck Injuries in Football: Mechanisms, Treatment, and Prevention. Baltimore: Williams & Wilkins, 1973.
[c]JS Torg, JJ Vegso, B Sennet. The National Football Head and Neck Injury Registry: 14-year report on cervical quadriplegia (1971–1984). Clin Sports Med 1987;6:61.

Football helmets were improved in response to an unacceptably high rate of head injuries, intracranial hemorrhage, and death. From 1959 to 1963, Schneider found 139 episodes of intracranial hemorrhage for an incidence of 3.39 per 100,000 and 65 deaths (1.58 per 100,000).[11] By 1971–1975, the incidence of intracranial hemorrhage had dropped 66% to 1.15 per 100,000, and deaths dropped 42% to 0.92 per 100,000.[21] The decrease is attributed largely to better helmet design. However, improved helmets allowed playing techniques to develop that place the cervical spine at greater risk. Cervical spine fractures or dislocations were reported as 56 injuries (1.36 per 100,000) with 30 cases of quadriplegia (0.73 per 100,000) in 1959–1963. From 1971 to 1975, 259 of these injuries were reported (4.41 per 100,000), with 99 cases of quadriplegia (1.58 per 100,000).[22] The rate of both cervical spine injuries and quadriplegia had jumped dramatically, whereas the rate of head injuries dropped (Table 7-2).

Torg et al. noted 12 cervical spinal cord injuries in high school players in New Jersey and Pennsylvania in the 1975 season. This prompted him to develop the National Football Head and Neck Injury Registry to document the incidence of these injuries nationwide and provide data for preventive rule changes.[22, 23] Torg and the Registry have provided football governing bodies and the medical profession with important data and have prompted rule changes that have made football safer for the athlete. Axial loading of the cervical spine is considered the highest-risk action. It usually occurs when a defensive back lowers his head to strike his opponent with the top or crown of the helmet. In 1976, the National Collegiate Athletic Association (NCAA) football rules committee banned this activity with three rules changes: "(1) no player shall intentionally strike a runner with the crown or top of the hel-

met, (2) spearing is the deliberate use of the helmet in an attempt to injure an opponent, and (3) no player shall deliberately use his helmet to butt or ram an opponent."[24] At the 12-year point of the National Football Head and Neck Injury Registry, the incidence of cervical fractures and quadriplegia has decreased 70% for high school and 65% for college athletes.[23]

Spear-Tackler's Spine

Tremendous forces must be dissipated in the milliseconds after contact between colliding players. Simple physics shows that a 300-lb defensive lineman running 15 miles per hour strikes a 250-lb fullback running 25 miles per hour with the same energy as a car striking a brick wall at 13 miles per hour. Only physical conditioning, technique, and adequate equipment make it possible to sustain that much contact without severe injury.

The most important energy-absorbing mechanism for the cervical spine is its inherent flexibility. When the spine is loaded in such a way as to minimize its ability to flex or extend to absorb energy, the energy must be concentrated in a brief moment. When forced into flexion or extension, the cervical musculature dissipates the energy over a greater time and area. This spreads a smaller amount of stress over more segments, stopping the motion before it exceeds the physiologic limit of the spine.

The cervical musculature has a mechanical advantage over the vertebrae and ligaments by virtue of greater distance from the axis of rotation. The muscles are thus in an ideal position to dissipate energy through controlled motion. On the other hand, when the cervical spine is flexed approximately 30 degrees, the normal cervical lordosis is lost, and the spine is straight. If the spine is loaded from the vertex of the skull in that position, there is no flexion or extension readily available to dissipate energy; all the energy is therefore transmitted down the spine by axial loading through the vertebrae and disks. This loading mechanism is responsible for most football-induced injuries: 52.5% of the quadriplegias and 49% of the cervical fractures overall.[21]

"Spear-tackler's spine" was described in 1993 after permanent neurologic injury was identified in four athletes with similar characteristics: (1) developmental narrowing of the cervical canal, (2) straightening or reversal of the normal cervical lordosis, (3) pre-existing post-traumatic bony or ligamentous injury, and (4) documentation of having used spear-tackling techniques.[25] Many experts think that an athlete with spear-tackler's spine should be precluded from contact or collision sports.[26] Others think that if the normal lordosis is restored and athletes refrain from spear-tackling techniques, they may return.[3]

Prevention requires a change in high-risk behavior. Players preventing injuries are decreasing their own chances of a permanent impairment. Every player must understand that to avoid spearing is to save himself from catastrophic injury as well as to protect his opponent and abide by the rules. A strengthening program for the cervical musculature is as important as strength training for the entire athlete. Finally, the helmet and shoulder pads should provide the best-possible fit and protection.

Spinal Shock and Spinal Cord Injury

Acute quadriplegia after trauma may represent spinal shock. For the first 24–48 hours after a spinal cord injury, the cord may be in "shock." During this period, no prognosis for long-term recovery can be given. A patient may recover fully, or a complete cord lesion may exist. Spinal shock is considered to be present if the bulbocavernosus reflex is absent, and the return of that reflex heralds the end of spinal shock. Once the reflex has returned, the degree of spinal cord injury may be assessed.

A complete spinal cord injury is present if no useful motor or sensory function exists below the level of injury. Partial spinal cord injuries may be anterior cord syndrome, central cord syndrome, posterior cord syndrome, or Brown-Séquard syndrome. The area of the cord that is injured determines the clinical picture. Anterior syndromes involve motor weakness with sensory sparing, central lesions involve more upper-extremity than lower-extremity paralysis, and the rare posterior lesion is primarily sensory. The Brown-Séquard syndrome involves ipsilateral motor paralysis with contralateral sensory deficit. All of the partial spinal cord injuries have some

capacity for improvement in function with time, whereas complete cord lesions have very little, if any, chance of improvement.

Steroids and Spinal Cord Injuries

Data suggest that as many as two cervical levels of function may be preserved with immediate administration of high-dose methylprednisolone after cervical spinal cord injury.[27] This protocol has become the standard in most emergency rooms. The medication must be given within 8 hours of injury and must continue for 23 hours. Dosage regimen is as follows: methylprednisolone 30 mg/kg intravenous bolus, then continuous intravenous infusion of 5.4 mg/kg per hour for 23 hours.

INTERVERTEBRAL DISK HERNIATION

Acute disk herniation in the cervical spine is considered to be as much as 10 times less common than acute disk herniation in the lumbar spine. Compression of a cervical nerve root can occur either from acute rupture of the disk with extrusion of disk material into the nerve foramen or, more commonly, from chronic degeneration of the disk with a combination of disk and osteophytic encroachment on the nerve foramen. In either case, nerve compression results in burning pain, weakness, or sensory changes in the distribution of the individual nerve root.

Neck pain is a feature of this problem, and it may be an acute or a chronic process. The distinguishing feature is that neurologic symptoms—motor weakness, loss of deep-tendon reflexes, or sensory disturbances—are restricted to the distribution of one nerve root. Nerve root compression is manifested by burning dysesthesia in the arm or hand, pain in the shoulder, numbness or tingling, weakness of a corresponding muscle group (see Table 7-1), or loss of a deep-tendon reflex. A common feature is referred pain to the inferior angle of the ipsilateral scapula or the center of the thoracic spine between the scapulae. This diagnosis should also be kept in mind when an athlete presents with primary shoulder pain or pain in the upper thoracic spine. The most common root affected is the C6 nerve exiting between the C5 and C6 vertebral bodies.

In the acute setting, the diagnosis is difficult to establish. The athlete may present with acute C6 radiculopathy and neck pain. A stinger usually resolves in minutes, whereas radiculopathy from nerve compression resolves in days or weeks. Likewise, cervical strain resolves in 1–2 weeks, whereas a herniated disk usually takes somewhat longer. If the painless range of motion does not promptly return to normal, the athlete should not return to the activity, and radiographs should be obtained. Once cervical fracture or instability is ruled out, symptomatic treatment may begin.

The presumptive diagnosis of herniated cervical disk is based on the clinical symptoms of radicular pain in the distribution of a cervical nerve root with or without neck pain, and on the findings of loss of reflex or motor weakness matching the sensory disturbance. The diagnosis can be confirmed only by MRI or cervical myelography, but these diagnostic tests should be reserved until the symptoms have been present for at least 6 weeks, unless there is a marked neurologic deficit or progression of a neurologic deficit. Eighty to 90% of cervical radiculopathies resolve with conservative care, generally in less than 6 weeks.[28] It is both prudent and responsible to follow the patient closely before recommending detailed imaging studies. Cervical myelography is invasive and carries some risk of complications. MRI has the considerable advantage of being noninvasive and providing excellent imaging, but it is expensive and may not be helpful if the symptoms are likely to resolve in a few weeks.

Treatment should consist of gentle active range of motion, a burst (6 to 7-day course) of oral steroids or a nonsteroidal anti-inflammatory agent (if well tolerated), and rest. Cervical traction and manipulative treatment are often used, but there is no scientific proof that either treatment speeds healing or a return to activity. In the acute setting, manipulative treatment should be avoided until muscle spasm has resolved, if it is used at all. Some physical modalities such as ice massage or electrical stimulation may be particularly useful if muscle spasm is present. A cervical epidural steroid injection may be useful in patients not responding to traction and therapy.[28] Symptomatic treatment should continue until a full painless range of motion of the neck has been achieved. The athlete should not return to contact sports until restrengthening has been achieved to protect the neck from further injury. The athlete should not return to sports while a neurologic deficit or symptom remains unresolved.[5]

If the symptoms or neurologic deficit remain after 6 weeks of symptomatic treatment and rest, further evaluation with MRI or orthopedic or neurosurgical consultation should be considered. Surgery is rarely required for herniated cervical disks, but when necessary it offers good relief of radicular pain and neurologic recovery. Several options for surgery are available, and the reader is referred to spine surgery texts for further details.

The question of whether an asymptomatic athlete who has had cervical fusion for intervertebral disk herniation should return to contact sports is difficult to answer.

Watkins[5] believed that these athletes should be counseled that they are at mild increased risk of a cervical spine injury based on the decreased ability of the spine to dissipate energy with motion. An athlete with fusion at C3–C4 is at higher risk than one with fusion from C6 to C7 because of the potential effects on the upper cervical spine. Athletes with fusion at C3–C4 should be counseled that they are at moderately increased risk. Athletes with more than one fused level should avoid contact sports altogether.

Torg and Ramsey-Emrhein[26] believed that an asymptomatic athlete with a stable single-level fusion and full range of motion may participate in contact activities. A more-than-three–level fusion is an absolute contraindication, and a two- to three-level fusion is a relative contraindication for contact sports. Any fusion that does not result in full range of motion is a contraindication.

CERVICAL SPINE FRACTURES AND DISLOCATIONS

The list of possible cervical fractures is long and confusing. This section organizes the many types of cervical fractures and dislocations into two categories based on the biomechanics of the upper and lower cervical spine. The first section is on upper cervical spine lesions—those occurring from C0 (the occiput) to C2. The second section covers the lower cervical spine from C3–T1. Some authors believe that C3 and C4 constitute a transition zone that is biomechanically unique, and that athletic injuries in this region have a distinct pattern as well as prognosis.[29] These injuries are included in the lower cervical spine in this discussion; nevertheless, C3–C4 injuries are common and often devastating.

A key concept in understanding cervical fractures is the mechanism of injury. White and Panjabi[29] have used the biomechanical term *maximum injury vector* (MIV) to describe the resultant force, direction, and point of application that causes the injury. The mechanism of injury, or the MIV, is generally consistent with the pattern of injury. Likewise, the pattern of injury is often strongly associated with the likelihood of neurologic injury, mechanical instability, and prognosis (see Figures 7-4 and 7-6). A working knowledge of these patterns minimizes the chances of missing an important lesion on the radiographs.

Upper Cervical Spine

Injuries to the upper cervical spine seldom cause neurologic deficit because of the space available in the canal to accommodate displacement of the vertebrae. On the other hand, a neurologic injury in the upper cervical spine may be fatal because of paralysis of the respiratory muscles. A complete description of these injuries is beyond the scope of this text, and the reader is referred to spine surgery texts. Figure 7-6 summarizes the types of injuries expected from application of force at various points in the sagittal plane. The three most common patterns are the odontoid fracture, hangman's fracture, and Jefferson fracture.

Odontoid Fracture

Fracture of the odontoid process usually occurs with hyperextension of the neck. The ring of C1 strikes the odontoid process, shearing it off at the base. Three types have been identified based on the location of the fracture: type 1 is an avulsion of the tip of the odontoid process and is inherently stable; a type 2 fracture has sheared off the process at its base and is inherently unstable; a type 3 fracture extends down into the body of C2—it is less unstable than a type 2 but still requires diligent protection. Type 2 fractures have the most difficulty and often go on to nonunion, requiring surgical treatment. The open-mouth odontoid radiograph most clearly demonstrates these fractures.

Hangman's Fracture

A great deal of writing has been done on this injury. Excellent medieval (and recent) texts exist advising the executioner on exactly how to produce this fracture fatally. In medical practice, however, this fracture rarely produces neurologic deficit or death. The MIV in this fracture is hyperextension. The posterior elements of C2 are separated from the body by fracture of the pars interarticularis bilaterally. Treatment is generally nonoperative. The lateral radiograph best demonstrates this fracture.

Jefferson Fracture

The MIV for this fracture is axial loading. The ring of C1 is broken in four places, two anterior and two posterior. This is difficult to visualize radiographically, and the CT scan shows it most clearly. However, the open-mouth odontoid view offers the clue to diagnosis. The lateral masses of C1 and C2 should line up smoothly, and there should be no step-off laterally. If the overhang on both sides adds up to greater than 7 mm, injury should be suspected. This fracture can usually be treated without surgery.

Lower Cervical Spine

Fractures of the lower cervical spine are often associated with profound neurologic injury because of the limited space available in the spinal canal for the spinal cord to adapt to displacement. Although numerous fracture patterns exist based on the MIV (see Figure 7-4), two fractures deserve special mention because of their incidence in athletics and the imperative nature of their diagnosis: the teardrop fracture and the burst fracture. The lateral radiograph is the key to diagnosis of most lower cervical spine fractures.

Teardrop Fracture

This injury is so named both for its characteristic appearance on lateral radiograph and for the often dismal prognosis. Radiographically it appears as if a small teardrop-shaped fragment has been chipped off the superior-anterior corner of one vertebral body. The size of the fragment belies the significance of the injury. The MIV is usually axial load and flexion on a flexed spine. The posterior ligamentous support, the posterior longitudinal ligament, and the intervertebral disk structures are disrupted. Significant displacement at the time of fracture often produces spinal cord injury, but occasionally the cord is spared. This injury is extremely unstable. The radiographic clues also include widening of the interspinous space posteriorly and an acute angulation between vertebral bodies (see Figure 7-4).

Burst Fracture

This is another axial-loading injury. If the neck is flexed approximately 30 degrees (as if to spear another player with the top of the athlete's helmet), all of the cervical lordosis is removed and the vertebral bodies are aligned. Axial loading in this position may produce a burst fracture. Again, the radiographic appearance belies the extent of the underlying damage. On the lateral radiograph, the vertebral body looks only slightly enlarged, and the trabecular pattern is disrupted. Often, a small chip of bone is avulsed from the upper or lower vertebral body. At the time of injury, however, the vertebral body is widely displaced and may severely damage the spinal cord. By the time the radiograph is taken, the fragments have been pulled back into alignment by the ligamentous attachments (see Figure 7-4). Awareness of the possibility of this injury makes its diagnosis easier.

Return-to-Play Guidelines After Cervical Spine Fracture

Before an athlete with a spinal fracture can be considered for return to play, two criteria must be met: (1) the fracture must be documented to have healed, and (2) the healed fracture must not pose an undue risk of catastrophic injury. Assessment of healing generally involves a full cervical spine series, flexion and extension views, and often a CT

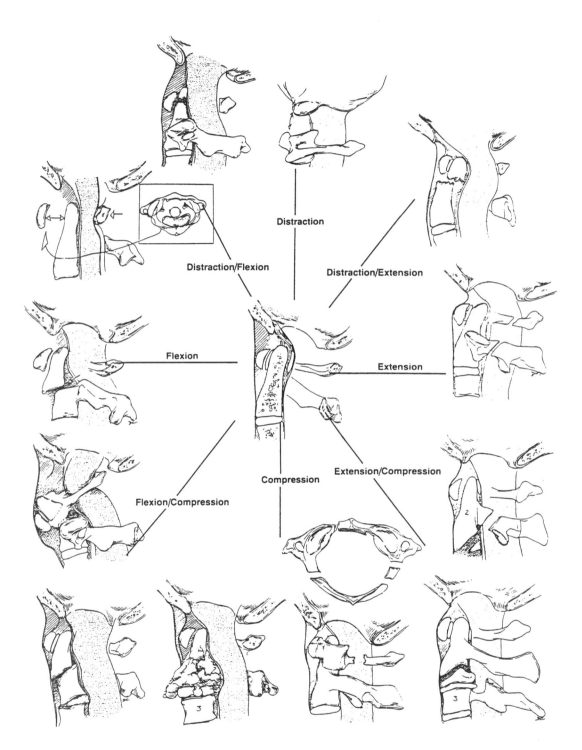

Distraction

Distraction/Flexion

Distraction/Extension

Flexion

Extension

Flexion/Compression

Compression

Extension/Compression

scan or tomograms. Certain fracture patterns, when healed, may be stable, and once full range of motion and strength have returned, some affected athletes may safely return to contact sports. Reasonable return-to-play guidelines have recently been promulgated by Torg and Ramsey-Emrhein[26] and are outlined in Table 7-3.

INTERPRETATION OF CERVICAL SPINE RADIOGRAPHS

Any physician involved in the care of athletes should be familiar with interpretation of cervical radiographs. Help is usually available from consultants and emergency physicians, but in a time of need some quick reference rules and

diagrams make it safer and easier. The following simple rules serve as a checklist and are designed to identify the athlete with a potentially dangerous instability or fracture.

Lateral Radiograph

See Figures 7-2, 7-3, and 7-7.

1. A clear radiograph of the entire cervical spine, including the entire body of C7 and the top of T1, should be done. Never read bad films.

◄ **FIGURE 7-6**

Cervical spine fractures can be related to the mechanism of injury (i.e., flexion, extension, compression, and distraction). This diagram illustrates fractures of the upper cervical spine as a "clock" of injuries and associated maximum injury vector. The vector of force at 12 o'clock is distraction, at 9 o'clock is forced flexion, at 6 o'clock is compression, and at 3 o'clock is forced extension.

At 12 o'clock, pure distraction is applied to the head. This results in atlanto-occipital dislocation, usually a fatal injury. At the 2 o'clock position, distraction is combined with extension to produce a type 1 or type 2 odontoid fracture (see text). At the 3 o'clock position, pure extension produces a fracture of the posterior elements of C2 or C1. At C2 this may take the form of a hangman's fracture. At the 4 o'clock position, extension combined with compression may produce a classic hangman's fracture with displacement of the body of C2 anteriorly or may produce a fracture of the body of C2.

Pure compression at the 6 o'clock position produces the classic Jefferson fracture pattern where the ring of C1 is burst, usually with three or four fractures in the ring and widening of the lateral masses. Pure compression may also result in crush of the body of C2 shown at the 6:30 position.

The 7 o'clock position demonstrates two versions of the type 3 odontoid fracture with the fracture line extending into the body of C2. The 9 o'clock position shows the most common odontoid fracture pattern, the type 2 odontoid fracture. In this fracture, the odontoid is sheared off at its base (see text).

At the 10 o'clock position, distraction combined with flexion may produce ligamentous injury at C1, allowing the odontoid to slide posteriorly and widening the atlantodens interval without fracture of the bony elements. This purely ligamentous injury is best diagnosed on the lateral or flexion and extension radiographs (see text). The 11 o'clock position demonstrates the rare type 1 odontoid fracture. (Adapted from PC McAfee. Cervical Spine Trauma. In JW Frymoyer, TB Ducker, NM Hadler, et al. [eds], The Adult Spine. New York: Raven, 1991;1068–1069.)

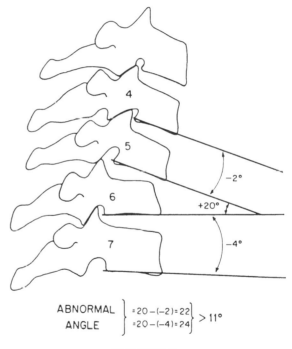

ABNORMAL ANGLE $\left.\begin{matrix} =20-(-2)=22 \\ =20-(-4)=24 \end{matrix}\right\} > 11°$

FIGURE 7-7

Abnormal sagittal angulation on the lateral radiograph of the cervical spine is defined as angulation between segments that is greater than 11 degrees more than angulation between adjacent segments. In this diagram, clockwise angulation is considered positive, and counterclockwise angulation is considered negative. In evaluating the C5–C6 level, angulation is measured between lines along the inferior border of each vertebral body from C4 to C7. The angle between C5 and C6 is 20 degrees clockwise. The angle between C4 and C5 is 2 degrees counterclockwise (–2 degrees) for an angular difference of 22 degrees. Likewise, the angle between C6 and C7 is counterclockwise 4 degrees (–4 degrees) for an angular difference of 24 degrees. Radiographic instability is considered if either of these angular differences exceeds 11 degrees. (Adapted from AA White, MM Panjabi [eds]. Clinical Biomechanics of the Spine. Philadelphia: Lippincott, 1990;57.)

TABLE 7-3
Return-to-Play Guidelines After Healed Cervical Spine Fracture

No Contraindication	Relative Contraindication	Absolute Contraindication
Stable compression fractures of the vertebral body without a sagittal component on AP view and no ligamentous instability or involvement of posterior elements	Stable displaced compression fractures of the vertebral body without a sagittal component on AP view (propensity to settle with increased deformity)	Vertebral body fracture with a sagittal component
Stable end-plate fracture without sagittal component on AP view and no ligamentous instability or involvement of posterior elements	Healed, stable fractures of the posterior neural ring (a rigid ring cannot break in only one location—paired healing must be demonstrated)	Fracture of the vertebral body with or without displacement with associated posterior arch fractures or ligamentous laxity
Healed spinous process fracture ("clay shoveler")		Comminuted fractures of the vertebral body with displacement into the spinal canal
		Any healed fracture with associated pain, neurologic findings, and limited range of motion
		Healed, displaced fractures involving the lateral masses with resulting facet incongruity

AP = anteroposterior.

2. Smooth, continuous lines should connect the posterior aspect of each vertebral body. A step-off of greater than 3.5 mm denotes either instability or dislocation of facets. Similar smooth lines should connect the anterior vertebral bodies and the facets.

3. The soft tissue shadow anterior to C3 should be less than 5 mm thick, and that anterior to C7 should be less than 22 mm. Various numbers have been proposed, as low as 3 mm at C3 and 17 mm at C7.

4. Look for widening of the space between spinous processes posteriorly.

5. Look for widening of the space between the odontoid and the ring of C1. It should be 3 mm. Greater than 5 mm is clearly abnormal, even in a child. This space should not change with flexion and extension views.

6. Abrupt changes in angulation between vertebral bodies may indicate instability or fracture. The amount of angulation difference should be less than 11 degrees on the static lateral radiograph (see Figure 7-7).

7. Spinal stenosis may be assessed using the Torg ratio (see Figure 7-3). This is calculated by dividing the sagittal diameter of the vertebral body by the distance from the spinolaminar line to the posterior aspect of the vertebral body. It should be 1.0 or greater. Less than 0.80 suggests spinal stenosis. An MRI to assess functional spinal stenosis is a more accurate method (see Figure 7-5).

Anteroposterior Radiograph

1. The alignment of the spinous processes should be along a continuous and unbroken line. All spinous processes should be in the midline.

2. The patient's head should not be tilted to one side (torticollis).

3. The patient's trachea should be in the midline position.

Open-Mouth Odontoid View

1. Look for the three types of odontoid fractures.

2. The lateral border of C1 should line up directly with the lateral border of C2. If overhang on both sides adds up to more than 7 mm, it is abnormal.

3. The space between the odontoid and the lateral masses of C1 should be equal on both sides.

This quick checklist may help in diagnosis of cervical spine instability or fracture, but the radiographs should also be reviewed by a qualified consultant. Flexion and extension views are indicated when there has been significant trauma before return to competition. They may also be helpful if pain or loss of motion persists. A qualified attendant should accompany the patient, and flexion or extension should not exceed the painless range of motion. The patient should be cautioned not to push beyond that range and to stop if any tingling or paresthesias develop. An attendant should never help the patient flex or extend, and these radiographs should never be attempted if the patient is not completely awake and cooperative.

REFERENCES

1. Garrett WE, Tidball J. Myotendinous Junction: Structure, Function, and Failure. In SL-Y Woo, JA Buckwalter (eds),

Injury and Repair of the Musculoskeletal Soft Tissues. Park Ridge, IL: AAOS, 1988;171–212.

2. White AA, Johnson RM, Panjabi MM, et al. Biomechanical analysis of clinical stability in the cervical spine. Clin Orthop 1975;109:85–95.

3. Wilberger JE. Athletic spinal cord and spine injuries. Clin Sports Med 1998;17:111–120.

4. Cantu RC. Stingers, transient quadriplegia, and cervical spinal stenosis: return to play criteria. Med Sci Sports Exerc 1997;29(suppl 7):233–235.

5. Watkins RG. Neck injuries in football players. Clin Sports Med 1986;5:215–238.

6. Jackson DW, Lohr FT. Cervical spine injuries. Clin Sports Med 1986;5:373–380.

7. Bailes JE, Hadley MN, Quigley MR, et al. Management of athletic injuries of the cervical spine. Neurosurgery 1991; 29:491–497.

8. Cervical Spine Research Society Editorial Committee. The Cervical Spine (2nd ed). Philadelphia: Lippincott, 1989;442–461.

9. Cibulka MT. Evaluation and treatment of cervical spine injuries. Clin Sports Med 1989;8:691–701.

10. Ladd AL, Scranton PE. Congenital cervical stenosis presenting with transient quadriplegia. J Bone Joint Surg Am 1986;68:1371–1374.

11. Schneider RC. Head and Neck Injuries in Football: Mechanisms, Treatment, and Prevention. Baltimore: Williams & Wilkins, 1973.

12. Torg JS, Pavlov H, Genuario SE, et al. Neurapraxia of the cervical spinal cord with transient quadriplegia. J Bone Joint Surg Am 1986;68:1354–1370.

13. Torg JS, Pavlov H. Cervical spinal stenosis with cord neurapraxia and transient quadriplegia. Clin Sports Med 1987;6:115–133.

14. Torg JS, Vegso JJ, O'Neill MJ, Sennet B. The epidemiologic, pathologic, biomechanical and cinematographic analysis of football induced cervical spine trauma. Am J Sports Med 1990;18:50–57.

15. Torg JS. Cervical spinal stenosis with cord neurapraxia and transient quadriparesis. Clin Sports Med 1990;9:279–296.

16. Torg JS, Corcoran TA, Thibault LE, et al. Cervical cord neurapraxia: classification, pathomechanics, morbidity, and management guidelines. J Neurosurg 1997;87:843–850.

17. Herzog RJ, Weins JJ, Dillingham MF, et al. Normal cervical spine morphometry and cervical spinal stenosis in asymptomatic professional football players. Spine 1991;16:178–186.

18. Cantu RC. The cervical spinal stenosis controversy. Clin Sports Med 1998;17:121–126.

19. Matsuura P, Waters RL, Adkins RH, et al. Comparison of computerized tomography parameters of the cervical spine in normal control subjects and spinal cord–injured patients. J Bone Joint Surg Am 1989;71:183–188.

20. Cantu RC. Functional cervical spinal stenosis: a contraindication to participation in contact sports. Med Sci Sports Exerc 1993;25:46–52.

21. Vegso JJ, Lehman RC. Field evaluation and management of head and neck injuries. Clin Sports Med 1987;6:1–15.

22. Torg JS, Quendenfeld TC, Burstein A, et al. National Football Head and Neck Injury Registry: report on cervical quadriplegia 1971–1975. Am J Sports Med 1979;7:127–132.

23. Torg JS, Vegso JJ, Sennet B. The National Football Head and Neck Injury Registry: 14 year report on cervical quadriplegia (1971–1984). Clin Sports Med 1987;6:61–72.

24. Torg JS, Vegso JJ, O'Neill J, Sennet B. The epidemiologic, pathologic, biomechanical, and cinematographic analysis of football-induced cervical spine trauma. Am J Sports Med 1990;18:50–57.

25. Torg JS, Sennett B, Pavlov H, et al. Spear tackler's spine: an entity precluding participation in tackle football and collision activities that expose the cervical spine to axial injury inputs. Am J Sports Med 1993;21:640–649.

26. Torg JS, Ramsey-Emrhein JA. Management guidelines for participation in collision activities with congenital, developmental, or postinjury lesions involving the cervical spine. Clin J Sport Med 1997;7:273–291.

27. Bracken MB, Shepard MJ, Collins WF, et al. National Acute Spinal Cord Injury Study. A randomized, controlled trial of methylprednisolone or naloxone in the treatment of acute spinal-cord injury: results of the second national acute spinal cord injury study. N Engl J Med 1990;322: 1405–1411.

28. Malanga GA. The diagnosis and treatment of cervical radiculopathy. Med Sci Sports Exerc 1997;29(suppl 7):236–245.

29. White AA, Panjabi MM. Clinical Biomechanics of the Spine (2nd ed). Philadelphia: Lippincott, 1990;210.

8

Shoulder Girdle Injuries

DAVID R. WEBB

Injuries to the shoulder girdle (sternoclavicular, acromio-clavicular, glenohumeral, and scapulothoracic joints and associated structures) perhaps account for no more than 5–10% of all sports injuries,[1] but they account for a disproportionately higher percentage of sports injury–related physician visits. That is, these injuries are generally perceived by athletes to be "serious" or disabling and thus requiring medical attention.

This chapter is organized as follows:

- Diagnosis and triage based on the typical clinical presentation
- Specific techniques of sorting out the presenting problem
  The problem-oriented history and physical examination
  Injection techniques
  Diagnostic imaging
- Acute, traumatic conditions
- Chronic conditions

PROBLEM-ORIENTED APPROACH TO DIAGNOSIS AND TRIAGE

Shoulder problems in athletes characteristically present in one or more of the following ways:

- Acute injury or the immediate sequelae of acute injury
- Acute painful episode
- Weakness
- Loss of motion
- Chronic activity-related pain or disability (overuse injury)
- Chronic or recurrent frank instability (dislocation or subluxation)

The following overview emphasizes diagnostic and therapeutic pitfalls to avoid and when consultation or referral is appropriate. The discrete diagnostic entities mentioned are discussed in greater detail in subsequent sections of this chapter.

Acute Injury or the Immediate Sequelae of Acute Injury

"I hurt my shoulder in the game last night." "I hurt my shoulder when I fell 3 weeks ago. The pain has gotten somewhat better, but I still can't. . . ."

Acute shoulder injuries, including contusions, sprains, strains, fractures, and dislocations, are especially common in football, skiing, and wrestling. Some of these injuries, such as anterior glenohumeral dislocation, will be clinically obvious. Others, such as posterior glenohumeral dislocation, are liable to be misdiagnosed even after radiographic examination. Most, at least on the first go-round, do not require operative treatment, and some aspects of nonoperative treatment will be common to all.

Injuries to the clavicle and its articulations may be considered "occupational risks" of participation in those sports in which falls sometimes occur at considerable speeds or from considerable heights onto unyielding surfaces. Bicycling, horseback riding, rock climbing, and skateboarding are notable examples. Clavicular injuries are also relatively common in those sports in which "piling on" sometimes occurs, especially in sandlot football, which lacks both referees and shoulder pads. The functional and clinical significance of these injuries is twofold. First, use of the upper limb in sports will be, at least temporarily, impaired. Second, associated injuries to the airway or great vessels, although rare, can be life threatening.

Diagnostic Pitfalls

Of primary importance is the establishment of a precise diagnosis. Appropriate initial treatment, indications for referral, definitive treatment, and rehabilitative treatment will logically follow. The differential diagnosis of concern includes

- Fractures of the acromion, clavicle, scapula, and proximal humerus
- Sternoclavicular sprains (and dislocations)
- Acromioclavicular sprains ("shoulder separation")
- Acute, traumatic glenohumeral dislocation or subluxation
- Acute or acute on degenerative tears of the rotator cuff
- Acute or acute on degenerative tears of the tendon of the long head of the biceps

For the most part, given careful clinical assessment and appropriate radiographic examination, diagnosis is straightforward. The diagnostic pitfalls of greatest consequence are failure to recognize initial, acute, traumatic, glenohumeral subluxation; extensive rotator cuff tear; and posterior glenohumeral dislocation.

The first, even the first few, occurrences of glenohumeral subluxation are likely to be dismissed by the athlete, by his or her coaches, and oftentimes by the physician as inconsequential. Once a pattern of recurrent subluxation has been established, however, the chance of success with nonoperative treatment is considerably diminished. Accordingly, any shoulder injury in which there is a history of forced abduction, external rotation mechanism of injury, perceived frank instability, or "dead arm" symptoms, should be considered as probable acute anterior glenohumeral subluxation and treated accordingly.

Isolated acute rotator cuff tears with the classic presentation of profound weakness after abrupt forceful loading of the shoulder is unlikely to be missed. However, rotator cuff tear associated with other injury is liable to be overlooked. For example, weakness after acute anterior glenohumeral dislocation may be the result of pain inhibition of normal muscle function, associated axillary nerve neurapraxia, or associated rotator cuff tear. It is most important to maintain a high index of suspicion. The differential diagnosis of profound weakness is discussed in the section Weakness.

Posterior glenohumeral dislocation is likely to be missed because it is rare and because the anteroposterior (AP) radiographic findings are subtle. The hallmark physical finding is that the arm is held adducted and internally rotated, and any attempt to rotate the shoulder externally will be painfully resisted. The lateral scapular radiograph is diagnostic (Figure 8-1).

A common, but less consequential, diagnostic pitfall is underestimating the severity of acromioclavicular sprains ("shoulder separations"). The classic "high-riding clavicle" deformity of grade III sprains is typically most obvious subacutely, after any hematoma, soft tissue swelling, and muscle spasm associated with the acute injury have subsided. Because grades I–III acromioclavicular sprains may be satisfactorily treated the same, the precise initial gradation of the injury is not critical. However, the physician who has authoritatively reassured the athlete that he or she has only a low-grade acromioclavicular sprain, only to have the athlete become aware of a pronounced deformity a couple of weeks later, will have (deservedly) experienced some loss of credibility.

The examining physician should also be aware that in the skeletally immature, physeal fractures of the acromion or distal clavicle may be difficult to differentiate from acromioclavicular sprain. However, they can generally be treated similarly.

By far, the therapeutic pitfall of greatest consequence is undertreatment of initial, acute, traumatic glenohumeral dislocation and subluxation. Many first-time anterior dislocations and subluxations can be definitively treated by nonoperative means, specifically immobilization (i.e., strict limitation of abduction and external rotation) and subsequent, complete shoulder rehabilitation. It is important to appreciate that rigorous nonoperative treatment does not equate with symptomatic treatment. The clinical outcomes of mere symptomatic treatment of acute shoulder dislocation are abysmal, with as much as a 90% recurrence rate in young male athletes. In contrast, with appropriate protective and rehabilitative treatment, the probability of success can be essentially reversed, with a 60–70% or better nonrecurrence rate. The essential therapeutic task is to convince the athlete that his or her only good chance of success with nonoperative treatment is to comply strictly with the treatment protocol. The primary treating physician is critically important in initiating this intervention.

Displaced fractures, intraarticular fractures, unreduced glenohumeral dislocations, suspected extensive tears of the rotator cuff, and musculoskeletal injuries with associated neurovascular injury are relatively common, unambiguous indications for orthopedic referral. The rare grade IV, V, or VI acromioclavicular injuries are also indications for orthopedic referral.

Referral to an appropriate facility on an emergent basis is indicated for fractures or dislocations complicated by

FIGURE 8-1

Importance of the lateral scapular view. A. Anteroposterior (AP) view of a normal (reduced) shoulder. B. AP view of posteriorly dislocated shoulder. The humerus is internally rotated, the humeral head does not fill the glenoid to the usual extent, and the humeral head may seem slightly smaller than usual, as it lies closer to the x-ray film. These findings are not striking, however, and the films could easily be misinterpreted as normal. (R = right.)

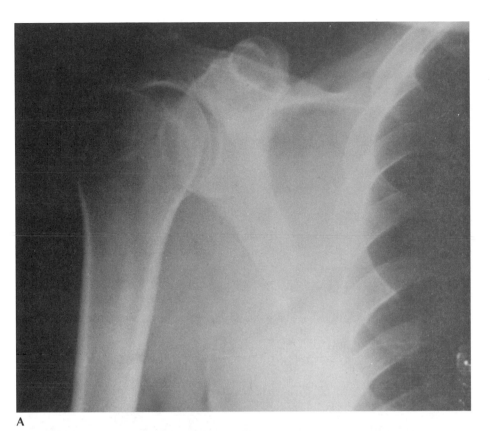

A

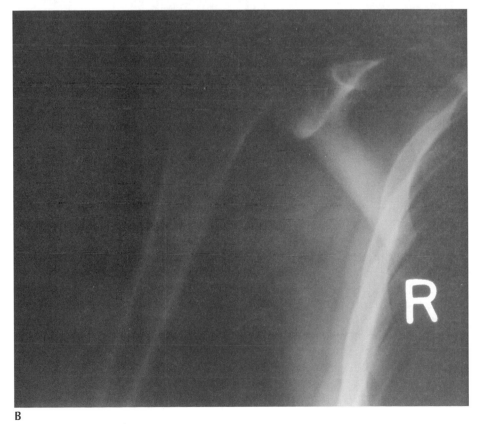

B

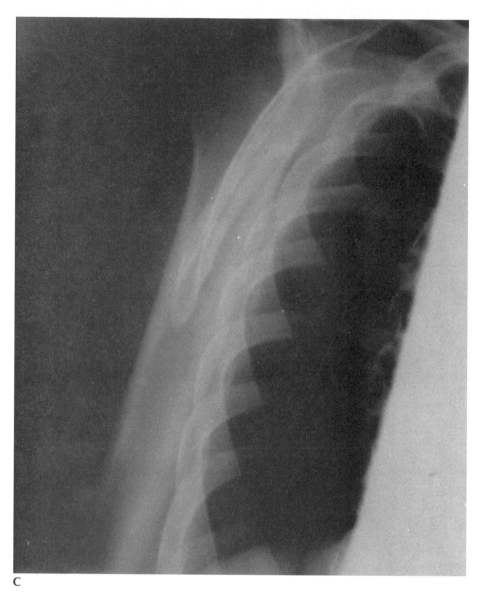

C

FIGURE 8-1 *(continued)*
C. Lateral scapular view, clearly revealing posterior displacement of the head of the humerus with respect to the glenoid. D. Lateral scapular view of an anteriorly dislocated shoulder for comparison. The humeral head is anteriorly displaced relative to the glenoid.

vascular impairment. On a less urgent basis, orthopedic consultation or referral is also recommended for dislocations complicated by nerve injury. Although most such injuries would appear to be neurapraxias and surgical exploration is generally not indicated, rehabilitation is more complicated, and it would be prudent in these cases to defer management to the specialist.

Nondisplaced fractures, grade III acromioclavicular sprains, and tears of the tendon of the long head of the biceps are possible indications for orthopedic referral.

Some primary care physicians may choose to manage some shoulder fractures themselves. Fractures of the proximal humerus with less than 1 cm displacement of any fragment, less than 45 degrees angulation of any

fragment, and less than 20% impression defect of the articular surface are amenable to nonoperative treatment.[2] Extraarticular scapular fractures are treated nonoperatively, as are minimally or nondisplaced fractures of the distal clavicle. Fractures not meeting these criteria should be referred to an orthopedist.

Fractures of the greater tuberosity of the humerus are frequently associated with anterior dislocations and are usually anatomically reduced when the dislocation is reduced. If they remain more than 1 cm displaced after reduction of the dislocation, orthopedic referral is indicated.[2, 3]

Fractures of the distal clavicle are managed differently from the more common midshaft fractures. Use of a figure-of-eight clavicle strap is relatively contraindicated;

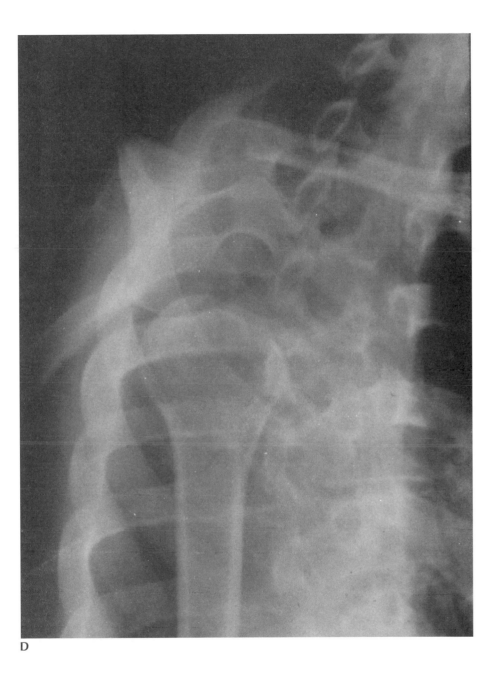

D

it would tend to displace, not to reduce, the fracture. Referral would generally be appropriate.

The management of grade III acromioclavicular sprains is as controversial as any topic in sports medicine. The athlete with acromioclavicular injury should be informed of the possible sequelae of the injury (deformity, degenerative joint disease) and the options regarding primary or delayed surgical treatment. The athlete should be referred if he or she is unwilling to accept the cosmetic deformity of an overly prominent distal clavicle or unwilling to allow the shoulder to recover from the acute injury and then see if it still hurts.

As always, for acute injuries in which the precise diagnosis is uncertain after initial evaluation, consultation or referral is indicated.

Acute Painful Episode

"I woke up in the middle of the night with my shoulder hurting. Since then, it's just gotten worse. I can't raise my arm, do my work, sleep. . . ."

Acute, atraumatic shoulder pain is a common presenting symptom in both the general and athletically active populations. In general, intrinsic musculoskeletal causes can be readily differentiated from extrinsic causes (referred pain) on the basis of the shoulder position and activity-relatedness of the pain and confirmatory physical examination findings. The differential diagnosis of usual greatest concern includes

- Rotator cuff overuse strain or tendinitis
- Calcific subacromial bursitis or rotator cuff tendinitis
- Brachioplexitis

Common sources of referred pain include

- Diaphragmatic (irritation from abdominal process)
- Cardiac (ischemia)
- Gastrointestinal (ulcer, gastrointestinal bleed)
- Pulmonary (pneumonia, embolism)

In the appropriate clinical settings—such as postintraarticular injection or procedure (joint replacement, arthrography)—inflammatory or septic acromioclavicular or glenohumeral arthritis should also be considered.

"Acute overuse injury" would seem to be an oxymoron. Semantics notwithstanding, episodes of acute, quite severe shoulder pain after unaccustomed shoulder-strenuous activity are common. This is especially true for "weekend warriors" and sedentary adults undertaking "honey do" projects. Youth, however, are not immune. Such problems are not uncommon in school-age athletes starting new sports seasons, especially in swimming, baseball, and volleyball.

The common historical finding is an abrupt, marked change in the type, amount, or intensity of shoulder-strenuous work—that is, an egregious "training error." Symptoms, tenderness, and pain with provocative tests may be moderate to severe. With rest (sling as required [prn]), intermittent icing, and nonsteroidal anti-inflammatory medication, pain usually subsides within a few days. Narcotics and intraarticular corticosteroids are usually not required. The main key to prevention of recurrence is recognition and avoidance of training error.

Common causes include biceps tendinitis, supraspinatus and other rotator cuff tendinitis, subacromial bursitis, and entrapment. These can be differentiated by palpation and by reproduction of pain by specific maneuvers (Yergason test for biceps, isolating and testing strength of supraspinatus, resisted external rotation or internal rotation for rotator cuff tendinitis.) Specific rest and icing of involved structures while maintaining range of motion and isometrics of uninvolved muscles will provide best outcome.

Calcific subacromial bursitis and rotator cuff tendinitis may be idiopathic or associated with acute overuse. The heterotopic precipitation of calcium in soft tissues may be both cause and effect of the inflammation. The associated pain is characteristically quite severe. Patients not uncommonly present in tears, having been unable to sleep or raise the affected arms, and with "touch-me-not" tenderness on examination. Radiographic examination is confirmatory (Figure 8-2). Nonsteroidal anti-inflammatory medication is usually insufficient for pain relief, and corticosteroid injection is generally indicated. For most acute cases, injection followed by a series of pulsed ultrasound treatments in physical therapy affords definitive treatment. I have been singularly unimpressed by attempting to aspi-

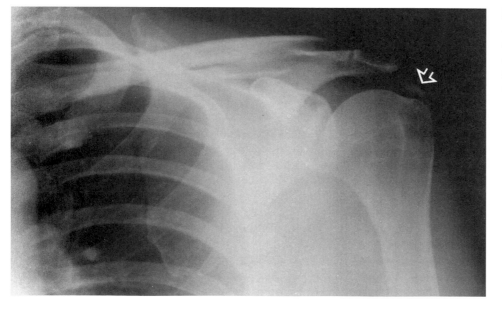

FIGURE 8-2

Anteroposterior radiograph of the shoulder demonstrating heterotopic soft tissue calcification in the subacromial bursa and rotator cuff tendon.

rate the precipitate, which is of the consistency of old glue. For recalcitrant cases with persistent pain, referral for surgical debridement is recommended.

Brachioplexitis is a less common cause of severe shoulder pain and profound shoulder weakness. There may or may not be a history of acute overuse or of an antecedent acute febrile (viral) illness. Pain is usually the initial presenting symptom. Brachioplexitis will not respond well to a trial of rest, intermittent icing, and nonsteroidal anti-inflammatory medication. Typically, it will worsen over time before abating. It can be unrelenting and severe for many days. Narcotic analgesics are usually indicated, and sometimes even these may not be completely pain relieving. As discussed in the next section, consultation or referral is probably indicated.

Weakness

"I can't bench [press] anymore." "I can't even lift my arm up."

Weakness is seldom a sole presenting symptom. It is usually associated with acute injury or acute or chronic pain conditions. Nonetheless, it is often the symptom that is most disconcerting to the patient, prompting him or her to seek medical attention, and it is frequently the finding of greatest concern to the examining physician.

The differential diagnosis of profound weakness includes

- Mechanical musculotendinous disruption
- Neuromuscular weakness
- Pain inhibition of normal muscular function

To some extent, these can be differentiated on physical examination. Smooth giving-way on manual muscle testing (i.e., uniform weakness throughout the range of motion) is characteristic of neuromuscular weakness. In contrast, abrupt or ratchetlike (cogwheel) giving-way is more characteristic of mechanical musculotendinous disruption or pain inhibition.

Differentiation is more reliably accomplished by selective local anesthetization as discussed in Injection and Aspiration. Possible results are as follows: Relief of pain but persistence of profound weakness after intraarticular injection is indicative of mechanical musculotendinous disruption. Pain relief and improved strength does not rule out intraarticular structural injury (e.g., labral tear), but does effectively rule out extensive full-thickness rotator cuff tear. Neither pain relief nor improved strength, assuming technically satisfactory injection, is indicative of an extraarticular problem such as brachioplexitis.

Other causes of weakness include moderate weakness attributable to handedness or muscular disuse atrophy, tran-

sient weakness (dead arm syndrome) associated with brachial plexus traction or compression injuries (stingers), acute glenohumeral subluxation, and nonphysiologic weakness.

Orthopedic referral is indicated if extensive rotator cuff tear is suspected or cannot be ruled out as the cause of the weakness. Further workup will likely include magnetic resonance imaging (MRI) arthrography, but a decision to obtain this study is best done in consultation with or deferred to the orthopedic surgeon.

Specialty (orthopedic or neurologic) referral is also recommended for profound weakness, probably attributable to brachioplexitis. Early on, there will be severe pain and weakness on the basis of pain inhibition. Subsequently, as the acute, severe pain begins to subside, a profound, neuromuscular weakness will become evident. Treatment options are actually quite limited. Nonetheless, these conditions are typically very distressing to the patient and even more so to the parents if the patient is a child. Reassurance that everything possible is being done is usually appropriate. Further workup, for both confirmatory diagnostic and prognostic purposes, may include electromyography, usually at approximately 6 weeks after the onset of symptoms.

Loss of Motion

"I can't reach. . . ." "I can't hook my bra."

Because of compensatory scapulothoracic motion, loss of glenohumeral motion (frozen shoulder) is generally unnoticed by patients until it gets to the point of limiting customary daily, occupational, or athletic activities. It is virtually always a sequela of constrained active motion secondary to injury, neuromuscular weakness, pain, inflammation, or prescribed treatment (e.g., immobilization for glenohumeral dislocation). Accordingly, the most important diagnostic and therapeutic challenge is to determine and to address the primary underlying problem(s).

The mainstays of treating frozen shoulder per se are physical therapy (mobilization treatment) and often intraarticular corticosteroid injection (to mute any counterproductive inflammatory response to the mobilization therapy). I do not recommend manipulation of the shoulder under anesthesia, a possible result of which is the creation of a soft tissue Bankart lesion (see discussions of glenohumeral instability problems).

Chronic Activity-Related Pain or Disability (Overuse Injury)

"My shoulder's hurt ever since the start of 'two-a-days.'" "It hurts to serve or spike." "I don't even try bench press or overhead press anymore, because it always hurts afterwards." "I can't put anything on the ball now when I throw."

Chronic shoulder pain is a very common clinical problem in both the general and athletically active populations. In general, intrinsic, mechanical, musculoskeletal problems (i.e., overuse injuries) can be readily differentiated from other intrinsic and extrinsic causes of shoulder pain on the basis of the history (especially the shoulder position and activity relatedness of the pain) and confirmatory physical examination findings. Overuse injuries are especially common in baseball, gymnastics, swimming, tennis, volleyball, and weight training, as well as in occupations requiring strenuous or prolonged overhead use of the hand. There are important diagnostic and therapeutic pitfalls and caveats to consider.

As is generally true for overuse injuries, especially early in the course of the problem, activity-related pain is more likely to be noted after rather than during the activity. Soreness, stiffness, and difficulty robing and disrobing the day after the provoking activity are common symptoms. Also, delayed soreness and overall trends are more important criteria as guidelines for treating and resuming activity than are the odd twinges of pain during activity.

Sometimes, functional impairment, rather than frank pain, is the primary symptom. For example, a coach may notice that a player is "serving funny," or a thrower may notice a loss of accuracy or velocity in his or her throws.

Shoulder overuse injuries represent maladaptations to the repetitive stresses of an activity or activities. Typically, there will be both structural and functional components of the problem, and there will be more than one structure or functional mechanism involved. Conversely, simple, isolated bursitis, tendinitis, or impingement problems are uncommon. In all cases, therefore, the examiner should assess each of the following possible components of the problem:

- Scapular stabilizing muscle insufficiency or dysfunction, or both
- (Structural) glenohumeral laxity (commonly, anterior laxity and posterior contracture)
- Rotator cuff overuse strain, tendinitis, tendinosis, degenerative tear, insufficiency (functional glenohumeral laxity)
- Long head of biceps overuse strain, tendinitis, tendinosis, degenerative tear, tendon subluxation, insufficiency
- Acromioclavicular degenerative joint disease or distal clavicular osteolysis
- Primary impingement (acromial, acromioclavicular, coracoclavicular, coracoid)
- Secondary impingement (anterior, posterior, and lateral; secondary to glenohumeral laxity and contracture or rotator cuff insufficiency, or both)
- Glenohumeral degenerative joint disease and cuff arthropathy

Less severe, shorter duration problems may respond to basic intervention comprising relative rest, anti-inflammatory measures, home program rehabilitation exercises, and gradual resumption of activity avoiding training error. Unless the patient has the luxury of avoiding the pain-provoking activity altogether, however, anti-inflammatory treatment alone (e.g., the ubiquitous cortisone shot) will likely prove insufficient. As is true for all overuse injuries that do not resolve promptly and completely with basic intervention, the essential therapeutic task is to identify and to reverse as many of the causative factors as possible.

In most cases, patients do not present promptly after onset of symptoms, but rather after symptoms and function have worsened over time. During this time, secondary problems (failed compensatory mechanisms) are likely to have developed. In virtually all such cases, intensive hands-on physical therapy will be necessary for successful resolution of the problem and return to shoulder-strenuous activity.

Structural injury does not necessarily imply a need for surgical intervention. Depending on the severity of the structural injury and the demands to be placed on the shoulder, many structural problems (e.g., partial-thickness and small full-thickness rotator cuff tears) can be well compensated if appropriate functional rehabilitation is carried out.

Physician follow-up is essential and should be scheduled every 3 weeks or so. Sports medicine or orthopedics consultation or referral is indicated for problems not demonstrably improving over time. Some structural problems (e.g., acromioclavicular arthrosis, primary impingement, rotator cuff tear, labral tears, glenohumeral laxity, glenohumeral arthrosis, and intraarticular osteochondral loose bodies) may require surgical intervention. Special diagnostic imaging, such as MRI arthrography, may be required but may be deferred to the consultant's discretion. Complex problems, such as rotator cuff tear associated with glenohumeral instability, are probably best managed by orthopedic surgeons subspecializing in shoulder problems.

Chronic or Recurrent Frank Instability (Dislocation or Subluxation)

"My shoulder went out again." "Sometimes it seems to go out of place, and I can't use the arm. Then I shake it or something, and it seems OK again."

Recurrent shoulder dislocations and subluxations may be attributable to congenital or acquired joint laxity or simply to being in the wrong place at the wrong time. Of these, acquired laxity—that is, failure of treatment of the initial injury—is the most common and preventable cause.

The probability of success (nonrecurrence) with non-operative treatment is not as good with recurrent as with initial instability episodes. A true pattern of chronic instability is established if there are multiple recurrences; if the recurrence(s) occur with increasing ease—that is, if less force is required to produce the dislocation or subluxation(s), if reduction(s) are achieved with increasing ease, and if associated symptoms become less severe. In such cases, the prognosis without surgical treatment is indeed poor.

If the recurrent dislocation or subluxation would appear to be a truly recurrent, acute, traumatic injury, then a trial of protective or rehabilitative treatment is recommended (see following section). Otherwise, especially for athletes intending return to shoulder-strenuous activities, referral for surgical treatment is recommended.

HISTORY

A careful history is the examiner's most important diagnostic tool. It provides data critical to establishing an accurate diagnosis, determining the etiology of the problem, and assessing the clinical significance of the diagnosed anatomic problem in the individual patient athlete. Physical examination and diagnostic imaging are essentially confirmatory or not confirmatory of hypotheses generated on the basis of the history.

Acute Injury

The athlete is asked about the mechanism of injury, his or her perception of the severity of injury, the extent of the disability, any associated symptoms, his or her postinjury course, and past history of any shoulder injuries or problems. The mechanism of injury provides important diagnostic clues. Direct trauma—for example, a direct blow to the acromion such as may occur in a fall or in being struck by an opponent's helmet—may produce a contusion (shoulder pointer), an acromioclavicular sprain (shoulder separation), or a fracture of the acromion or distal clavicle. Less commonly, direct trauma to the anterior or posterior shoulder may produce glenohumeral dislocation. Indirect trauma—for example, forced abduction and external rotation of the arm such as may occur in arm tackling—is the usual mechanism of anterior glenohumeral subluxation or dislocation and may result in injury to any of the static or dynamic anterior stabilizers of the shoulder. A fall onto the adducted, internally rotated arm or

a direct blow to the forearm or elbow with resultant force along the long axis of the humerus may produce a posterior glenohumeral subluxation or injury to the bony or cartilaginous glenoid. Sudden loading of the partially abducted arm is a common cause of rotator cuff strain in the middle-aged.

A tearing sensation at the time of injury is diagnostically nonspecific but is characteristic of more severe soft tissue injury. The athlete's perception of the shoulders having "come out of place" is probably accurate. Inability to move the arm or to lift the arm immediately postinjury is characteristic of rotator cuff tears, dislocations, and subluxations. Both holding the arm a bit away from the side externally rotated and unwillingness to have the arm internally rotated across the torso is characteristic of unreduced anterior dislocation. Similarly, holding the arm internally rotated across the torso and unwillingness to have it externally rotated is characteristic of posterior dislocation. A transiently "dead arm" with perceived loss of sensation and inability to use the arm with quick recovery is characteristic both of acute glenohumeral subluxations and stinger nerve injuries.

Overuse Injury

As is true for overuse injury in general, successful treatment and prevention of recurrence with shoulder overuse injury depends as much on determining the etiology of the problem as on establishing a precise diagnosis.

The etiology of chronic shoulder problems (activity-related pain, weakness, loss of motion, functional impairment, or frank instability) is virtually always multifactorial. The two most common causes are (1) physiologic—abrupt increase in physical demand on the shoulder that, at least in retrospect, would be considered a "training error," and (2) anatomic—the residuals of undertreated or incompletely rehabilitated prior acute injury. Accordingly, the athlete is asked about changes in the type, frequency, duration, and intensity of exercise and any other circumstances that might have been changing before onset of symptoms. He or she is also asked about any antecedent injury and the mechanism of that injury.

More often than not, activity-related pain occurs after rather than during the activity. If there is pain during activity, however, determining the precise circumstances in which pain occurs can provide important diagnostic clues, analogous to determining the mechanism of injury for acute injuries. Pain with overhead use of the hand—for example, with throwing; serving or overhead shots in volleyball or racquet sports; freestyle, butterfly, and backstroke swimming; and with certain weight lifts—is characteristic of shoulder overuse syndrome. Similarly,

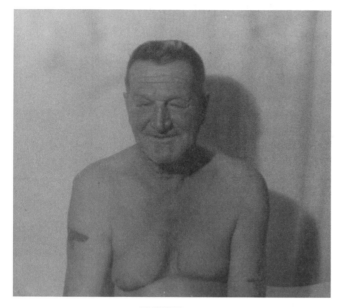

FIGURE 8-3

Clinical signs of anterior glenohumeral dislocation. The acromion process is quite prominent with an indentation beneath it, giving the shoulder a shortened, squared-off appearance. The arm is held in slight abduction.

activities of daily living and occupation involving repetitive use of the elevated arm—for example, painting, plastering, cello playing, and so forth—are characteristic of this problem. Pain with daily, athletic, or occupational activities, involving horizontal flexion of the shoulder—such as that which occurs when swinging a baseball bat or a golf club—is typical of acromioclavicular degenerative joint disease. Also, a painful arc of motion with certain weight lifts—especially overhead press, bench press, bench flies, and dips—is typical of acromioclavicular pain.

Lateral arm pain extending distally to mid-arm level, approximately the level of deltoid insertion, is a very common referral pattern for rotator cuff pain. Pain that extends further distally, or that is associated with paresthesias, or that is more related to position or motion of the head and neck or shoulder girdle as opposed to the shoulder joint, is more typical of nerve impingement. Pain at rest may be attributable either to inflammation produced by a mechanical injury or any of the nonmechanical intrinsic or extrinsic causes of shoulder pain. A toothache-quality pain at night is quite characteristic of rotator cuff pain.

Perception and admission of pain are quite individually variable. Sometimes, functional impairment, rather than frank pain, may be the primary symptom.

The athlete is also asked about any previous treatment he or she may have received. Often, treatment will have been directed at relief of pain, swelling, and inflammation, and rehabilitation will have been neglected. The athlete may have had some temporary relief of symptoms, only to have them recur with resumption of activity.

PHYSICAL EXAMINATION

The principal caveat is to be gentle. Obviously, parts of the examination will cause the patient some discomfort: tenderness on palpation of injured or inflamed structures and provocation of pain and apprehension with various tests. The examiner, however, should control the examination in such a way that the information being sought is elicited with minimal discomfort to the patient. Accordingly, examination of the acutely injured or severely painful shoulder will differ considerably from that for subacute injuries or chronic problems. The specific objectives and techniques of the components of the examination are discussed in the following sections.

Screening Examination of the Acutely Injured Shoulder

Physical examination begins with simple observation of the athlete and the position of the injured limb. With acute, traumatic, first-time anterior glenohumeral dislocation, the athlete will be in obvious distress. The injured arm will be held in an abducted, externally rotated position, supported if possible by the uninjured arm. Any shoulder motion, particularly internal rotation, will be painful and resisted by the athlete. The normal rounded contour of the shoulder will be lost. The acromion will be inordinately prominent, with an indentation beneath it, as shown in Figure 8-3. Examination will usually also reveal an anterior fullness caused by the anteriorly displaced humeral head. These findings can usually be appreciated by palpation—for example, under shoulder pads—as well as by inspection.

The clinical findings with acute posterior glenohumeral dislocation are not as obvious. Pain is likely to be greater than with anterior dislocation.[4] In slender individuals, the coracoid process may be unusually prominent, and a posterior fullness may be appreciated. However, these two findings are likely to be obscured in the heavily muscled athlete. The key to making the clinical diagnosis is that the arm is held adducted and internally rotated, and any attempt at abduction or external rotation will be blocked and painful.[4]

An acromioclavicular sprain with complete rupture of the coracoclavicular ligaments (grade III or higher sprain) may present with obvious deformity ("high-riding clavicle" or, more correctly, "low-riding scapula"). Absence of this sign does not rule out grade III sprain, however, as muscle spasm can minimize the extent of acromioclavicular separation.

Complete rupture of the tendon of the long head of the biceps is usually readily apparent on initial inspection. There may be dependent ecchymosis, and the retracted muscle belly of the biceps will be prominent distally.

If none of these injuries are evident, examination continues with systematic inspection and palpation of possibly injured structures (anteriorly: sternoclavicular joint, clavicle, acromion, acromioclavicular joint, coracoid process, coracoclavicular space, lesser tuberosity, bicipital groove; laterally: acromion, subacromial space, greater tuberosity; posteriorly: spine and medial border of scapula, muscle bellies of supraspinatus and infraspinatus). Joint effusion may be detectable as visible or palpable swelling over the anterior joint line—that is, just lateral to the coracoid process. Inspection can be facilitated by having the patient sit on a low stool.

Assessment of the neurovascular status of the limb is particularly important if any deformity is present. Any of the nerves of the brachial plexus may be injured with anterior dislocation of the shoulder; however, the axillary nerve is particularly at risk. Although sensory testing is usually carried out as shown in Figure 8-4, Blom and Dahlback[5] have shown that this is an unreliable predictor of axillary nerve injury. Motor function of the nerve can be satisfactorily assessed by gentle isometric testing of the deltoid muscle.

Further examination of the injured shoulder is usually deferred until indicated radiographic examination has been carried out. If radiographic examination is negative, gentle muscle testing may be carried out to confirm the diagnosis of musculotendinous injury.

As a quick screening test for active motion, the patient is simply asked to raise his or her arms forward, raise his or her arms to the side, put his or her hands behind his or her head, and put his or her hands behind his or her back, testing flexion, abduction, external rotation, and internal rotation, respectively. Any dyssymmetry or limitation of motion, pain, or apprehension is noted.

Loss of normal synchronization of glenohumeral and scapulothoracic motion with abduction is characteristic of rotator cuff injury. Normally, with full abduction, the scapula rotates outwardly approximately 60 degrees. Scapulothoracic motion begins at 30 degrees of abduction, after which abduction comprises 2 degrees of glenohumeral motion for every degree of scapulothoracic motion. With rotator cuff injury, however, scapulotho-

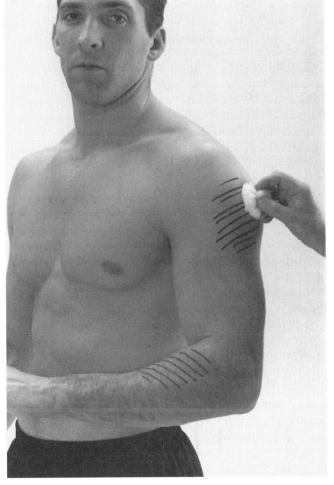

FIGURE 8-4

Testing for sensation in the distribution of the axillary and musculocutaneous nerves, as described by Rockwood.[4]

racic motion begins sooner, and abduction comprises relatively more scapulothoracic motion. With acute rotator cuff tears, the patient may be unable to initiate glenohumeral abduction at all, but may be able to maintain the position of the arm that has been passively abducted beyond 90 degrees.

As appropriate, additional testing may be carried out as discussed in the following sections.

Standard Shoulder Examination

Screening Examination of the Cervical Spine

In the general population, shoulder pain is a common presenting symptom of intrinsic neck problems. Perhaps even more commonly in the athletic population, neck and scapulovertebral pain are the result of an intrinsic shoulder problem. In either case, screening examination of the cervical and upper thoracic spine is an appropriate part of the standard shoulder examination.

Tenderness to palpation is sought over the vertebral spinous processes and over the paraspinous muscles. Active motion and flexion, extension, left and right rotation, and left and right lateral bending is then observed. The examiner looks for abnormal limitation of motion, quality of motion, and pain or sensation of "tightness" with motion. Quality of atlantooccipital motion is assessed by having the patient nod his or her head. Commonly, contracture of the short cervical extensors will be manifested by stiffness or jerkiness in nodding.

The Spurling test is a screen for radicular irritation or impingement. The patient is guided in extending and then rotating the cervical spine, which narrows the neuroforamina. If the position causes no symptoms, the examiner can then gently place longitudinal compression on the spine by gently pressing down on the patient's head. The examiner notes whether this test provokes any pain or paresthesias and if so, whether it reproduces the patient's presenting symptoms.

As indicated by the history and the preceding screening tests, the examiner may proceed with a more detailed examination of the cervical spine and neurologic examination or continue with the shoulder examination as described in the following sections.

Scapular Stabilizing Muscle Function

In virtually all handed activities, the shoulder joint functions as one mechanical link between the axial skeleton and the hand. Dysfunction at any link in the kinetic chain, especially adjacent links, can adversely affect the shoulder. Accordingly, assessment of the muscles that position and stabilize the scapula is an important part of the basic shoulder examination.

The Kibler test (Figure 8-5) is a test of scapular stabilizing muscle function that meets the criteria of simplicity, reliability, and relevance. Kibler test is a static test of scapular stabilizing muscle function in which the position of the scapulae relative to the spine are noted in each of three test positions as shown in Figure 8-5. A lateral slide or winging of the scapula is the hallmark sign of scapular stabilizing muscle dysfunction. Scapular dyssymmetry, however, may also result from thoracic scoliosis or frozen shoulder. Pain or inability to attain test positions two and three is commonly noted with rotator cuff injury or inflammation.

Additional tests include forward flexion of both shoulders, observing for lateral slide or winging of the scapulae, and the "wall push-up"—the classic diagnostic test for long thoracic nerve and serratus anterior.

In most cases, the specific dysfunction is overactivity of the upper trapezius relative to the lower trapezius. This problem, if identified, can be readily and appropriately addressed by physical therapy, including McConnell techniques and biofeedback.

The Kibler test should be incorporated in the preparticipation examinations of throwing and racquet sport athletes. Addressing the problem of scapular stabilizing muscle dysfunction in the preseason can obviate clinical problems during season.

Range and Quality of Shoulder Motion

What is generally considered to be shoulder motion is actually a complex of sternoclavicular, acromioclavicular, scapulothoracic, and glenohumeral motion. Depending on the purposes of the examination, it may be appropriate to measure either total combined motion or isolated glenohumeral joint motion. For example, for a worker who has to reach overhead shelves, total range of combined flexion would be useful in assessing his or her ability to carry out that task. Conversely, in assessing and following the course of a clinical problem, such as frozen shoulder, measurement of isolated glenohumeral motion is critical.

Standard orthopedic measurements are of combined motion in the cardinal planes: flexion, abduction, extension, and internal and external rotation with the shoulder adducted to the side. Another common test of combined motion is the internal rotation reach test, measured by the highest vertebral level to which the patient can bring his or her thumb, as shown in Figure 8-6. A difference of up to two vertebral levels less on the dominant-hand side relative to the nondominant-hand side is considered normal. These measurements are probably most useful in disability assessments.

Measurement of isolated glenohumeral range of motion is generally more clinically useful. This is most readily accomplished with the patient seated or lying supine with the scapula and shoulder girdle stabilized by the examiner's hand or the examining table as shown in Figure 8-7.

Although arguably less "objective," quality of motion is probably more significant than precise range of motion. The first part of the shoulder examination—which is carried out with the patient standing, facing away from the examiner—concludes with observation of combined glenohumeral and scapulothoracic abduction. The examiner looks for abnormal limitation of motion, a painful arc of motion, early onset of scapulothoracic motion, or other dyssymmetric patterns of motion. Pain with motion is associated with many diagnostic entities. Pain occurring at about 90 degrees of combined motion or a painful arc from 90 degrees upward is commonly found with acromioclavicular conditions. Increased pain with the

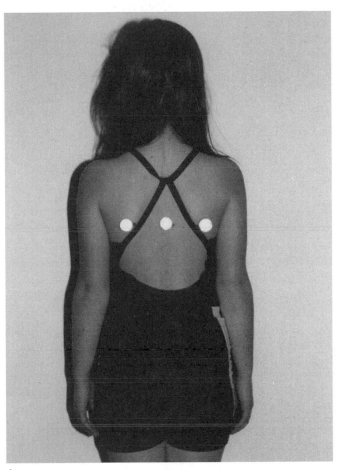

A

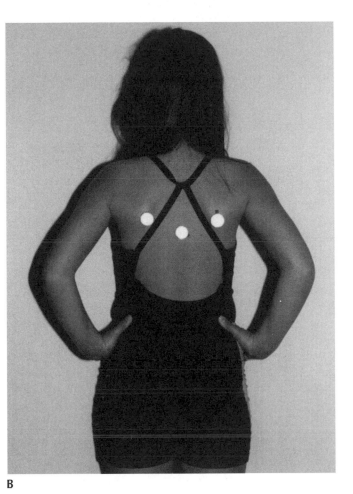

B

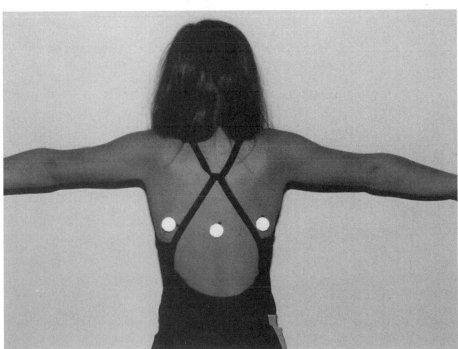

C

FIGURE 8-5

Kibler test of scapular stabilizing muscle function. A–C. Test positions 1–3 in an asymptomatic, 10-year-old, right-handed, nonthrowing athlete (normal). In test position 1, the patient is asked to stand with her arms by her side; in position 2, with her hands on her hips; and in position 3, with her hands straight out to the side with the thumbs rotated down. In going from 1 to 3, greater muscular action is required to position the scapula properly on the thoracic cage. (Markers are positioned over the tips of the scapulae and an intermediate vertebral spinous process.)

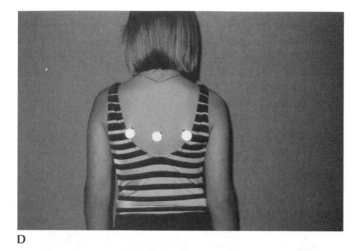

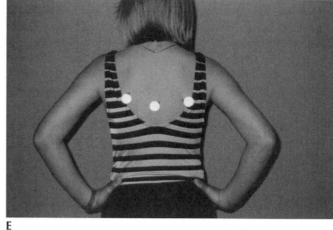

D

E

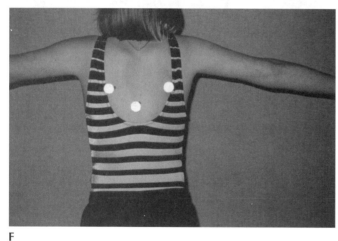

F

FIGURE 8-5 (continued)

D–F. Test positions 1–3 in an asymptomatic, 10-year-old, right-handed tennis player who had played competitively for 5 years (lateral slide of right scapula in all three positions). In such cases, the lateral scapular slide is thought to represent a mal-adaptation of the scapular stabilizing muscles to the stresses of repetitive overhead use of the arm and to predispose to shoulder overuse injury.

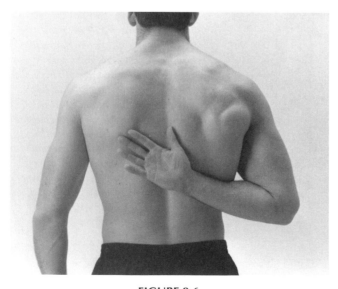

FIGURE 8-6

Internal rotation reach test. Reach of the dominant hand to within two vertebral levels of the nondominant is considered normal.

shoulder in neutral, or internal rotation and less or no pain with the shoulder externally rotated, is characteristic of subacromial impingement (of the bursa, rotator cuff, and long head of the biceps tendon). Conversely, greater pain or apprehension with the shoulder externally rotated, and less or no pain with it internally rotated, is characteristic of any of the internal derangements associated with anterior glenohumeral instability. Early onset of scapulothoracic motion is seen with scapular stabilizing muscle dysfunction and with abnormal limitation of glenohumeral motion, such as may be caused by rotator cuff injury or frozen shoulder. Dyssymmetry, especially a "glitch" associated with pain, has similar implications as a painful arc of motion.

Point Tenderness

Shoulder examination proceeds with inspection and palpation with the patient seated facing the examiner. Tenderness to palpation is sought over possibly injured or painful structures, including sternoclavicular joint, acromioclavicular joint, coracoid process, coracoacromial arch, coracoclavicular space, anterior glenohumeral joint line, posterior glenohumeral joint line, greater and lesser humeral tuberosities, and the bicipital groove (Figure 8-8). Examination then continues with assessment of isolated passive glenohumeral range of motion.

Impingement Testing

Impingement tests are best considered a means of eliciting tenderness of structures not readily accessible to direct palpation. A positive impingement test does not imply a diagnosis of primary impingement. Rather, it implies only that one or more of the structures lying between the humerus and the coracoacromial arch, namely the subacromial bursa, the rotator cuff, and the long head of the biceps tendon, are sensitive to being compressed between the greater tuberosity of the humerus and the arch. Thus, a positive impingement test (impingement sign) can be elicited with any inflammatory condition of or injury to these structures. The recommended impingement test described by Hawkins and Kennedy is shown in Figure 8-9.[6]

Neer[7] uses the terms "impingement sign" and "impingement test" somewhat differently. His *impingement sign* refers to pain elicited with passive abduction of the glenohumeral joint with the scapula stabilized by the examiner's hand. His *impingement test* refers to abatement of such pain after subacromial injection of a local anesthetic. The more common and more intuitive usage of these terms is as presented in the text.

Acromioclavicular and Sternoclavicular Compression Tests

In addition to a painful arc of motion, pain with compression of the acromioclavicular and sternoclavicular joints is a characteristic but not pathognomonic finding of injury to or inflammation of these joints. Compression of the joints is achieved by passive horizontal flexion of the shoulder, resisted active horizontal extension of the horizontally flexed shoulder, and resisted elevation of the horizontally flexed shoulder as shown in Figure 8-10. Pain localized discretely to the top of the shoulder (acromioclavicular joint) or to the sternoclavicular joint is highly specific. Diffuse shoulder pain, or pain localized to the posterior aspect of the shoulder with these maneuvers, is nonspecific and is not uncommonly seen with internal derangement of the shoulder, glenohumeral instability, and muscular injury.

Manual Muscle Testing

With manual muscle testing, the examiner looks for pain or weakness relative to the contralateral side, the cause of which then should be differentiated. The principal

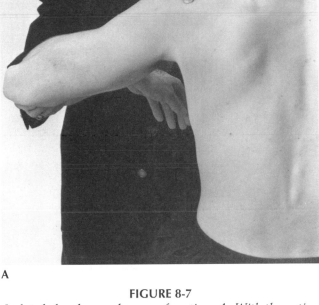

A

FIGURE 8-7
Isolated glenohumeral range of motion. A. With the patient seated, the examiner stabilizes the shoulder girdle with his hand. True glenohumeral flexion, abduction, and external rotation in adduction are measured.

caveat is to do no further harm. The desired information can be safely and reliably elicited by isometric manual muscle testing in positions within the patient's pain-free range of motion. It is important that the examiner control the position of the patient's arm and the amount of muscular force generated by the patient and resisted by the examiner. This is accomplished by the examiner's specific instructions to the patient (i.e., "Don't let me push your hands down" or "Don't let me push your hands together") as opposed to "Push up against my hands" or "Push out against my hands." The examiner can then begin with very light pressure, increase it gradually, and stop either at the point at which good strength and no pain are clearly demonstrated or as soon as any pain or weakness is demonstrated. Specific manual resistance tests for

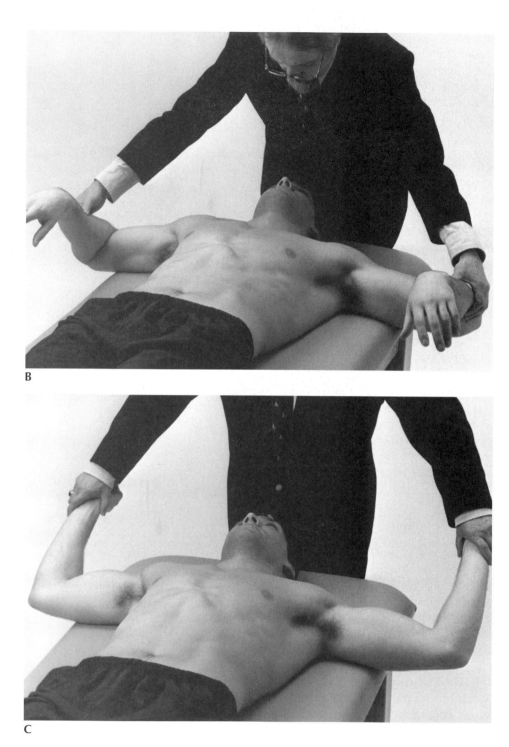

B

C

FIGURE 8-7 *(continued)*
B and C. With the patient supine, the shoulder girdle is stabilized by the table, and the examiner controls shoulder position and motion. Internal and external glenohumeral rotation in 90 degrees abduction are measured.

anterior, middle, and posterior leaves of the deltoid, supraspinatus, external and internal rotators, and biceps are shown in Figures 8-11 and 8-12.

With testing of the anterior deltoid or supraspinatus muscles, the clavicular part of pectoralis major may be observed to substitute for them. Protraction of the shoul-

der girdle and fasciculation of the anterior deltoid may also be noted.

With supraspinatus testing, a drop arm sign is elicited when the patient is able to hold the shoulder in 90 degrees of elevation (scaption, see Figure 8-11A) against gravity, but with slight additional manual pressure, the shoulder

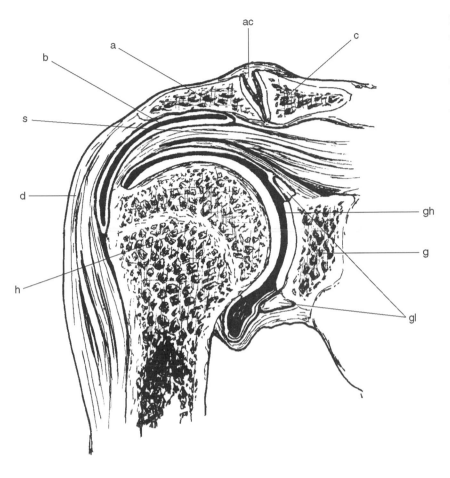

FIGURE 8-8
Shoulder anatomy: acromion (a), clavicle (c), acromioclavicular joint (ac), head of humerus (h), (bony) glenoid (g), glenohumeral (shoulder) joint (gh), glenoid labrum (gl), supraspinatus muscle and tendon (s), subacromial bursa (b), deltoid muscle (d).

abruptly gives way, and the arm drops. In my experience, this finding may be elicited with any of the conditions causing profound weakness (see Weakness) and is not pathognomonic of rotator cuff tear.

Smooth giving-way on manual muscle testing—that is, uniform weakness throughout the range of motion—is characteristic of neuromuscular weakness. In contrast, abrupt or ratchetlike (cogwheel) giving-way is more characteristic of mechanical musculotendinous disruption or pain inhibition.

Tests of Glenohumeral Instability
Various instability tests have been described, many of which seem unnecessarily draconian; they entail an unnecessary risk of causing the patient at least undue pain if not actual injury, and the information they offer the examiner can be obtained as readily by other means. Any such test should be used cautiously, if at all, by very experienced examiners and not at all by primary care physicians. The following four tests meet the criteria for simplicity, reliability, clinical relevance, and above all, safety.

1. *Sulcus test.* With the patient seated facing the examiner, and with the patient's shoulders adducted with his or her arms by his or her sides, the examiner grasps the patient's arms with one hand just above the elbow and gently exerts a downward force. With inferior instability, the examiner and patient may appreciate the head of the humerus slipping inferiorly relative to the glenoid, and a sulcus between the acromion and head of the humerus may become visible (Figure 8-13). The sulcus test is as likely to be positive with functional as structural instability of the shoulder. It may be elicited even with rotator cuff insufficiency caused by fatigue (e.g., after isokinetic shoulder exercise to exhaustion). In "normal" shoulders, some inferior subluxation can usually be demonstrated. The extent is probably a measure of how "loose-jointed" the individual is. Dyssymmetry, however, probably represents "abnormal laxity."

2. *Apprehension test.* The seated patient is asked to abduct his or her shoulders to 90 degrees and then to externally rotate the 90-degree abducted shoulders. Any symptoms of pain or apprehension, or simply unwillingness to carry out the maneuver, constitutes a positive test. If the

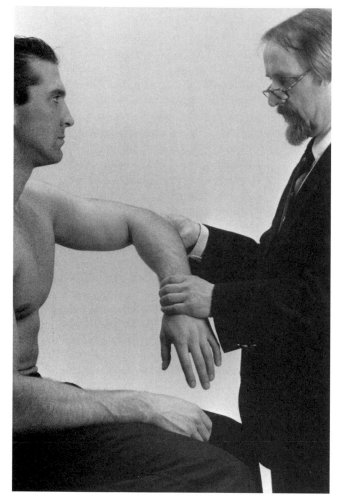

FIGURE 8-9
Impingement test, as described by Hawkins and Kennedy.[6] With passive flexion and internal rotation of the shoulder, the rotator cuff, the tendon of the long head of biceps, and the subdeltoid bursa can be impinged between the greater tuberosity and the coracoacromial arch. A positive test (i.e., pain and grimacing) is characteristic of inflammation of the impinged structures.

patient is able, without symptoms, to rotate the abducted shoulder to 90 degrees of external rotation, he or she may then be asked to "flick" his or her arm backwards from that position, thus imparting a mild external rotation impact stress to the shoulder.

3. Containment (Jobe relocation) test.[8] The patient is asked to lie supine on the examining table with his or her shoulders 90 degrees abducted, as described for assessing range of internal and external rotation in 90 degrees of abduction (Figure 8-14). If there is pain during or at the limits of external rotation, the examiner, now standing beside the patient and examining just the affected shoulder, uses one hand to control the position and motion of the patient's arm and the other hand to "contain" the head of the humerus reduced in the glenoid socket. This may be accomplished either by direct manual pressure over the head of the humerus or indirectly by pressure over the neck of the humerus. A positive test comprises pain with passive external rotation of the 90 degrees of abducted shoulder, abatement of pain with containment, and recurrence of pain as the examiner slowly lifts the hand exerting the containing force. The containment test is not pathognomonic of any specific structural injury, but is probably the most sensitive test for any functional or structural anterior glenohumeral instability problem.

4. (Iowa) shoulder shift test. If the containment test is negative or equivocal, and minimally or not pain provoking, a moderately more strenuous instability test may be carried out as follows: Anterior translation of the humeral head relative to the glenoid is effected by gentle anterior force applied by the examiner's hand beneath the patient's humeral head. The patient, with his or her hand on the examiner's chest, is asked to push the examiner toward the foot of the bench (resisted internal rotation of the shoulder), both when the shoulder is subluxed forward anteriorly and when it is reduced. A positive test constitutes pain or relative weakness with the effort when the shoulder is subluxed anteriorly.

The results of instability testing may depend in large measure on the skill, experience, and enthusiasm of the examiner. As is always the case, if there is clinical suspicion of joint instability, and this possibility cannot be confirmed or not confirmed by the primary physician, then consultation or referral is recommended. Pain and apprehension, as well as frank subluxation, should be considered positive signs of instability.

Neurovascular Examination
When the patient presents with symptoms or signs of shoulder weakness or radicular symptoms, neurovascular examination of the upper limb is critical. Screening neurologic examination comprises deep tendon reflexes, manual muscle testing, tactile sensation, and two-point discrimination of the palmar surfaces of the digits. Screening examination for thoracic outlet syndrome includes Allen, Wright, and Roos tests.

INJECTION AND ASPIRATION

In sports medicine, occasions requiring diagnostic arthrocentesis of the shoulder are decidedly rare. The most likely

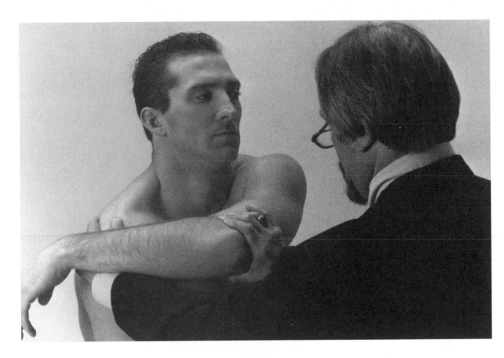

FIGURE 8-10
Acromioclavicular and sternocla-vicular compression tests comprise passive horizontal flexion of the shoulder, resisted active horizontal extension of the horizontally flexed shoulder, and resisted elevation of the horizontally flexed shoulder. These maneuvers also stretch posterior glenohumeral structures.

indication is suspected septic arthritis, such as in an immunocompromised individual with atraumatic shoulder pain.

In contrast, local anesthetic injection at sites of tenderness, the acromioclavicular and glenohumeral joints, or the subacromial bursa is frequently useful. As discussed in Weakness, it can help differentiate weakness secondary to pain inhibition of normal muscular function from other causes of shoulder weakness. It can also help precisely localize the source(s) of a patient's pain—for example, it can help in sorting out the relative importance of acromioclavicular degenerative joint disease versus rotator cuff tendinosis in a patient with activity-related shoulder pain. This is particularly important if surgery for pain relief is being considered.

Sometimes, combining a corticosteroid with local anesthetic injection can be both diagnostic and therapeutic. Typically, if the injection is appropriately placed, the patient will experience prompt offset of pain when the painful structure is anesthetized, recurrence of pain when the anesthetic has worn off, and then offset of pain again a day or more later, when the corticosteroid has exerted its full effects. It is important to advise the patient beforehand of this expected course.

The duration of pain relief after corticosteroid injection is quite variable. For the individual able to limit or to modify the pain-provoking activity, the pain relief may be indefinite. For the patient who is unable or unwilling to comply with activity and rehabilitation recommendations, pain may recur within a week or two.

All injections are carried out after the skin has been cleansed and prepared (e.g., with povidone-iodine solution) and using sterile technique. For diagnostic injections, 1% lidocaine with epinephrine is used. For diagnostic and therapeutic injections, a 1 to 1 mixture of betamethasone and 0.25% bupivacaine (1 to 2 for the shoulder joint) is used.

Provocative tests—for example, impingement test, manual muscle test—are carried out before and after injection, and the extent of postinjection pain relief or strength gain is noted. The patient is asked to attend carefully to pain and pain relief he or she experiences, especially during the first few hours postinjection. Patients are encouraged to keep a log of activities found to be painful or pain free for comparison with preinjection symptoms. As a rule, patients are then seen again in follow-up in 1 week.

Patients are cautioned that after corticosteroid injection, they might not have reliable protective pain sensation for 1–2 months postinjection. Accordingly, for the first several weeks postinjection, they are asked to limit their activities to the type, frequency, duration, and intensity that were fairly well tolerated preinjection.

Acromioclavicular Joint

A superior approach, as shown in Figure 8-15, is preferred. This permits, if desired, injection of the underlying subacromial bursa, as well as the acromioclavicular joint, with one needle stick. An AP radiograph of the shoulder will define the obliquity of the individual patient's acromioclavicular joint and thereby guide direction of the needle.

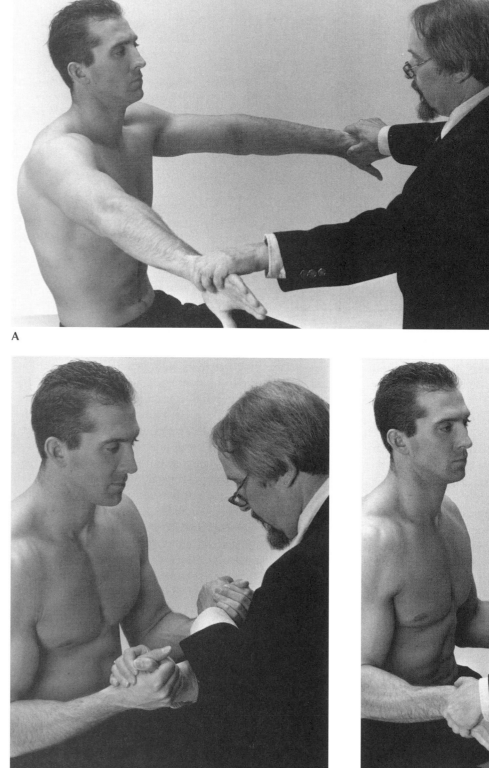

A

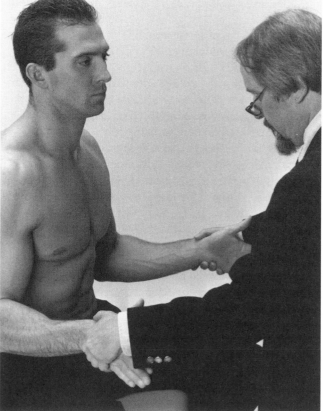

FIGURE 8-11
Selective testing of the supraspinatus (A) and the internal (B) and external (C) rotators of the shoulder.

B

C

FIGURE 8-12

Testing of the biceps.
A. Speed test. The shoulders are flexed and externally rotated, the elbows extended, and the forearms supinated. The patient tries to resist the examiner's downward pressure on his forearms. B. Yergason test.[58] The elbow is flexed to 90 degrees and the forearm is pronated. The patient attempts to supinate the forearm against the examiner's resistance.

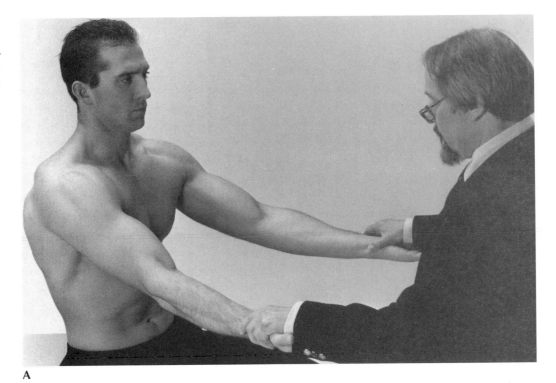

A

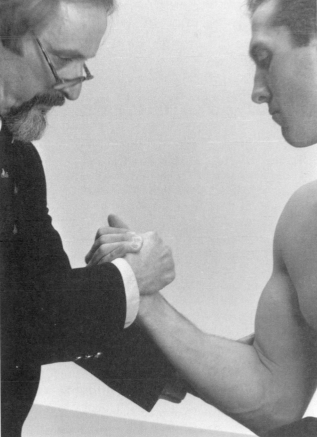

B

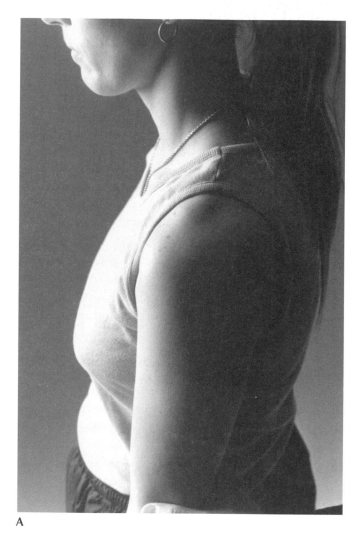
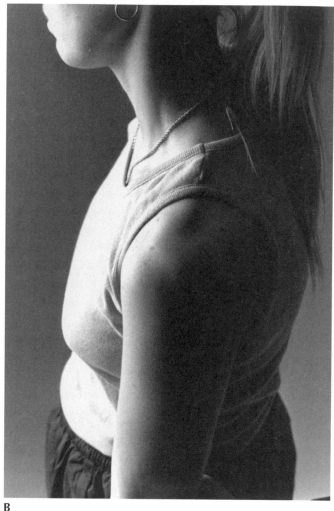

A   B

FIGURE 8-13

Sulcus test. The examiner places gentle downward traction on the arm as in (A). A click may be felt as the shoulder subluxes inferiorly, and a subacromial indentation will be apparent as in (B). With supraspinatus strain or tendinitis, this motion may produce pain and may be voluntarily or involuntarily resisted.

In some individuals, marked osteophytosis may preclude easy superior needle entry, in which case an anterior approach may be used. The intact adult acromioclavicular joint will accommodate a volume of 3–4 ml, after which pressure limits further injection. The needle may then be advanced to inject the bursa. Promptly postinjection, there should be relief of acromioclavicular pain with compression tests, horizontal flexion of the shoulder, and so forth.

Shoulder (Glenohumeral) Joint

The shoulder joint can reliably be entered anteriorly or posteriorly as shown in Figure 8-16. I generally use an anterior approach with needle entry in the anterior joint line approx-

imately one finger breadth inferior to and one finger breadth lateral to the tip of the coracoid. The intact adult shoulder joint will accommodate some 30 ml, but generally approximately 10 ml of fluid is instilled. The patient is then asked to move the shoulder (e.g., Codman or "fungo" active motion exercises as described elsewhere) to help distribute the fluid within the joint. Promptly postinjection, there should be relief of pain from intraarticular structures with impingement testing, manual muscle testing, and so forth.

Subacromial Bursa

The subacromial bursa is generally injected using a posterior approach as described above. However, the bursa

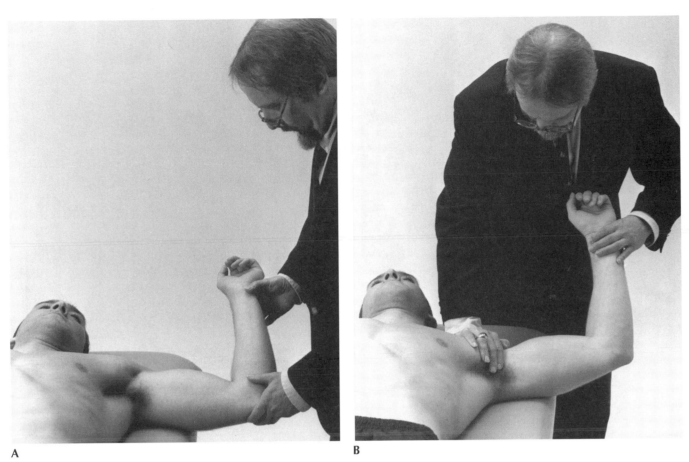

A   B

FIGURE 8-14

Containment test for anterior glenohumeral instability. A positive test comprised pain with passive external rotation of the 90 degrees of abducted shoulder (A) and abatement of pain with "containment" of the humeral head in the glenoid by the examiner's manual pressure (B).

may be selectively injected using an anterolateral approach with needle entry beneath the edge of the acromion and above the anterior aspect of the greater tuberosity of the humerus. It will accommodate several milliliters of fluid.

DIAGNOSTIC IMAGING OF THE SHOULDER

Trauma Series Radiographs

With acute shoulder injuries, radiographic examination is generally indicated. A trauma series, consisting of AP and lateral scapular views, is recommended. (The lateral scapular view is variously referred to as a *true lateral view of the shoulder*, a *transscapular lateral view of the shoulder*, or a *Y view of the shoulder*.) These views can

and should be obtained as is—that is, without moving the arm or removing it from a sling. The patient may be standing, sitting, or lying.

The trauma series has some important advantages over "standard" radiographic examination of the shoulder. First, because the views are obtained as is, discomfort and risk of further injury to the patient are minimized. Second, these views will reveal all of the skeletal injuries of concern: fractures of the distal clavicle, fractures of the proximal humerus, and both anterior and posterior glenohumeral dislocations (see Figure 8-16).

Radiographic examination is not always required before reduction of glenohumeral dislocations. If the clinical diagnosis of anterior dislocation can be made, then gentle reduction may be attempted on the playing field or in the locker room.[3, 9] If there is possible growth plate injury (elementary or junior high school athlete), or if the injury is a first-time posterior dislocation, then radiographic

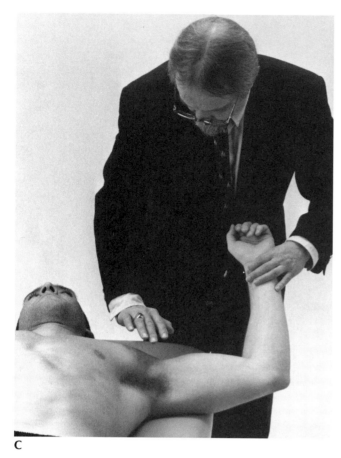

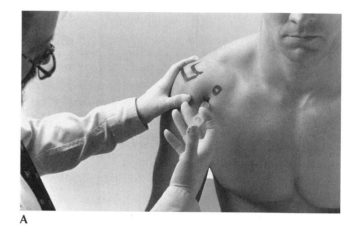

A

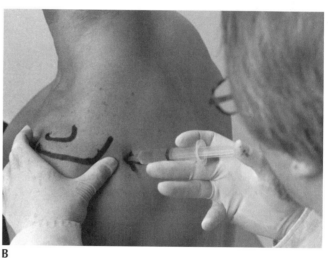

B

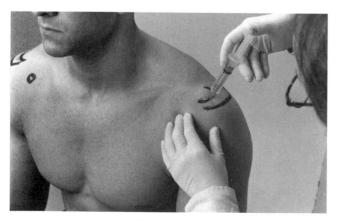

C

FIGURE 8-14 (continued)
and recurrence of pain as the examiner slowly lifts the hand exerting the containing force (C).

FIGURE 8-15
Injection of the acromioclavicular joint and underlying sub-acromial bursa, superior approach. The distal clavicle and lateral margin of the acromion are outlined. Coronal plane orientation of the needle follows the obliquity of the joint as would be demonstrated on an anteroposterior radiograph of the shoulder.

FIGURE 8-16
Injection of the glenohumeral joint. A. Anterior approach. The tip of the coracoid, distal clavicle, and anterolateral margin of the acromion are outlined. Needle entry is a finger breadth inferior and medial to the tip of the coracoid. B. Posterior approach. The distal clavicle and posterolateral margin of the acromion are outlined. Needle entry is a thumb's breadth inferior to the posterior margin of the acromion. The needle is directed anteriorly toward the tip of the coracoid.

examination before reduction is recommended. In all cases, postreduction radiographic examination is indicated.

Acromioclavicular Stress Radiographs

Many orthopedists and radiologists recommend stress views of the acromioclavicular joints whenever the clinical findings are suggestive of grade III or higher acromioclavicular sprains. These AP views of the acromioclavicular joints should be obtained with 5–15 lb of weight suspended from the patient's wrists (not held). The coracoclavicular

FIGURE 8-17
Acromioclavicular stress radiographs incorrectly obtained with the weight held not suspended from the wrists. The separation is greater in (A), "without weights," than in (B), "with weights." Deltoid muscle action and spasm has reduced the grade III sprain.

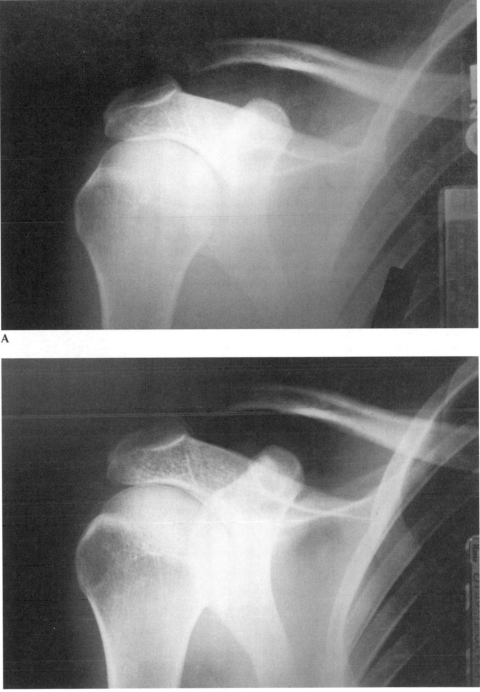

A

B

distance is measured on the injured and uninjured sides. A difference of 5 mm or more is considered diagnostic of complete disruption of the coracoclavicular ligaments (grade III sprain).

In common practice, radiographs are obtained with handheld (as opposed to wrist-suspended) weights, in which case protective deltoid muscle action can "reduce" the acromioclavicular separation and result in a false-negative diagnostic test, especially if the shoulder is still painful (Figure 8-17). I generally treat grades I–III acromioclavicular sprains the same, so I do not routinely order these films.

Shoulder Series Radiographs

Radiographic examination of the shoulder is generally indicated both for acute injury and for any problem of more than a few weeks' duration. If shoulder joint motion is not contraindicated or is very painfully limited, a standard shoulder series—comprising internal and external rotation AP views and an axillary view—may be ordered instead of the trauma series.

Classic signs of anterior glenohumeral instability are the Bankart lesion,[10] a defect of the anteroinferior aspect of the glenoid rim, and the Hill-Sachs lesion,[11] an impression defect of the posterolateral aspect of the humeral head. The Bankart lesion is best evidenced radiographically in a West Point axillary view.[12] The patient is positioned prone with his or her shoulder abducted 90 degrees. The x-ray beam is directed 25 degrees inferiorly and 25 degrees medially. The Hill-Sachs lesion is best visualized in an AP view with the shoulder internally rotated.

With posterior instability, there may be an impression defect of the anteromedial part of the humeral head. The defect is best visualized in a standard axillary view (Figure 8-18). It corresponds to the Hill-Sachs lesion with anterior dislocation and is sometimes referred to as a "reverse Hill-Sachs lesion." A more common finding with posterior instability is a defect or irregularity of the posterior glenoid rim, seen best on AP views.

Shoulder Arthrography

This former test of choice for diagnosis of full thickness rotator cuff tears has now been virtually replaced by MRI, which provides more accurate and more complete information.

Radionuclide Scintigraphy

Indications are rare. A bone scan may be useful as a screening test for ruling out uncommon shoulder girdle problems, such as stress reaction of bone, osteochondrosis ("Little Leaguer's shoulder"), and bone tumors.

Magnetic Resonance Imaging and Magnetic Resonance Imaging Arthrography

MRI with gadolinium arthrography is, with certain caveats, the (nonsurgical) diagnostic test of choice for sorting out internal derangements of the shoulder and for assessing structural glenohumeral instability. Partial- and full-thickness rotator cuff tears, rotator cuff tendinitis or tendinosis, glenoid labral tears, SLAP (mnemonic for

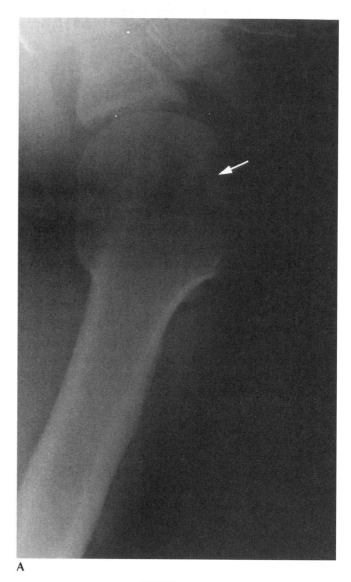

A

FIGURE 8-18
Axillary radiograph (A) and MRI arthrogram axial section (B) demonstrating a reverse Hill-Sachs lesion (arrows), an impression defect of the anteromedial part of the humeral head.

superior *l*abrum, *a*nterior to *p*osterior) lesions, bony and fibrocartilaginous Bankart lesions, long head of biceps tendon rupture or dislocation, acromioclavicular arthrosis, and various bone lesions can all be well demonstrated (Figures 8-19 and 8-20).

The clinical usefulness of the MRI is not limited to preoperative planning. Information obtained can help with decisions regarding operative versus nonoperative treatment and the specifics of nonoperative rehabilitative treatment. The decision to order this test versus some other test or no test is probably best made in consulta-

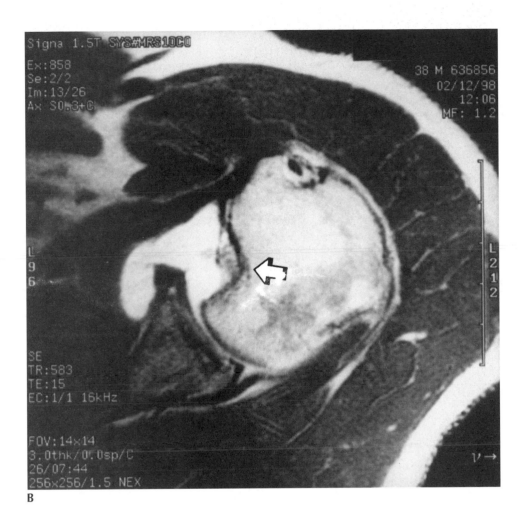

B

tion with or deferred to the sports medicine or orthopedic consultant.

ACUTE TRAUMATIC CONDITIONS

For an algorithm for evaluation of acute shoulder injuries, see Figure 8-21.

Sternoclavicular Sprains

The sternoclavicular joint is the only true articulation of the shoulder girdle with the axial skeleton. Some sternoclavicular motion occurs with virtually all motions of the shoulder and shoulder girdle. The joint has little inherent bony stability. Motion is constrained mainly by the surrounding ligaments—namely, the articular disk ligament, the costoclavicular ligament, the anterior and posterior sternoclavicular ligaments, and the interclavicular ligament. The fact that dislocation is uncommon attests

to the strength of these ligaments, most or all of which must be completely disrupted for dislocation to occur.[13]

The brachiocephalic, jugular, and subclavian veins; the brachiocephalic, carotid, and subclavian arteries; the trachea; the esophagus; the lungs and pleurae; and the brachial plexus lie just deep to the sternoclavicular joint and proximal clavicle. Posterior dislocation can cause compression or laceration of any of the underlying structures. Such complications reportedly occur in roughly one-fourth of cases of traumatic posterior dislocation.[13]

Sternoclavicular injury may be produced by either direct or indirect trauma. The most common mechanism is lateral compression of the shoulder girdle as a result of force applied to the shoulder or upper limb.

The hallmark symptom is pain, which is well localized and roughly proportional to the severity of injury. With mild and moderate sprains, the pain is likely to become progressively more limiting during the first 24 hours or so postinjury. With dislocation, especially posterior dislocation, the pain will be immediate and quite severe.

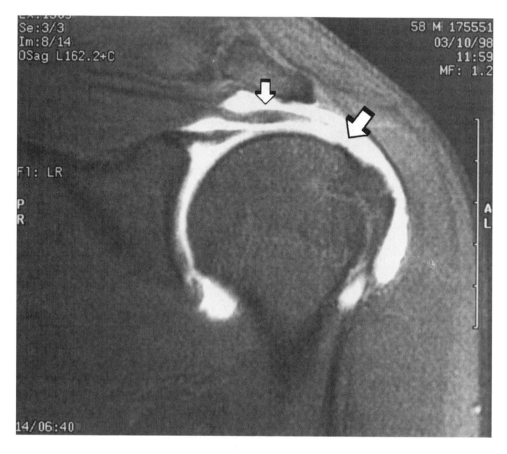

FIGURE 8-19
Magnetic resonance imaging arthrogram coronal section demonstrating a full thickness acute on degenerative tear (large arrow) of the supraspinatus in a 57-year-old retired miner and recreational league basketball player. Note that the contrast medium injected into the joint fills the subacromial bursa (small arrow).

With posterior dislocation, there may be symptoms of associated injury to underlying vital structures. The most ominous symptoms are those of airway obstruction and ventilatory impairment (e.g., dyspnea, dysphonia, stridor, choking, and coughing). Compression of the esophagus may cause dysphagia, and compression of the subclavian artery or brachial plexus may cause upper limb pain and paresthesias.

Treatment. Attention is first directed to ruling out life- or limb-threatening injury. After vital functions have been stabilized, attention can then be directed to diagnosing the specific musculoskeletal injury. With all sternoclavicular sprains, there will be point tenderness over the joint. With anterior dislocation, the clavicle will be visibly or palpably displaced anterior to the manubrium. With posterior dislocation, the usual prominence of the proximal clavicle will be lost. Although all of these signs can be more or less obscured by obesity or swelling, careful palpation will usually establish the diagnosis. (Before closure of the proximal clavicular growth plate, which occurs at approximately age 25 years, it will be practically impossible to differentiate clinically sternoclavicular dislocations from fractures through the growth plate. Indeed, before ossification of the proximal epiphysis,

which occurs at approximately age 18 years, it will be impossible even to do so radiographically. As both injuries are treated the same, however, the differentiation is not clinically important.)

Radiographic examination of the sternoclavicular joint can be difficult to interpret. If the clinical diagnosis is uncertain, however, fractures of the sternum or proximal clavicle can be ruled out by the appropriate studies. Computerized axial tomography or MRI may be useful to confirm the diagnosis of dislocation and to reveal the extent of impingement of underlying structures.[14]

Vital functions are supported as indicated. Definitive treatment on an emergent basis is seldom necessary. However, immediate treatment of a complication (e.g., thoracentesis for decompression of a tension pneumothorax) might be required.

Reduction of dislocations, particularly complicated posterior dislocations, is indicated on an urgent basis. In nearly all cases, closed reduction is the treatment of choice. A possible contraindication might be suspected perforation—as opposed to compression—of a major blood vessel.

Closed reduction of sternoclavicular dislocations can be achieved in several ways, all of which involve direct or

FIGURE 8-20
Magnetic resonance imaging arthrogram axial (A) and sagittal (B) sections demonstrating an acute, traumatic fibrocartilaginous Bankart lesion (arrows), the result of a snowmobiling accident.

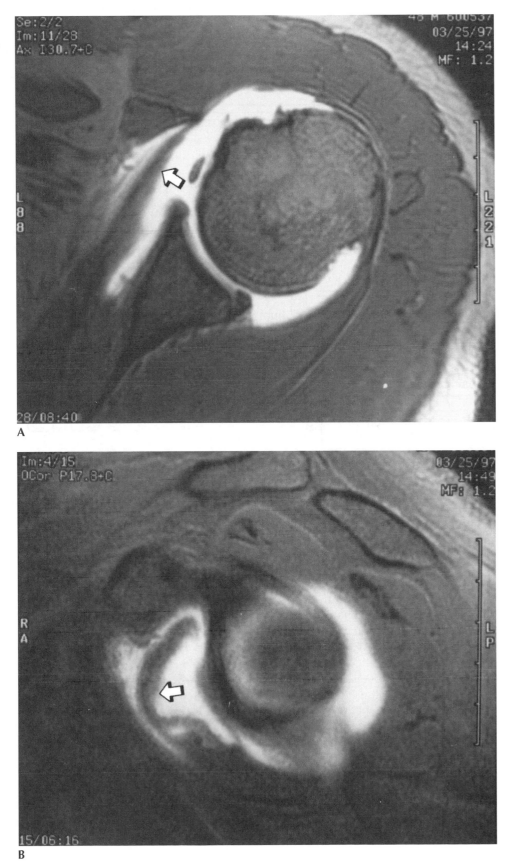

A

B

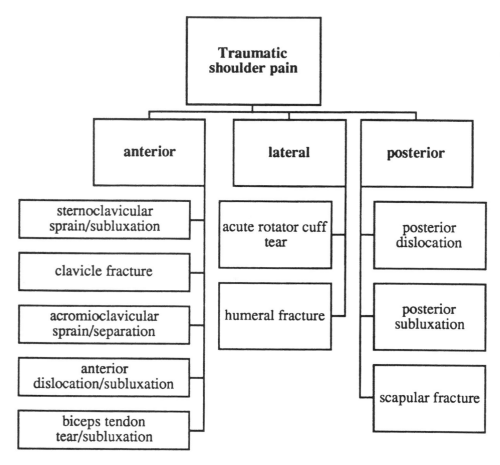

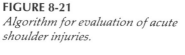
FIGURE 8-21
Algorithm for evaluation of acute shoulder injuries.

indirect retraction of the shoulder girdle. Both anterior and posterior dislocations are reduced by this mechanism. Before significant swelling and muscle spasm have occurred, it may be possible to achieve reduction simply by placing a knee between the seated athlete's scapulae and pulling back on his or her shoulders. In the standard method of closed reduction, the athlete is supine with a sandbag placed between the scapulae. Lateral traction is applied to the abducted and slightly extended upper limb. With anterior dislocation, anterior pressure over the proximal clavicle may also be required. With posterior dislocation, anterolateral traction on the proximal clavicle with the fingers or a sterile towel clip may be required. An alternative method for reducing posterior dislocations is to apply caudal traction to the adducted upper limb while direct anterior pressure is applied to both shoulders. Reportedly, less force is required to effect reduction, and manipulation of the clavicle with a towel clip is usually unnecessary.[15]

Postreduction, a figure-of-eight clavicle strap is applied to maintain retraction of the shoulder girdle. As a rule, reductions of posterior dislocations will be stable. Closed

reductions of anterior dislocations may or may not be stable. Even with the shoulders held back, the joint may sublux anteriorly.

Posterior dislocations should be considered much the same as penetrating wounds of the neck. Even if stable reduction has been achieved and all signs and symptoms of associated injury have resolved, the athlete should still be admitted to the hospital and closely observed for signs of delayed complications.

Orthopedic referral on an urgent basis is indicated for all unreduced acute dislocations. Open reduction of acute posterior dislocations is required if stable closed reduction cannot be achieved. Severe vascular injury may require surgical exploration. If such injury is suspected, referral should be made on an emergent basis to a major center with angiographic and cardiovascular or thoracic surgical capabilities.

Fractures of the Proximal and Middle Thirds of the Clavicle

As with sternoclavicular sprains, injury may be produced by either direct or indirect trauma. The mechanisms of injury are much the same. With fractures, however, the most common mechanism would appear to be falls onto the outstretched hand.

Symptoms are for the most part those usually associated with long bone fractures: a snapping or cracking sensation at the time of injury, immediate and well-localized pain, rapid swelling, crepitus on motion, increased pain on motion, and limitation of motion. There may also be symptoms of associated injury to underlying vital structures. Pneumothorax may cause dyspnea, and brachial plexus injury may cause upper limb pain and paresthesias.

Even though the skeletal injury may be strikingly evident, attention must first be directed to ruling out associated life- or limb-threatening injury. Lying just deep to the clavicle are the pleurae and dome of the lung, the subclavian vessels, and the brachial plexus. Serious and sometimes fatal complications can and do occur as a result of laceration of underlying structure(s) by a fracture fragment. The most common serious complication is laceration of the subclavian artery, which will be evidenced by a large, rapidly expanding or pulsatile hematoma. The pulsatile nature of the mass can sometimes best be demonstrated by holding a tongue depressor on top of it to amplify the movement.

There may be obvious deformity with anterior and superior angulation and possibly penetration of the skin by a fracture fragment. Other physical findings are for the most part those usually associated with long bone fractures: point tenderness over the fracture site, false motion, crepitus with motion, and pain with motion.

Radiographic examination is indicated initially to assess position and alignment and in follow-up to assess the extent of healing.

Treatment. Immediate treatment of life-threatening complications—such as thoracentesis for decompression of a tension pneumothorax—might be required. Such measures are undertaken as the problems are identified. Open fractures should be debrided of gross contamination, covered with a moist saline dressing, and immobilized as is. Tetanus prophylaxis should be undertaken according to standard guidelines. Prophylactic antibiotics should be administered only as directed by the consulting orthopedist.

With displaced, angulated, comminuted, or overriding closed fractures of the proximal and middle thirds of the clavicle, the position and alignment can usually be improved—although not always completely corrected—by retraction of the shoulder girdles. This should be done with care, particularly if a fracture fragment is tenting the skin, so as not to convert the closed fracture to an open one.

A figure-of-eight clavicle strap is then used to keep the shoulders back. A clavicle strap is contraindicated for fractures distal to the point at which the strap crosses the clavicle. It will tend to displace, rather than reduce, such fractures.

Initial treatment may also include use of a sling (in addition to the clavicle strap) and intermittent icing until swelling has stabilized.

Orthopedic referral on an urgent basis is indicated for all open fractures. Otherwise, orthopedic referral is required only for complications (e.g., nonunion). Severe vascular injury may require surgical exploration. If such injury is suspected, referral should be made on an emergent basis to a major center with angiographic and cardiovascular or thoracic surgical capabilities.

The standard treatment of proximal and middle third clavicle fractures is closed reduction by retraction of the shoulder girdle(s), "immobilization" in a figure-of-eight clavicle strap for 6 weeks or so, and complete rehabilitation of the shoulder before resumption of strenuous activity.

When clinical union has occurred and some callus has formed, the clavicle strap is discontinued. A sling is used for an additional week or so. The athlete is then allowed to resume noncontact, nonthrowing activities as tolerated. Complete shoulder rehabilitation is recommended before resumption of throwing and racquet sports, swimming, and related activities. Complete shoulder rehabilitation and radiographic union are recommended before resuming contact and collision sports (including bicycle racing and horseback riding) as well as football and wrestling.

Open reduction and internal fixation may seem tempting in the case of the athlete who "must" return to competition as soon as possible, but it is fraught with complications. Nonunion, which is rare with closed treatment, is not uncommon with open treatment. Other possible complications include infection and even death (e.g., as a result of migration of a Steinmann pin or Kirschner wire into the heart or one of the great vessels).

Less than anatomic reduction is primarily of cosmetic, rather than functional, significance. With appropriate rehabilitation, return without impairment to strenuous and demanding use of the upper limb (e.g., baseball pitching and gymnastics) is the rule.

Acromioclavicular Sprains (Shoulder Separations)

The typical mechanism of injury is a direct blow to the superior aspect of the acromion, such as may occur in a fall onto the point of the shoulder or in being struck there by an opponent's helmet. The force thus produced tends

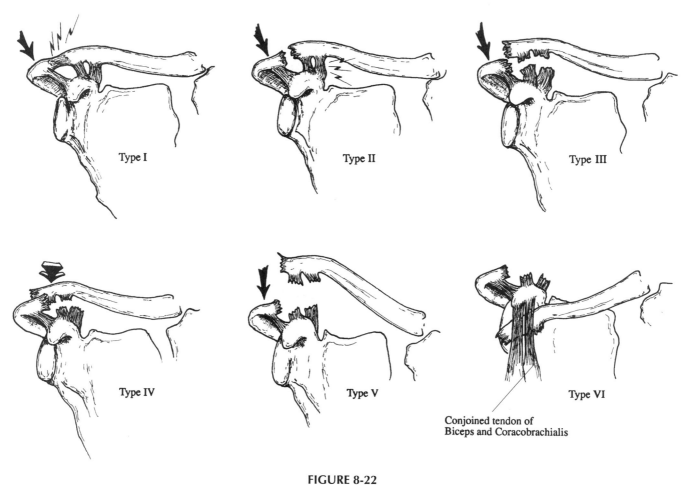

FIGURE 8-22
Classification of acromioclavicular sprains, as described by Allman[16] and Rockwood.[17]

to drive the scapula inferiorly away from the clavicle. This force is resisted mainly by the coracoclavicular ligaments. Acromioclavicular injury is less commonly produced by direct blows to the clavicle or by indirect forces, such as those that may occur with falls onto the elbow or outstretched hand.

The extent of acromioclavicular separation will depend on the amount of force applied and the corresponding degree of injury to the coracoclavicular ligaments. Allman[16] classified acromioclavicular sprains as grades I, II, and III, representing, respectively, no involvement, partial tearing, and complete disruption of the coracoclavicular ligaments. More recently, Rockwood[17] has further classified the more severe injuries as grades III–VI, depending on the direction and amount of acromioclavicular displacement and the extent of associated injury to the deltoid and trapezius muscles (Figure 8-22).

The hallmark physical finding is point tenderness over the acromioclavicular joint. Tenderness over the cora-coclavicular space is characteristic of grade II and III injuries and differentiates these injuries from grade I injuries and contusions (shoulder pointers).

With complete disruption of the coracoclavicular ligaments (grade III sprains), there may be obvious deformity ("high-riding clavicle" or, more correctly, "low-riding scapula"). However, absence of this sign does not rule out grade III sprain, as muscle spasm can minimize the extent of acromioclavicular separation.

Radiographic examination is indicated to differentiate acromioclavicular sprain from distal clavicle fracture. A trauma series will suffice for this purpose, although acromioclavicular views would be equally appropriate.

Many orthopedists and radiologists recommend stress views of the acromioclavicular joints whenever the clinical findings are suggestive of grade III or higher acromioclavicular sprains. These AP views of the acromioclavicular joints should be obtained with 5–15 lb of weight, not held, but rather suspended from the patient's wrists. The coracoclavicular distance is measured on the injured and uninjured sides. A difference of 5 mm or more is considered diagnostic of complete disruption of the coracoclavicular ligaments (grade III sprain). Because of the likelihood of false-negative radiographs that are due to incorrect technique, and because all acromioclavicular sprains may be treated the same, these films need not be routinely ordered.

Initial treatment is symptomatic and consists of rest (sling or shoulder immobilizer prn), ice, and analgesics as required. Urgent treatment is required only in the rare event of neurovascular impairment or grade IV–VI sprains. Rehabilitation entails range of motion and progressive resistance exercises for the intrinsic shoulder muscles, as well as specific strengthening exercises for the upper trapezius, such as shoulder shrugs with Thera-Band or weights.[18]

Treatment. Definitive treatment is, to say the least, controversial. I concur with Nicol[19] and others[18, 20] that nonoperative treatment cannot achieve the unattainable (restoration of a normal joint) and that primary operative treatment is rarely justified. Acromioclavicular injuries of all grades are associated with some risk of subsequent degenerative joint disease and chronic pain.[17, 21] This complication can be satisfactorily treated by resection of the distal clavicle, however, which need not be done a priori.[22] Furthermore, failure to reconstruct the acromioclavicular joint has not been found to result in impaired strength or functional use of the arm.[18, 20, 23] Indeed, it would appear that the only significant differences in operative and nonoperative treatment of grade III sprains are a longer recovery time with operative treatment, a decreased risk of chronic pain if the distal clavicle is resected, and a trade-off between deformity and surgical scar.

The athlete should be informed of the possible sequelae of acromioclavicular injury (deformity, degenerative joint disease) and the options regarding primary or delayed surgical treatment.[22] The patient should be referred to an orthopedist if he or she is unwilling to accept the cosmetic deformity of an overly prominent distal clavicle or to allow the shoulder to recover from the acute injury and then see if it still hurts.

Acute, Traumatic, Anterior Glenohumeral Dislocation

The characteristic mechanism of injury is indirect trauma: forced abduction and external rotation, such as that which may occur in arm tackling in football or in falls onto the abducted, externally rotated arm. Direct trauma to the shoulder is a less common mechanism of injury.

Especially with first-time dislocations, the athlete will be in obvious distress. He or she will invariably be quite unwilling to continue any athletic activity and may or may not be aware that the shoulder is out of place.

The injured arm will be held in an abducted, externally rotated position, supported if possible by the uninjured arm. Any shoulder motion, particularly internal rotation, will be painful and resisted by the athlete. The normal rounded contour of the shoulder will be lost. The acromion will be inordinately prominent, with an indentation beneath it, as shown in Figure 8-3. Examination will usually also reveal an anterior fullness caused by the anteriorly displaced humeral head. These findings can usually be appreciated by palpation (e.g., under shoulder pads) as well as by inspection.

Assessment of the neurovascular status of the limb is important. Blom and Dahlback[5] reported a 33% incidence of nerve injury with acute anterior dislocations. In patients older than 50 years, the incidence was nearly 50%.[5] Any of the nerves of the brachial plexus can be injured; however, the axillary nerve is particularly at risk. The most reliable clinical test for axillary nerve function is gentle isometric testing of the deltoid muscle. The significance of nerve injury complicating anterior dislocation would appear to be that rehabilitation is likely to be prolonged. With diligent rehabilitation, eventual full recovery should be expected.

Assessment for possible associated rotator cuff injury is also very important.

Trauma series radiographs, consisting of AP and lateral scapular views, should be obtained as is—that is, without moving the arm.

Prereduction films are not always required. If the clinical diagnosis of anterior dislocation can be made, and if growth plate injury is unlikely (high-school–age or older athlete), then gentle reduction may be attempted on the playing field or in the locker room.[3, 9] In all cases, postreduction films are indicated.

Acutely, MRI is indicated only if an extensive, surgically treatable rotator cuff tear is suspected.

Treatment. Acute glenohumeral dislocations should be reduced as quickly, gently, and safely as possible. Early reduction minimizes the amount of muscle spasm that must be overcome to effect reduction and thereby minimizes discomfort and risk of further injury.

Before any attempted reduction, the physician must be certain that the dislocation is acute. This is not always as obvious in the office or emergency room as it is on the playing field. Chronically dislocated shoulders may present after other acute injury.

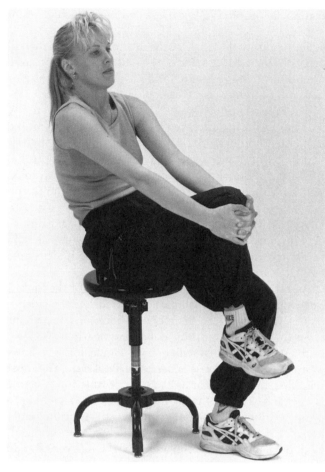

FIGURE 8-23

The technique of self-reduction of anterior dislocation of the shoulder, as described by Aronen.[24] With her hands clasped about her (ipsilateral) knee, the patient herself applies gentle in-line traction to the dislocated shoulder by extending her hip.

Reduction of uncomplicated anterior dislocations can usually be achieved using the techniques of Aronen,[24] Stimson,[25] or Rockwood.[4] Each of these techniques is based on the principle of traction and countertraction, and all are safe. Leverage techniques, such as the Kocher maneuver,[26] entail unacceptable risk of further injury to the soft tissues and the articular surface of the humerus.[4, 27] The primary care physician who is unfamiliar with any of the recommended techniques should defer the reduction of the shoulder to an orthopedist.

Of the three recommended techniques, those of Aronen and Stimson are logistically quite simple. They are most useful when reduction is relatively easily achieved. This is usually the case with multiply recurrent dislocations or immediately after injury, before much swelling and muscle spasm have occurred. Both techniques have

the advantage of sometimes enabling patients to carry out the reductions by themselves. It is prudent to teach the Aronen technique to patients who have sustained shoulder dislocations, as self-reduction may be the only method available to them in certain situations (e.g., solo sailing, backpacking, or cross-country skiing).

In the technique described by Aronen, the patient is instructed to clasp his or her hands about the (ipsilateral) knee and then to relax the shoulder muscles, allowing the weight of the lower limb to provide gentle in-line traction on the upper limb as the hip is extended (Figure 8-23). Countertraction is provided by the patient's own (paraspinous) muscles.

In the Stimson technique, the patient lies prone on a flat surface (examining table, automobile hood, boulder, and so forth) with the injured limb hanging over the side. Traction is applied by weight suspended from the wrist; countertraction is provided by the flat surface. It is important that the weight be tied to the wrist (two half-hitch knots), as opposed to being held by the patient (which would preclude desired relaxation of the muscles of the upper limb). The amount of weight suspended from the wrist depends on the size of the patient. Five pounds is usually sufficient.

With difficult reductions (e.g., a first-time dislocation in a heavily muscled athlete), the Stimson technique tends to be, at best, rather time-consuming. Standard advice is that the patient be left undisturbed for at least 20 minutes. This does not imply, however, that the patient be heavily sedated and then left unattended. If reduction is achieved, there will be a dramatic reduction in the level of pain. Without that stimulus, the heavily sedated patient may very well lose consciousness (see discussion below).

In the Rockwood technique, the patient is supine. A swathe (towel, stockinet, or folded sheet) is placed around his or her torso and as high up in the (ipsilateral) axilla as possible. An assistant (on the opposite side) holds the free ends. Manual in-line traction on the patient's injured limb is then gently applied and gradually increased against the countertraction provided by the axillary swathe. With adequate analgesia or muscle relaxation, reduction is usually readily achieved. Sometimes, in addition to this basic maneuver, very slight internal and external rotation or lateral traction may be required.

Whereas Rockwood's technique does require more "manpower," in most situations—on the playing field, in the locker room, in the office, or in the emergency department—an assistant or two capable of holding a swathe is usually not hard to find. The technique is safe, effective, and expedient. That the patient is not "left alone" is probably an advantage.

Shortly after injury, reduction may be attempted without medication. If reduction cannot be readily achieved, however, or if more than 1 hour has elapsed after injury, analgesia and sedation are indicated. Usual adult dosages are meperidine 50 mg intravenously or morphine 5 mg intravenously. Intravenous midazolam (Versed) may be administered to attain conscious sedation or muscle relaxation. Usual adult dosage is 1.0–2.5 mg titrated slowly to desired effect. After reduction has been achieved and the pain stimulus is no longer present, the patient may be excessively sedated. Naloxone should be available to reverse the sedative effects of the narcotic analgesic, if necessary.

Postreduction, the neurovascular status of the limb is reassessed, the arm is placed in a sling or Velpeau-type shoulder immobilizer, and the radiographic examination of the shoulder is repeated. (Shoulder immobilization— that is, strict limitation of abduction and external rotation—is continued as discussed below.)

Unreduced dislocations should be padded and splinted as is. Slings are inappropriate for unreduced anterior dislocations, because their application requires internal rotation of the shoulder.

Intermittent icing (application of crushed ice for 20 minutes at least once every 4 waking hours) is appropriate, whether reduction has been achieved. It is continued until any swelling stabilizes.

Referral to an appropriate facility on an emergent basis is indicated for fractures or dislocations complicated by vascular impairment. Orthopedic referral on an urgent basis is indicated for unreduced glenohumeral dislocations.

Orthopedic referral is also recommended for dislocations complicated by nerve injury. Although most such injuries would appear to be neurapraxias, and surgical exploration is generally not indicated, it would seem prudent to defer their management to a specialist.

Fractures of the greater tuberosity of the humerus are frequently associated with anterior dislocations and are usually anatomically reduced when the dislocation is reduced. If they remain more than 1 cm displaced after reduction of the dislocation, orthopedic referral is indicated.[2, 3]

Many first-time anterior dislocations can be definitively treated by immobilization (i.e., strict limitation of abduction and external rotation) and complete shoulder rehabilitation, as discussed below.

The principal overall objective of treatment is to prevent chronic or recurrent instability. Specific, sequential, intermediate objectives are

- To keep the avulsed or torn tissues approximated so as to permit healing

- To strengthen the muscles, especially subscapularis, that act as dynamic restraints against hyperabduction and external rotation
- To restore normal glenohumeral and scapulothoracic patterns of motion
- To strengthen all intrinsic shoulder and scapular-stabilizing muscles

All of these objectives should be accomplished before return to shoulder-strenuous activity is attempted. (The principal objective of treatment notwithstanding, all patients who have sustained an acute dislocation should be taught the Aronen technique of self-reduction, should there be a recurrent injury.)

Based on known principles of wound healing, knowledge gained from arthroscopic treatment of chronic or recurrent shoulder instability, and various outcome studies,[28-33] immobilizing the shoulder for 6 weeks postinjury would seem to afford the best chance of healing. This is in fact recommended for athletic patients younger than 20 years old. With increasing age, there is decreasing risk of recurrent instability and increasing risk of frozen shoulder. Accordingly, for 20–30 year olds, the shoulder is immobilized 5 weeks; for 30–40 year olds, 4 weeks; for 40–50 year olds, 3 weeks; and for patients older than 50, the shoulder is mobilized as soon as symptoms permit. During the period of immobilization, the immobilizer may be removed only for prescribed isometric exercises (in which the shoulder is kept adducted and internally rotated) or bathing. It should not be removed for sleeping.

Usually within a few days of the injury, the athlete will no longer be in much pain and will be reluctant to stay in the immobilizer. The essential therapeutic task is to convince him or her that the only good chance of success with nonoperative treatment is to comply strictly with the rehabilitation protocol. Everyone involved—primary care provider, athletic trainer, team physician, physical therapist, and coach—should reinforce this.

It has been commonly held that the young athlete who has sustained an anterior dislocation is at very high risk for recurrent dislocation. McLaughlin and MacLellan[34] and Rowe and Sakellarides[35] reported 80–95% recurrence rates in patients younger than 20 years old.

Recurrence is perhaps related in part to pathoanatomy. It has been reported that recurrent dislocation is more likely with labral detachment types of injury than with capsular tear types.[36] It has also been reported that recurrence is less likely in dislocations associated with fractures of the greater tuberosity.[37]

It would appear, however, that the likelihood of recurrence is also related to the specifics of treatment and rehabilitation. In contrast to the studies noted above are the excellent results reported by Yoneda and coworkers[33] and Aronen and Regan,[29] who have emphasized specific strengthening exercises, as well as avoidance of abduction. These authors have shown that with appropriate rehabilitation, even the young athlete who intends to return to vigorous athletic activity should have a 75% or better chance of having no subsequent instability.

Ideally, return to sports participation is simply the final step in the sequence of rehabilitation. There should be full restoration of motion without pain, apprehension, or instability; there should be full restoration of strength as determined by isokinetic testing; and, finally, there should be a gradual resumption of activity as tolerated.

With shoulder injuries, the physician should resist letting the athlete return to his or her sport before full rehabilitation has been carried out. Particularly with dislocations, the risk of reinjury and the consequences of reinjury are too great. At best, the athlete only invites overuse injury if he or she attempts strenuous use of the shoulder before sufficient strength and flexibility have been restored.

With anterior dislocations, abduction and external rotation–limiting harnesses are sometimes used when, for example, football line play is resumed. These should be used in addition to, rather than in substitution for, adequate rehabilitation.

Recurrent shoulder dislocation is definitively treated by surgical reconstruction of the shoulder. Indications are discussed below.

In most handed sports, recurrent shoulder dislocation would be unacceptable. In some, such as rock climbing, it could be life threatening. The athlete at substantial risk for recurrent dislocation would seem to have but two logical choices: limit or modify athletic activity or undergo surgical treatment.

However, not all authors agree as to which athletes are at substantial risk for recurrent dislocation. I do not share the opinion of those who believe that a single dislocation in a young athlete most likely dooms him or her to recurrent dislocations. I would submit that the extent to which a second dislocation implies substantial risk of recurrence depends on individual circumstances.

A second dislocation is less likely to pose significant risk if more than 1 year has elapsed since the initial dislocation, if there was inadequate rehabilitation after the first dislocation, or if the recurrent dislocation was the result of significant trauma (force greater than or equal to that which produced the original injury). On the other hand, a true pattern of instability is established if recurrent dislocation(s) occur with increasing ease—if less force is required to produce the dislocation(s), if reduction(s) are achieved with increasing ease, and if associated symp-

toms become less severe. A radiographically or MRI-confirmed Bankart or Hill-Sachs lesion would also imply an increased likelihood of recurrence.

Acute or Recurrent Anterior Glenohumeral Subluxation

Subluxation is perhaps best defined as transient displacement of the head of the humerus with respect to the glenoid fossa, associated with momentary disruption of shoulder function.[3] Since first described by Blazina and Satzman,[37] it has been increasingly recognized as an important problem in athletes.[38–41] Any shoulder injury in which there is a history of forced abduction, external rotation mechanism of injury; perceived frank instability; or "dead arm" symptoms should be considered as probable acute anterior glenohumeral subluxation and treated accordingly.

The mechanism of injury is the same as previously noted for acute, traumatic anterior dislocation: forced abduction and external rotation. Pain associated with the acute injury is usually not very severe or prolonged and may be quite transient.

A perception of frank instability—"My shoulder went out of place and then popped back in"—is, in my experience, virtually always accurate. (Patients do not always volunteer this information and should be specifically asked about it.) However, absence of frank instability symptoms does not rule out the possibility of acute subluxation. Some patients will be aware only that they somehow hurt their shoulders or arms.

A characteristic, but not pathognomonic, associated symptom is the sensation of "the arm's going dead."[37, 40] This symptom may also occur with cervical spine or brachial plexus injury or with thoracic outlet syndrome.[40, 42]

Symptoms of recurrent subluxation are positional pain, apprehension, or frank instability. Instability is likely to be perceived and described as painful "clicking" or "slipping out of place."

As the shoulder becomes increasingly unstable, the athlete is likely to become increasingly apprehensive about those motions that reproduce his or her symptoms. Symptoms occurring with repetitive abduction, external rotation motions—such as the cocking phase of throwing or serving—is characteristic of anterior instability.

With acute injury, appreciable swelling and ecchymosis are uncommon, and anterior tenderness is usually not very marked. The hallmark physical finding of anterior instability is a positive containment test (see Figure 8-14). With the typical "thrower's shoulder," there will be increased external rotation reflecting anterior laxity and

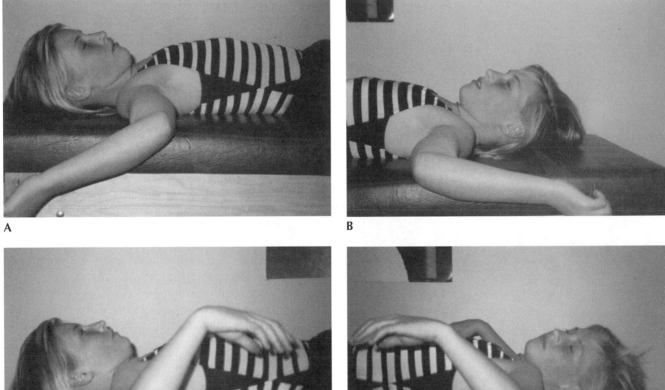

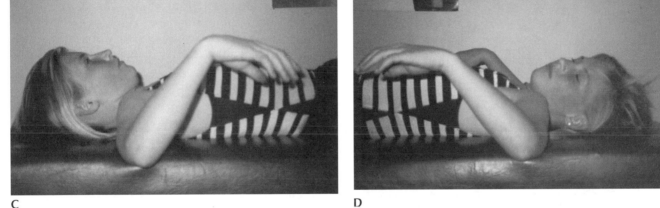

FIGURE 8-24

Range of external and internal glenohumeral rotation in a 10-year-old, right-handed girl who had played competitive tennis since age 5 years, demonstrating anterior laxity and posterior contracture of the shoulder of the dominant arm. A. External rotation, right shoulder. B. External rotation, left shoulder. C. Internal rotation, right shoulder. D. Internal rotation, left shoulder.

decreased internal rotation reflecting posterior contracture (Figure 8-24). There may be pain, apprehension, or frank instability with combined abduction and external rotation or with horizontal extension of the shoulder. There may also be a painful arc of combined glenohumeral or scapulothoracic abduction, more so with the shoulder externally rotated than with it internally.

Radiographic examination is indicated. The radiographic findings associated with anterior instability are the Bankart lesion (a defect of the anteroinferior aspect of the glenoid rim) and the Hill-Sachs lesion (an impression defect of the posterolateral aspect of the humeral head).

The diagnostic imaging test of choice for chronic or recurrent instability is MRI arthrography (see Figure 8-20). The decision to order MRI, however, is most appropriately deferred to the surgical consultant.

Treatment. Rehabilitative treatment follows precisely that discussed above for shoulder dislocation. Many first-time anterior subluxations can be definitively treated by nonoperative means. The essential therapeutic task is to convince the athlete that his or her only good chance of success with nonoperative treatment is to comply strictly with the treatment protocol—a difficult task indeed, given the paucity of symptoms and signs and the general underappreciation of the injury. The primary treating physician is critically important in initiating appropriate intervention.

If disabling pain, apprehension, or frank instability persists despite complete rehabilitation, then orthopedic referral is indicated. Operative treatment is essentially the same as for recurrent dislocation. It may include both labral debridement and Bankart repair and is guided by the MRI arthrographic and intraoperative findings.

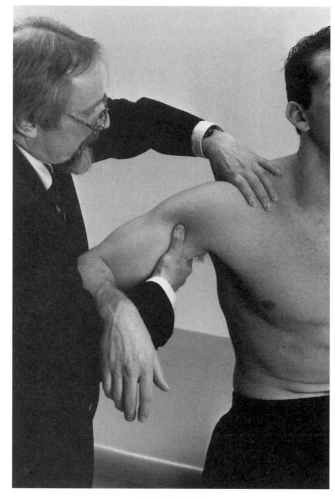

FIGURE 8-25

Examination of the (right) shoulder for posterior instability, the posterior drawer test.[59] The athlete is seated with his right forearm resting comfortably on the examiner's right forearm. The scapula is stabilized by the examiner's left hand. The shoulder is in 90 degrees abduction and neutral rotation. With his right hand, the examiner applies backward pressure on the proximal arm, noting any symptoms or subluxation produced. The pressure is slight, comparable to that used in the Lachman test of the knee.

Acute, Traumatic, Posterior Glenohumeral Subluxation

In contrast to posterior glenohumeral dislocation, which is rare in sports, posterior subluxation is not uncommon. The principal mechanism of injury is axial loading of the arm with the shoulder flexed or horizontally flexed. The force may be applied to the olecranon or ulnar forearm, such as may occur with blocking in football, or it may be applied further distally, such as with a fall onto the outstretched hand.

Pain associated with the acute injury is typically more severe than with acute anterior subluxation and is usually sufficient to cause the athlete to seek medical attention. A perception of frank instability is, in my experience, virtually always accurate, but the absence of frank instability symptoms does not rule out the possibility of acute subluxation. Recurrent instability is typically perceived and described as "clicking" or "slipping out of place" with horizontal flexion movements.

A painful click may be appreciated with active or passive motion. There is likely to be pain—localized posteriorly, not superiorly—with acromioclavicular compression tests (see Figure 8-10). Pain, click, and frank subluxation may be found with a posterior drawer test (Figure 8-25).

Radiographic examination is indicated. With posterior instability, there may be an impression defect of the anteromedial part of the humeral head. The defect is best visualized in a standard axillary view. It corresponds to the Hill-Sachs lesion with anterior dislocation and is sometimes referred to as a *reverse Hill-Sachs lesion*. A more common finding with posterior instability is a defect or irregularity of the posterior glenoid rim—the reverse Bankart lesion—seen best on AP views (Figure 8-26).

The diagnostic imaging test of choice for chronic or recurrent instability is MRI arthrography. The decision to order this test, however, is most appropriately deferred to the surgical consultant.

Treatment. Initial and rehabilitative treatment is similar to that previously discussed for anterior shoulder dislocation and subluxation.

With posterior instability, the shoulder is unstable with horizontal flexion. If it is kept adducted, however, it is not usually unstable with internal rotation. Accordingly, the acute injury is immobilized in adduction and internal rotation just as for anterior instability.

If disabling pain, apprehension, or frank instability persists despite complete rehabilitation, then orthopedic referral is indicated. Operative treatment is similar to that discussed for recurrent anterior dislocation. A reverse Bankart lesion may be repaired similarly to the anterior fibrocartilaginous Bankart lesion.

Acute or Acute on Degenerative Tears of the Rotator Cuff

The rotator cuff comprises four muscles (subscapularis, supraspinatus, infraspinatus, and teres minor) and their tendons. Acting as a force coupled with larger muscles that insert further distally on the humerus (deltoid, pectoralis major, and latissimus dorsi), the rotator cuff and

FIGURE 8-26
Anteroposterior radiograph (A) and magnetic resonance imaging arthrogram axial section (B) demonstrating an intraarticular fracture of the posterior glenoid (arrows) associated with acute, traumatic posterior shoulder subluxation in an 18-year-old high school football down lineman.

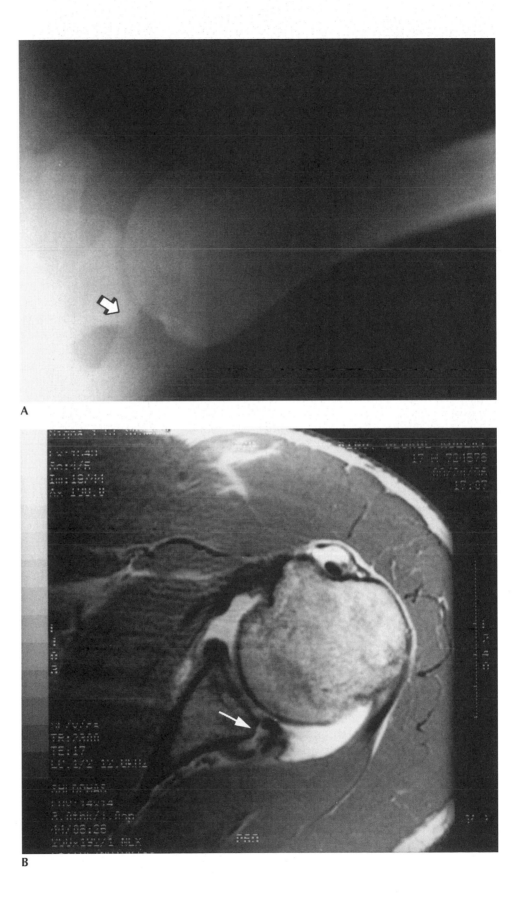

A

B

long head of biceps maintain the axes of shoulder motion centered at the glenohumeral joint.

Tears of the cuff are best described as acute versus degenerative, full thickness versus partial thickness, and large or extensive versus small. The term "complete" as applied to cuff tears is ambiguous. Although it has been used synonymously with "full thickness" to describe tears extending from the articular (deep) surface of the tendon completely through to the bursal (superficial) surface, it also seems to connote extensive tearing, which is not always the case.

Large, full-thickness tears typically occur with abrupt, forceful, eccentric loading of the cuff. A classic example is that of an individual on a ladder, stairs, rock face, or gymnastics apparatus who starts to fall and attempts to arrest the fall by maintaining a handhold. Violent trauma like this may cause extensive tears in the young or old.

Somewhat less forceful "yanking" on the shoulder, such as may occur with attempting to lift up a heavy suitcase or having a grandchild tug on one's outstretched hand, may be sufficient to cause extensive tearing in an older individual who already has tendinosis (tendon degeneration) or partial-thickness tearing.

Partial-thickness tearing may result from less forceful acute trauma but is typically the result of repetitive trauma.

The preceding mechanisms pertain mainly to the supraspinatus and infraspinatus. Tearing typically occurs just proximal to the insertion, or the cuff may be avulsed from its insertion. Tearing of the subscapularis is typically caused by forced abduction and external rotation. Cuff tear or avulsion or avulsion of the greater tuberosity may be associated with shoulder dislocations.

Injuries to the rotator cuff are not all easily dichotomized as acute or overuse. Attrition from aging, overuse, chronic inflammation, and tendinosis predisposes to acute injury (acute on degenerative tear). Conversely, chronic inflammation is often simply a sequela of acute injury that has been neglected, abused, or inadequately rehabilitated. Either acute injury or chronic inflammation may lead to the vicious cycle of muscular insufficiency, functional instability, and secondary impingement, which in turn may lead to further injury and inflammation.

The characteristic presentation of acute rotator cuff tears is abrupt onset of pain and weakness (inability to elevate the arm) after forceful loading of the shoulder.

Note that rotator cuff tear associated with other injury is liable to be overlooked. For example, weakness after acute anterior glenohumeral dislocation may be the result of pain inhibition of normal muscle function, associated axillary nerve neurapraxia, or associated rotator cuff tear. It is most important to maintain a high index of suspicion. (The differential diagnosis of profound weakness is discussed above.)

The hallmark physical findings are provoked pain and weakness with manual muscle testing (see Figure 8-11). In the acute setting, with large full-thickness tears of supraspinatus, the patient will typically be unable to initiate shoulder abduction even against gravity resistance.

A drop arm sign is elicited with supraspinatus testing when the patient is able to hold his or her shoulder in 90 degrees of elevation (scaption) against gravity, but with slight additional manual pressure, the shoulder abruptly gives way, and the arm drops. This finding may be elicited with any of the conditions causing profound weakness (see above) and is not pathognomonic of rotator cuff tear.

Abrupt or ratchetlike (cogwheel) giving-way on manual muscle testing is more characteristic of either cuff tear or pain inhibition, whereas smooth giving-way—that is, uniform weakness throughout the range of motion—is more characteristic of neuromuscular weakness.

Point tenderness is typically localized to the greater tuberosity with acute supraspinatus and infraspinatus tears, and to the lesser tuberosity with subscapularis tears. Soft tissue swelling and ecchymosis are inconsistent findings. Especially with acute on degenerative tears, even with extensive tearing, there may be very little bleeding.

Subacutely, even with extensive tears, the patient may regain ability to elevate the arm somewhat, albeit with a grossly abnormal pattern of motion. A characteristic compensatory pattern is to use scapulothoracic motion and lateral bending of the torso to sling the arm upwards. Some patients may be able to attain and hold a position of more than 90 degrees of combined glenohumeral or scapulothoracic abduction in this manner. However, they are unlikely to be able to attain a full range of active combined abduction.

With subscapularis tears, there will be pain and weakness with resisted internal rotation of the shoulder. In the acute setting, there is likely to be tenderness, swelling, and ecchymosis localized anteriorly. With isolated infraspinatus tears, there will be pain and weakness with resisted external rotation of the shoulder.

Radiographic examination is indicated. Avulsion of the greater tuberosity as opposed to cuff tear may be demonstrated. Also, if the cuff injury is associated with acute shoulder dislocation or subluxation, any of the radiographic findings associated with those injuries may be present. With extensive cuff tears, a high-riding humeral head (superior subluxation of the humeral head relative to the glenoid fossa with diminished subacromial space) may be noted (Figure 8-27).

Shoulder weakness can often be differentiated by selective local anesthetization as discussed above. Relief of pain but persistence of profound weakness after intraarticular injection is characteristic of large cuff tears.

FIGURE 8-27
Anteroposterior radiograph of the shoulder, status postextensive, full-thickness rotator cuff tear. Note superior subluxation of the humeral head relative to the glenoid fossa and marked glenohumeral osteophytosis.

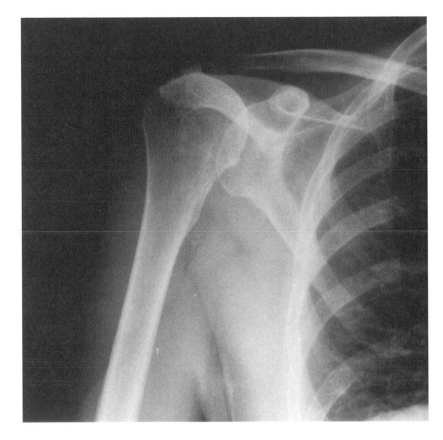

The diagnostic imaging test of choice for demonstrating subtle or gross cuff tears is MRI arthrography. Gross tears can also quite reliably be demonstrated with plain arthrography or plain MRI. The decision regarding diagnostic imaging may be deferred to the surgical consultant.

Treatment. Initial treatment comprises standard symptomatic and protective measures for musculotendinous injury: relative rest (use of sling or shoulder immobilizer prn), intermittent icing, nonsteroidal anti-inflammatory or analgesic medication, and gentle active or active-assisted range of motion exercises as tolerated (Figure 8-28).

Cuff tear does not necessarily imply a need for surgical intervention. Depending on the demands to be placed on the shoulder, many partial-thickness and small full-thickness rotator cuff tears can be adequately treated with appropriate functional rehabilitation. Nonoperative, rehabilitative treatment also can be helpful in reducing pain and maintaining functional motion in patients with large tears who for whatever reason are not candidates for surgery.

Very severe injury (e.g., complete cuff avulsion) is a clear indication for surgery in virtually any active patient. Referral on recognition of the problem is appropriate.

Large, full-thickness tears with profound weakness are generally best treated surgically. Injury to the dominant side, intended or desired return to shoulder-strenuous occupation or sport, and younger age are factors that would favor surgical referral early on. If these factors do not pertain, or if the patient is averse to surgery, or if the patient is a poor surgical risk, a cautious "wait and see" approach may be elected. In a month or so, the acute effects of the injury should have subsided; if considerable pain or disability persists, referral is indicated.

A caveat with respect to a "wait and see" approach is that over time, the torn cuff will retract proximally, the gap between the torn ends will widen, and repair will become technically more difficult. As this occurs, some patients will develop worsening of their symptoms, further functional impairment, and eventually arthropathy. They (and in some cases their physicians) may belatedly come to the conclusion that surgery would have been appropriate. There is no reliable way to predict which patients will do well and which will not. Certainly, surgical options are greater and outcomes better if surgery is carried out before irreversible changes have occurred. For the primary physician, probably the best way out of this conundrum is to advise patients of the

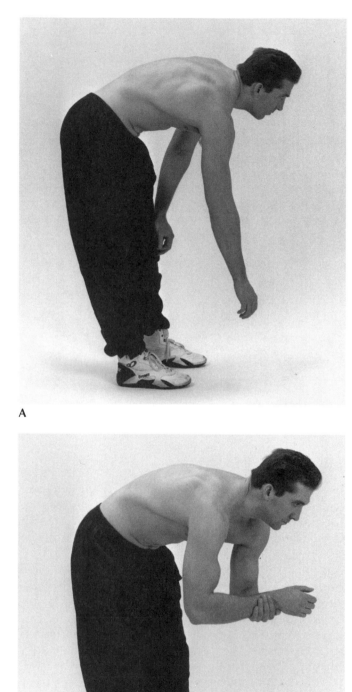

A

B

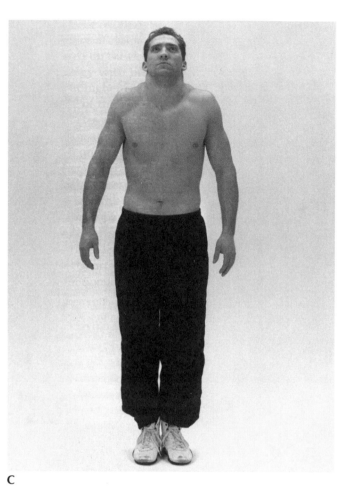

C

FIGURE 8-28
A–E. Gravity-resisted, endurance, and range of motion exercises for the shoulder. A and B. Codman pendulum exercises: unassisted (A) and assisted by the other limb (B). C–E. Additional fungo exercises (shrugs, saws, and swings, respectively).

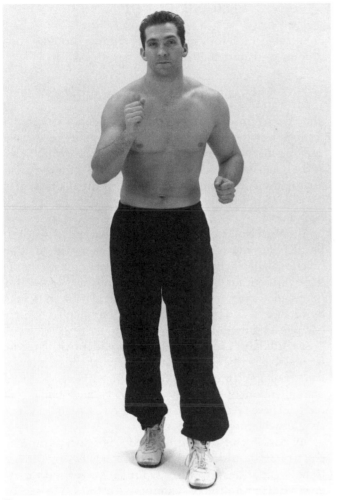

D

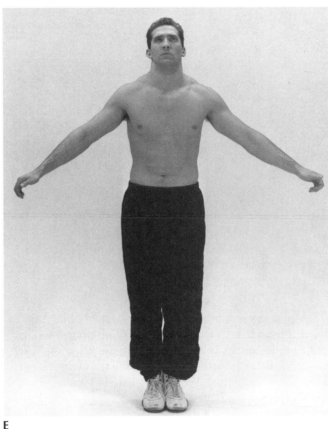

E

natural history and the uncertain prognosis and to consult early on if surgical treatment might ever seem to be a consideration.

Surgical repair of cuff tears most often entails sewing the proximal edge of the torn cuff down into the humerus as opposed to sewing the tendon stumps together. Typically, to protect the repair, coracoacromial arch decompression would be done at the same time. It would also be important to have identified and to address any instability problem, such as a fibrocartilaginous Bankart lesion.

Many cases of partial-thickness tears will do well with nonoperative treatment. If the patient is unable to resume a desired level of activity without recurrence of symptoms and is willing to consider surgical treatment, he or she should be referred. Surgery for partial-thickness tears is more likely to include cuff debridement (as opposed to cuff repair), with arch decompression and Bankart repair as may be indicated.

Acute or Acute on Degenerative Tears of the Tendon of the Long Head of the Biceps

Acute tears of the tendon of the long head of the biceps typically occur with abrupt, forceful, eccentric loading (resisted elbow extension), such as may occur with attempting to catch a heavy object slipping from one's (supinated forearm) grasp. As with rotator cuff tears, acute on degenerative tears can occur with lesser external forces.

The acute rupture is commonly associated with a perceptible "pop" or tearing sensation. There may be pain associated with the acute injury, or pain relief with acute tears of an inflamed tendon. Typically, the patient will be aware of the characteristic ecchymosis and deformity.

The hallmark physical finding is a "Popeye" deformity of the anterior arm (Figure 8-29). The distal bunching up of the long (lateral) head muscle belly is accentuated with resisted elbow flexion.

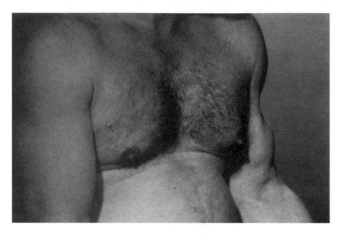

FIGURE 8-29
Complete rupture of the tendon of the long head of the biceps with prominent retracted muscle belly of the biceps.

Because the tendon is no longer attached at its origin, manual muscle testing is not especially pain provoking, and because of the action of synergistic muscles, there may be little or no weakness with resisted elbow flexion or forearm supination. There is likely to be weakness with Speed test (see Figure 8-12).

In the acute setting, dependent ecchymosis of the anterior and medial arm is common. Radiographic examination and other diagnostic tests are not required.

Initial treatment is symptomatic. Specific treatment is not usually required. Any residual disuse shoulder girdle or upper limb motion or strength deficits can usually be readily and adequately addressed with home program exercises. In the overhand athlete, shoulder overuse symptoms on return to activity may require physical therapy emphasizing shoulder stabilization.

Referral and definitive treatment are indicated if the patient is concerned about cosmesis or if there is residual symptomatic glenohumeral instability unresponsive to rehabilitative treatment. Strength deficit is seldom a problem, even in individuals doing heavy manual labor, and is not an indication for surgical intervention. Surgical treatment typically entails tenodesis of the distal stump to the proximal humerus, not reattachment to the superior glenoid.

As discussed below, conditions causing degenerative tears of the tendon of the long head of the biceps are also liable to cause degenerative tears of the rotator cuff. The disabling effect of the combined injury has long been appreciated.[27, 43] Thus, for the patient who has sustained an acute on degenerative tear of the long head of the biceps, referral for assessment of the status of the cuff may be appropriate.

CHRONIC CONDITIONS

For an algorithm for evaluation of chronic shoulder conditions, see Figure 8-30.

Shoulder Overuse Syndrome

Shoulder overuse injuries represent maladaptations to the repetitive stresses of an activity or activities. The maladaptations may be structural or functional or both. Any of the bones and joints of the shoulder girdle, the dynamic neuromusculotendinous units acting at these joints, and the static fibrocartilaginous stabilizers of the joints may be involved.

Although isolated problems (e.g., rotator cuff tendinitis) do occur, much more commonly, several structures or functional mechanisms are involved. The "typical" shoulder overuse injury, therefore, is a composite of several things gone awry, including structural injuries, muscular dysfunctions, and failed compensatory mechanisms, each complicating the other.

Accordingly, I prefer the term "shoulder overuse syndrome" to describe the clinical problem. Labeling the problem "tendinitis," "bursitis," or "impingement" tends to focus one's attention too narrowly, too quickly, and often incorrectly. These terms should not be used as synonyms for shoulder overuse syndrome.

My concept of the pathophysiology and pathomechanics of shoulder overuse injury has evolved over time. Neer's[7] description of clinical stages with progressive deterioration of symptoms, function, and pathologic changes remains valid; however, it now seems clear that not all shoulder pain related to overhand activity is necessarily attributable to impingement of the cuff and long head of the biceps against the coracoacromial arch. Accordingly, I choose not to label overuse strain or tendinitis of the rotator cuff as "stage 1 impingement." The term "primary impingement" corresponds closely to Neer's (stage 2 and 3) "impingement lesions." The term "secondary impingement" follows the terminology of Jobe.[44]

The terms "thrower's shoulder," "swimmer's shoulder," "weight lifter's shoulder," and so forth do not denote any specific diagnostic entities. These terms simply connote the sports settings in which shoulder overuse injuries commonly occur.

Semantics notwithstanding, the multiple possible components of the clinical problem should be appreciated and, as discussed below, treated in proper sequence. The examiner should look for each of the following:

FIGURE 8-30
Algorithm for evaluation of chronic shoulder conditions. (C-spine = cervical spine; DJD = degernerative joint disease.)

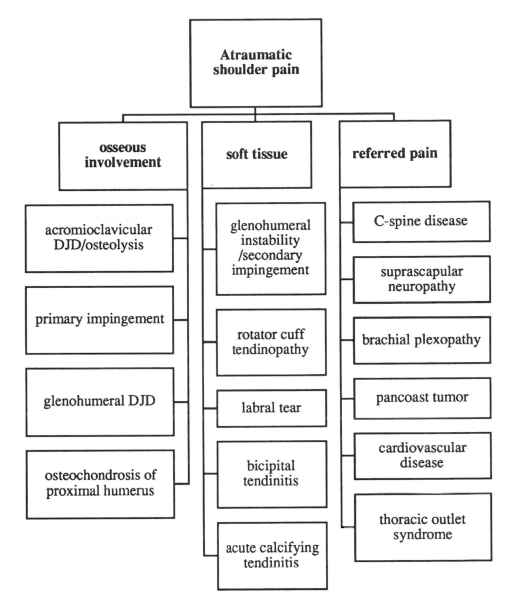

- Scapular stabilizing muscle insufficiency or dysfunction
- (Structural) glenohumeral laxity or contracture (most commonly, anterior laxity or posterior contracture)
- Rotator cuff overuse strain, tendinitis, tendinosis, degenerative tear, insufficiency (functional glenohumeral laxity)
- Long head of biceps overuse strain, tendinitis, tendinosis, degenerative tear, tendon subluxation, insufficiency
- Acromioclavicular degenerative joint disease or distal clavicular osteolysis
- Primary impingement (acromial, acromioclavicular, coracoclavicular, coracoid)

- Secondary impingement (anterior, posterior, and lateral; secondary to glenohumeral laxity or contracture or rotator cuff insufficiency)
- Glenohumeral degenerative joint disease or "cuff arthropathy"

As is true for overuse injury in general, successful treatment and prevention of recurrence depends as much on determining the etiology of the problem as on establishing a precise diagnosis. The etiology of overuse injury is virtually always multifactorial, and three broad categories of causes are sought:

- Physiologic—usually an abrupt increase in physical demand on the shoulder, which, at least in retrospect, would be considered a "training error"
- Anatomic—frequently the residual of undertreated or incompletely rehabilitated prior acute injury
- Mechanical

For most shoulder overuse injuries, and certainly for any injury that does not resolve promptly and completely with initial basic treatment, the essential diagnostic and therapeutic task is to identify and to reverse as many of the causative factors as possible.

Structural injury does not necessarily imply a need for surgical intervention. Depending on the severity of the structural injury and the demands to be placed on the shoulder, many structural problems (e.g., partial-thickness and small full-thickness rotator cuff tears) can be adequately compensated if appropriate functional rehabilitation is carried out.

Acromioclavicular Degenerative Joint Disease or Distal Clavicular Osteolysis

Acromioclavicular degenerative joint disease is commonly a sequela of acute injury. As discussed in the previous section dealing with acute injuries, degenerative changes may follow any acute acromioclavicular sprain, regardless of grade.[16-23]

In weight lifters and male gymnasts, degenerative changes may also occur without definite antecedent injury.[45] With these activities, the joint is subject to repetitive, high, combined sheer and compression loads.

The hallmark symptom of acromioclavicular arthritis is activity-related, aching *pain* localized to the top of the shoulder. Pain with daily, athletic, or occupational activities involving horizontal flexion of the shoulder—such as that which occurs with swinging a baseball bat or a golf club—is characteristic. A painful arc of motion with certain weight lifts—especially overhead press, bench press, bench flies, and dips—is also typical but by no means pathognomonic. With any of these activities, the patient may note crepitation and pain. Positional night pain with inability to sleep on the affected side is very common.

In addition, whether or not the joint itself is painful, acromioclavicular swelling and osteophytosis may be a cause of shoulder impingement pain.

The hallmark physical findings are point tenderness over the acromioclavicular joint and pain provocation with acromioclavicular joint compression tests (see Figure 8-13). There may also be deformity from antecedent injury, palpable enlargement (effusion or osteophytosis) of the joint, or crepitation with motion.

Radiographic examination is indicated. Degenerative changes of the acromioclavicular joint will usually be well demonstrated on standard shoulder views and acromioclavicular views. Depending on the stage of the degenerative joint disease, as well as on the effects of antecedent acute injury, the joint may appear abnormally widened or narrowed. A common finding in young strength athletes is concave erosion (osteolysis) of the distal clavicle, as opposed to the osteophytosis and gonarthrosis (joint space narrowing) more typically seen in older athletes.

The extent to which a given patient's shoulder pain is attributable to acromioclavicular arthritis can be confirmed by selective local anesthetic injection of the joint. A caveat for the clinician is that although postinjection pain relief is diagnostic, the converse is not true. That is, lack of pain relief after injection of the acromioclavicular joint does not rule out acromioclavicular degenerative joint disease as a possible cause of shoulder impingement pain.

Treatment. The mainstay of initial treatment is relative rest. This often involves avoidance or modification of certain offending activities, such as push-ups, bench press, overhead press, and so forth. If there is pain with activities of daily living and occupation, then complete rest (i.e., use of a sling) is recommended. Other initial treatment measures include nonsteroidal anti-inflammatory medication, ice massage, and physical therapy modalities.

Local anesthetic or corticosteroid injection may be used as a diagnostic and possibly therapeutic measure. Because the definitive treatment for chronic acromioclavicular pain is resection of the distal clavicle,[22] there is little cause for concern regarding the use of intraarticular corticosteroids when simpler measures have not afforded satisfactory relief of symptoms.

The duration of pain relief after corticosteroid injection is quite variable. For the individual who is able to limit or to modify the pain-provoking activity (e.g., a strength athlete who has pain only with overhead press at 90 degrees of shoulder abduction), the pain relief may be indefinite. For the patient who is unable or unwilling to comply with activity and rehabilitation recommendations (e.g., an individual whose occupation requires strenuous or prolonged overhead work), pain may recur within a week or two.

Associated shoulder motion and (especially deltoid and trapezius) strength deficits are rehabilitated.

In most cases, symptomatic treatment and activity modification will permit the athlete to return to sports participation. If the athlete is unable to resume a desired level of activity without recurrence of symptoms and is willing to consider surgical treatment, he or she should be referred to an orthopedist. Chronic acromioclavicular pain is definitively treated by resection of the distal clavicle as described by Mumford.[22] Postoperatively, patients are generally able to resume heavyweight wrestling and weight training, football line play, and other shoulder-strenuous activities without symptoms or functional impairment.

Structural Glenohumeral Instability (Anterior Laxity or Posterior Contracture)

As an overuse injury, abnormal glenohumeral laxity occurs when repetitive stresses are applied to the stabilizing structures of the shoulder at a rate exceeding that of tissue repair.[8] Over time, the capsule and ligaments become attenuated and lax. Degenerative tearing of the glenoid labrum or detachment of the labrum and capsule from the glenoid (Bankart and SLAP lesions) may occur.

This mechanism of injury pertains mainly to throwing, racquet sports, and swimming. The direction of the resultant instability is anterior. In throwing, the anterior stabilizing structures are subject to repetitive high stress during the late cocking and acceleration phases of the throwing motion; in swimming, during the catch and early pull phases of the strokes.

Laxity of the static (fibrocartilaginous) anterior stabilizing structures has the effect of permitting anterior subluxation of the shoulder during overhand activities if not compensated by action of the dynamic (musculotendinous) stabilizers of the joint. These structures, however, are also liable to overuse injury with the same activities. As compensatory mechanisms fail and subluxation becomes chronic, contracture of the posterior ligaments and capsule can occur. This has the effect of forcing the anterior subluxation.

Anterior glenohumeral laxity can be exacerbated by ill-advised strength training and stretching techniques. Push-ups, bench press (including incline and decline presses), bench flies, and dips place similar stresses on the anterior stabilizing structures, as does throwing. Use of the inverted bar for bench pressing or doing deep push-ups between chairs are especially bad in this regard. Classic pectoralis stretches (e.g., corner push-ups, wall stretches, door-jamb stretches, and buddy stretches), which use the upper limb as a lever arm, actually stretch or stress the anterior shoulder much more than the pectorals (Figure 8-31).

Abnormal glenohumeral laxity may also be congenital or the result of acute trauma. The clinical significance for the throwing athlete or swimmer is the same as for that resulting from repetitive trauma.

Frank instability symptoms—"My shoulder goes out of place"—are uncommon. Pain with overhand activities is most often attributable to rotator cuff overuse strain, tendinitis, or secondary impingement. Pain associated with labral tear or detachment is characteristically intermittent and positional. For example, in throwing, pain is most likely to be noted at the end of late cocking or start of acceleration, when there is maximal horizontal extension and external rotation of the shoulder. The athlete may also be aware of a click associated with such pain.

The range of internal and external rotation of the 90-degree abducted shoulder is the best measure of structural glenohumeral laxity. With the typical "thrower's shoulder," there will be increased external rotation reflecting anterior laxity and decreased internal rotation reflecting posterior contracture (see Figure 8-24).

In throwing athletes and swimmers, what constitutes abnormal anterior laxity versus physiologic adaptation to the activity is not always clear. Up to 120 degrees of external rotation of the 90-degree abducted shoulder is probably within normal limits for these athletes. Any limitation of internal rotation or any pain at the limit of external rotation is, however, clearly abnormal.

In the skeletally immature, or in the skeletally mature who began throwing or swimming at an early age, an increased range of external rotation and decreased range of internal rotation may be the result, in part, of bony torsion, as opposed to capsuloligamentous changes.

A painful arc of combined glenohumeral or scapulothoracic abduction with the shoulder externally rotated and positive apprehension and containment tests are characteristic, but not pathognomonic, of structural injury, such as labral tear or detachment (see Figure 8-14).

Shoulder series radiographs are indicated if symptoms have been present for more than a few weeks. Bony Bankart lesions and glenohumeral degenerative changes are sought. The diagnostic imaging test of choice is the MRI arthrogram (see Figure 8-21).

Isokinetic testing can sometimes corroborate a positive containment test. If the isokinetic device is set up properly so its axis of rotation is centered on the center of the glenohumeral joint, there may be provoked pain and demonstrable weakness on manual muscle testing, but little or no pain and good strength with isokinetic testing. This is indicative of abnormal glenohumeral laxity and secondary impingement.

The clinical significance of structural instability is twofold:

- The ligamentous, capsular, or labral injury may be painful in and of itself.
- More commonly, the abnormal laxity will result in secondary impingement problems.

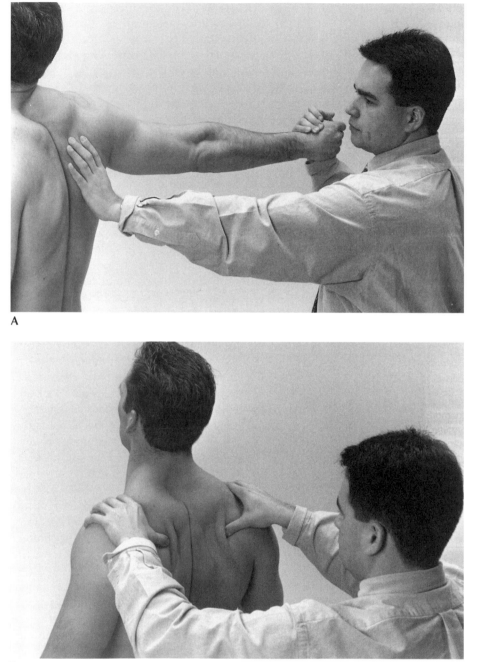

A

B

FIGURE 8-31
*A. "Buddy" stretch. Stretches such as
this, which use the upper limb as a
lever arm, place undue stress on the
anterior stabilizing structures of the
shoulder. They are generally ill-
advised, especially for throwing athletes. For individuals with secondary
impingement, they are contraindicated.
B. Appropriate stretching techniques
for the anterior chest muscles do not
use the upper limb as a lever arm.*

Treatment. Structural anterior laxity cannot be changed nonoperatively. However, the ability to compensate for it can be markedly improved by physical therapy (supervised rotator cuff endurance and functional stability training). Posterior capsular contracture can (and should) be readily addressed with an appropriate stretching program.

Referral and definitive treatment is indicated in case of failure of nonoperative treatment. Surgical treatment may include both labral debridement and Bankart repair and is guided by the MRI arthrographic and intraoperative findings.

Preventive Measures. Throwing athletes and swimmers should be instructed to avoid other activities that place undue stress on the anterior stabilizers of the shoulder (e.g., wall stretches and full-arc bench press). They should be encouraged to maintain flexibility of posterior capsule and maintain rotator cuff endurance to minimize the clinical consequences of any anterior laxity that may be present.

Rotator Cuff Overuse Strain, Tendinitis, Tendinosis, Degenerative Tear, Insufficiency

The rotator cuff comprises four muscles (subscapularis, supraspinatus, infraspinatus, and teres minor) and their tendons. Acting as a force coupled with larger muscles that insert further distally on the humerus (deltoid, pectoralis major, and latissimus dorsi), the rotator cuff and long head of biceps maintain the axes of shoulder motion centered at the glenohumeral joint.

The supraspinatus and infraspinatus are particularly liable to overuse strain and associated muscle soreness and tendinitis with repetitive or prolonged overhand activities. As discussed above, the cuff is subject to high tensile loads during the late cocking, acceleration, and especially the deceleration phases of throwing. When repetitive stresses are applied at a rate exceeding that of tissue repair, tendinosis (tendon degeneration) occurs. Over time, tendon changes may become irreversible, and degenerative tearing may occur.

In addition, the cuff is liable to abrasion injury with primary and secondary impingement problems. Over time, this also may lead to tendinosis and degenerative tearing.

As a very general rule, cuff failure that is due to excessive tensile loading is first manifested as fraying of the articular (deep) surface of the tendon(s), whereas failure that is due to anterior and lateral impingement is manifested as fraying of the bursal (superficial) surface. Failure that is due to posterior impingement involves the posterosuperior aspect of the articular surface.

The hallmark symptom of rotator cuff tendinitis is toothache-quality pain related to (i.e., during or after) overhand activities of daily living, occupation, and sports. As for other overuse injuries, there is often a progression of symptoms. At first, there may be moderate postexercise pain only. Subsequently, there may be increasing pain during athletic activity. By the time the athlete presents for treatment, there may be constant, aching pain, exacerbated even by routine activities of daily living (e.g., lifting a carton of milk).

Characteristically, the pain is not well localized to the shoulder, but rather referred to the lateral arm, as far distally as the insertion of the deltoid. Pain at night with inability to sleep on the affected side or with the arm overhead is a common symptom.

The hallmark physical findings of musculotendinous overuse injury are point tenderness over the involved muscles and tendons and pain reproduced with specific muscle testing (see Figure 8-11). Point tenderness is sought over the muscle bellies of supraspinatus and infraspinatus, the greater tuberosity (supraspinatus and infraspinatus insertion), and the lesser tuberosity (subscapularis insertion). Impingement testing is likely to be positive (see Figure 8-9). There is also likely to be a painful arc of combined glenohumeral or scapulothoracic abduction.

Shoulder series radiographs are indicated if symptoms have been present for more than a few weeks or if pain is especially severe. With calcific tendinitis or bursitis, heterotopic calcification may be demonstrated. The diagnostic imaging test of choice is the MRI arthrogram (see Figure 8-19).

Isokinetic testing provides a quantitative assessment of muscle power and, as discussed above, may permit muscle testing to be carried out without impingement pain.

Treatment. The mainstay of initial treatment is relative rest. If there is pain with activities of daily living and occupation, then complete rest (i.e., use of a sling) is recommended. Other initial treatment measures include nonsteroidal anti-inflammatory medication, ice massage, physical therapy modalities, and McConnell techniques. For calcific tendinitis or bursitis, corticosteroid injection is recommended.

Treatment consisting solely of symptomatic and anti-inflammatory measures for tendinitis and bursitis will be doomed to failure. The pain is bound to recur when the athlete attempts to return to sports. The key to successful treatment is identification and correction of the specific muscular insufficiencies. A trial of rehabilitative treatment is generally indicated, even with MRI-confirmed, full-thickness cuff tears.

The athlete who is unable to resume a desired level of activity without recurrence of symptoms should be counseled regarding the risks of continuing the activity (e.g., worsening of the tendinitis or tendinosis, worsening of functional instability, wear and tear on the articular surfaces). The recreational or fitness athlete should be advised of alternative activities that do not place as much stress on the shoulder. A swimmer, for example, may be able to swim breaststroke rather than freestyle. A weight lifter may be able to substitute limited arc lifts for bench press, dips, and flies. If, despite appropriate rehabilitation and realistic activity modification, disabling symptoms persist, then orthopedic referral is indicated.

A surgical caveat is that unless the associated gleno-humeral instability (secondary impingement) and primary impingement problems are appropriately addressed, cuff repair is likely to fail. Preoperative and intraoperative assessment of glenohumeral stability is therefore critical. Therefore, operative treatment may entail, in addition to debridement and repair of the rotator cuff, a Bankart repair and coracoacromial arch decompression.

Preventive Measures. For swimmers and throwing, racquet sports, and strength athletes, "prehabilitation" rotator cuff progressive resistance exercises, identical to the rehabilitation exercises discussed below, should be incorporated into the year-round training regimen. Frequency, duration, and intensity of exercise should be kept within the limits of relative rest. Athletes should anticipate increased demands (e.g., start of team practice), allot adequate time for preparation and adaptation, and thereby avoid training error problems. Mechanical and technical problems predisposing to injury should be identified and corrected; for this, working with a knowledgeable coach is most helpful. Coaches and parents of young athletes should emphasize participation, fun, and motor skill learning over winning—if for no other reason, to lessen the temptation of overusing the shoulders of the most talented young athletes.

Long Head of Biceps Overuse Strain, Tendinitis, Tendinosis, Degenerative Tear, Tendon Subluxation, Insufficiency

Similar mechanisms apply as with overuse injury of the rotator cuff. In addition, the long head of biceps, more so than the rotator cuff, is liable to overuse injury in fast-pitch softball pitching. (The acceleration phase of the underhand pitching motion entails rapid, forceful shoulder flexion from a cocked position of extreme shoulder extension.)

The hallmark symptom of tendinitis is activity-related pain, characteristically localized to the anterior shoulder and arm. In addition to pain with overhand activities and softball pitching, there may be pain with activities, especially lifting, that entail forceful shoulder or elbow flexion or forearm supination. Subluxation of the tendon of the long head of the biceps out of the bicipital groove typically presents as painful anterior snapping with shoulder motion.

The hallmark physical findings are point tenderness over the bicipital groove and anterior arm and pain reproduced with specific muscle testing (Speed and Yergason tests; see Figure 8-12). Impingement testing is likely to be positive (see Figure 8-9). Tendon subluxation may be

reproduced with a modified Yergason test in which, concomitantly with supinating the forearm against resistance, the patient also attempts to externally rotate the shoulder against the examiner's resistance.

If symptoms have been present for more than a few weeks or if pain is especially severe, shoulder series radiographs are indicated as part of the general workup. Other diagnostic tests are not required unless surgical treatment of tendon subluxation or tear is being considered, in which case the clinical diagnosis may be confirmed by MRI.

Initial and rehabilitative treatment follow the same general plan as for tendinitis in general and as for rotator cuff overuse injury as discussed. Referral or definitive treatment is indicated for chronic, painful tendon subluxation or possibly for tendon rupture.

Primary Impingement (Acromial, Acromioclavicular, Coracoclavicular, Coracoid)

The term "impingement" may properly be used to describe a physical examination finding, a structural abnormality (primary impingement), or a mechanical dysfunction (secondary impingement). Primary impingement implies bony or ligamentous encroachment on the subacromial space capable of impinging on the subacromial bursa, the rotator cuff, and the tendon of the long head of the biceps and causing or exacerbating injury, inflammation, or pain.

As previously discussed, there is not a one-to-one correlation between activity-related shoulder pain and primary impingement. Rather, the diagnosis of primary impingement is made when characteristic physical, radiographic, and MRI findings (e.g., osteophytosis) are noted in an appropriate clinical setting (e.g., pain with overhand activities or a positive impingement test).

Primary impingement may be congenital or acquired. The latter is by far the more common, usually the result of degenerative bone and joint changes occurring over years of shoulder-strenuous activity. Encroachment may be from the lateral or anterior aspect of the acromion, the acromioclavicular joint, the coracoacromial ligament, and the coracoid process (Figure 8-32).

Treatment. Treatment options are essentially twofold: (1) activity modification or limitation (relative rest) and (2) surgical intervention (coracoacromial arch decompression). A typical operative procedure might include acromioplasty, resection of the distal clavicle (Mumford procedure), and resection of the coracoacromial ligament.

Secondary Impingement (Anterior, Posterior, and Lateral; Secondary to Glenohumeral Laxity or Contracture or Rotator Cuff Insufficiency)

Activity-related shoulder pain may be the result of musculotendinous overuse strain or tendinitis; an internal derangement, such as a glenoid labral tear; or impingement of inflamed tendons and bursae between the humeral head and the coracoacromial arch. That impingement occurs does not necessarily imply that there is insufficient space to accommodate the impinged structures. Especially in the athletically active, impingement pain is commonly secondary to (1) structural glenohumeral laxity or contracture (most commonly anterior laxity or posterior contracture); or (2) insufficiency of the stabilizing muscles of the shoulder, which result in functional instability of the shoulder (i.e., subluxation during activity).

This mechanism of injury pertains especially to ballistic overhand activities, such as throwing. During the acceleration phase of throwing, anterior laxity permits anterior subluxation of the shoulder. If uncompensated by action of the rotator cuff or if exacerbated by posterior contracture, the axis of humeral rotation will move anterior to the center of the glenohumeral joint. The eccentric rotation, in turn, may result in impingement of the bursal surface of the cuff anteriorly against the unyielding coracoacromial arch. It may also cause impingement of the articular surface of cuff posteriorly against the sharp posterosuperior edge of the glenoid rim. Abrasion injury of the cuff (mainly to supraspinatus and infraspinatus) is a predictable sequela, given the speed of humeral rotation (up to 7,000 degrees per second) and the repetitiveness of the activity (often more than 100 pitches per day). In swimming, glenohumeral subluxation may similarly lead to cuff impingement anteriorly and laterally against the acromion during the recovery phases of the crawl and butterfly strokes.

In addition, as with other overuse syndromes, a vicious cycle may ensue, whereby pain leads to disuse, which leads to muscular atrophy and dysfunction, which leads to increased vulnerability to injury and recurrence of pain on attempted resumption of activity. Rotator cuff tendinitis or insufficiency is often thus both effect and cause of secondary impingement.

In contrast to primary impingement, which is more common in the older athlete, secondary impingement may affect athletes of any age and should be a primary consideration in evaluating younger individuals.

The hallmark presenting symptom of secondary impingement is pain related to overhand activities: throwing, racquet sports, swimming, weight training, and man-

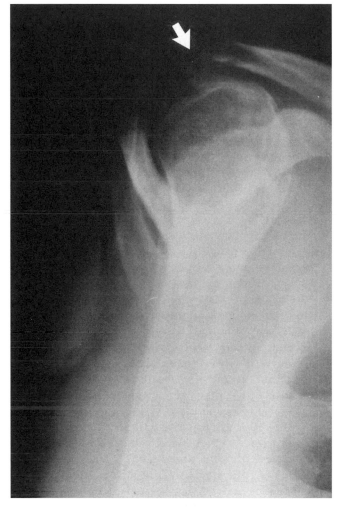

FIGURE 8-32

Lateral scapular radiograph demonstrating acromial osteophytosis (arrow) causing primary impingement of the underlying rotator cuff in a 69-year-old man with full-thickness cuff tear.

ual work. Other symptoms of glenohumeral instability or rotator cuff injury may also be present.

Muscular atrophy and dysfunction, particularly of the rotator cuff, are not always as obvious to the athlete. Attempted return to functional use of the arm before full recovery and rehabilitation can result in recurrence of symptoms.

The hallmark physical finding of symptomatic functional anterior instability is a positive containment test. It is not, however, pathognomonic of any particular structural abnormality. The Iowa shoulder shift test has the same implications. Other findings related to glenohumeral instability or rotator cuff injury may also be present.

Sorting out the following relative contributions of impingement versus tendinitis can help guide both rehabilitative and operative treatment:

- A positive impingement test with little or no pain or weakness on manual muscle testing within a pain-free range of motion suggests the problem is mainly impingement.
- A negative impingement test and pain and weakness with manual muscle testing suggest the problem is mainly rotator cuff strain or tendinitis.
- A positive impingement test with acromioclavicular tenderness and positive acromioclavicular compression tests suggest primary acromioclavicular impingement is likely.
- A positive containment test or shoulder shift test indicates that the problem is attributable at least in part to secondary impingement and that injury to anterior stabilizing structures is likely.

Indications for radiographic examination and MRI arthrography are as discussed for structural glenohumeral laxity, rotator cuff overuse injury, and acromioclavicular degenerative joint disease (see Figure 8-20).

Initial and rehabilitative treatment is discussed below. Most cases of secondary impingement, not complicated by advanced degenerative changes causing primary impingement or extensive structural injury, can be successfully treated by nonoperative means.

Treatment. Referral and definitive treatment is indicated mainly for structural glenohumeral laxity that remains inadequately compensated after an appropriate trial of rehabilitative treatment.

Glenohumeral Degenerative Joint Disease or "Cuff Arthropathy"

After extensive full-thickness tear of the rotator cuff, action of the deltoid causes superior subluxation of the glenohumeral joint before initiation of arm elevation. Dynamically, the shoulder joint thus becomes an acromiohumeral joint.

Some individuals seem to tolerate this condition quite well for many years. Once the effects of acute injury have subsided and any residual frozen shoulder symptoms have resolved, they may have little or no pain and little or no functional impairment with customary activities of daily living. The shoulder does, however, remain weak, and strenuous overhand activities (e.g., throwing or racquet sports) are likely to be at least somewhat painful or impaired.

Others seem to do exceedingly poorly, having constant pain (especially night pain) and marked functional impairment. Typically, advanced glenohumeral degenerative changes can be confirmed on radiographic examination (see Figure 8-27).

Treatment. The arthropathy would seem related to functional instability of the shoulder, as opposed to the cuff tear per se. Instability from capsuloligamentous laxity can also lead to arthropathy over time.

In either case, treatment is surgical and would ideally be carried out before marked symptomatic and functional deterioration and radiographically demonstrated degenerative changes have occurred.

A surgical caveat relates to decompression of the coracoacromial arch. If the torn cuff is repairable, then decompression to protect the repair is generally indicated. If, however, the cuff is not repairable, then decompression is contraindicated; it would render the functional acromiohumeral joint unstable, more likely exacerbate than alleviate activity-related pain, and limit future surgical (arthroplasty) options.

Rehabilitative Treatment of Shoulder Overuse Injuries

Most cases of shoulder overuse syndrome can be adequately treated with appropriate functional rehabilitation as presented in the following paragraphs. This is true, within certain limits of severity of injury and demands to be placed on the shoulder, even for cases in which structural injuries (e.g., glenoid labral tears and partial- or small, full-thickness rotator cuff tears) may be present.

Sequential objectives to be achieved are as follows:

- Reduction of pain and inflammation
- Restoration of scapular stabilizing muscle function
- Restoration of range of (glenohumeral) motion
- Restoration of normal glenohumeral scapulothoracic patterns of motion
- Restoration of (rotator cuff and long head of biceps) muscular endurance
- Restoration of strength
- Return to full function and shoulder-strenuous occupational and athletic activities

Experience has shown that carrying out rehabilitative treatment in the proper sequence is critical. For example, attempting strength training before a normal pattern of motion has been reestablished simply reinforces the abnormal pattern. A recommended treatment and rehabilitation sequence with specific treatment objectives and techniques for each step and criteria for advancement to the next step is presented in outline form in Table 8-1. Specific techniques and rehabilitation exercises are also illustrated in Figures 8-28 and 8-33.

TABLE 8-1
Rehabilitation Protocol for the Shoulder Overuse Syndrome

Level 0 (acute painful episode,* continuous or severe rest pain, severe night pain)
Objectives:
  Reduce pain, swelling, inflammation
Rx:
  Rest; sling or shoulder immobilizer prn
  Local anesthetic or corticosteroid injection(s)—intraarticular (glenohumeral and acromioclavicular), bursal, peritendinous, trigger point
  Analgesics, anti-inflammatory medication prn
  Modalities to reduce pain and limit and reduce swelling
  Gentle glenohumeral oscillatory mobilization techniques
  Gentle active-assisted range of motion (e.g., limited-arc, assisted Codman) as tolerated
  Static posture correction, isometric "scap sets," as tolerated
Activities permitted:
  Necessary manual activities of daily living and occupation as tolerated
  Active arm elevation limited to <45 degrees
  No prolonged or repetitive arm elevation or shoulder horizontal flexion
  No lifting >10 lb (shoulder adducted)
Criteria for advancement:
  Rest and night pain substantially reduced
  Able to sleep
Level I (activity-limiting pain)
Objectives:
  Reduce pain, swelling, inflammation
  Restore or maintain scapular stabilizing muscular endurance, strength, and function
  Restore or maintain glenohumeral motion
Rx:
  Relative rest; occasional sling prn postactivity pain, fatigue
  Analgesics, anti-inflammatory medication prn
  Local anesthetic or corticosteroid injection(s) prn with precaution in regards to activity
  Modalities to reduce pain and limit and reduce swelling
  McConnell taping
  Gentle active range of motion (e.g., Codman) exercises, as tolerated
  Moderate active-assisted range of motion exercises (e.g., cane and wall-climb exercises), as tolerated
  Isometric "scap sets"
  Osteopathic and "muscle energy" techniques for thoracic dysfunctions
Activities permitted:
  Necessary manual activities of daily living and occupation as tolerated
  Active arm elevation limited to <60 degrees
  No prolonged or repetitive arm elevation or shoulder horizontal flexion
  No lifting >20 lb
  Noncontact sports or exercise involving essentially sagittal plane shoulder motion (e.g., running) as tolerated
Criteria for advancement:
  Activity-related pain substantially reduced
  Rest and night pain virtually abated
Level II (activity-related pain, performance impairment)
Objectives:
  Reduce pain, swelling, inflammation
  Restore or maintain scapular stabilizing muscular

endurance, strength, and function
  Restore or maintain glenohumeral motion
  Restore normal basic patterns of glenohumeral and scapulothoracic motion
  Restore or maintain intrinsic shoulder muscular endurance
Rx:
  Relative rest
  Anti-inflammatory medication
  Modalities to reduce pain and limit and reduce swelling
  McConnell taping
  Active range of motion exercises, as tolerated
  Mobilization techniques (especially posterior capsular stretching), as indicated and tolerated
  Isometric "scap sets"
  Manual and biofeedback techniques for dynamic scapular stabilizing muscular function
  Thera-Band and dumbbell progressive resistance exercises for scapular stabilizing muscles, biceps, and triceps as tolerated
  Upper limb endurance exercise (e.g., upper-body exercise, rowing, rope skipping) as tolerated
Activities permitted:
  Active arm elevation limited to <90 degrees
  No prolonged or repetitive arm elevation
  No lifting >50 lb
Criteria for advancement:
  Pain virtually abated
  Negative Kibler test
  Glenohumeral range of motion comparable to contralateral side
  Pain-free, symmetrical arc of combined motion
Level III (performance impairment)
Objectives:
  Maintain scapular stabilizing muscular endurance, strength, and function
  Maintain glenohumeral motion
  Restore normal complex patterns of glenohumeral and scapulothoracic motion
  Restore or maintain intrinsic shoulder muscular endurance and strength
Rx:
  Relative rest
  McConnell taping
  Stretching as indicated (attention to avoid anterior stretch)
  Isometric "scap sets"
  Manual techniques for dynamic scapular stabilizing muscular function
  Thera-Band progressive resistance exercises for scapular stabilizing muscles, as tolerated
  Upper limb endurance exercise (e.g., upper-body ergometer, rowing, rope skipping) as tolerated
  Thera-Band and dumbbell resistance exercises (flexion, abduction, extension, scaption, 90/90) for intrinsic shoulder muscles, as tolerated
  Fungo return to throwing, serving program
Activities permitted:
  Tennis ground stroke practice, breaststroke swimming, etc.
  No overhead sports or exercise
Criteria for advancement (to full activity):
  Fungo program completed
  Strength on manual muscle testing comparable to contralateral shoulder

*For example, calcific subacromial bursitis and rotator cuff tendinitis.

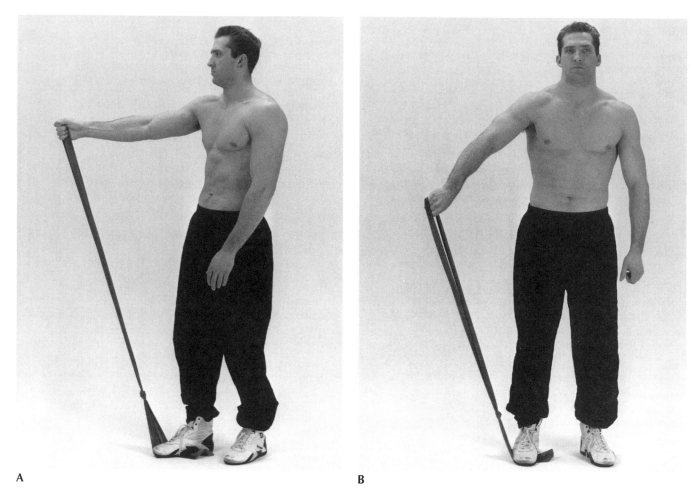

A　　　　　　　　　　　　　　　　　　　　　　　　　B

FIGURE 8-33

A–D. Specific Thera-Band exercises for the anterior deltoid, supraspinatus, and middle and posterior deltoid, respectively.

In most cases of shoulder overuse syndrome, the single most important aspect of rehabilitative treatment is neuromuscular reeducation: "unlearning" abnormal postures and patterns of motion and relearning proper mechanics. Most patients, even athletes with very good "body sense," do not come by this easily. Hands-on motor skill coaching by a physical therapist is indispensable in this regard.

A caveat for the physician and therapist is that the frequency, duration, and intensity of rehabilitative exercise, as well as manipulative treatment and other activities, should be kept within the limits of relative rest. Attention should be paid to any symptoms during or after every session. The odd twinge of pain during activity is perhaps permissible but should be regarded with caution. Pain that persists for more than an hour afterward or is present the following day should be taken as an indication that the activity was excessive.

This is especially true regarding mobilization therapy. Any pain after treatment is probably indicative of an inflammatory response to tissue injury. The patient's response to increased pain will be limitation of active motion, and the net effect of treatment is more likely to be a further decrease rather than increase in range of motion.

Sport-specific functional drills are not begun until full and pain-free shoulder motion has been achieved. For return to baseball pitching, the fungo program described by Kerlan[46] is highly recommended. It can also be readily adapted to other overhand activities (e.g., serving in tennis or volleyball). The fungo program for throwers and a modified fungo program for tennis players are presented in outline form in Table 8-2.

Ideally, there will be a gradually progressive return to full activity as symptoms permit. Absence of symptoms

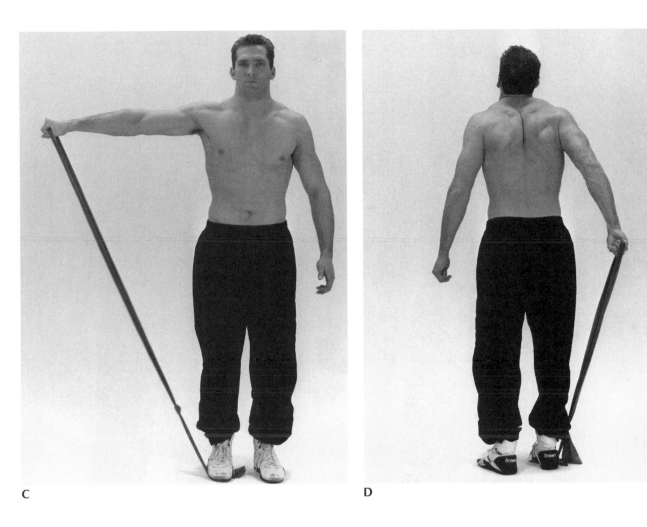

C

D

with an attempted level of activity is the criterion for advancement to that level of activity.

Osteochondrosis of the Proximal Humeral Epiphysis ("Little Leaguer's Shoulder")

The differential diagnosis of "thrower's shoulder syndrome" in the skeletally immature includes injury (osteochondrosis) of the proximal humeral epiphysis, humeral stress fracture, glenoid osteochondrosis,[47] and elastofibroma,[48] all of which are rare.

Given the well-recognized and devastating problem of humeral capitellar osteochondrosis ("Little Leaguer's elbow"), there has been understandable concern about the possibility of similar injury to the shoulders of young throwing athletes. Indeed, overuse injury of the proximal humeral epiphysis—variously described in the lit-

erature as "epiphysitis," "epiphysiolysis," "false osteochondrosis," "fracture," "Little Leaguer's shoulder," "osteochondritis," and "stress fracture"—has been reported. All would appear to be the same entity and to be clinically quite similar to the other repetitive trauma-related osteochondroses (e.g., "Little Leaguer's elbow," Osgood-Schlatter disease [traction apophysitis of the anterior tibial tubercle], and Sever disease [traction apophysitis of the posterior calcaneus]).

To put the problem in perspective, one should note that since it was first described by Dotter in 1953, there have been but 17 reported cases of "Little Leaguer's shoulder" in the English-speaking literature, and as late as 1990, a single case was considered reportable in a refereed journal.[49-56] In contrast, Kibler[57] reported that in his large series of young tennis players with shoulder overuse problems, 90% had the typical findings of

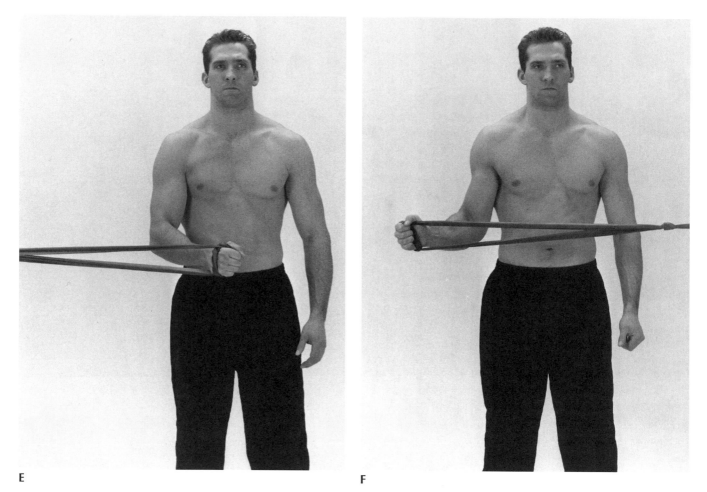

E

F

FIGURE 8-33 *(continued)*

E and F. Specific Thera-Band exercises for internal and external rotation. G and H. The "90/90" dumbbell resistance exercise for the rotator cuff, a recommended position-specific; and muscle action-specific rehabilitation and "prehabilitation" exercise for throwing athletes. From a start position (G), with the shoulder abducted 90 degrees, the dumbbell is lowered to horizontal (H) and raised back up. As the weight is lowered, internal rotation of the shoulder is resisted by eccentric action of the rotator cuff.

"thrower's shoulder syndrome," as presented in the preceding section.

In my experience, virtually all young athletes with throwing-related shoulder pain have essentially the same problems as do skeletally mature athletes. As discussed, the finding of an increased range of external glenohumeral rotation and decreased range of internal rotation in the skeletally immature may be in part the result of bony torsion, as opposed to capsuloligamentous changes. The clinical significance of this is uncertain.

The basic approach for young athletes with "thrower's shoulder syndrome" is the same as for older athletes. The possibility of bony or physeal injury should simply be kept in mind. If, after an appropriate trial of rehabilitative treat-

ment, pain persists or promptly recurs with attempted return to activity, further work-up—including radionuclide scintigraphy or MRI examination—is indicated.

One unique aspect of caring for young athletes is that there is appropriately a greater emphasis on injury prevention. There is a greater opportunity for this as well. Recommended measures for prevention of "thrower's shoulder" problems in young athletes are as follows:

- A preparticipation examination, in which treatable conditions such as posterior glenohumeral capsular contracture and rotator cuff insufficiency are sought
- Rehabilitation of subclinical (asymptomatic) conditions identified on the preparticipation examination

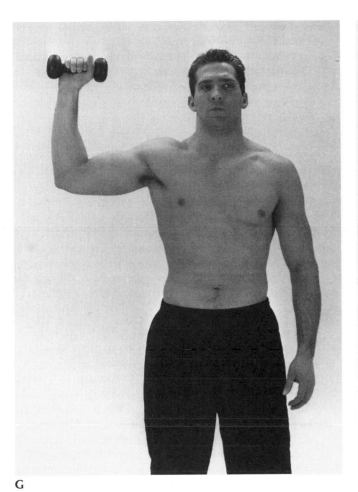

G

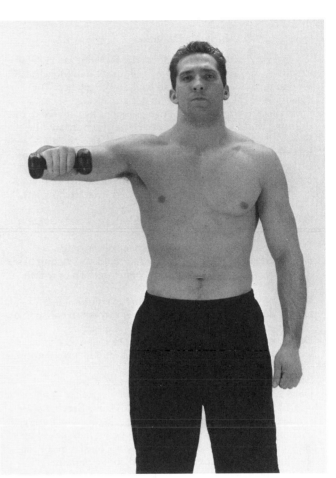

H

- Incorporation of "prehabilitation" stretching and strengthening exercises, identical to the rehabilitation exercises already discussed, into the year-round training regimen
- Keeping frequency, duration, and intensity of all exercise within the limits of relative rest
- Anticipating increased demands (e.g., start of team practice) and allotting adequate time for preparation and adaptation
- Limiting total amount of pitching (especially individual practice additional to games and team practice)
- Learning and practicing proper throwing techniques
- Emphasizing participation, fun, and motor skill learning over winning

Of all of these, parents' deemphasizing winning is probably most important. If Little League moms and dads continually complain, "We lost because you put in Jimmy instead of Johnny," coaches will respond; Johnny will see more time on the mound. How does Johnny then continue to be the team's number-one pitcher or Jimmy try to work his way back into the lineup? Besides natural talent, it is "practice, practice, practice"—a setup for overuse injury.

The effect of throwing different pitches probably also has more to do with competitiveness than technique. To be more competitive, a less talented young pitcher might try to learn to throw a curve ball or slider in addition to his or her fast ball and change-up. More pitches imply

TABLE 8-2
Fungo Return to Throwing Program

The program derives its name from the fact that as originally described, a baseball pitcher would throw to a fungo hitter, who in turn would hit the ball back to the pitcher. The essentials of the fungo program are as follows:

To minimize overuse, the throwing sessions are limited to 30 minutes, and a single ball is used. After each throw, the ball is hit or thrown back to the pitcher. The pitcher is instructed to throw with a full, easy, and painless motion. If there is any pain with attempted throwing, he or she refrains from throwing for 5 days. The sessions are preceded by stretching exercises and followed by stretching and ice massage.

Days 1 and 2: pitcher in center field; throws ball so that it barely rolls to home plate

Day 3: no throwing; continues other exercises

Days 4 and 5: pitcher between center field and second base; throws so ball arrives at home plate on third or fourth bounce

Day 6: no throwing, continues other exercises

Days 7 and 8: pitcher at second base; throws so ball arrives at home plate on the fly (1–2 ft off ground)

Day 9: no throwing; continues other exercises

Days 10 and 11: pitcher on pitcher's mound; throws normal pitches

Day 12: no throwing; continues other exercises

Days 13 and beyond: returns to normal activity

Modified Fungo Program for Return to Tennis Serving

The player selects a court with a high backstop. Only one of three balls is used. The balls must be hit and picked up before they are hit again. All serving is done from the service line. All other conditions noted above pertain.

Days 1 and 2: serves to hit backstop at eye level (5–6 ft off ground)

Day 3: rest; continues other exercises

Days 4 and 5: serves to hit at or near junction of fence and ground

Day 6: rest; continues other exercises

Days 7 and 8: serves to hit backcourt boundary line

Day 9: rest; continues other exercises

Days 10 and 11: serves normally

Day 12: rest; continues other exercises

Days 13 and beyond: returns to normal activity

Source: Adapted from RK Kerlan, FW Jobe, ME Blazina, et al. Throwing injuries of the shoulder and elbow in adults. Curr Pract Orthop Surg 1975;6:41–48.

more practice required to perfect the pitches, which in turn implies greater risk of overuse injury.

REFERENCES

1. Garrick JG, Requa RK. Medical care and injury surveillance in the high school setting. Phys Sportsmed 1981;9:115–120.
2. Neer CS II. Displaced proximal humeral fractures, part 1: classification and evaluation. J Bone Joint Surg Am 1970;52:1077–1089.
3. Matsen FA III, Zuckerman J. Anterior glenohumeral instability. Clin Sports Med 1983;2:319–338.
4. Rockwood CA Jr, Wirth MA. Subluxations and Dislocations About the Glenohumeral Joint. In CA Rockwood Jr, DP Green, JD Heckman, RW Bucholz. (eds), Rockwood and Green's Fractures in Adults (4th ed). Philadelphia: Lippincott–Raven, 1996;1193–1339.
5. Blom S, Dahlback LO. Nerve injuries in dislocations of the shoulder joint and fractures of the neck of the humerus. Acta Chir Scand 1970;136:461–466.
6. Hawkins RJ, Kennedy JC. Impingement syndrome in athletes. Am J Sports Med 1980;8:151–158.
7. Neer CS II. Impingement lesions. Clin Orthop 1983;173: 70–77.
8. Kvitne RS, Jobe FW. The diagnosis and treatment of anterior instability in the throwing athlete. Clin Orthop 1993; 291:107–123.
9. Rowe CR. Acute and recurrent anterior dislocations of the shoulder. Orthop Clin North Am 1980;11:253–270.
10. Bankart ASB. The pathology and treatment of recurrent dislocation of the shoulder joint. Br J Surg 1938;26:23–29.
11. Hill HA, Sachs MD. The grooved defect of the humeral head: a frequently unrecognized complication of dislocations of the shoulder joint. Radiology 1940;35:690–700.
12. Rokous JR, Feagin JA, Abbott HG. Modified axillary roentgenogram. A useful adjunct in the diagnosis of recurrent instability of the shoulder. Clin Orthop 1972;82:84–86.
13. Rockwood CA Jr., Wirth MA. Injuries to the Sternoclavicular Joint. In CA Rockwood Jr, et al. (eds), Fractures in Adults. Philadelphia: Lippincott–Raven, 1996;1415–1471.
14. Selesnick FH, Jablon M, Frank C, Post M. Retrosternal dislocation of the clavicle. Report of four cases. J Bone Joint Surg Am 1984;66:287–291.
15. Buckerfield CT, Castle ME. Acute traumatic retrosternal dislocation of the clavicle. J Bone Joint Surg Am 1984;66:379–385.
16. Allman FL Jr. Fractures and ligamentous injuries of the clavicle and its articulation. J Bone Joint Surg Am 1967;49:774–784.
17. Rockwood CA Jr, Williams GR, Young CD. Injuries to the Acromioclavicular Joint. In CA Rockwood Jr, et al. (eds), Fractures in Adults. Philadelphia: Lippincott–Raven, 1996; 1341–1413.
18. Glick JM, Milburn LJ, Haggerty JF, Nishimoto D. Dislocated acromioclavicular joint: follow-up study of 35 unreduced acromioclavicular dislocations. Am J Sports Med 1977;5:264–270.
19. Nicol EE. Miners and mannequins. J Bone Joint Surg Br 1954;36:171–172.
20. Imatani RJ, Hanlon JJ, Cady GW. Acute complete acromioclavicular separation. J Bone Joint Surg Am 1975;57A:328–332.
21. Bergfeld JA, Andrish JT, Clancy WG. Evaluation of the acromioclavicular joint following first- and second-degree sprains. Am J Sports Med 1978;6:153–159.
22. Mumford EB. Acromioclavicular dislocation. J Bone Joint Surg Am 1941;23:799–802.
23. Walsh WM, Peterson DA, Shelton G, Neumann RD. Shoulder strength following acromioclavicular injury. 1985;13: 153–158.

24. Aronen JG. Anterior shoulder dislocations in sports. Sports Med 1986;3:224–234.

25. Stimson LA. An easy method of reducing dislocations of the shoulder and hip. Medical Record 1900;57:356–357.

26. Kocher T. Eine neue Reductionsmethode fur Schulterverrenkung. Klin (Berlin) 1870;7:101–105.

27. Codman EA. The Shoulder. Boston: Thomas Todd & Co., 1934.

28. Arciero RA, Wheeler JH, Ryan JB, McBride JT. Arthroscopic Bankart repair versus nonoperative treatment for acute, initial anterior shoulder dislocations. Am J Sports Med 1994;22:589–594.

29. Aronen JG, Regan K. Decreasing the incidence of recurrence of first time anterior shoulder dislocations with rehabilitation. Am J Sports Med 1984;12:283–291.

30. Broström LA, Kronberg M, Nemeth G, Oxelback U. The effect of shoulder muscle training in patients with recurrent shoulder dislocations. Scand J Rehabil Med 1992;24:11–15.

31. Protzman RR. Anterior instability of the shoulder. J Bone Joint Surg Am 1980;62:909–918.

32. Rowe CR. The Bankart procedure: a long-term end-result study. J Bone Joint Surg Am 1978;60:1–16.

33. Yoneda B, Welsh RP, MacIntosh DL. Conservative treatment of shoulder dislocation in young males. J Bone Joint Surg Br 1982;64:254–255.

34. McLaughlin HL, MacLellan DL. Recurrent anterior dislocation of the shoulder, II: a comparative study. J Trauma 1967;7:191–201.

35. Rowe CR, Sakellarides HT. Factors related to recurrences of anterior dislocations of the shoulder. Clin Orthop 1961;20:40–47.

36. Kuriyama S, Fujimaki E, Katagiri T, Uemura S. Anterior dislocation of the shoulder sustained through skiing. Arthrographic findings and prognosis. Am J Sports Med 1984;12:339–346.

37. Blazina ME, Satzman JS. Recurrent anterior subluxation of the shoulder in athletes—a distinct entity. J Bone Joint Surg Am 1969;51:1037–1038.

38. Aronen JG. Problems of the upper extremity in gymnastics. Clin Sports Med 1985;4:61–71.

39. Pappas AM, Goss TP, Kleinman PK. Symptomatic shoulder instability due to lesions of the glenoid labrum. Am J Sports Med 1983;11:279–288.

40. Rowe CR, Zarins B. Recurrent transient subluxation of the shoulder. J Bone Joint Surg Am 1981;63:863–871.

41. Warren RF. Subluxation of the shoulder in athletes. Clin Sports Med 1983;2:339–354.

42. Strukel RJ, Garrick JG. Thoracic outlet compression in athletes. Am J Sports Med 1978;6:35–39.

43. Gilcreest EL. The common syndrome of rupture, dislocation, and elongation of the long head of the biceps brachii: an analysis of one hundred cases. Surgery, Gynecology and Obstetrics 1934;58:322–340.

44. Jobe FW, Kvitne RS, Giangarra CE. Shoulder pain in the overhand or throwing athlete: the relationship of anterior instability and rotator cuff impingement [published erratum appears in Orthop Rev 1989;18:1268]. Orthop Rev 1989;18:963–975.

45. Cahill B. Osteolysis of distal part of clavicle in male athletes. J Bone Joint Surg Am 1982;64:1053–1058.

46. Kerlan RK, Jobe FW, Blazina ME, et al. Throwing injuries of the shoulder and elbow in adults. Curr Pract Orthop Surg 1975;6:41–48.

47. Stanley DJ, Mulligan ME. Osteochondrosis dissecans of the glenoid. Skeletal Radiol 1990;19:419–421.

48. Haney TC. Subscapular elastofibroma in a young pitcher: a case report. Am J Sports Med 1990;18:642–644.

49. Adams JE. Little League shoulder osteochondrosis of the proximal humeral epiphysis in boy baseball pitchers. Calif Med Assoc J 1966;105:22.

50. Adams JE. Bone injuries in very young athletes. Clin Orthop 1968;58:129–140.

51. Albert MJ, Drvaric DM. Little League shoulder: case report. Orthopedics 1990;13:779–781.

52. Barnett LS. Little League shoulder syndrome: proximal humeral epiphysiolysis in adolescent baseball pitchers. J Bone Joint Surg Am 1985;67:495–496.

53. Cahill BR. Little League shoulder: lesions of the proximal humeral epiphyseal plate. J Sports Med 1974;2:150–152.

54. Dotter WE. Little Leaguers' shoulder: a fracture of the proximal epiphyseal cartilage of the humerus due to baseball pitching. Guthrie Clinic Bulletin 1953;23:68–72.

55. Torg JS. The Little League pitcher. Am Fam Physician 1972;6:71–76.

56. Tullos HS, Fain RS. Little League shoulder: rotational stress fracture of the proximal humeral epiphysis. J Sports Med 1974;2:152–153.

57. Kibler WB. The Sport Preparticipation Fitness Examination. Champaign, IL: Human Kinetics Books, 1990.

58. Yergason RM. Supination sign. J Bone Joint Surg 1931;13:160.

59. Gerber C, Ganz R. Clinical assessment of instability of the shoulder, with special reference to the anterior and posterior drawer tests. J Bone Joint Surg Br 1984;66:551–556.

9

Elbow and Forearm Injuries

Francis G. O'Connor, Carl O. Ollivierre, and
Robert P. Nirschl

Primary care physicians are frequently called on to evaluate and manage injuries of the upper extremity. The elbow, arguably the most complex joint in the upper extremity, frequently does not receive the attention in training programs that is devoted to the shoulder and hand. Although the elbow joint is more stable than the shoulder or hand, its detailed anatomy and central positioning in the upper extremity kinetic chain predispose it to an array of overuse and traumatic injuries. This chapter illustrates and reviews the pertinent functional anatomy (Figures 9-1 through 9-4) and clinical examination of the elbow, and details effective diagnostic and management strategies for common elbow disorders seen by the primary care physician. Overuse injuries have been subdivided by anatomic distribution (Figure 9-5), whereas traumatic injuries are categorized by the nature of the disorder (Figure 9-6). Injuries unique to the pediatric athlete are considered separately (Figure 9-7).

FUNCTIONAL ANATOMY

The elbow joint is inherently stable and consists of three articulations: humeroulnar, radiohumeral, and radioulnar (see Figure 9-1). These articulations accommodate two types of motion: The humeroulnar joint resembles a hinge and provides flexion and extension, and the radiohumeral and radioulnar joints allow axial rotation, or pronation and supination. The normal elbow moves from 0 degrees to 135 degrees of flexion and accommodates 80 degrees of both pronation and supination. Additional stability is provided by the joint capsule and the surrounding ligaments.

The medial or ulnar collateral ligament complex (see Figure 9-2C) consists of three bundles: anterior, posterior, and transverse. The anterior bundle is the major portion of the medial ligament complex, providing the majority of the ligament's functional integrity. The ulnar collateral ligament is the primary valgus stabilizer of the elbow, with the radiocapitellar joint offering secondary stability. The lateral ligament complex is not as well defined as the medial ligament complex (see Figure 9-2B). This complex consists of the radial collateral ligament and the annular ligament, and it functions primarily to prevent posterolateral rotatory instability of the elbow.

The brachialis, brachioradialis, and biceps muscles are the primary muscles of elbow flexion (see Figure 9-4). The biceps additionally functions as a strong supinator when the elbow is in a pronated position. The major elbow extensors are the triceps and anconeus (see Figure 9-3). Pronation is accomplished by the pronator teres and the more distal pronator quadratus. Supination is best described as an elastic recoil initiated by pronation, continued by the supinator muscle, and then augmented by the biceps.[1] The muscles of wrist flexion have their origin (common flexor tendon) on the medial epicondyle. The extensors originate on the lateral epicondyle (common extensor tendon) and lateral supracondylar ridge.

The three principal nerves that cross the elbow joint complex are the median, ulnar, and radial nerves. The median nerve crosses the anterior elbow medial to the biceps tendon and the brachial artery before entering the pronator teres (see Figure 9-4). The median nerve is responsible for pronation; not uncommonly, the nerve

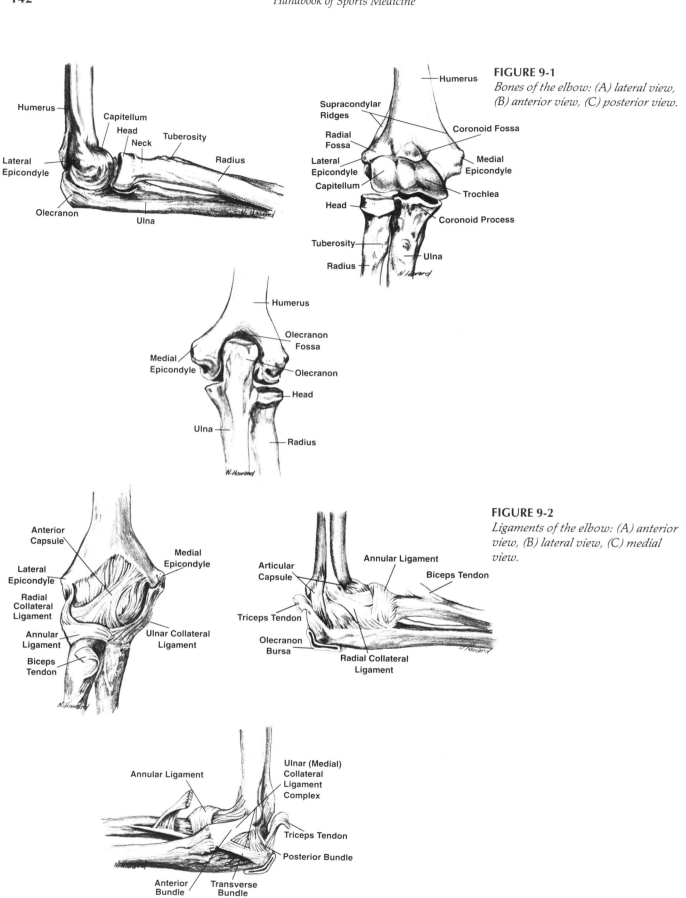

FIGURE 9-1

Bones of the elbow: (A) lateral view, (B) anterior view, (C) posterior view.

FIGURE 9-2

Ligaments of the elbow: (A) anterior view, (B) lateral view, (C) medial view.

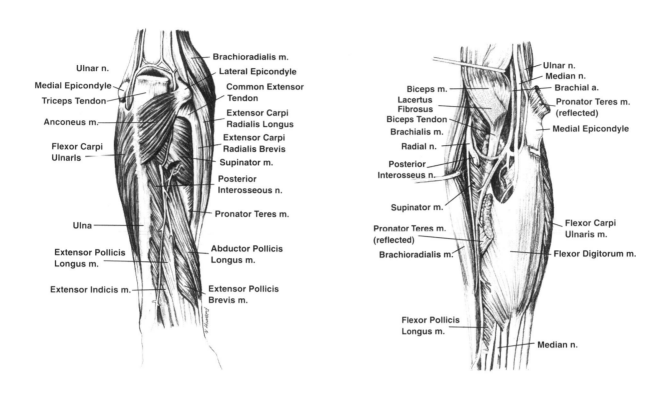

FIGURE 9-3
Nerves and muscles of the forearm, posterior view.

FIGURE 9-4
Nerves and muscles of the forearm, anterior view.

FIGURE 9-5
Algorithm for overuse injuries.
(UCL = ulnar collateral ligament;
PIN = posterior interosseous nerve.)

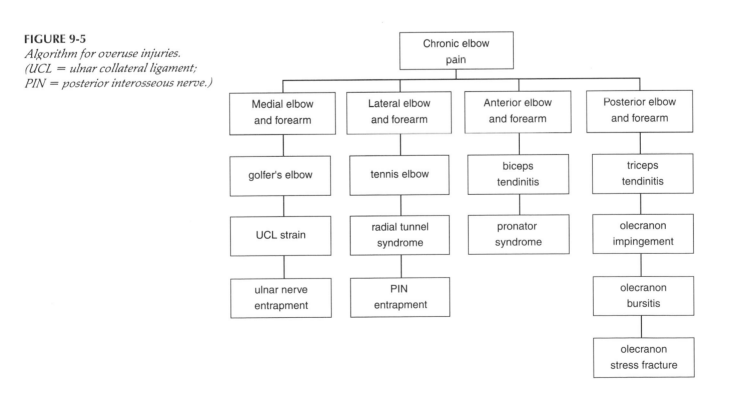

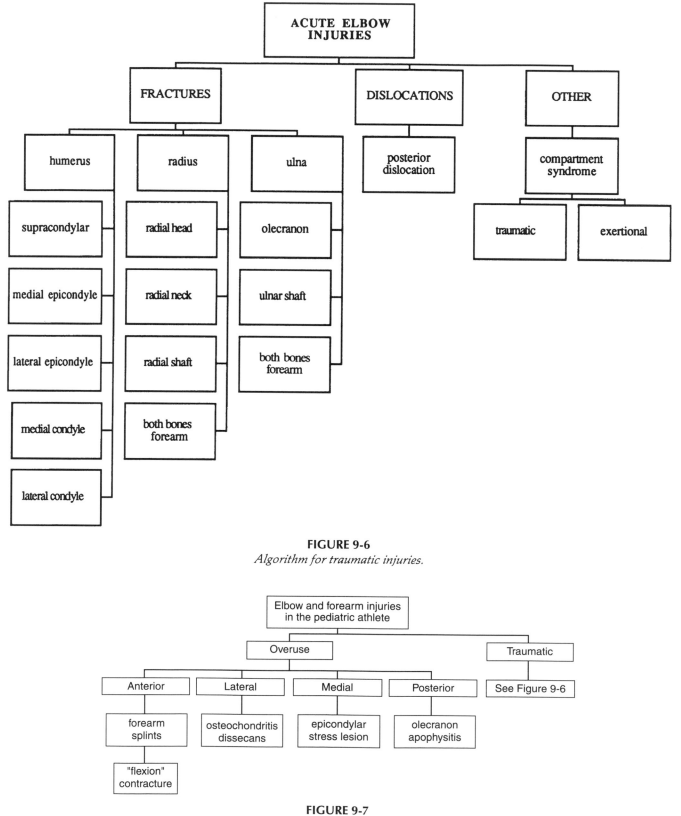

FIGURE 9-6
Algorithm for traumatic injuries.

FIGURE 9-7
Algorithm for pediatric injuries.

can become entrapped between the two heads of the pronator teres. The ulnar nerve passes posterior to the medial epicondyle in the cubital tunnel before entering the flexor carpi ulnaris (see Figure 9-3). The cubital tunnel is the most common site for ulnar nerve compression. The radial nerve emerges from the radial groove behind the humerus to pass anterior to the lateral epicondyle before dividing into superficial (sensory component) and deep (motor component–posterior interosseous) branches. The radial nerve is responsible for the extensor muscles of the arm; the nerve is vulnerable to injury at the arcade of Frohse as it passes under the proximal edge of the supinator (see Figure 9-4).

CLINICAL EXAMINATION

A thorough examination of the elbow is accomplished by a systematic evaluation that includes inspection, palpation, range of motion, neurologic assessment, special tests, and examination of related areas. A complete review of the examination of the elbow is beyond the scope of this chapter, and the reader is referred to texts by Magee and Hoppenfeld.[2, 3] Several points and clinical tests, however, deserve special attention.

The elbow, secondary to its central positioning, is a common site for referred pain. The pain of cervical radiculopathy, acromioclavicular disorders, rotator cuff disease, and carpal tunnel syndrome can all refer pain to the elbow. In addition, overuse injuries to the elbow are frequently associated with concomitant pathology in the shoulder girdle. Examination of related areas should always accompany a site-specific examination of the elbow. This examination offers the greatest opportunity to diagnose and identify all structures requiring further diagnosis and management.

Several special tests are included in the examination of the elbow and assist the clinician in making an accurate pathoanatomic diagnosis. The most common tests incorporated in the examination of the elbow involve provoking the pain of tennis elbow and assessing instability.

Tennis Elbow Test

The patient's extended elbow is stabilized by the examiner's hand, with the thumb resting on the lateral epicondyle. The patient is then asked to make a fist, pronate the forearm, and radially deviate and extend the wrist while the examiner resists the motion. A positive test reproduces pain in the area of the lateral epicondyle. In more advanced cases, there will be reproduction of pain

with the elbow flexed to 90 degrees. Resisted extension of the third digit of the hand, distal to the proximal interphalangeal joint, with pain provocation over the extensor muscle mass in the proximal forearm suggests radial tunnel syndrome.

Ligamentous Instability Test

Valgus and varus stress testing should be performed at 20 degrees of flexion, unlocking the olecranon from its fossa and relaxing the anterior capsule, with the forearm in relaxed supination. The examiner should note any laxity, decreased mobility, apprehension, or pain that may be present compared with the uninvolved side.

Posterolateral Rotatory Instability Test

With the patient in a supine position and the clinician standing at the head of the examining table, the test is performed by axial loading the elbow. The elbow is taken from an extended and supinated position and slowly flexed while applying a valgus force. A positive test produces a rotatory subluxation of the humeroulnar articulation and a dislocation of the radial head. Flexion beyond 40 degrees facilitates a reduction. This test is best performed under anesthesia; while awake, posterolateral rotatory instability can be suspected if the patient is apprehensive with this maneuver.[4]

DIAGNOSTIC IMAGING

The standard radiographic series of the elbow includes anteroposterior (AP) and lateral views. The AP view is taken with the elbow extended and the forearm supinated, and the lateral view is taken with the elbow flexed at 90 degrees and the forearm in neutral position. Special views can be ordered to help better define specific symptomatic areas, including oblique, axial, radial head, and stress views. Specific radiographic indications and clinical findings for selected pathoanatomic conditions are reviewed individually throughout this chapter.

The AP view (Figure 9-8) demonstrates the humeroradial, humeroulnar, and proximal radioulnar articulations, as well as the medial and lateral epicondyles. The carrying angle of the elbow can be measured from the AP view, with normal values for males ranging from 5 to 10 degrees and for females from 10 to 15 degrees.

The lateral view (Figure 9-9) best demonstrates the coronoid process of the ulna and the tip of the olecranon. The

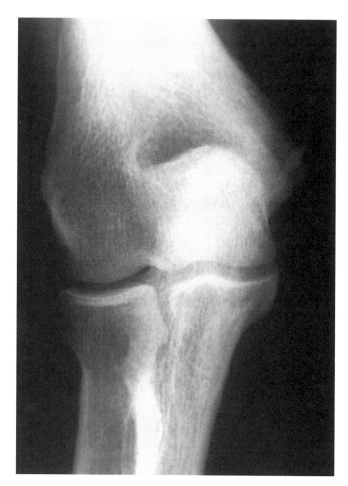

FIGURE 9-8
Radiograph demonstrating normal anteroposterior view.

articular surface of the humerus normally projects anteriorly, forming an angle of 140 degrees with the midshaft of the humerus. The radial head normally articulates with the capitellum, and a line bisecting the proximal radial shaft should always pass through the capitellum on any radiographic view. Absence of this relationship indicates fracture or dislocation.

Additional ancillary special imaging includes arthrography, computerized tomography (CT), and magnetic resonance imaging (MRI). Arthrography involves injection of a radiopaque contrast material into the elbow and can be helpful in outlining articular surfaces, loose bodies, and capsular contractions or defects. CT can be helpful in defining bony abnormalities such as tumors, bony ankylosis, and articular relationships after fractures. MRI, in particular with intraarticular contrast material (gadolinium) enhancement, provides better definition of the soft tissues and articular cartilage and assists in the diagnosis

of ligament and tendon injuries, as well as osteochondritis dissecans.

OVERUSE INJURIES

Overuse syndromes represent the majority of sports medicine injuries seen in the primary care setting.[5, 6] These injuries are the result of repetitive loading culminating in tissue microtrauma. Repetitive tissue loading can result in a self-perpetuating chronic inflammatory process that predisposes to tissue degeneration or necrosis. Further abusive overload can ultimately lead to macrotrauma with subsequent tissue failure in the form of rupture, dislocation, or fracture.

The etiology of overuse injuries is well described in the sports medicine literature.[7, 8] Principal risk factors include intrinsic and extrinsic factors. Intrinsic factors are unique to the athlete, and they generally consist of problems related to muscular imbalance, instability, or malalignment. Overuse elbow injuries are frequently the result of forearm or shoulder muscular insufficiency. Extrinsic factors include training errors and inadequate equipment. Overload phenomena from excessive weightbearing (gymnastics) or improper technique in throwing and racket sports are the most important reversible risk factors for injury. Vulnerability to extrinsic overload varies with intrinsic characteristics.

Anterior Elbow and Forearm Injuries

Biceps Tendinitis
Biceps tendinitis is the result of overuse microtrauma of the biceps tendon unit secondary to repetitive flexion or supination. This disorder generally occurs in athletes who engage in repetitive activities involving the biceps mechanism, such as weight lifters, bowlers, boxers, and gymnasts. The athlete with biceps tendinitis reports anterior elbow pain and weakness. Physical examination demonstrates that the patient's pain is exacerbated by direct palpation over the biceps tendon and provoked by resisted flexion and supination. X-ray findings are generally unremarkable.

Treatment follows the general principles of *p*rotection and *p*revention, *r*est, *i*ce, *c*ompression, *e*levation, *m*edications, and *m*odalities to include therapeutic exercise (PRICEMM). Therapeutic exercise should focus on increasing strength and flexibility of the flexor mechanism. Attention should be additionally directed at modifying training errors to include technique and training patterns. Steroid injections should be avoided because of the risk of tendon rupture. Biceps tendinitis is generally successfully

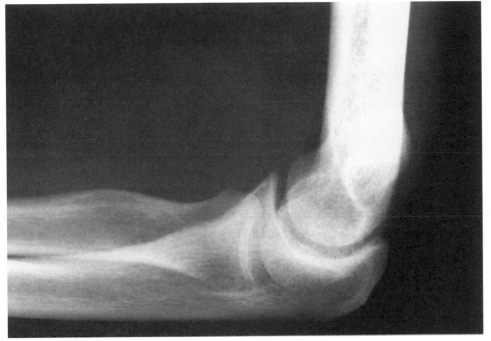

FIGURE 9-9
Radiograph demonstrating normal lateral view.

managed by the primary care physician. Refractory cases, which may suggest a musculotendinous tear or nerve entrapment, mandate referral.

A distal biceps rupture, as opposed to the more common and less debilitating proximal long head rupture, requires immediate referral for surgical repair. Diagnostic clues suggesting a full rupture include sudden and profound pain, marked swelling, and a history of heavy exertion against a major resistance.

Pronator Syndrome

Pronator syndrome is the result of median nerve entrapment distal to the elbow joint. As the nerve crosses the antecubital fossa of the elbow joint, there are three common sites for compression: the bicipital aponeurosis, the two heads of the pronator teres, and the fibrous arch of the flexor digitorum superficialis (see Figure 9-4). The pronator syndrome is generally seen in sports in which repetitive pronation and gripping is involved, such as the throwing and racket sports, weight lifting, archery, rowing, and arm wrestling. Hypertrophy seen in the pronator teres in these athletes may predispose to this entrapment.

The athlete presents with insidious onset of pain in the anterior elbow (antecubital fossa or proximal forearm), often activity related and with a radiating character. There is often a positive Tinel sign in the proximal forearm, where the median nerve passes under the pronator teres. Numbness distal to the entrapment in the forearm and hand

can be detected by sensory testing; however, sensory symptoms are not as common as in carpal tunnel syndrome. The patient's pain can be provoked or aggravated by resisted pronation. Index- and long-finger active flexion may be compromised in chronic cases (papal sign). Nerve conduction studies can be useful in demonstrating decreased conduction in the upper forearm and in ruling out carpal tunnel entrapment. Negative electromyogram (EMG) and nerve conduction velocity testing, however, does not rule out the pronator syndrome. X-ray findings are normal.

The treatment of pronator syndrome is initiated with rest and nonsteroidal anti-inflammatory drugs (NSAIDs). The rehabilitative exercise program is designed to increase flexibility and balance the strength of the forearm, with particular attention to the forearm pronators. Surgical exploration with decompression is indicated in cases that fail to respond to conservative treatment after 3–6 months, show an axonal loss by EMG, or exhibit a persistent decrease in function.[9]

Posterior Elbow and Forearm Injuries

Triceps Tendinitis or Tendinosis

Triceps tendinitis is the result of triceps tendon overload from repetitive extension of the elbow. The athlete with triceps tendinitis generally reports posterior elbow pain that becomes worse with forceful extension. Triceps tendinitis occurs in sports that involve repetitive elbow extension, such as competitive weight lifting, boxing, gymnastics, throwing, and racket sports. The athlete has tenderness at or above the insertion of the triceps tendon at the olecranon. The pain is worse with resisted extension of the elbow. X-ray films of the elbow are generally unremarkable but may demonstrate calcification in the tendon. Associated olecranon osteoarthritis may demonstrate olecranon spurs or loose bodies in the olecranon fossa.

Conservative therapy for triceps tendinitis should follow the principles of PRICEMM. Exercise therapy should be directed at strengthening the triceps mechanism, as well as improving flexibility. Modification of exercise techniques is an important aspect of treatment. Steroid injections generally should be avoided because of the risks of tendon rupture. Referral is indicated in refractory cases, but triceps tendinitis generally responds to conservative therapy.

A rupture or avulsion of the triceps tendon is a rare event. The patient most often presents with a history of a fall on an outstretched arm. Examination will demonstrate significant pain, swelling, and a palpable depression just proximal to the olecranon. Immediate surgical referral is recommended.

Olecranon Impingement Syndrome

Olecranon impingement syndrome results from the repetitive impingement of the olecranon in the olecranon fossa, as commonly occurs with valgus stress in throwing sports. Resultant stress occurs to the articular surfaces of both osseous structures. Loose bodies and osteophyte formation commonly result secondary to repetitive overload. Athletes with olecranon impingement syndrome report posterior elbow pain and clicking or symptoms consistent with mechanical blockade.

Olecranon impingement occurs in racket and throwing athletes as well as in boxers and basketball players. Associated triceps tendinitis is a common companion injury. Examination reveals that the patient's pain is worse with extension of the elbow. Palpation during elbow range of motion may reveal crepitation and major limitation of full extension secondary to mechanical blockade. A careful examination may reveal subtle instability. X-ray films generally reveal osteophytes or loose bodies; however, MRI or CT arthrography may be required.

Treatment of olecranon impingement is dependent on the nature of the blockade. If no loose bodies are present, a trial of conservative therapy is warranted. In addition to NSAIDs and modification of activities, therapeutic exercise should be directed toward increasing the strength and flexibility of the elbow musculature. Continued pain despite conservative therapy, the presence of loose bodies, and mechanical blockade, are all indications for sur-

gical referral. Surgical excision of osteophytes and loose bodies can be performed with an arthroscopic technique.

Olecranon Bursitis

Irritation to the olecranon bursa, through repetitive friction or direct contact, results in bursal swelling. The athlete reports painless swelling of the posterior elbow. Olecranon bursitis is not uncommon in football players (defensive players and wide receivers), wrestlers, and basketball players, who may land on hard surfaces. The bursal swelling is well localized to the olecranon and is generally nontender. Joint motion is usually not limited, except when flexion produces skin tension. Painful swelling associated with erythematous tissue warrants aspiration, gram stain, and culture to rule out septic bursitis. The clinician should additionally include gout, pseudogout, and other rheumatic disorders in the differential diagnosis. X-ray films are generally unremarkable, but they may reveal a spur on the tip of the olecranon.

Treatment should involve prevention with a liberal use of elbow pads in high-risk sporting activities. The distended or uncomfortable bursa may be sterilely aspirated, with fluid sent for culture, gram stain, cell count, and crystal analysis. Light dressings should be applied for 48–72 hours with intermittent cold packs to minimize rebleeding into the bursal sac. Undue compression or Ace wraps should be avoided, as distal swelling is an unwanted complication. A short course of NSAIDs administered orally can be helpful. Steroid injections for acute or subacute olecranon bursitis are of limited value.[10] A minimally distended and nontender olecranon bursitis does not necessarily require aspiration. Secondary infection requires systemic antibiotics and aggressive aspiration or open drainage. Recurrent bursal swelling or the presence of cartilaginous chips warrants referral for possible bursectomy.

Olecranon Stress Fracture

Depending on the age of the bone, repetitive overload may result in olecranon stress fracture or separation of the olecranon apophysis. The athlete reports gradually increasing pain in the posterior elbow. These disorders are generally seen in the throwing or racket sports, most commonly in baseball pitchers. The patient generally reports tenderness over the olecranon and increased pain with extension against resistance. The x-ray findings may be negative in stress fracture, and a bone scan may be required.

Olecranon stress fractures are treated nonoperatively. Sporting activities are precluded until clinical and radiographic evidence of healing are present. Activities of daily living are permitted as tolerated; those individuals with significant pain with activities of daily living may initially require an elbow immobilizer.

Medial Elbow and Forearm Overuse Injuries

Golfer's Elbow

Repeated microtrauma to the medial epicondyle and the flexor-pronator muscle group results in tendon degeneration. Medial tennis elbow, or golfer's elbow, is seen in sports that require wrist snap and forearm pronation. Activities that require this motion include the late forehand stroke in tennis or squash, volleyball spiking, baseball throwing, and the golf swing. The athlete generally reports tenderness over the medial elbow and proximal forearm that is aggravated by activity. Examination reveals localized pain to palpation predominantly at the tip of the medial epicondyle and distally approximately 1–2 in. along the track of the pronator teres and the flexor carpi radialis. The examiner should assess instability and ulnar nerve pathology. X-ray findings are generally unremarkable; however, there may be extraarticular calcification.

Initial treatment involves control of inflammation by means of the standard concepts of PRICEMM. Steroid injections should be used only after a trial of NSAIDs and with the intent of providing pain relief only to allow compliance with a rehabilitative exercise program. When performing this injection, one must remain anterior to the medial epicondyle to avoid injuring the ulnar nerve. The athlete is then encouraged to begin rehabilitative exercise to enhance collateral circulation, to encourage collagen production, and to increase strength and flexibility of the flexor pronator muscle group. Attention is also directed at controlling abusive overload by reviewing proper technique, modifying equipment as necessary, and using appropriate medial elbow counterforce bracing. Failure to respond to a 3-month trial of quality rehabilitation is an indication for surgical referral rather than for multiple steroid injections.

Ulnar Collateral Ligament Strain

Repeated valgus overload to the ulnar collateral ligament results in overuse microtrauma. This injury is most frequently seen in throwing athletes, most commonly pitchers. The athlete generally presents with vague medial elbow pain that becomes worse with activity. On physical examination, the athlete has palpable tenderness inferior to the medial epicondyle, along the anterosuperior section of the ligament. Valgus stress testing of the elbow at 20 degrees confirms the diagnosis by provoking the pain or demonstrating instability. X-ray films may demonstrate traction spurs and loose bodies. In addition, there may be heterotopic ossification of the ulnar collateral ligament. MRI has been demonstrated to be effective in identifying both partial and complete tears.

The ulnar collateral ligament strain generally responds to conservative therapy that includes rest, ice, and NSAIDs. Attention should also be directed at modifying the sport technique. Chronic ligamentous strains that fail to respond to rehabilitative exercise may require surgery, in particular if accompanied by heterotopic ossifications, traction spurs, or loose bodies. Rupture of the ulnar collateral ligament requires surgical repair or reconstruction.

Ulnar Nerve Entrapment and Subluxation

Ulnar nerve entrapment is the second most common compressive neuropathy in the upper extremity. The nerve in this location is vulnerable to injury by compression, traction, and friction. Ulnar nerve pathology is often found in throwing athletes, but can also be seen in racquet sport athletes, skiers, and weight lifters.

Nirschl has divided the medial epicondyle groove into three zones: zone I—proximal to the medial epicondyle; zone II—the level of the medial epicondyle; and zone III—below the level of the medial epicondyle. Repetitive overuse, particularly from overarm activities, can result in compression of the ulnar nerve by a tight flexor carpi ulnaris sling in the cubital tunnel (see Figure 9-3). Zone III ulnar nerve tension entrapment can be precipitated by a subluxating ulnar nerve, a cubitus valgus deformity in zone I or zone II, or an entrapment of the medial intermuscular septum in zone I.

The athlete presents with medial elbow discomfort associated with distal paresthesias in the distribution of the ulnar nerve. Reports of grip weakness, early fatigue of the hand, and clumsiness may be noted. Physical examination can demonstrate a positive Tinel sign or tenderness over the ulnar nerve in any of the three zones dependent on the pathoanatomy, as well as hypothenar atrophy and index pinch weakness. Zone III (cubital tunnel or flexor ulnaris arcade) is the most common area involved with nerve dysfunction. Full flexion of the elbow may provoke subluxation of the ulnar nerve with sudden symptoms noted. X-ray findings are unremarkable. EMG and conduction tests may demonstrate decreased conduction velocity at zone III and motor abnormalities in distal ulnar innervated muscles. False-negatives are not uncommon.

Initial conservative treatment involves rest, NSAIDs, and therapeutic exercise directed at increasing general strength and flexibility at the elbow. Night splinting with the elbow in 45 degrees of flexion and the forearm in neutral position may be helpful. A cortisone injection alongside the nerve in zone III may prove helpful. Penetration of the nerve is to be avoided, as this could prove harmful. Failure to respond to conservative therapy within 3–4 months, evidence of subluxation, ligamentous instability, or progressive motor or sensory deficits mandate surgical referral. Surgical options include decompression and anterior transposition of the ulnar nerve.

Lateral Elbow and Forearm Overuse Injuries

Lateral Tennis Elbow

Tennis elbow, the most common overuse injury of the elbow, is the result of repetitive loading of the wrist. The principal site of degenerative tendinosis is the extensor carpi radialis brevis (see Figure 9-3). Tennis elbow is most commonly seen in racket sports. The athlete presents with aching lateral elbow pain that generally becomes worse with activity. The pain can radiate into the proximal forearm and can progress to the point of interfering with sleep. On physical examination, there is localized tenderness immediately anterior, medial, and distal to the lateral epicondyle, directly over the extensor brevis. The pain is worse with resisted wrist extension, especially with the elbow in full extension and pronation at the time of testing. X-ray findings, although generally unremarkable, are needed to rule out other pathologies in those cases that fail to respond to initial conservative therapy. X-ray findings can occasionally demonstrate calcific deposits and spurring (20% in the Nirschl series).

The initial conservative treatment of tennis elbow involves activity modification; a short course of NSAIDs; and a trial of high-voltage electrical stimulation, iontophoresis, or phonophoresis for relief of pain and inflammation. The patient is then started in a tennis elbow rehabilitation program, concentrating on restoring normal range of motion, followed by progressive strengthening. Isometric exercises are initially introduced with a gradual progression to submaximal isotonics. Strengthening exercises should not cause symptoms. Lateral counterforce bracing is used during rehabilitation, as well as a graduated return to sports activity. Steroid injections should be used sparingly and always with intent of providing pain relief only to allow progression of the rehabilitation effort. Steroid injections have been demonstrated to provide short-term relief, but their long-term efficacy is unproved.[11] When we choose to use an injection, we have found the following to be helpful: 2.5 ml of 0.5% lidocaine (Xylocaine) mixed with 20 mg of triamcinolone, instilled below the extensor brevis just anterior and slightly distal to the lateral epicondyle into a triangular fatty recess that occupies this area. Healing occurs through rehabilitation, not with a steroid injection. Surgical referral is warranted only after a trial of quality rehabilitation of at least 3–4 months in duration.

Radial Tunnel Syndrome

The most common compressive neuropathy of the radial nerve occurs at the radial tunnel. In the radial tunnel syndrome, the motor branch of the radial nerve (posterior interosseous nerve) becomes entrapped under the fibrous arcade of the supinator muscle during forearm pronation or resisted supination (see Figure 9-3). Radial tunnel syndrome is often the diagnosis in recalcitrant cases of tennis elbow and may coexist with this disorder in 10% of cases.

The athlete reports lateral elbow pain that radiates into the dorsal forearm. The pain is aggravated by activities that involve pronation and supination (especially resisted supination). This disorder is seen in weight lifters, bowlers, rowers, swimmers, golfers, and those athletes that participate in racquet sports. The patient feels tenderness over the anterolateral elbow, where the radial nerve crosses the radial head 2–4 cm distal to the lateral epicondyle. The point of maximal tenderness is not over the common extensor tendon or extensor brevis as it is in tennis elbow. The patient may additionally have finger and wrist extensor weakness. A positive Tinel sign distal and anterior to the lateral epicondyle over the radial nerve can occasionally be demonstrated. X-ray findings are generally unremarkable. The patient with radial tunnel syndrome often exhibits pain with resisted supination of the extended forearm, or with resisted extension of the long finger. Night pain is not uncommon.

Nerve conduction studies can demonstrate a delay of radial nerve conduction across the elbow. EMG studies may demonstrate a muscle motor dysfunction of radial innervated distal muscles. Normal electrodiagnostic studies do not necessarily exclude the diagnosis. A diagnostic block of 1 ml of 1% lidocaine four finger breadths distal to the lateral epicondyle that relieves pain and is accompanied by a deep radial palsy, plus a complementary injection more proximal in the region of the lateral epicondyle (usually given 24–48 hours later) that does not relieve the patient's symptoms, assists in confirming the diagnosis of radial tunnel syndrome.[12]

Initial treatment involves relative rest, NSAIDs, and wrist splinting. A comprehensive rehabilitation of the elbow musculature concentrating on flexibility, strength balance, and endurance should be initiated. If the patient fails to respond to conservative therapy after 3–6 months, surgery should be considered for nerve decompression.

Posterior Interosseous Nerve Entrapment

The literature frequently refers to a variant of the radial tunnel syndrome known as the *posterior interosseous nerve entrapment syndrome.* The main difference with this disorder is that the patient presents with weakness in wrist extension as the predominant feature. In the radial tunnel syndrome, the principal symptom is pain. The management and treatment for the two conditions is essentially the same.

TRAUMATIC INJURIES

Traumatic injuries of the elbow and forearm can be challenging to the most experienced of clinicians. Injuries involving the elbow have a propensity for stiffness if immobilized for extended periods and for developing heterotopic ossification if irritated during the immediate postinjury period. Most traumatic injuries resulting in fracture are best treated initially by splinting in the presenting position and then by seeking definitive management by an orthopedic surgeon.

Minor injuries can produce subtle fractures. It is imperative, therefore, that proper radiographs be taken. This usually means that in addition to standard AP and lateral views, obliques and x-rays of the opposite elbow are often required for accurate assessment. The posterior fat pad sign can be a radiographic clue to a subtle elbow fracture. Because the posterior fat pad is located deep within the olecranon fossa, it is not normally visible on the lateral view. Capsular distention caused by hemarthrosis (occult fracture) or effusion displaces the fat pad into the radiographic plane and is seen as a radiolucency. Elevation of the normal anterior fat pad with a hemarthrosis results in the classic "sail sign" (Figure 9-10).

Fractures

Supracondylar Fracture of the Humerus

Although these fractures are most commonly seen in children, they can also occur in adults. Typically, the mechanism involves falling on an outstretched arm. Incomplete or minimally displaced fractures may be difficult to diagnose, but careful palpation of the bony landmarks about the elbow along with radiographic assessment usually reveals the extent of the injury. Oblique radiographic views may be useful in visualizing more subtle fractures. The Gartland classification of supracondylar fractures provides guidelines as to the proper course of treatment. Type I nondisplaced fractures are treated with splinting with a sling or a collar and cuff for 2–3 weeks. Type II partially displaced fractures must be carefully assessed to determine the true position of the fragments. If the fragments are in an acceptable position, splinting or casting is sufficient. With extensive angulation, however, reduction and pinning is the treatment of choice. For type III or completely displaced fractures, reduction is carried out either by closed or open means with or without internal fixation and subsequent immobilization. The preferred method, if possible, is closed reduction and percutaneous pinning.

FIGURE 9-10
Radiograph demonstrating fat pads. Arrow demonstrates the classic "sail sign."

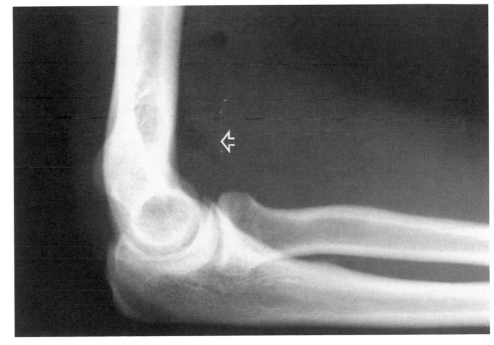

The most serious complication of supracondylar fractures are injuries to the brachial artery. This can occur as a result of arterial spasms, lacerations of the artery, and kinking of the artery by soft tissues along the fracture site. It is imperative that the distal pulses are meticulously monitored after a supracondylar humeral injury so that an arterial injury will not be missed. Ulnar nerve injuries can also occur with internal fixation, and this is best avoided by placing all fixation devices through a lateral approach. In approximately 10% of these fractures, cubitus varus can occur, usually as a result of malunion of the fracture. Most often, the deformity is only cosmetic with little functional impairment.

Volkmann ischemic contracture and compartment syndrome can also occur as a result of supracondylar humeral fractures. Meticulous observation is recommended for at least 24 hours after such injuries. The most important clinical finding for an impending compartment syndrome is severe pain with passive extension of the digits. The clinician should keep in mind that good pulses and capillary refill are often present in patients with muscle ischemia and compartment syndromes. If compartment syndrome is suspected, the splint or cast must be removed immediately and the injury site inspected. If the clinical examination and compartment pressure measurements indicate compartment syndrome, forearm and elbow fasciectomies are indicated.

Medial Epicondyle Fracture

These injuries occur most often in children who fall on an arm or occasionally in athletes involved in throwing sports. The medial epicondyle may be avulsed by the attached medial collateral ligament or the common flexor origin. The fragment occasionally becomes trapped in the elbow joint. The patient presents with pain and local tenderness. Occasionally, ulnar nerve symptoms may be present. X-ray films must be carefully analyzed, as the normal growth plate may be confused with an acute fracture in the skeletally immature patient. Comparison views of the opposite elbow may be helpful.

Minimally displaced fractures (<1 cm) require short-term immobilization (2–3 weeks) in a long-arm cast with the elbow and wrist flexed; progressive rehabilitation follows. Displaced or entrapped fragments usually require manipulation or open reduction by an orthopedic surgeon.

Lateral Condyle Fracture

This is a serious injury because the joint surface is disrupted. The patient presents with local pain and tenderness and without gross deformity. Careful assessment of routine AP and lateral x-ray findings may reveal the degree of articular surface involvement, but oblique views and x-ray films of the noninjured elbow are needed to define the injury more clearly.

Open reduction and internal fixation are needed if there is any degree of displacement. Late arthritic changes, ulnar nerve neuropathy, cubitus valgus, and instability may occur if accurate reduction is not achieved. Avascular necrosis and growth disturbance are additional complications that can be associated with this injury.

Radial Head and Neck Fractures

Fractures of the radial head and neck result from a fall on the outstretched hand with the elbow extended. These fractures generally present with tenderness over the radial head, local swelling, and pain on flexion and rotation of the elbow. The Mason classification is very useful in treatment of isolated radial head fractures. When associated with other fractures or ligamentous injuries (complex fractures), the management principles differ.

Simple radial head fractures are those that occur without any associated injury. Mason I (undisplaced fractures) should be treated nonsurgically because of the excellent prognosis. Treatment consists of a sling for pain control and early motion. In cases in which there is intense painful hemarthrosis, aspiration and injection in the posterolateral triangle with a local anesthetic may be helpful. There is a 90–95% chance of an excellent result with a nondisplaced Mason I type fracture. Complications can occur, however, and these include nonunion, loss of elbow extension, loss of rotation, and occasionally, persistent aching with use of the arm.

The treatment of Mason II (displaced fractures of the radial head) is somewhat controversial. The method of treatment is best determined after careful examination, usually after anesthetic injection into the elbow joint. Most musculoskeletal physicians agree that if 20–140 degrees of flexion along with 70% of the forearm rotation is obtainable, nonsurgical treatment is preferred. In these cases, the elbow is typically immobilized for 3 weeks, then active and active-assisted range of motion is begun. The previous method of early radial head excision is no longer acceptable as the results are unpredictable. In patients with an inadequate range of motion, open reduction and internal fixation of the radial head is recommended. In patients who are seen late after the injury or who have residual discomfort after initial nonsurgical treatment, delayed radial head excision may be indicated.

For type III (comminuted fractures of the radial head), early excision (within 48 hours) is preferred. Studies have shown that there is maintenance of stability about the elbow with simple radial head excision provided by the intact ligaments. Studies have also shown that early excision is preferred to delayed excision in terms of functional outcome.

For complex fractures (i.e., fractures with associated ligamentous bony injuries), treatment principles follow those of simple fractures, which are usually preceded by surgical or nonsurgical stabilization of the associated injury. It is rare that a ligamentous injury should be surgically repaired when associated with a fracture dislocation of the elbow.

Radial replacement with a silicone implant has been used in the past. Because of the complications associated with the use of silicone, however, this has been abandoned for the most part. Metal implants are being developed as a replacement device for the treatment of unstable radial head fractures.

Overall, for uncomplicated radial head fractures, prognosis is good. With associated injuries, however, long-term stiffness, chronic aching, and osteoarthritis may develop.

Olecranon Fractures

This injury occurs in isolation or as a part of a fracture dislocation of the elbow. As an isolated injury, direct trauma is the most common mechanism of injury. The patient generally presents with an effusion as a result of the intraarticular component of this fracture. The patient is unable to extend the elbow, and neurologic (ulnar nerve) symptoms may be present.

Undisplaced fractures may be treated by immobilization in a posterior splint or elbow immobilizer with the elbow flexed at 90 degrees. Pronation and supination are started at 2–3 days, and easy flexion and extension motions begin at 2 weeks. Protective immobilization should continue until there is evidence of union (approximately 6 weeks). Displaced fractures should be referred to an orthopedic surgeon and are most effectively treated with anatomic reduction, rigid internal fixation, and early motion to avoid elbow stiffness. Smaller displaced fractures (<30% of the olecranon) can be treated by surgical excision and firm reattachment of the triceps insertion.

Radial and Ulnar Shafts

These are common upper extremity fractures, caused indirectly by a fall on the arm or by direct violence. For a displaced fracture of the radius shaft to occur alone, the distal end of the ulna must subluxate (Galeazzi fracture); for a displaced ulnar fracture to occur in isolation, the radial head must subluxate (Monteggia fracture). The more common occurrence, however, is fractures of both bones of the forearm.

The clinical examination varies with the degree of displacement. Initial displacement may be unremarkable,

but these fractures are prone to severe displacement, resulting in long-term elbow and wrist instability with loss of motion—that is, pronation and supination. The x-ray films must include the joints above and below the fracture, as associated injuries are often present.

The goal of treatment is accurate alignment to permit pronation and supination. In children, whose fractures are often no more than greenstick fractures with minimal angulation, manipulation by an orthopedic surgeon and long-arm casting are usually definitive management. Six weeks of total immobilization is usually sufficient. In adults, open reduction and internal fixation with plates and screws is the treatment of choice. With rigid fixation, mobilization of the wrist and forearm is allowed at 2–3 weeks. These fractures are usually well united in 12–14 weeks. Most complications related to these fractures result from the magnitude of the comminution, vascular compromise, or less than ideal fixation.

Posterior Elbow Dislocation

This occurs typically as a result of a fall on an outstretched arm. The patient presents with an elbow that is swollen and held in a flexed position. The ulna is posteriorly positioned on the distal humerus. The coronoid process of the ulna or the radial head may be fractured in association with the dislocation. X-ray findings demonstrate the direction of the displacement: directly posterior (most common), posterolateral, or posteromedial. Complete x-ray evaluation includes a lateral of the elbow and AP views of the humerus and forearm.

Reduction, which usually requires anesthesia for muscle relaxation, is achieved by gentle traction in line with the forearm, with the elbow flexed approximately 45 degrees. Complete motion should be possible after reduction if no fracture has occurred. Postreduction x-ray films are mandatory, as they help determine management. Incomplete reduction resulting from bony or soft tissue interposition of associated fractures mandates referral to an orthopedic surgeon for open reduction. Stability after reduction and the presence or absence of associated fractures will determine the length of time for immobilization. A stable reduction warrants an elbow immobilizer at 90 degrees continuously for 1 week and intermittently for another 1–2 weeks. Graduated rehabilitation starts at 1 week. Rehabilitation can be challenging, and prompt referral is recommended if steady progress is not occurring.

Limited motion (usually extension) is the most common complication seen after an elbow dislocation. Rarely, peripheral nerve (most commonly ulnar) or brachial artery injuries may occur. Myositis ossificans (brachialis in antecubital fossa) can also occur as a result of trauma to the surrounding soft tissue. Adhesive capsulitis and compromised mobility can be treated by surgical release or quality rehabilitation undertaken by experienced elbow surgeons.

Other Traumatic Injuries: Compartment Syndrome

A compartment syndrome occurs when increased pressure within the space compromises the circulation to the contents of that space. Other terms that have been used to describe this syndrome include exercise ischemia, Volkmann ischemia, and traumatic tension in muscles. In the upper extremity, the most common locations are the volar and dorsal compartments of the forearm.

Trauma increases pressure within a compartment by bleeding or by increasing capillary permeability. Muscle hypertrophy or an infiltrated infusion can also cause a compartment syndrome. Chronic exertional compartment syndrome during athletic activity is a rare entity, resulting from excessive intermittent pressure reducing blood flow to the compartment.

Intense pain, sensory symptoms, or muscle weakness should raise suspicion of a compartment syndrome. The patient at risk must be followed closely with serial examinations. Severe pain with passive muscle stretch is the classic finding for muscle ischemia within the compartment. Absence of pulse may be a late sign; presence of a pulse does not necessarily rule out compartment syndrome. Several simple compartment measuring devices are available for confirming the clinical suspicion. Pressures exceeding 35–40 mm Hg are strongly suggestive of a compartment syndrome. Surgical decompression of the involved compartment should be performed urgently once the diagnosis is made.

THE PEDIATRIC ATHLETE

The increasing involvement of children in sports has led to a parallel increase in sports-related childhood injuries. The elbow is one of the most common sites for both traumatic and overuse injuries in the pediatric athlete.[13] The unique nature of the pediatric elbow with immature articular cartilage, and the presence of epiphyseal and apophyseal plates, necessitates knowledge of injury patterns to the pediatric elbow to promote early injury identification and obviate potential permanent disability.

The elbow has been consistently demonstrated to be one of the most common sites of overuse injury in the young throwing athlete with a constellation of injuries known as "Little Leaguer's elbow." The throwing motion in the young athlete creates four areas of overload: tension overload of the medial elbow restraints, compression overload on the lateral articular surface, posterior shear forces on the posterior articular surface, and extension overload on the lateral restraints. The term *Little Leaguer's elbow* includes a constellation of injuries: medial epicondylar fragmentation and avulsion, delayed or accelerated apophyseal growth of the medial epicondyle, osteochondritis dissecans of the capitellum, osteochondritis of the radial head, hypertrophy of the ulna, and olecranon apophysitis with or without delayed closure of the olecranon apophysis.[14]

Medial Elbow and Forearm Injuries: Medial Epicondyle Apophysitis

The most common presentation of medial epicondyle apophysitis (Little Leaguer's elbow) is medial elbow pain. Repetitive valgus stress of the medial elbow before closure of the apophyseal growth plate can result in avulsion of the ossification center. The athlete generally reports intense medial elbow pain that is worse with athletic activity. The patient has tenderness over the medial epicondyle with occasional swelling. X-ray findings may demonstrate widening of the apophyseal line with complete separation or partial fragmentation of the apophysis. Contralateral radiographs are frequently required for comparison.

In the young athlete in whom the apophysis is separated less than 5 mm, the treatment involves rest for approximately 2–3 weeks. Avulsion with displacement greater than 5 mm may require open reduction and internal fixation. A full separation with entrapment into the joint is an absolute indication for surgery. In athletes treated with rest and NSAIDs, a rehabilitative program should be combined with reeducation in proper throwing mechanics. The athlete may resume throwing when pain free with activities of daily living and when the injury is nontender to palpation; this period of activity modification may be 2–3 months. Indications for referral include apophyseal separation of more than 5 mm, failure of response to conservative therapy for those separations less than 5 mm, or associated ulnar nerve symptoms.

Anterior Elbow and Forearm Injuries

Forearm Splints

Forearm or wrist splints are almost exclusively seen in young gymnasts, particularly in male gymnasts training on the pommel horse. The injury is somewhat analogous to shin splints; Aronen hypothesized that wrist splints were the result of overuse and strain at the origin of the extensor carpi ulnaris.[15] The athlete generally presents with a history of forearm overuse, with lateral forearm pain that is worse with activity. Relief of symptoms is achieved with ice before and after practice. Taping of the wrist and wrapping the affected forearms can assist in an early return to activity. A forearm strengthening program with attention to the wrist extensors, as well as careful attention to technique and overtraining, can help with both treatment and prevention.

Flexion Contracture

The throwing pediatric and adolescent elbow is particularly susceptible to hyperextension forces secondary to muscle tendon imbalances and poor mechanics. Anterior elbow pain in the young athlete can be non pecific, but often presents with elbow flexion contracture. The differential diagnosis may include anterior capsulitis, osteochondritis dissecans capitellum, biceps strain, myositis ossificans, or the pronator syndrome. Radiographs may demonstrate trochlear hypertrophy, osteophytes, fragmentation, loose bodies, or coronoid osteophytes. Treatment is relative rest from abusive activity, as well as focused attention on mechanical abnormalities. Flexion contractures without demonstrable mechanical and radiographic abnormalities can be treated with range-of-motion exercises and dynamic extension splinting specifically designed to passively increase the flexibility of the anterior capsule.

Lateral Elbow and Forearm Injuries: Osteochondritis Dissecans of the Capitellum

Repetitive valgus overload at the elbow results in lateral compressive stress. In young athletes with open epiphyses, osteochondritis dissecans can result. In athletes with closed epiphyses, radiocapitellar chondromalacia can ensue with subsequent degeneration of articular cartilage and the formation of loose bodies. The athlete reports lateral elbow pain that becomes worse with activity. In addition, the athlete can relate a history of clicking, catching, or locking. The radiocapitellar joint is tender to palpation, as well as with forearm pronation and supination. Range-of-motion testing may also reveal palpable and audible crepitus and a partial loss of supination; occasionally a loose body can be palpated. X-ray findings may demonstrate loose bodies and radiolucent defects in the capitellum (Figure 9-11). Elbow arthrography with selected tomography or MRI may be required. Distortion of the radial head is sometimes noted.

The management of osteochondritis and radiocapitellar chondromalacia requires the involvement of an ortho-

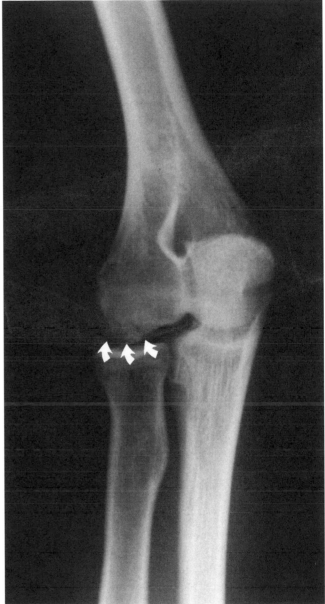

FIGURE 9-11

Radiograph demonstrating osteochondritis dissecans. Arrows identify capittelar osteochondritis dissecans.

pedic surgeon. Although prolonged relative rest is required, the possibility of significant elbow morbidity and the evolving criteria for surgical intervention warrant surgical consultation. Athletes who do not require surgery should be involved in elbow rehabilitative exercise, including passive flexibility to improve and maintain full extension and pronation and supination. Young baseball pitchers should be moved to a position involving less throwing, such as first base, when symptoms are resolved. Osteochondritis dissecans requires surgery when loose bodies are present or when the patient has large symptomatic osteochondral defects that have not responded to conservative therapy.

Posterior Elbow and Forearm Injuries: Olecranon Apophysitis

Musculotendinous imbalance and rapid growth can put stresses on the olecranon apophysis similar to that seen with Osgood-Schlatter disease. A separated olecranon apophysis can persist into adulthood. Additional complications include fragment avulsion and heterotopic ossification at the tip of the olecranon that may lead to a loss of extension.

Treatment is entirely symptomatic and focused on relative rest to promote revascularization and repair while discouraging muscle atrophy and deconditioning. In those young athletes with evidence of epiphyseal widening, the elbow may require immobilization for 4–6 weeks with a 90-degree elbow immobilizer and daily intermittent gentle range-of-motion exercises. After 4–6 weeks, the elbow may begin progressive resistance rehabilitation if x-ray findings and clinical examination support appropriate healing. In those athletes in whom avulsion or clear evidence for a nonunion is diagnosed, orthopedic referral for surgical fixation is recommended.

SUMMARY

Elbow injuries are commonly encountered by primary care providers and present with a complete spectrum of overuse and traumatic injuries. Primary care clinicians can successfully diagnose and manage these injuries by combining a knowledge of anatomy and biomechanics with a carefully performed history and physical examination. With an adequate understanding of elbow disorders, the clinician can return athletes to competition intelligently and safely and facilitate appropriate referrals to orthopedic specialists when required.

REFERENCES

1. Basmajian JV, Travill A. Electromyography of the pronator muscle of the forearm. Anat Rec 1961;139:45–49.
2. Magee DJ. Orthopedic Physical Assessment (3rd ed). Philadelphia: Saunders, 1997.
3. Hoppenfeld S. Physical Examination of the Spine and Extremities. New York: Appleton-Century-Crofts, 1976.
4. O'Driscoll SW, Bell DF, Morrey BF. Posterolateral rotatory instability of the elbow. J Bone Joint Surg Am 1991;73:440–446.
5. Herring SA, Nilson KC. Introduction to overuse injuries. Clin Sports Med 1987;6:225–233.
6. Butcher JA, Zukowski CA, Brannen SJ, et al. Patient profile, referral sources, and consultant utilization in a primary care sports medicine clinic. J Fam Pract 1996;43:556–560.
7. Leadbetter WB. Cell-matrix response in tendon injury. Clin Sports Med 1992;11:533–578.
8. O'Connor FG, Howard TM, Fieseler CM, Nirschl RP. Managing overuse injuries. Phys Sports Med 1997;25:88–113.
9. Plancher KD, Peterson RK, Steichen JB. Compressive neuropathies and tendinopathies in the athletic elbow and wrist. Clin Sports Med 1996;15:331–371.
10. Larson RL, Ostering LR. Traumatic bursitis and artificial turf. J Sports Med 1974;2:183–188.
11. Assenfeldt WJ, Hay EM, Adshead R, et al. Corticosteroid injections for lateral epicondylitis: a systematic review. Br J Gen Pract 1996;46: 209–216.
12. Cabrera JM, McCue FC. Nonosseous athletic injuries of the elbow, forearm and hand. Clin Sports Med 1986;5:681–700.
13. Wilkins KE, Beaty JH, Chambers HG, et al. Fractures and Dislocations of the Elbow Region. In CA Rockwood, KE Wilkins, JH Beaty (eds), Fractures in Children (4th ed). Philadelphia: Lippincott–Raven, 1996;653–904.
14. Bradley JP. Upper Extremity: Elbow Injuries in Children and Adolescents. In CL Stanitski, JC DeLee, D Drez (eds), Pediatric and Adolescent Sports Medicine. Philadelphia: Saunders, 1994;242–261.
15. Aronen JG. Problems of the upper extremity in gymnasts. Clin Sports Med 1985;4:61–71.

SUGGESTED READING

Behr CT, Altcheck DW. The elbow. Clin Sports Med 1997;16:681–704.
Cabanela ME, Morrey BF. Fractures of the Proximal Ulna and Olecranon. In BF Morrey (ed), The Elbow and Its Disorders (2nd ed). Philadelphia: Saunders, 1993;405–428.
Crawford AH. Operative management of fractures of the shaft of the radius and ulna. Orthop Clin North Am 1990;21:245–250.
Gartland JJ. Management of supracondylar fractures of the humerus in children. Surg Gynecol Obstetr 1959;109:145–154.
King FJ, Evans DC, Kellan JF. Open reduction and internal fixation of radial head fractures. J Orthop Trauma 1991;5:21–28.
Knight DJ, Rymaszewski LA, Amis AA, et al. Primary replacement of the fractured radial head with a metal prosthesis. J Bone Joint Surg Br 1993;75:572–576.

Larsen E, Jensen CM. Tension-band wiring of olecranon fractures with nonsliding pins: report of 20 cases. Acta Orthop Scand 1991;62:360–362.

Mehlhoff TL, Bennett JB. Elbow Injuries. In MB Mellion, WM Walsh, GL Shelton (eds), The Team Physicians' Handbook. Philadelphia: Hanley and Belfus, 1990;334–345.

Morrey BF. Fracture of the Radial Head. In BF Morrey (ed), The Elbow and Its Disorders (2nd ed). Philadelphia: Saunders, 1993;383–404.

Morrey BF. Current concepts in the treatment of fractures of the radial head, the olecranon and the coronoid. Instructional Course Lectures 1995;44:175–185.

Morrey BF, Regan WD. Tendinopathies About the Elbow. In JC DeLee, D Drez (eds), Orthopaedic Sports Medicine. Philadelphia: Saunders, 1994;860–881.

Nirschl RP. Soft-tissue injuries about the elbow. Clin Sports Med 1986;5:637–652.

Parkes JC. Overuse Injuries of the Elbow. In JA Nicholas, EB Hershman (eds), The Upper Extremity in Sports Medicine. Baltimore: Mosby, 1990;337–346.

Rang ME. Children's Fractures. Philadelphia: Lippincott, 1983.

Tullos HS, Bennett J. Acute Injuries to the Elbow. In JA Nicholas, EB Hershman (eds). The Upper Extremity in Sports Medicine. Baltimore: Mosby, 1990;321–334.

Woods EW, Tullos HS. Elbow instability and medial epicondyle fractures. Am J Sports Med 1977;5:23–30.

10

Wrist Injuries

WADE A. LILLEGARD

The magnitude of a wrist injury is often underestimated by the athlete and clinician because of its generally non-weightbearing nature, the tendency to label it as a sprain, and the pressure to continue playing. The misdiagnosis of a sprain is potentially harmful, because it may overlook an osseous or ligamentous injury, which could lead to chronic instability or pain. This chapter serves to guide the reader in evaluating and treating common wrist injuries. Some wrist injuries can be quite complex, and early referral is warranted when the diagnosis is in question.

FUNCTIONAL ANATOMY

No tendons originate from or insert into the carpal bones, except for the sesamoidal pisiform (Figure 10-1). Wrist motion is therefore purely passive, with the carpal bones functioning as an intercalated segment.

The scaphoid is the only carpal bone to cross the midcarpal joint. This position provides stability by preventing the proximal row from collapsing in a zigzag configuration under compressive loads.[1] This position and function also place the scaphoid at the greatest risk of injury.

LIGAMENTOUS ANATOMY

The general configuration of the wrist is a double inverted V (Figure 10-2). The distal inverted V is formed by the two components of the deltoid ligament (capitoscaphoid and capitotriquetral ligaments); these are intracapsular and intrinsic.[2] The proximal inverted V is formed by two intracapsular extrinsic ligaments: the radiolunate and ulnolunate.[2] Between these two Vs is an area frequently devoid of ligamentous support over the capitolunate articulation. This is a potentially weak space called the *space of Poirier*,

which may allow perilunate instability in hyperextension injuries.[3] Dermatomes are shown in Figure 10-3, and motor nerve function and testing are shown in Table 10-1.

TRAUMATIC WRIST INJURIES

Significant pain or swelling after trauma to the wrist implies a significant injury. Osseous and ligamentous injury that may lead to instability must be carefully investigated and ruled out before the injury is classified as a wrist sprain (Figure 10-4).

History

The history is generally the same for most of these injuries. Usually, the athlete falls on or strikes a dorsiflexed wrist, experiences rotational stress, or does not remember the mechanism. Pain and swelling are often noted immediately.

Physical Examination

The wrist has a variable degree of swelling. Generally, greater swelling is associated with a worse injury. Tenderness can be diffuse or localized over the general area of injury. Range of motion is limited by pain, swelling, or instability. The neurovascular status must be assessed in all injuries (see Table 10-1). Other specific tests and findings are mentioned under specific injuries.

Radiography

Initial radiographs for the acutely injured wrist should include posteroanterior (PA) in neutral and ulnar deviation, true lateral, oblique, and PA in 45 degrees pronation from neutral (Figure 10-5). Additional views or imaging

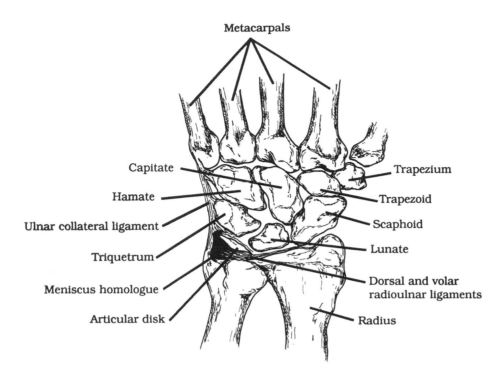

Metacarpals

Capitate

Hamate

Ulnar collateral ligament

Triquetrum

Meniscus homologue

Articular disk

Trapezium

Trapezoid

Scaphoid

Lunate

Dorsal and volar
radioulnar ligaments

Radius

FIGURE 10-1
The carpal bones and the triangular fibrocartilage complex (triangular fibrocartilage, ulnar meniscus homologue, ulnar collateral ligament, dorsal and volar radioulnar ligaments, ulnolunate and ulnotriquetral ligaments, extensor carpi ulnaris tendon sheath).

techniques may be necessary and are mentioned where indicated under specific injuries. Technetium 99 scintigraphy (bone scan) is useful for evaluating suspected fractures not visualized on plain radiography. If there is focal increased uptake on the bone scan, computed tomography (CT) or tomograms of the area should follow to define small frac-

tures. Magnetic resonance imaging (MRI) of the wrist has a high rate of false-positive and false-negative results for many instabilities, whereas arthrography can be very useful.[4] The decisions regarding more detailed radiographic imaging for suspected serious injuries are probably best left with the surgical consultant.

FIGURE 10-2
Ligaments of the wrist.

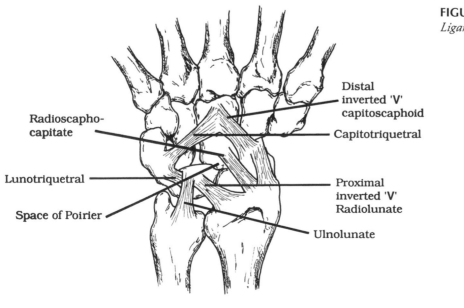

Radioscapho-
capitate

Lunotriquetral

Space of Poirier

Distal
inverted 'V'
capitoscaphoid

Capitotriquetral

Proximal
inverted 'V'
Radiolunate

Ulnolunate

Treatment

Treatment is based on the specific injury. If no gross fracture or instability is noted on initial examination and x-ray findings, but significant pain or swelling is present, the wrist should be immobilized and reexamined in 2 weeks. The algorithm in Figure 10-4 illustrates a systematic method to assist the clinician in considering and identifying the more significant traumatic injuries.

Radial Osseous Injuries: Scaphoid Fractures

Scaphoid fracture accounts for 70% of all carpal bone injuries in adults and is the most common carpal fracture in athletes (Table 10-2).[5] The scaphoid is vulnerable because of the key stabilizing role it plays as it bridges the proximal and distal carpal rows. Avascular necrosis (AVN) is not uncommon because of the scaphoid's dependence on a single interosseous blood supply that enters distally and runs proximally.[6] More proximal fractures have more delayed healing and a higher risk of AVN.

Most scaphoid fractures result from a fall on a dorsiflexed wrist or a sudden blow to the palm. Physical exam-

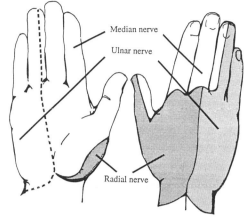

FIGURE 10-3
Dermatomes of the wrist and hand.

TABLE 10-1
Motor Nerve Function at the Wrist

Nerve	Muscle Innervated	Test for Function
Radial	Extensor carpi radialis, brevis, and ulnaris	Resist wrist extension*
	Extensor pollicis brevis/longus	Push against extended thumb
	Abductor pollicis longus	Push against abducted thumb
	Extensor digitorum communis	Wrist neutral; extend MCP with flexed PIP (prevents use of intrinsics)
	Extensor indicis	
	Extensor digiti minimi	
Median	Flexor digitorum superficialis	Hold all fingers in extension (isolates superficialis); patient flexes isolated PIP
	Flexor pollicis longus	Patient holds flexed thumb against hypothenar eminence; examiner attempts to pull it away
	Abductor pollicis longus	Patient abducts thumb against resistance
	Opponens pollicis	Patient apposes small finger and thumb; examiner attempts to separate them
	Flexor pollicis brevis—lateral portion	Patient makes O with thumb and index finger; examiner pulls them apart*
	Radial two lumbricals	
Ulnar	Flexor digitorum profundus (ulnar two digits)	Stabilize MCP and PIP in extension; patient actively flexes DIP
	Dorsal interossei (DAB: *dorsal abducts*)	Patient fans extended fingers; examiner forces each pair together*
	Palmar interossei (PAD: *palmar adducts*)	Patient holds extended fingers together; examiner attempts to force them apart
	Adductor pollicis	Patient adducts thumb against resistance
	Opponens digiti minimi	Test as for opponens pollicis (under Median)
	Flexor pollicis brevis—medial portion	
	Abductor digiti minimi	Patient attempts to abduct small finger against examiner's resistance (most specific for ulnar nerve)
	Flexor carpi ulnaris	

*Most commonly used screening test.
MCP = metacarpophalangeal (joint); PIP = proximal interphalangeal (joint); DIP = distal interphalangeal (joint).

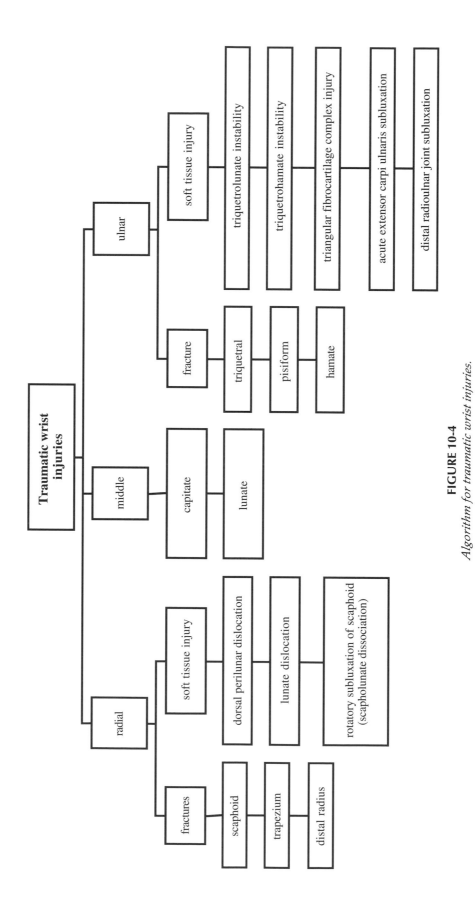

FIGURE 10-4
Algorithm for traumatic wrist injuries.

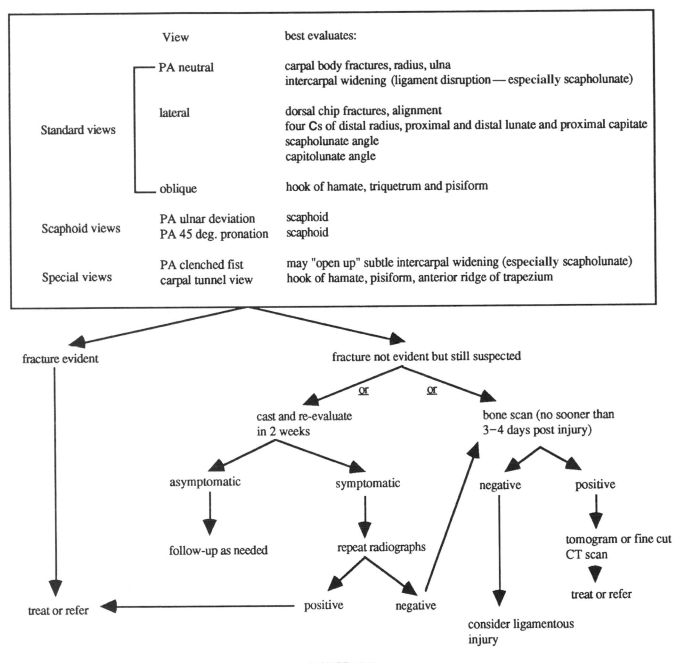

FIGURE 10-5

Algorithm for radiologic evaluation of the acutely injured wrist. (PA = posteroanterior; CT = computed tomography.)

ination reveals pain or swelling in the "anatomic snuff box" and the dorsoradial aspect of the wrist. Radiographs should include a PA, true lateral, PA in 45 degrees pronation, and PA in ulnar deviation (scaphoid series).[7] If no fracture line is visualized on the initial radiographs but clinical suspicion remains, the wrist should be immobilized in a thumb spica cast and repeat radiographs taken in 10 days to 2 weeks (see Figure 10-5). If a more expedient diagnosis is

necessary, a day-4 bone scan is 100% sensitive and 92% specific for scaphoid fractures with a positive predictive value of 65% and a negative predictive value of 100%.[8]

Fractures at high risk for delayed union, nonunion, and AVN include displaced fractures (>1 mm separation or both cortices involved on PA views), fractures of the proximal one-third pole, and any fracture presenting 2–3 weeks or more after the injury.[9] Consideration should be made

TABLE 10-2
Summary of Carpal Bone Fractures

Carpal Bone	Best Views or Studies	Fracture	Treatment
Scaphoid	Scaphoid series (PA, PA ulnar deviation, PA 45 degrees pronation, lateral) Bone scan or screening MRI if x-rays equivocal	**Distal ⅓** Tuberosity Distal ⅓ extraarticular Intraarticular/displaced **Middle ⅓** Acute nondisplaced	SAC-TS × 4–6 wks LAC-TS × 6 wks, then SAC ORIF LAC-TS × 6 wks, then SAC-TS until clinical and radiographic union (2–4 mos)
		Acute displaced **Proximal ⅓** Acute nondisplaced	ORIF LAC-TS × 6 wks, then SAC-TS, consider referral due to prolonged casting or possible ORIF
		Displaced	ORIF
Lunate	PA, lateral Bone scan or MRI if Kienböck disease (AVN) suspected	Main body fractures Dorsal or marginal chip fractures Kienböck disease (AVN)	Refer (high risk) SAC × 4–6 wks Refer
Triquetrum	PA, oblique, lateral	Dorsal chip Body nondisplaced Body displaced	SAC × 4 wks SAC × 4–6 wks Refer for possible ORIF or associated CMC injury
Trapezium	Oblique, lateral, and carpal tunnel views Bett's view Consider CT	Dorsal cortical (trapezio-metacarpal) Body displaced	SAC-TS × 4 wks Refer, may be associated with first CMC Subluxation/dislocation
		Body nondisplaced Trapezial ridge, distal Trapezial ridge, proximal	SAC-TS × 4 wks Refer SAC-TS × 4 wks
Capitate	PA, lateral, oblique Consider CT, MRI	Body	Refer (high-risk AVN)
Hamate	PA, lateral, 45 degrees oblique supinated, carpal tunnel view, CT scan	Body nondisplaced Body displaced Hook	SAC × 4–6 wks Refer Refer for possible early excision
Pisiform	Lateral with wrist 20–45 degrees oblique supinated, carpal tunnel view Consider CT or bone scan	Pisiform	SAC with wrist 30 degrees flexed and mild ulnar deviation × 4 wks Excision if still painful

PA = posteroanterior; SAC = short arm cast; TS = thumb spica; LAC = long arm cast; ORIF = open reduction (with) internal fixation; CMC = carpometacarpal; CT = computed tomography; MRI = magnetic resonance imaging; AVN = avascular necrosis.

to refer individuals with these risk factors to an orthopedic surgeon for management.

Acute nondisplaced distal fractures have a union rate of between 90% and 100%, with an average immobilization time of 10 weeks.[7, 10, 11] Approximately 80–90% of waist fractures heal after 10–12 weeks.[12] Proximal pole fractures have a healing rate of 60–70% after 12–20 weeks of immobilization.[13] Nondisplaced distal or waist fractures (Figure 10-6) should be placed in a long arm thumb spica cast for 6 weeks followed by a short arm thumb spica cast until clinical and radiographic healing is evident.[14] The cast should be replaced and x-ray films of the injury

taken every 2–3 weeks to ensure good fit and confirm proper fracture healing.[15] Excessive use of even the casted hand can cause compression at the fracture site and should be avoided. Impact loading should be avoided for 3 months after cast removal. For certain sports, however, consideration may be given to allow the return to play a week after cast removal, if the athlete is given a short arm thumb spica orthosis and understands the risks.[14] Silicone rubber casts have appropriate hardness and impact-absorbing qualities and are generally well tolerated.[16] Fractures of the proximal pole can be treated as described but will require prolonged immobilization and

FIGURE 10-6
Scaphoid fracture. Subtle appearance of a nondisplaced transverse fracture of the waist of the scaphoid (arrow).

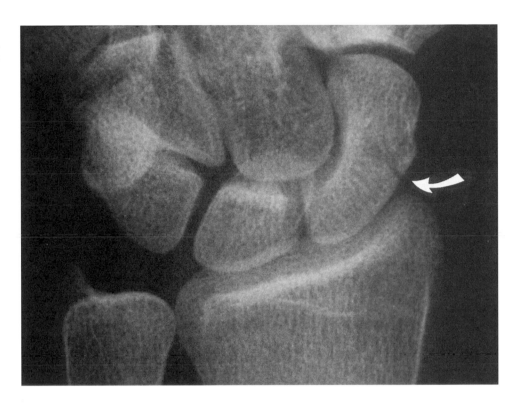

still may result in nonunion or AVN. For this reason, referral to a surgeon may be advisable.

The prolonged immobilization time necessary for healing of even nondisplaced fractures may be unacceptable to some athletes, and it is reasonable in these circumstances to refer for consideration of Herbert-Whipple screw fixation.[17] This technique has been shown to allow athletes to return to play in 7 weeks with a 100% union rate of middle third fractures.[9]

SPECIAL CONSIDERATIONS IN THE PEDIATRIC ATHLETE
In children, 87% of scaphoid fractures are of the distal third, whereas 70% of adult fractures are at the waist.[18] The nondisplaced distal one-third fractures respond well to short arm thumb spica casting for 6–10 weeks, and all others should be treated similar to adults.[19]

Other Carpal Fractures

Lunate
Acute fractures of the lunate are unusual and include marginal chip, dorsal pole, sagittal and transverse body, and volar pole fractures.[20] Fractures of the main body of the hamate may progress to carpal instability, nonunion, or AVN.[21] Displaced volar pole and any body fractures should be referred for consideration of open reduction, internal

fixation (ORIF), because distraction by important volar stabilizing ligaments may interfere with healing. Marginal and dorsal fractures are inherently more stable and can be treated with casting for 4–6 weeks.[20]

Kienböck disease refers to idiopathic AVN of the lunate. This is generally atraumatic in origin, although trauma may precipitate symptoms. Patients present with wrist pain, stiffness, and variable swelling, and tenderness is localized over the dorsum of the lunate. The diagnosis is generally made radiographically. Plain radiographs frequently demonstrate a negative ulnar variance (the articular surface of the ulna aligns proximal to the articular surface of the radius). The lunate may appear normal in early stages but will eventually progress to a linear compression fracture, increased sclerosis, and carpal collapse. If clinical suspicion is strong with normal radiographs, a bone scan or MRI should be considered. Patients with diagnosed or suspected Kienböck disease should be referred, because the treatment may involve complex joint leveling procedures, proximal row carpectomy, or joint fusion.

Triquetral Fractures
Fractures of the triquetrum can be to the body or, more commonly, a dorsal cortical chip fracture (Figure 10-7). Dorsal chip fractures are likely caused by the ulnar styloid

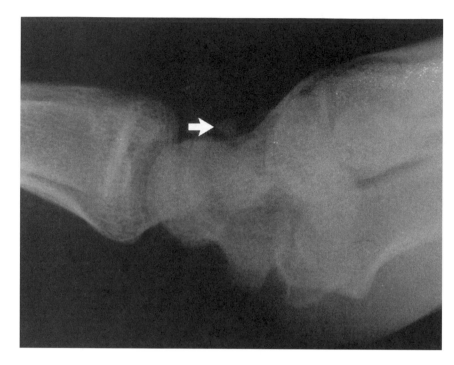

FIGURE 10-7
Dorsal triquetral chip fracture (arrow).

impacting the dorsal triquetrum during forced dorsiflexion of the wrist. The fracture is best visualized on lateral and oblique views. The body fractures with direct trauma and is generally nondisplaced. Both dorsal chip fractures and nondisplaced body fractures can be treated with a short arm cast for 4–6 weeks.[20] Displaced body fractures should be referred for evaluation of associated ligamentous injury and consideration of surgery. Dorsal chip fractures, which do not heal and are symptomatic, can be treated with a local injection and possibly excision of the fragment.

Trapezium Fractures

The trapezium is fractured directly when the base of the thumb metacarpal is axially driven into the articular surface or indirectly from ligamentous or capsular avulsion.[21] Isolated trapezial fractures are rare and can be one of three types: body, marginal trapeziometacarpal, and trapezial ridge (volar).[20] Trapezial ridge fractures are suspected with point tenderness just distal to the scaphoid tuberosity. Body fractures and trapeziometacarpal fractures are tender dorsally proximal to the thumb carpometacarpal joint. Thumb range of motion may be painless, but pinch strength is weak. Radiographic views should include PA, lateral, oblique, carpal tunnel, and Bett view (thumb extended and abducted, wrist slightly pronated, hypothenar eminence on cassette, and the beam centered on the scapho-trapeziotrapezium joint).

Nondisplaced body, marginal trapeziometacarpal, and trapezial ridge fractures at the base (proximal) can be treated with a short arm thumb spica cast for 4 weeks.[20]

Displaced body and distal trapezial ridge fractures should be referred for possible surgical treatment.

Capitate Fractures

Isolated capitate fractures are rare and predisposed to AVN or nonunion. PA and lateral radiographs may show a transverse fracture through the waist. If these views are normal and suspicion remains, a bone scan, CT, tomogram, or MRI should be ordered. These fractures should be splinted and referred for management because of the high complication rate.

Hamate Fractures

There are two main types of hamate fractures: (1) body and (2) hook of the hamate (hamulus). Body fractures occur with direct trauma, but hook fractures may be more insidious. The base of a bat, racket, or golf club may abut the hook of the hamate at the end of a swing, causing a fracture. Hook fractures may be missed unless strongly suspected. Ulnar and volar wrist pain is aggravated when the patient attempts to swing a club or racket. Deep palpation over the hook of the hamate in the base of the palm is painful, and there may be tenderness over the dorsoulnar aspect of the hamate. Radiographs should include PA, lateral, carpal tunnel, and 45-degree supinated oblique views. Tomograms or CT may be necessary to demonstrate fractures at the base of the hook. Nondisplaced body fractures can be treated with a short arm cast for 4–6 weeks, and displaced body fractures should be referred for possible ORIF.[20] The treatment for acute hook fractures is somewhat more controversial, because only approximately 50% will heal with prolonged casting (6 weeks to 4 months or longer).[22] Adults with an acute injury can be given the option of a trial of casting (if they present within 2 weeks of injury) or early excision. Many authors recommend early excision and rehabilitation, because athletes can generally return to full, painless activity by 3 months.[15, 20] Fractures older than 2 weeks should undergo excision of the hook.

SPECIAL CONSIDERATIONS IN THE PEDIATRIC ATHLETE
Children with hook of the hamate fractures should initially be treated for 6 weeks with a short arm cast incorporating the fourth and fifth metacarpophalangeal joints in flexion and the base of the thumb included.[15] If there is no sign of union or if symptoms persist, excision is indicated.

Pisiform Fractures

Pisiform fractures are uncommon but can occur with a direct blow to the hypothenar eminence or with repetitive microtrauma. Affected individuals will have tenderness over the pisiform on the proximal volar hypothenar eminence. Radiographs should include 20- to 45-degree supinated oblique and carpal tunnel views, and a bone scan or CT may be necessary to confirm the fracture. Initial treatment is a short arm cast for 4–6 weeks.[20] Patients with symptomatic nonunions or subsequent pisotriquetral arthritis can be treated with a pisiform excision.

Distal Radius Fractures

The initial determination should be whether the fracture is in an acceptable position or needs reduction. For young or active individuals, there should be no more than 2 mm of radial shortening, 2 mm displacement of an articular fragment, or 15 degrees dorsal angulation of the distal fragment.[20] Nondisplaced extraarticular fractures can be treated with a sugar tong splint for 3 weeks followed by 3 weeks of short arm casting[20] or short arm casting for 6 weeks.[21] It is prudent to repeat radiographs through the cast weekly for 2–3 weeks to assure the alignment is maintained. Fractures requiring reduction are inherently unstable and should be treated with a well-molded long arm cast for 6 weeks, with weekly radiographs for the first 3 weeks to assure the reduction is maintained. Most displaced, angulated, or intraarticular fractures should probably be managed by a surgeon, because he or she can perform the ORIF if closed treatment fails.

SPECIAL CONSIDERATIONS IN THE PEDIATRIC ATHLETE
The generally softer bone and open growth plates in children are responsible for different patterns of injury than in adults. Epiphyseal injuries can occur with loads as small as 55% of a child's body weight.[23] A Salter-Harris I fracture is

a clinical diagnosis whereby there is tenderness over the growth plate in a traumatized wrist with normal radiographs.[24] In a Salter-Harris II fracture, there is a fracture through the growth plate that extends into the metaphysis, and the joint space is not involved. Salter-Harris III and IV fractures involve the joint space. All displaced or angulated fractures and all Salter-Harris III and IV fractures should be referred for anatomic reduction and close follow-up because of the risk of premature growth plate closure. Nondisplaced Salter-Harris I and II fractures can be treated with short arm casting for 3 and 5 weeks respectively.[19, 25] Parents should be cautioned that there is a still a possibility of premature growth arrest with the grade I and II injuries.

Torus fractures involve buckling of the soft cortex (generally dorsal) and are relatively stable (Figure 10-8A). Greenstick fractures are caused by greater forces and involve buckling of one cortex associated with disruption of the opposite cortex; they can be quite subtle and unstable (Figure 10-8B). Careful inspection should be made of the lateral radiographs to look for a crack of the cortex opposite the buckling. All displaced or angulated fractures should be referred for reduction, casting, and close follow-up.

Nonangulated true torus fractures (disruption or buckling of only one cortex) can be treated with a short arm cast or volar splint for 3–4 weeks.[26] It is probably prudent to repeat radiographs in a week to assure proper alignment. Greenstick fractures (both cortices involved) are more problematic. Angulations more than 10 degrees should be reduced and are at high risk of reangulation, even in a cast.[26] If alignment is anatomic, these can be treated with a well-molded long arm cast for 4 weeks, followed by a wrist splint for 1–2 weeks.[26] Radiographs must be repeated weekly for the next 2 weeks to make sure the fracture has not angulated in the cast. If there is any question regarding acceptable position or management, these are best referred to an orthopedic surgeon.

Radial Ligamentous Injuries

Radial instabilities center around injuries to the ligaments surrounding the scaphoid and include scapholunate dissociation (rotatory subluxation of the scaphoid), dorsal perilunate dislocation, and lunate dislocation[3] (see Figures 10-2 and 10-4).

Scapholunate Dissociation (Rotatory Subluxation of the Scaphoid)

The mechanism of injury is similar to that of scaphoid fractures (dorsiflexion injury to the wrist). In the absence of associated scaphoid fracture, these can be easily missed unless there is a high index of suspicion and radiographs are carefully interpreted. Early diagnosis and treatment

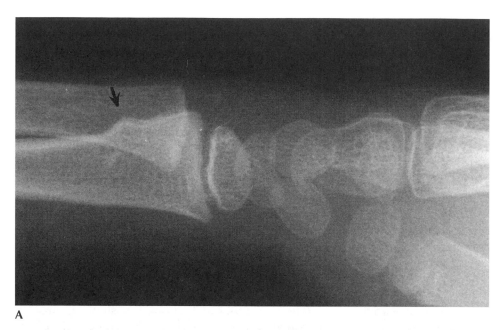

A

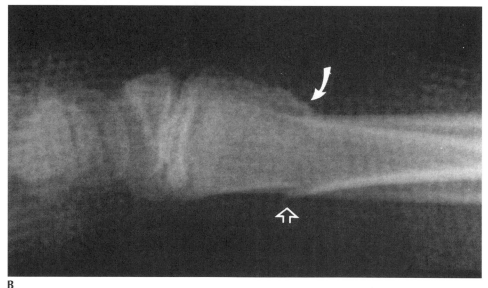

B

FIGURE 10-8
*Distal radius fractures in children.
A. Torus fracture. There is cortical
buckling of the dorsal cortex
(arrow), but the volar cortex is
intact (making this fracture stable).
B. Greenstick fracture. Note the
dorsal cortex buckling (closed
arrow) and the volar cortical disruption (open arrow). This fracture has a high propensity toward
angulating, even in a cast.*

of this injury are imperative to prevent future static instabilities and degenerative changes.

An understanding of normal wrist mechanics is necessary to interpret physical examination and radiographic
findings. The scaphoid normally moves out of the way
by palmar flexing (becoming more vertical) with radial
deviation. An intact scapholunate ligament forces the
lunate to move with the scaphoid—that is, the lunate will
palmar flex with radial deviation. If the scapholunate ligament is ruptured, the scaphoid will still palmar flex with
radial deviation, but the lunate will go with its natural
tendency to dorsiflex. The result is a vertical scaphoid

(rotatory subluxation) and a dorsiflexed lunate (dorsal
intercalated segment instability [DISI]) (Figures 10-9 and
10-10A).

Physical examination reveals a tender, swollen wrist
with limited range of motion. The tenderness is concentrated over the volar and dorsal aspects of the scapholunate joint (just distal to the midradius). Watson scaphoid
test[27] may be positive. In this test, the patient's hand is
placed in ulnar deviation (making the scaphoid horizontal and neutral). The examiner's thumb is placed on the
scaphoid tuberosity and the four fingers of the same hand
placed on the dorsal aspect of the distal radius. The thumb

pushes on the scaphoid in an attempt to keep it from becoming vertical as the patient's hand is radially deviated. If the scapholunate ligaments are ruptured, the thumb will effectively prevent the scaphoid from palmar flexing, which will force the proximal pole to move dorsally and cause pain or a painful click.

PA radiographs will show the scapholunate space to be more than 3 mm, or greater than the other carpal spaces (Figure 10-10B), and may show a ring sign (the scaphoid appears short, and the end-on projection of the rotated scaphoid gives a ringed appearance). Bilateral PA clenched-fist view will occasionally reveal a more subtle scapholunate widening not appreciated on regular PA views. Lateral views (see Figures 10-9 and 10-10A) show the lunate is dorsiflexed (DISI pattern) with a capitolunate angle more than 15 degrees, and the scapholunate angle will be more than 60–70 degrees.[28] These injuries should be referred to an orthopedic surgeon. Treatment involves closed reduction and percutaneous pinning within 3–4 weeks of injury or ORIF with ligament repair or capsulorrhaphy in more chronic cases.[29]

Perilunate and Lunate Dislocations

A severe hyperextension injury to the wrist causes the scaphoid to extend and strike the dorsal lip of the radius. This ruptures the volar radioscaphoid and scapholunate ligaments, freeing the proximal pole of the scaphoid while compressive forces wedge the capitate between the scaphoid and lunate. Continued dorsiflexion essentially causes the distal carpal row to "peel" away from the lunate and come to rest dorsal to the lunate and radius, resulting in a perilunate dislocation. Further force ruptures the dorsal restraining radiocarpal ligament, allowing the lunate to "flip" palmward (spilled teacup sign) as the remaining carpal bones relocate. This results in a lunate dislocation.[30]

On physical examination, the neurovascular status must be assessed, with particular attention to the median nerve (see Table 10-1 and Figure 10-3). On PA radiographs, the lunate appears triangular rather than in its normal trapezoidal configuration. Lateral views show the distal carpal row lies dorsal to the lunate and radius with a perilunate dislocation and a spilled teacup sign (the lunate faces palmward and rests volar to the radius and distal carpal row) with a lunate dislocation. Patients with these injuries should be referred to an orthopedic surgeon for closed or open reduction.

Ulnar Side Ligament Injuries

Ulnar side instabilities are due to a rupture of the stabilizing triquetrolunate or triquetrohamate ligaments (see Figure 10-2).

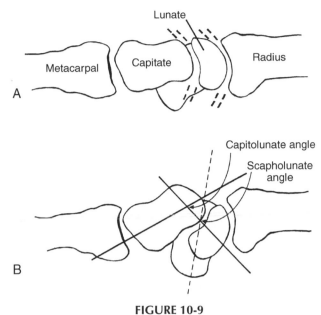

FIGURE 10-9
Carpal bone alignment, lateral view. A. Normal alignment. The four Cs of the distal radius, proximal lunate, distal lunate, and capitate should line up (be parallel). The angle between the horizontal axis of the capitate and lunate (capitolunate angle) should be 0 ± 15 degrees. The scapholunate angle should be 30–60 degrees. B. Dorsal intercalated segmental instability pattern with an increase in both the scapholunate and capitolunate angles.

Triquetrolunate Instabilities

In the normal wrist, ulnar deviation causes the triquetrum to dorsiflex. This causes the lunate and scaphoid to also dorsiflex because of the triquetrum's ligamentous attachments to the rest of the proximal carpal row. With rupture of the triquetrolunate ligament, the triquetrum will still dorsiflex with ulnar deviation, but the lunate and scaphoid will now be volar flexed. This results in a volar intercalated segment instability (VISI).

Physical examination reveals a painful click as the wrist is compressed and moved from ulnar to radial deviation. Tenderness is concentrated over the ulnar aspect of the carpus. The lunotriquetral ballottement test is done as follows: The lunate is stabilized with the examiner's thumb and index finger. With the other hand, the examiner grasps the patient's pisiform and triquetrum and moves them in a volar and dorsal direction, checking for laxity, crepitus, and pain.[31]

Static radiographic views are often normal. PA views may show a break in the carpal arc between the lunate and triquetrum, and lateral views may show a dorsiflexed triquetrum with a volar flexed scaphoid and lunate (VISI pattern). The scapholunate angle (see Figure 10-5) remains less than 70 degrees, but there is a volar tilt to the lunate

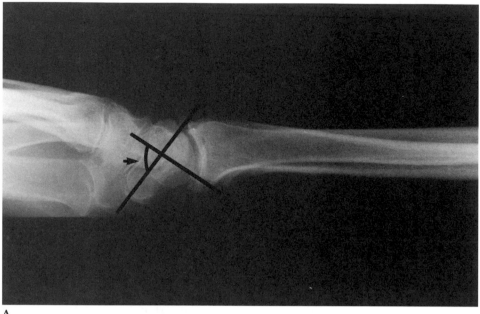

A

FIGURE 10-10
*Scapholunate dissociation.
A. Lateral view demonstrating an
increased scapholunate angle
(arrow) of approximately 85
degrees (normal is <60–70
degrees). B. Posteroanterior view
of the same wrist demonstrating
the widened intercarpal space
between the lunate and scaphoid
(arrow).*

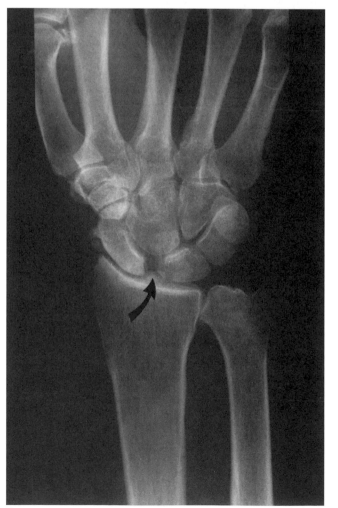

B

relative to the distal radius. Careful inspection of PA views may reveal a small avulsion fracture off the radial aspect of the volar surface of the triquetrum. This small fleck is easily missed but is strongly associated with triquetrolunate ligament disruption.[32] If clinical suspicion remains, an arthrogram or arthroscopy may be necessary. MRI is not very accurate for triquetrolunate disruptions because of the relatively small size of the ligament.[4]

Treatment depends on the severity of injury. Acute injuries with obvious instability (positive ballottement test and VISI deformity) should be referred to a hand surgeon for consideration of ligament repair.[33] Less severe injuries can be treated with a trial of long arm casting followed by ligament repair if this fails.[29, 33]

Triquetrohamate Instability

In triquetrohamate rupture, the loss of the hamate's bony geometric influence on the triquetrum allows for a VISI pattern.[34] On physical examination, there is often a painful click with ulnar deviation and pronation.

These ulnar instabilities are often dynamic and not identified on plain static views. Lateral x-ray films may show a volar flexed lunate (VISI) pattern. Videofluoroscopy is the most useful tool in evaluating dynamic instabilities. Suspected injuries should be referred to a hand surgeon, because these are difficult to diagnose and treat.

Triangular Fibrocartilage Complex Injuries

The triangular fibrocartilage complex (TFCC) is composed of a triangular fibrocartilage, meniscus homologue, articular disk, ulnar collateral ligament, dorsal and volar radioulnar ligaments, and the extensor carpi ulnaris sheath (see Figure 10-1). It "suspends" the carpal bones from the radius, serves as a major stabilizer of the radioulnar joint, and functions as a cushion for ulnar axial loads.[34] The height or thickness of the TFCC depends on ulnar variance (ulnar head in relation to the radial articular surface). In individuals with positive ulnar variance (articular surface of the ulnar head distal to the articular surface of the radius), the TFCC is thinner and more prone to injury. TFCC tears may be posttraumatic (fall on a dorsiflexed and ulnar-deviated wrist) or degenerative. Affected individuals report ulnar side wrist pain aggravated by forearm supination and pronation.

The physical examination should address both the TFCC and the distal radioulnar joint (DRUJ). The press test is a simple office test that has been shown to be 100% sensitive for TFCC tears.[35] The seated patient grips both sides of the chair and lifts him- or herself up by pressing down on the chair. Pain on the ulnar aspect of the wrist is a positive test. The TFCC grind test assesses three components

of the TFCC and is positive with provocation of pain, with or without crepitus or a click.[36] Central or peripheral tears are stressed by placing the forearm in neutral rotation with the wrist ulnarly deviated. The wrist is then passively rolled from an ulnar dorsal position to ulnar volar and back. The volar radioulnar ligament is tested by repeating the preceding maneuver with the forearm fully supinated. The dorsal attachment is tested by performing the test with the forearm fully pronated.

Subluxation of the DRUJ must be evaluated in all suspected TFCC tears. Subluxations of the DRUJ are generally associated with a fracture of the radial head (Essex-Lopresti) or the shaft of the radius (Galeazzi) but rarely can occur in the absence of fracture. With DRUJ subluxations, the joint is generally swollen and tender, and active supination and pronation is painful. To evaluate DRUJ involvement in TFCC tears, the examiner applies a radioulnar squeeze proximal to the DRUJ, and the forearm is passively rotated. If the DRUJ is involved, the wrist will still be painful, but there is little to no pain with an isolated TFCC tear.[37]

PA radiographs should be taken with the shoulder abducted 90 degrees, elbow flexed 90 degrees, and hand flat.[38] Positive ulnar variance (ulna 1–5 mm longer than the radial articular surface[30]) is associated with TFCC injury and impingement.[34] The lateral radiograph should be taken with the shoulder at 0 degrees, elbow flexed to 90 degrees, and the x-ray beam at a right angle to the wrist. One should look for fracture or ulnar subluxation (the ulnar styloid normally should be in the center of the ulnar head). Bilateral CT may be necessary to assess for subtle radioulnar subluxation, and MRI is a more reliable method for evaluating for TFCC tears (90–95% accurate[10]) (Figure 10-11). Arthrography may be the best method of detecting tears of the TFCC but can be difficult to interpret.

Initial treatment for acute injuries is immobilization. If there is no ulnar subluxation, a long arm cast with the forearm in neutral position is worn for 4–6 weeks. With ulnar instability, the long arm cast is applied with the wrist rotated in the position of stability or reduction of the radioulnar joint.[29] The proper position may be difficult to determine in the acute setting, and referral should be considered. Casting is followed by splinting and progressive range of motion and strengthening exercises. A steroid injection may be attempted for persistent localized pain after immobilization. Those with persistent pain should be referred for possible surgical intervention.

Acute Subluxation of Extensor Carpi Ulnaris Tendon

Acute subluxation of extensor carpi ulnaris tendon is caused by tears of the retinaculum over the sixth com-

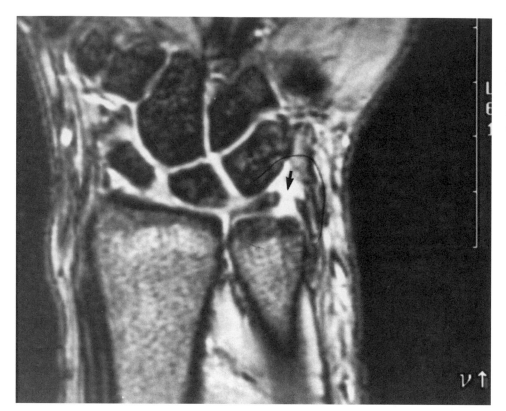

FIGURE 10-11
Triangular fibrocartilage complex (TFCC) tear. Magnetic resonance imaging demonstrates increased signal intensity within the TFCC (arrow) and a lack of attachment to the base or apex of the ulnar styloid.

partment, allowing the extensor carpi ulnaris (ECU) tendon to "snap" out of the groove (Figure 10-12). The mechanism of injury is generally forced wrist supination, flexion, and ulnar deviation.

On physical examination, there is tenderness dorsal and just distal to the ulnar head with the wrist pronated and over the ulnar aspect when supinated. There may be a painful snapping sensation over the dorsal ulnar aspect of the distal ulna when the supinated, flexed wrist is actively moved from radial deviation to ulnar deviation.[33] Relief of pain after injecting the sixth dorsal compartment with a local anesthetic may help confirm the diagnosis. The acutely injured patient is treated either with above-the-elbow casting with the wrist supinated and in radial deviation for 6 weeks, or with acute surgical repair of the retinaculum.[33] Chronic symptomatic subluxators may benefit from surgical reconstruction of the retinaculum.

OVERUSE INJURIES OF THE WRIST

Tendinitis (inflammation of the tendon itself) and tenosynovitis (inflammation of the tendon sheath) can involve any of the tendons about the wrist (see Figure 10-12). The common denominator in tendinitis is simply an overdemand on the involved tendon. The tendon responds in a characteristic sequential manner: inflammation or hemorrhage, cellular invasion, collagen production, maturation, and strengthening.[39] These injuries are overdemand injuries that are a result of repetitive microtrauma, and they are of insidious onset. Acute macrotrauma may aggravate an underlying chronic condition.

Specific overuse injuries of the wrist are listed in Figure 10-13.

Physical Examination

The involved tendon or group of tendons are tender to touch and painful with passive stretching or when working against resistance. Swelling and erythema are variable but most prominent with tenosynovitis.

Treatment Guidelines

Treatment guidelines are similar for all of the tendinitides and are based on the pathologic processes. Pain and inflammation are controlled with ice massage for 10 minutes 4 times a day for the first 48–72 hours, nonsteroidal anti-inflammatory drugs (NSAIDs), and relative rest from the

FIGURE 10-12
The six dorsal compartments of the wrist and the location of intersection syndrome. The synovial sheaths that enclose the tendons within the sheaths are not depicted.

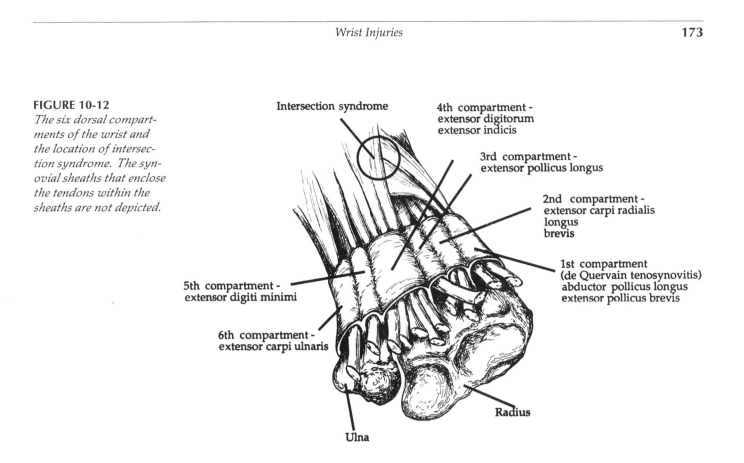

Intersection syndrome

4th compartment -
extensor digitorum
extensor indicis

3rd compartment -
extensor pollicus longus

2nd compartment -
extensor carpi radialis
longus
brevis

1st compartment
(de Quervain tenosynovitis)
abductor pollicus longus
extensor pollicus brevis

5th compartment -
extensor digiti minimi

6th compartment -
extensor carpi ulnaris

Radius

Ulna

inciting activity. The goal is for the athlete to participate only in activities during which the wrist is not painful. This may require any or all of the following: (1) continue the sport but protect the injured tendon with a wrist splint or brace, (2) decrease the intensity or duration of the activity, or (3) temporarily substitute another sport or activity that does not cause pain. Steroid injection in the tendon sheath for tenosynovitis is useful in resistant cases; the tendon itself should never be directly injected. The only exception to injection in the tendon sheath is the third dorsal compartment (extensor pollicis longus), where the risk of rupture precludes injection. Healing and range of motion are promoted using contrast baths after 72 hours or when the swelling subsides. The wrist is placed in a container of hot water (102°–105°F) for 4 minutes, during which active range of motion exercises are performed. The wrist is then placed in cold water (< 50°F) or ice water for 1 minute. This cycle is repeated four times, always ending with the ice water, and should be done two to three times a day.

Ultrasound or phonophoresis is useful at tendon-bone or tendon-muscle interfaces, primarily to provide a deep-heating action with possibly some anti-inflammatory benefit. Iontophoresis is possibly a more useful anti-inflammatory modality, because the inflamed tissue is relatively superficial. Relative rest or splinting is continued as necessary to allow pain-free activity. When pain is absent at rest and swelling has subsided, high-

repetition, low-resistance, and progressive-resistance exercises are initiated for wrist flexion, extension, supination, and pronation, using elastic therapy bands, surgical tubing, or free weights. The athlete begins the exercise sessions with 30-second stretches of the anterior and posterior forearm muscles three times, followed by three sets of 10–15 repetitions of each exercise. The amount of resistance is increased as pain resolves. The forearm stretches are repeated, and ice massage to the involved tendon for 10 minutes is applied.

Dorsal Radial Injuries

de Quervain Tenosynovitis
The tendons in the first dorsal compartment, the abductor pollicis longus and extensor pollicis brevis, are highly prone to tendinitis and tenosynovitis from repetitive wrist motion (see Figure 10-12). Physical examination reveals tenderness and variable swelling over the first dorsal compartment, lateral to the radial styloid. Finkelstein test is performed by having the patient grasp his or her thumb under the index and middle fingers of the same hand and making a clenched fist. The patient then actively deviates the wrist in an ulnar direction. This maneuver causes pain radially if the tendons are inflamed. Treatment is as outlined under the treatment guidelines for overuse injuries. Approximately 80% of patients respond to thumb spica

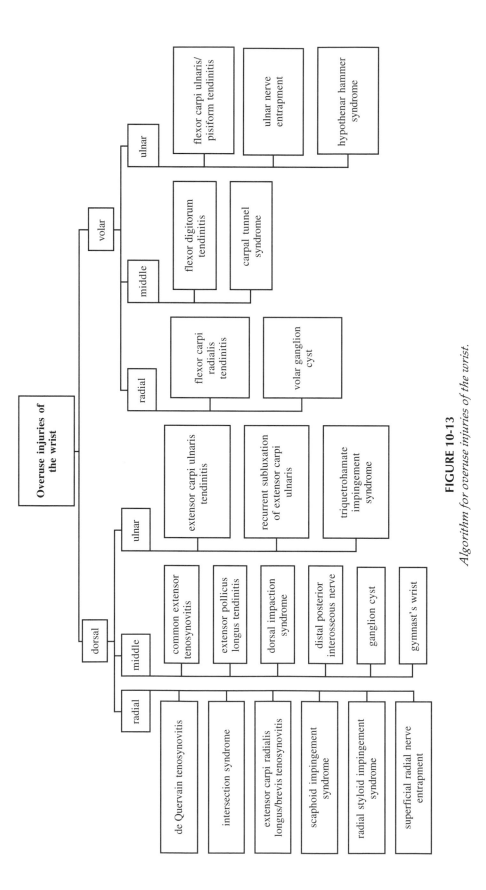

FIGURE 10-13

Algorithm for overuse injuries of the wrist.

splinting, NSAIDs, ice massage, and steroid injections.[40] There may be a longitudinal septum between the abductor pollicis longus and extensor pollicis brevis in 20–30% of individuals, and a second steroid injection more dorsally may prove useful.[11] Surgical release is indicated for patients who fail conservative treatment.

Intersection Syndrome

Intersection syndrome, described by Wood and Dobyns,[41] is similar to de Quervain disease but occurs more proximally, where the abductor pollicis longus and extensor pollicis brevis cross the radial wrist extensors (approximately 3 in. proximal to the radial styloid; see Figure 10-12). Pain and swelling may be due to a peritendinitis or an adventitial bursitis. This is common in sports such as weight lifting and rowing. Physical examination reveals tenderness, swelling, and crepitus approximately 3 in. proximal to Lister tubercle. Symptoms are aggravated by active wrist radial and ulnar deviation. Treatment is as outlined under the treatment guidelines for overuse injuries. Thumb spica splinting, ice, NSAIDs, and steroid injections are effective in 95% of cases.[42] Resistant cases should be referred for surgical exploration and debridement.

Extensor Carpi Radialis Longus and Brevis Tenosynovitis

The extensor carpi radialis longus and brevis tendons are contained in the second dorsal compartment and are frequently involved in overuse syndromes of the wrist (see Figure 10-12). This tenosynovitis is often seen in sports requiring repetitive wrist acceleration and deceleration. Treatment is as outlined under the treatment guidelines for overuse injuries.

Scaphoid Impingement Syndrome

In the scaphoid impingement syndrome, repetitive forced hyperextension of the wrist, such as in weight lifting or gymnastics, causes the proximal scaphoid and the radius to abut. This leads to damage to the capsule, ligament, or articular surface.[43] Physical examination reveals tenderness dorsally between the proximal scaphoid and radius, with the wrist slightly flexed and in ulnar deviation. Dorsiflexion of the wrist accentuates the pain. Lateral radiographs in chronic cases may show a hypertrophic ridge on the dorsal scaphoid rim. Treatment is as outlined under the treatment guidelines for overuse injuries. Splints or braces that limit wrist dorsiflexion are useful in gymnasts (Lions Paw, RBJ Athletics Specialties, Spanish Forks, UT). Steroid injection along the dorsal rim of the scaphoid may be attempted if conservative therapy fails. Resistant cases may require surgery.

Radial Styloid Impingement Syndrome

This syndrome is similar to scaphoid impingement (except for its location) and is usually caused by a mechanism similar to a golfer decelerating the club head during a backswing. Physical examination reveals tenderness on the dorsal aspect of the radial styloid, and pain is present with forced radial deviation. Radiographs may show degenerative changes in the radioscaphoid joint. Treatment is as outlined under the treatment guidelines for overuse injuries, including local steroid injection. Slowing or changing the mechanics of the backswing may also help.

Superficial Radial Nerve (Wartenberg) Syndrome

The superficial radial nerve may become either tethered between the extensor carpi radialis and brevis tendons from repetitive pronation and supination or damaged from direct trauma or extrinsic pressure (wrist bands).[44] Patients report numbness over the dorsoradial aspect of the wrist and hand, dorsal thumb, and index finger. There is a positive Tinel sign over the dorsoradial wrist, and symptoms are not aggravated by motion (this distinguishes it from tendinitis, arthritis, and impingement). Finkelstein test is negative unless there is a concomitant de Quervain tenosynovitis. Sensory nerve action potentials are helpful only if they are positive. Treatment involves splinting, NSAIDs, and avoiding any constrictive wrist bands. Surgery may be considered if symptoms last longer than 6–12 months, although surgery after 18 months offers little benefit.[44]

Dorsal Middle Injuries

Common Extensor Tenosynovitis

Common extensor tenosynovitis is also called *fourth compartment syndrome* and is characterized by a painful erythematous "goose-foot" swelling over the dorsum of the wrist (see Figure 10-12). Treatment is as outlined under the treatment guidelines for overuse injuries.

Extensor Pollicis Longus Tenosynovitis

The extensor pollicis longus (EPL) tendon courses through the third dorsal compartment and is relatively thin where it passes through a narrow curved tunnel around Lister tubercle (see Figure 10-12). Early diagnosis and treatment is necessary to prevent tendon rupture at Lister tubercle. EPL tendinitis or rupture is more common in patients with rheumatoid arthritis, after a distal radius fracture, and with repetitive motion (drummer boy palsy).[42] Physical examination reveals tenderness over the third dorsal compartment (next to Lister tubercle), which is aggravated by thumb extension. Treatment should include thumb spica splinting, ice, NSAIDs, and relative rest (as outlined under the treatment guidelines for overuse injuries). Steroid injections should not be performed because of the risk of rupture. Resistant cases should be referred to a surgeon for consideration of tunnel release and tendon transposition.

Dorsal Impaction Syndrome

Repetitive loading of the dorsum of the wrist (e.g., in gymnastics) can lead to localized synovitis or bony hypertrophy on the dorsum of the scaphoid, lunate, or capitate.[45] Physical examination reveals tenderness and variable soft tissue or bony changes over the middorsum of the wrist, particularly the lunocapitate area. Lateral radiographs may show bony hypertrophy of the involved carpal bones. Treatment involves a splint restricting dorsiflexion (lion's paw), wrist flexion exercises, and possibly a local steroid injection into the hypertrophied synovium.[46] More severe cases may require a static wrist splint and absolute wrist rest for 4–6 weeks, followed by gradual resumption of activities. Resistant cases may benefit from a limited synovectomy or cheilectomy.

Distal Posterior Interosseous Nerve Syndrome

Repetitive forced dorsiflexion of the wrist can lead to compression of the deep terminal branch of the posterior interosseous nerve as it passes dorsally over the distal radius and enters the wrist capsule.[47] This syndrome is generally a diagnosis of exclusion. Patients report a deep, dull ache in the wrist that may become worse with wrist extension. Symptoms may be reproduced with deep palpation of the dorsal distal forearm (over the fourth dorsal compartment) with the wrist flexed or with forceful extension. Relief of pain with a local anesthetic or steroid injection helps support the diagnosis. Treatment involves limiting wrist dorsiflexion (Lions Paw) and as outlined under the treatment guidelines for overuse injuries. Surgical excision of the nerve may be considered if all conservative measures fail.[48]

Dorsal Ganglion

Occult dorsal ganglion is one of the most common causes of dorsal radial wrist pain in tennis players.[33] There is generally mucinous degeneration of the dorsal aspect of the scapholunate ligament and dorsal wrist capsule. Approximately 15% of cases are associated with trauma, and the remainder occur insidiously.[29] Physical examination reveals normal wrist range of motion and tenderness over the dorsoradial aspect of the wrist, generally over the scapholunate joint. Masses are better visualized and palpated with the wrist held in flexion; however, occult ganglion may not be palpable at all. Pain is often inversely related to the size of the mass. Plain radiographs are generally normal. Special imaging is often unnecessary for a larger, characteristic ganglion. MRI may be useful to define occult ganglion cysts and to rule out other entities such as lipomas, giant cell tumors, or arteriovenous malformations.[29] Treatment involves splinting the wrist in neutral (especially at night) and cyst aspiration and steroid injection. A recurring ganglion may require surgical excision.

Gymnast's Wrist (Pseudorickets Growth Plate Abnormality)

Repetitive compressive and shearing forces across the wrist growth plate are thought to cause Salter-Harris I microfractures within the growth plate in the zone of hypertrophying cells.[49] The same forces may induce temporary ischemia, which inhibits normal calcification of the growth plate.[49] The athlete, typically a gymnast, reports dorsal wrist pain that is aggravated by loading the wrist. Physical examination reveals tenderness over the distal radial growth plate but generally no swelling or restricted range of motion. Radiographs may be normal in the early stages but will progress to physeal widening and metaphyseal haziness and irregularity ("pseudorickets").[50] MRI is generally unnecessary but will show a parallel isointense line proximal to the growth plate.[50] Treatment involves omitting the inciting activity and strengthening the wrist flexors until asymptomatic. Taping the wrist or using a splint that blocks full wrist extension (e.g., lion's paw) should be considered on return to activities. If there are no radiographic changes on initial radiographs, return to full activity can be anticipated within 4 weeks. With radiographic changes, however, it may take 3 months or longer.[51] Premature closure of the growth plate may occur with continued stress on the painful wrist. In the long run, this may lead to relative overgrowth of the ulna and ulnar side wrist pain.

Dorsal Ulnar Injuries

Extensor Carpi Ulnaris Tenosynovitis

After de Quervain tenosynovitis, ECU is the most common stenosing tenosynovitis of the wrist (see Figure 10-12).[41] It may be caused by repetitive wrist motion that is posttraumatic (forced flexion, supination, and ulnar deviation) or secondary to a TFCC tear.[40] Local pain and tenderness may not be limited to the ECU tendon sheath because of its close proximity to the TFCC, and TFCC pathology may mimic ECU tenosynovitis. Injection of the ECU tendon sheath with a local anesthetic may help differentiate tenosynovitis from TFCC pathology. Treatment is as outlined under the treatment guidelines for overuse injuries.

Recurrent Subluxation of Extensor Carpi Ulnaris Tendon

Recurrent subluxation of the ECU tendon is caused by tears of the retinaculum over the sixth compartment (see Figure 10-12), allowing the ECU tendon to "snap" out of the groove. This may initially occur after traumatic supination of the wrist. On physical examination, there is a snapping sensation over the dorsal ulnar aspect of the distal ulna with wrist supination, flexion, and ulnar deviation. Acute cases are treated with immobilization in a long arm cast with the wrist fully supinated and slight dorsiflexion for 4 weeks.[41] Chronic cases should be referred to an orthopedic surgeon for possible reconstruction.

Triquetrohamate Impingement Syndrome

Triquetrohamate impingement syndrome usually results from acute or chronic wrist extension and ulnar deviation[45] such as occurs in floor exercises, racket sports, and side horse routines. Pain is from impaction of the proximal pole of the hamate on the triquetrum or chondromalacia on the lunate facet.[33] Physical examination reveals tenderness over the triquetrohamate joint dorsally. Pain increases with wrist extension and ulnar deviation. Treatment is as outlined under the treatment guidelines for overuse injuries. Steroid injection along the triquetral ridge may be used in resistant cases. Arthroscopic debridement may benefit selected patients.

Volar Radial Injuries: Flexor Carpi Radialis Tendinitis

The flexor carpi radialis tendon crosses the volar radial wrist and enters a synovial tunnel bordered by the scaphoid, trapezial ridge, and transverse carpal ligament. It then deviates 30 degrees over the scaphoid to insert on the bases of the second and third metacarpals and the trapezial ridge.[52] This angulation predisposes the tendon to mechanical wearing and tenosynovitis. Inflammation in the scaphotrapezial and metacarpotrapezial joints may either cause or be caused by flexor carpi radialis inflammation. Occult ganglia or an anomalous slip from the flexor pollicis longus to the flexor digitorum profundus (Linberg syndrome) may mimic tendon inflammation. Tenderness is localized over the flexor carpi radialis just proximal to the wrist crease, and pain is increased with resisted wrist flexion and

radial deviation. Treatment is as outlined under the treatment guidelines for overuse injuries, in addition to splinting the wrist flexed at 30 degrees. Resistant cases may respond to surgical decompression of the fibroosseous tunnel.[53]

Volar Middle Injuries

Flexor Digitorum Tendinitis

The flexor digitorum tendons pass through the carpal tunnel and can both mimic and cause carpal tunnel syndrome, complete with median nerve compression. The tendinitis is more common in sports requiring repetitive pulling (e.g., rowing) or prolonged pressure on the palms (e.g., cycling). Physical examination reveals pain and limited mobility of the fingers with possible hypoesthesia in the median nerve distribution (see Figure 10-3). Intrinsic muscle weakness indicates motor damage to the median nerve (see Table 10-1). Treatment is as outlined under the treatment guidelines for overuse injuries, but if pain is resistant or motor weakness is noted, a carpal tunnel release and synovectomy may be necessary.

Carpal Tunnel Syndrome

The median nerve at the level of the carpal tunnel contains the sensory branches to the radial 3.5 digits and a motor branch to the thenar eminence. Swelling in the rigid tunnel causes compression of the median nerve with the associated sensory and motor deficits. On physical examination, Phalen wrist flexion test reproduces symptoms, and Tinel test is positive in approximately 45% of cases.[54] Decreased vibratory sensation in the radial 3.5 digits is noted early, followed by decreased two-point discrimination. Electromyograms may be normal in 25% of patients with carpal tunnel syndrome[54] but still can exclude other etiologies of neurogenic wrist pain. Median nerve entrapment at the elbow can mimic carpal tunnel syndrome and should be considered (see Chapter 9).

Treatment is conservative, consisting of splinting the wrist in 20–30 degrees of dorsiflexion (especially at night), NSAIDs, and relative rest of the wrist. A steroid injection may be given with persistent symptoms. This is performed with a long 25-gauge needle inserted just proximal to the distal flexion crease between the palmaris longus and flexor carpi radialis tendons. If the needle insertion induces median nerve paresthesias, it must be withdrawn and redirected. Refer resistant cases for electromyography and nerve conduction studies, because these will give useful information regarding chronicity, severity, and regeneration. A carpal tunnel release may be necessary.

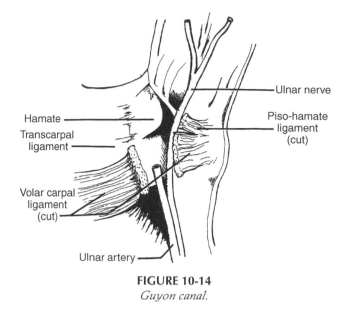

FIGURE 10-14
Guyon canal.

Volar Ulnar Injuries

Flexor Carpi Ulnaris and Pisiform Tendinitis

Flexor carpi ulnaris (FCU) and pisiform tendinitis is the most common wrist flexor tendinitis.[41] Repetitive wrist motion in racket sports, golf, and gymnastics leads to abnormal stress on the FCU and pisiform. The broad area of insertion into the pisiform and hypothenar fascia may allow for vague pain from the forearm to the ulnar side of the hand, but it is usually well localized. The ulnar nerve runs close to the tendon and is responsible for paresthesias in its distribution when the FCU is inflamed. Physical examination reveals moderate to marked swelling over the pisiform with increased pain on medial and lateral movement of the pisiform. Resisted wrist flexion and ulnar deviation makes the pain worse. An oblique radiograph will show the pisiform in profile and may reveal a calcific deposit near the insertion of the FCU.

Treatment is as outlined under the treatment guidelines for overuse injuries, in addition to a dorsal splint. A steroid injection can be directed into the calcific deposit or the tendon sheath. Surgery may be warranted if conservative measures fail.

Ulnar Nerve Compression

The ulnar nerve traverses Guyon canal between the pisiform and hamate and is divided into the superficial terminal branch (supplying sensation to the ulnar palm, fifth digit, and ulnar side of the fourth digit) and the deep terminal branch (innervating the interossei, hypothenar muscles, third and fourth lumbricals, adductor pollicis brevis, and the deep head of the flexor pollicis brevis)

(see Table 10-1 and Figure 10-14). The most common compression syndrome involves the deep terminal branch distal to the branch supplying the hypothenar muscles.[55] The second syndrome involves both the deep and superficial branches proximal to Guyon canal. This is most prevalent in sports such as cycling, weight lifting, and baseball (catchers) because of chronic repetitive insults to the hypothenar area.

Physical examination with deep terminal ulnar nerve involvement (most common) reveals weakness in the interossei, third and fourth lumbricals, adductor pollicis brevis, and flexor pollicis brevis. The hypothenar muscles may be spared, because the compression is usually distal to this nerve branch.[55] Proximal Guyon canal involvement results in weakness in all of the ulnar innervated muscles plus numbness in the ulnar 1.5 digits. Carpal tunnel views rule out hamate fractures or other osseous pathology.

Treatment involves protective padding over the hypothenar area and NSAIDs. Resistant cases should be referred for electromyography and nerve conduction studies, because these give useful information regarding chronicity, severity, and regeneration. Resistant cases or cases with evidence of motor loss should be referred to an orthopedic surgeon.

Hypothenar Hammer Syndrome (Ulnar Artery Injury)

The ulnar artery traverses Guyon canal and becomes relatively superficial for approximately 2 cm distal to the canal. It is covered at this point by the skin, the subcutaneous tissue, and the palmaris brevis muscle. A single blow or repetitive microtrauma in this vulnerable area (proximal ulnar palm) can cause spasm, thrombosis, or aneurysm of the ulnar artery.[56] Patients may report numbness in the ulnar 1.5 digits, ischemic pain, and possibly cold intolerance. Physical examination may reveal a mass in the hypothenar area indicative of an ulnar artery aneurysm. An Allen test will be positive if the ulnar artery is thrombosed, and intrinsic muscle cramping with repetitive finger flexion and extension indicates ischemia. Doppler ultrasonography may be helpful, and angiography is seldom needed but is diagnostic. Patients with these findings should be referred to a vascular surgeon.

Ganglions

Ganglions are benign tumor masses filled with viscous fluid. They arise most commonly from the dorsal scapholunate ligament, volar radioscaphoid ligament, and the sheath of the flexor carpi radialis tendon.[56] They are probably traumatically induced, allowing for fluid to pass through a rent in the potential weak spot and producing a cyst. They occur predominantly in young athletes and do not inhibit function. Physical examination reveals a variably sized cystic mass palpable on the volar or dorsal aspect of the wrist. Pain is variable but usually mild or absent. Treatment involves relative rest and splinting initially. Aspiration with or without steroid injection may be performed on larger, symptomatic cysts. Surgical excision may be necessary for recurrent cysts.

REFERENCES

1. Kauer J. Functional anatomy of the wrist. Clin Orthop 1980;149:9–20.
2. Taleisnik J. The ligaments of the wrist. J Hand Surg [AM] 1976;1:110–118.
3. Mayfield J, Johnson R, Kilcoyne R. Carpal dislocations: pathomechanics on progressive perilunar instability. J Hand Surg [AM] 1980;5:226–241.
4. Mooney J, Siegel D, Koman A. Ligamentous injuries of the wrist in athletes. Clin Sports Med 1992;11:129–139.
5. Zemel N, Stark H. Fractures and dislocations of the carpal bones. Clin Sports Med 1986;5:709–724.
6. Gelberman R, Panagis J, Taleisnik J, Baumgaertner M. The arterial anatomy of the human carpus. J Hand Surg [Am] 1983;8:367–375.
7. Brown B, Jupiter J, Levine A, et al. (eds), Skeletal Trauma. Philadelphia: Saunders, 1992.
8. Murphy D, Eisenhauer M, Powe J, Pavlofsky W. Can a day 4 bone scan accurately determine the presence or absence of scaphoid fracture? Ann Emerg Med 1995;26: 434–438.
9. Rettig A, Adsit W. Athletic Injuries of the Hand and Wrist. In L Griffin (ed), Orthopedic Knowledge Update: Sports Medicine. Rosemont, IL: American Academy of Orthopaedic Surgeons, 1994;205–224.
10. Fritz R, Brody G. MR imaging of the wrist and elbow. Clin Sports Med 1995;14:315–352.
11. Leslie B, Ericson W, Morehead J. Incidence of a septum within the first dorsal compartment of the wrist. J Hand Surg [Am] 1990;15:88–91.
12. Mastey R, Weiss A, Akelman E. Primary care of hand and wrist athletic injuries. Clin Sports Med 1997;16:705–724.
13. Cooney W, Dobyns J, Linscheid R. Fractures of the scaphoid: a rational approach to management. Clin Orthop 1980;149: 90–97.
14. Culver J, Anderson T. Fractures of the hand and wrist in the athlete. Clin Sports Med 1992;11:101–128.
15. Griggs S, Weiss A. Bony injuries of the wrist, forearm, and elbow. Clin Sports Med 1996;15:373–400.
16. Canelon M. Silicone rubber splinting for athletic hand and wrist injuries. J Hand Ther 1995;8:252–257.
17. Huene D. Primary internal fixation of carpal navicular fractures in the athlete. Am J Sports Med 1979;7:175–177.
18. Vahvanen V, Westerlund M. Fracture of the scaphoid in children. Acta Orthop Scand 1980;51:909–913.
19. Gill T, Micheli L. The immature athlete: common injuries and overuse syndromes of the elbow and wrist. Clin Sports Med 1996;15:401–423.
20. Amadio P, Taleisnik J. Fractures of the Carpal Bones. In D Green (ed), Operative Hand Surgery. New York: Churchill Livingstone, 1993;799–860.
21. Cooney W, Linscheid R, Dobyns J. Fractures and Dislocations of the Wrist. In C Rockwood, D Green, R Bucholz, J Heckman (eds), Rockwood and Green's Fractures in Adults. Philadelphia: Lippincott-Raven, 1996;745–868.
22. Carroll R, Lakin J. Fracture of the hook of the hamate. J Trauma 1993;34:803–805.
23. Weiss A, Sponseller P. Salter-Harris type I fracture of the distal radius due to weightlifting. Orthop Rev 1989;18: 233–235.
24. Salter R, Harris W. Injuries involving the epiphyseal plate. J Bone Joint Surg Am 1963;45:587–622.
25. Markiewitz A, Andrish J. Hand and wrist injuries in the preadolescent and adolescent athlete. Clin Sports Med 1992;11:203–225.
26. Wilkins K, Obren E. Fractures of the Distal Radius and Ulna. In C Rockwood, K Wilkins, J Beaty (eds), Fractures in Children. Philadelphia: Lippincott-Raven, 1996;451–515.
27. Brown D, Lichtman D. The evaluation of chronic wrist pain. Orthop Clin North Am 1984;15:183–192.
28. Dobyns J, Linscheid R, Chao E, et al. Traumatic instability of the wrist. American Academy of Orthopaedic Surgeons Instructional Course Lectures 1975;24:182–188.
29. Halikis M, Taleisnik J. Soft tissue injuries of the wrist. Clin Sports Med 1996;15:235–259.
30. Green D. Carpal Dislocation. In D Green (ed), Operative Hand Surgery (Vol 1). New York: Churchill Livingstone, 1982;703–742.
31. Reagan D, Linscheid R, Dobyns J. Lunotriquetral sprains. J Hand Surg [Am] 1984;9:502–514.
32. Smith D, Murray P. Avulsion fractures of the volar aspect of triquetral bone of the wrist: a subtle sign of carpal ligament injury. AJR Am J Reontgenol 1996;166:609–614.
33. Rettig A. Wrist problems in the tennis player. Med Sci Sports Exerc 1994;26:1207–1212.
34. Jennings J, Peimer C (eds). Ligamentous Injuries of the Wrist in Athletes (1st ed). St. Louis: Mosby, 1990.
35. Lester B, Halbrecht J, Levy I, Gaudinez R. "Press test" for office diagnosis of triangular fibrocartilage complex tears of the wrist. Ann Plast Surg 1995;35:41–45.
36. Savoie F, Whipple T. The role of arthroscopy in athletic injuries of the wrist. Clin Sports Med 1996;15:219–233.
37. Taleisnik J. Pain on the ulnar side of the wrist. Hand Clin 1987;3:51–68.
38. Bowers W (ed). The Distal Radioulnar Joint. New York: Churchill Livingstone, 1988.
39. Nirschl R. Elbow and shoulder injuries in the tennis player. Clin Sports Med 1988;7:289–308.
40. Osterman A, Moskow L, Low D. Soft tissue injuries of the hand and wrist in racquet sports. Clin Sports Med 1988; 7:329–348.

41. Wood M, Dobyns J. Sports related extra-articular wrist syndromes. Clin Orthop 1986;202:93–102.

42. Plancher K, Peterson R, Steichen J. Compressive neuropathies and tendinopathies in the athletic elbow and wrist. Clin Sports Med 1996;15:331–371.

43. Dobyns J, Franklin H, Linscheid R. Sports stress syndromes of the hand and wrist. Am J Sports Med 1978;6:236–254.

44. Dellon A, Mackinnon S. Radial sensory nerve entrapment in the forearm. J Hand Surg [Am] 1986;11:199–205.

45. Linscheid R, Dobyns J. Athletic injuries of the wrist. Clin Orthop 1985;198:141–151.

46. Aronen J. Problems of the upper extremity in gymnastics. Clin Sports Med 1985;4:61–71.

47. Carr D, David P. Distal posterior interosseous nerve syndrome. J Hand Surg [Am] 1985;10:873–878.

48. Dellon A. Partial dorsal wrist denervation: resection of the distal posterior interosseous nerve. J Hand Surg [Am] 1985;10:527–533.

49. Carter S, Aldridge M, Fitzgerald R, Davies A. Stress changes of the wrist in adolescent gymnasts. Br J Radiol 1988;61:109–112.

50. Liebling M, Berdon W, Ruzal-Shapiro C, et al. Gymnast's wrist (pseudorickets growth plate abnormality) in adolescent athletes: findings on plain films and MR imaging. AJR 1995;164:157–159.

51. Roy S, Caine D, Singer K. Stress changes of the distal radial epiphysis in young gymnasts. Am J Sports Med 1985;13:301–308.

52. Bishop A, Gabel G, Carmichael S. Flexor carpi radialis tendinitis: I. operative anatomy. J Bone Joint Surg Am 1994;76:1009–1014.

53. Gabel G, Bishop A, Wood M. Flexor carpi radialis tendinitis: II. results of operative treatment. J Bone Joint Surg Am 1994;76:1015–1018.

54. Pianka G, Hershman E. Neurovascular Injuries. In J Nichols, E Hershman (eds), The Upper Extremity in Sports Medicine. St. Louis: Mosby, 1990;691–722.

55. Hunt J. The thenar and hypothenar types of neural atrophy of the hand. Am J Med Sci 1911;141:224–227.

56. Johnson R. Soft tissue injuries of the forearm and hand. Clin Sports Med 1986;5:701–707.

11

Hand Injuries

PATRICK ST. PIERRE

Hand injuries in athletes are devastating injuries, preventing athletes from continuing to play. Because the hand is nonweightbearing, however, some athletes with a hand injury may still be able to perform. In those circumstances, hand injuries may be looked on by the athlete and physician as trivial, and mismanagement may lead to long-term morbidity. This chapter is a guide to diagnosis, treatment, and referral criteria for common hand injuries in athletes.

ANATOMY

The anatomy of the hand (Figures 11-1 and 11-2) is complex, and a detailed description is beyond the scope of this chapter. When the hand is injured, one needs to understand not only the bony and musculotendinous anatomy, but also the intricate neurovascular structures, the several compartments that may restrict fluid or edema, and the major ligaments that provide joint stability. A basic knowledge of hand anatomy is necessary for those who wish to treat hand injuries, and frequent referral to reference materials may be necessary.[1, 2] An algorithm of injuries to the hand is shown in Figure 11-3.

PHYSICAL EXAMINATION

A thorough and systematic physical examination of the hand is essential in evaluating a hand injury. Because visual structures to the hand are so superficial, a small wound may be an indicator of a much more serious injury. The outcome for patients with nerve, artery, and tendon injuries is usually much better when immediate treatment is provided.

Inspection and Range of Motion

Both hands should be examined simultaneously to assess for asymmetric dysfunction. Swelling and discoloration should be quantified and noted. The patient is asked to actively extend his or her fingers with palms facing the floor, then supinate and slowly make a fist. This latter test is critical in that it will pick up subtle rotational deformities that may otherwise be missed. After this screening examination, areas of pain and abnormal function are more closely examined.

Vascular Examination

The radial and ulnar arteries can be palpated at the wrist and should be a part of the hand examination. Capillary refill should be noted in each finger, and alteration of flow in the injured finger should alert the examiner to possible arterial injury.

Neurologic Examination

A motor and sensory examination should be performed distal to any injury. Specific dermatomes for the sensory branches are shown in Figure 10-3 (see Chapter 10). Light touch, pinprick, and two-point discrimination should be tested for each finger with possible injury to a digital nerve. Intact two-point discrimination (<5 mm) confirms that the digital nerve is intact.[3, 4]

The motor examination should be performed for each of the three major nerves (median, ulnar, and radial). Specific muscle function should then be tested to rule out laceration of individual motor branches or tendons. These are summarized in Table 10-1 (see Chapter 10).[2–4]

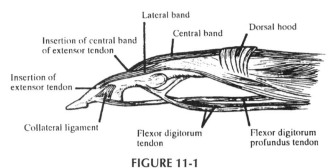

FIGURE 11-1

Lateral view of the flexor and extensor mechanisms.

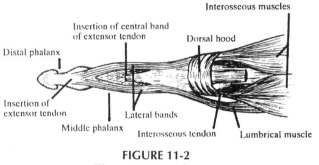

FIGURE 11-2

The extensor mechanism.

Radiographic Examination

Radiographs should be obtained for any specific bony tenderness or angulation. Mechanism of injury should be taken into account when x-ray studies are ordered; lacerations around a joint need films to rule out osteochondral fracture.

Anteroposterior, lateral, and oblique views of the hand are usually sufficient for most injuries. Similar views of specific fingers may be needed to evaluate finger injuries.[5]

Magnetic resonance imaging has been advocated for assessment of tendon injury in acute, closed injuries.[6] This requires a special coil and may prove to be beneficial in many cases; however, the most cost-effective use of this modality may be after consultation with an orthopedic specialist.

TREATMENT

Injuries involving the hand and digits are difficult problems to manage in athletes. Strict compliance with immobilization is often difficult to achieve with a high-level athlete who "needs" to return to competition. A certain amount of risk must be taken by the athlete and the physician to continue participation. In the younger, little league athlete, the solution is easier because no risk should be taken, and injuries should be allowed to heal fully. In a college or professional athlete, the situation is different. Cooperation among the athlete, physician, trainer, therapist, and orthotist is usually needed to arrive at an acceptable solution.

Three treatment principles apply to management of most hand injuries: splinting, ice, and elevation. The hand has little space to accommodate swelling, and management must be directed toward preventing the devastating results of compression injuries through compartment syndromes. Additionally, swelling contributes to increased pain, and it may also interfere with fracture reduction or skin closure if open reduction is necessary. Volar or dorsal splints, or uni- or bivalved casts should usually be used instead of circumferential casts to allow further swelling to occur. These may be converted or changed to a cast in a week when the swelling has decreased.[7, 8]

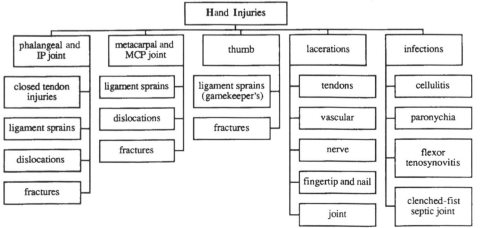

FIGURE 11-3

Algorithm for injuries to the hand. (MCP = metacarpophalangeal; IP = interphalangeal.)

Most fractures are nondisplaced and without malalignment. These fractures can usually be treated by closed methods, and because they are usually stable, an early, protected return to sports is usually achievable. Fractures that cannot be reduced, that are unstable after reduction, or that involve displacement of the articular surface should be referred to an orthopedic surgeon for management.

PHALANGEAL AND INTERPHALANGEAL INJURIES

Tendon Injuries

Rugger Jersey Finger

Rugger jersey finger is the closed rupture of the flexor digitorum profundus tendon from its insertion in the distal phalanx. The mechanism of injury is the forced extension of a finger that is being actively flexed with maximum force. In the usual scenario, the football or rugby player reaches out to tackle another player and a finger catches the jersey and is pulled away. The ring and long (middle) fingers are the ones most commonly affected. These injuries may be completely tendinous, or a small piece of bone may be avulsed from the volar surface of the phalanx (Figures 11-4 and 11-5).[9–11]

Physical Examination. The key to diagnosis is suspicion from the history followed by an adequate physical examination. The patient will have pain at the volar aspect of the distal interphalangeal (DIP) joint that cannot be casually disregarded as a sprain. Inability to actively flex the DIP joint while the proximal interphalangeal (PIP) joint is held in extension confirms the diagnosis.

Radiographs. A lateral radiograph may be helpful with the diagnosis if an avulsed fragment is present (see Figure 11-5). A smaller fragment may be caught at the PIP joint, whereas a larger fragment may be caught at the DIP joint by the A4 pulley.

Treatment. All flexor tendon ruptures or lacerations need surgical repair. A purely tendinous injury will retract into the palm, causing complete disruption of blood supply and scarring. These injuries should be repaired within 7 days. Bony avulsions are not as emergent because the blood supply is preserved, but early surgical repair is advised. The wrist and fingers should be splinted in slight flexion, iced, and elevated, and prompt referral should be made to an orthopedic surgeon.[9, 11]

Mallet Finger

Mallet finger is used for the bony or tendinous disruption of the extensor digitorum tendon from its insertion on the

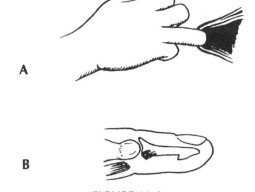

A

B

FIGURE 11-4
Pathogenesis of "rugger jersey finger." A. The actively flexed distal interphalangeal joint is forcibly extended by catching on a jersey. B. Avulsion of the flexor digitorum profundus.

dorsal aspect of the distal phalanx. There are three types of injuries (Figure 11-6):

- Type I—stretching of the tendon without complete disruption of the tendon; there may be a mild drop of the distal phalanx, but weak active extension remains.
- Type II—complete disruption of the tendon; no active extension persists; there is usually a 40- to45-degree flexion deformity.
- Type III—bony avulsion from the distal phalanx (Figure 11-7).

Treatment. All acute tendinous injuries may be treated nonoperatively. Prefabricated (mallet finger or stack) splints that hold the DIP joint straight or in slight hypertension work very well. The PIP joint does not need to be immobilized. The splint should be worn at all times for at least 6–8 weeks. If the DIP joint cannot be actively held

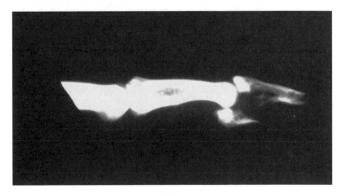

FIGURE 11-5
Bony "rugger jersey finger" avulsion.

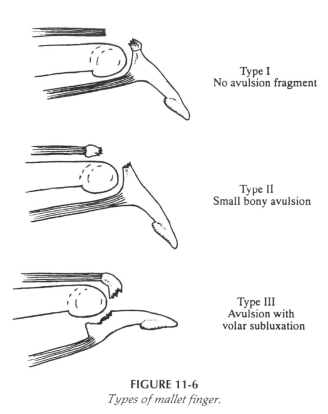

Type I
No avulsion fragment

Type II
Small bony avulsion

Type III
Avulsion with
volar subluxation

FIGURE 11-6
Types of mallet finger.

in extension at that time, another 4 weeks full-time wear may be required. Otherwise, 4 more weeks of nighttime wear is usually sufficient.[12]

Most bony avulsions are treatable by closed methods (as in treatment for ligamentous avulsions) for 4–6 weeks. If the avulsed fragment is large and the distal phalanx subluxates volarly, however, referral to an orthopedic or hand surgeon for operative repair is warranted.[7, 9, 12]

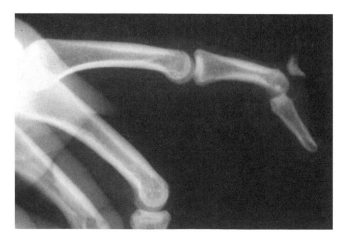

FIGURE 11-7
Type III mallet finger avulsion.

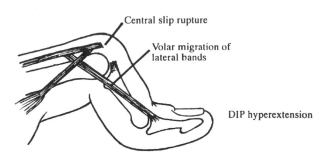

Central slip rupture

Volar migration of
lateral bands

DIP hyperextension

FIGURE 11-8
Rupture of the central slip of the extensor mechanism with volar migration of the lateral bands resulting in a boutonnière deformity. (DIP = distal interphalangeal [joint].)

Boutonnière Deformity

A traumatic boutonnière deformity (Figure 11-8) is a result of disruption of the extensor mechanism at the PIP joint. This may occur indirectly or may be secondary to a laceration or crush injury to the dorsum of the hand. Once the central slip of the extensor tendon is ruptured, the lateral bands are allowed to slip volarly and allow the PIP joint to herniate through the central slip. This gives the classic button-through-the-buttonhole appearance. This deformity, if allowed to progress, causes flexion at the PIP joint with extension at the metacarpophalangeal (MCP) and DIP joints (see Figure 11-8).[7, 9]

Treatment. Treatment of the acute injury is splinting the PIP in extension for 6–8 weeks. This should be followed by splinting during competition for the remainder of the season or 2 months, whichever is longer. Misdiagnosis and delayed treatment should be managed by a hand surgeon and may need operative correction.[7, 9]

Trigger Finger

Trigger finger is a nonspecific tenosynovitis of the flexor tendon sheath. In athletes, the most common cause is repetitive trauma that causes increased swelling within the tendon. The swollen tendon catches on the closely applied pulley system, causing the snapping sensation in either the flexed or the extended position. A tender nodule is generally palpable over the volar aspect of the MCP joint.

Treatment. Early on, splinting the finger straight at night along with nonsteroidal anti-inflammatory drugs may be effective. More chronic injuries, especially with repetitive triggering, may require injection of a mixture of local anesthetic and steroid into the tendon sheath. This is done by means of a midlateral approach at the level of the distal third of the proximal phalanx while the patient resists flexion. In unresponsive cases, surgery is needed to release the pulley.[8]

Climber's Finger

Rock climbing has enjoyed increasing popularity in recent years. Climbers are susceptible to many hand injuries, in particular to injuries of the flexor tendons and the tendon sheath. Rupture of the A2 pulley has been termed "climber's finger" and can lead to bowstringing of the flexor tendon. Referral to a hand specialist for possible reconstruction of the tendon is indicated.[13]

Ligamentous Injuries (Sprains): Interphalangeal Joints

Sprains of the fingers and thumb are common injuries in athletes. Most are relatively minor injuries and heal uneventfully. However, some are more involved and lead to delayed healing if not correctly managed. Early recognition and treatment of these injuries may prevent chronic disability. Sprains are usually graded in order of severity as follows[7, 14]:

- Grade I: pain at the joint is present with minimal swelling and no instability.
- Grade II: increased pain and swelling at the joint is present with mild laxity; complete instability is not present.
- Grade III: complete instability of the joint is present with complete disruption of the supporting ligaments.

Sprains of the interphalangeal joints are common and almost always amenable to closed treatment. Sprains are caused by either excessive lateral angulation at the joint, thereby stretching the collateral ligaments, or by hyperextension, causing injury to the volar plate.

The physical examination is characterized by local pain and swelling, often causing decreased range of motion. Active and passive range of motion should be tested and recorded. Laxity or locking with these movements may indicate instability. Lateral stress should be applied to the joint in full extension and 45-degree flexion to determine collateral ligament stability.

Treatment. For grade I sprains, buddy taping is usually sufficient. Treatment is continued until symptoms subside. Taping for the remainder of the competitive season is usually helpful to prevent reinjury. For grade II sprains, immobilization in a dorsal aluminum splint for 7–10 days in slight flexion is indicated. Buddy taping with range of motion exercises may start thereafter. Flexion should not exceed 90 degrees, and buddy taping should continue for the entire season. For grade III sprains, even complete tears should do well with nonoperative treatment. Treat as for grade II injuries; however, a full-finger splint should be used for 2–3 weeks followed by buddy taping to the finger adjacent to the injured side. For hyperextension

injuries to the volar plate manifested by volar pain, tenderness, and swelling, treat in slightly more flexion for 2–3 weeks and avoid hyperextension.

Acute ruptures with obvious angular deformity and gross instability on active motion or passive stretch may need early surgical repair. These patients should be referred to an orthopedic or hand surgeon.[7, 14]

Dislocations

Dislocations of the joints in the hand are fairly common among athletes. The most commonly involved joint is the PIP of the fingers. Almost as commonly, the dislocation is reduced by the patient or a teammate before formal medical attention is received. Proper identification and treatment help prevent prolonged stiffness of the joint.

Distal Interphalangeal Joint

Dislocation at the DIP joint is less common than at the PIP joint. The mechanism of injury is usually hyperextension, causing a dorsal or lateral dislocation. This injury is easily recognizable because of the dorsal prominence. The skin here is tightly applied to the joint, and open injuries are frequent and must be looked for.

Treatment. Reduction is accomplished through gentle traction on the distal phalanx and direct pressure over its dislocated base. At times, as with other dorsal dislocations, a hyperextension maneuver may be necessary to "unlock" the joint. Rarely, closed reduction is unsuccessful and operative reduction may be necessary.[15]

The joint should be immobilized with a dorsal aluminum splint for 2–3 weeks. Protection from hyperextension should continue for another month or the remainder of competition, whichever is longer. Range of motion should be started after the initial immobilization period ends, and the patient should be advised that the joint will be stiff for several months.[7, 14]

Proximal Interphalangeal Joint

PIP joint dislocations are the most common dislocations in the hand. The most frequent mechanism is hyperextension, causing a dorsal or lateral dislocation (Figures 11-9 and 11-10). This produces a disruption of the volar plate from the base of the middle phalanx. Frequently, this is accompanied by a tear of the proper and accessory collateral ligaments on either side of the joint.[7, 14] The joint should be examined after reduction for collateral ligament instability.

Treatment. Reduction is obtained by the same maneuver described earlier for DIP dislocations. After reduction, active flexion and extension should be tested to

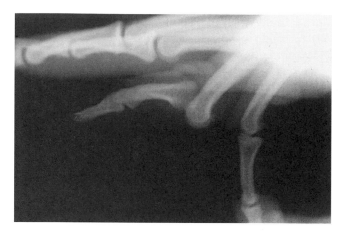

FIGURE 11-9
Proximal interphalangeal joint dorsal dislocation.

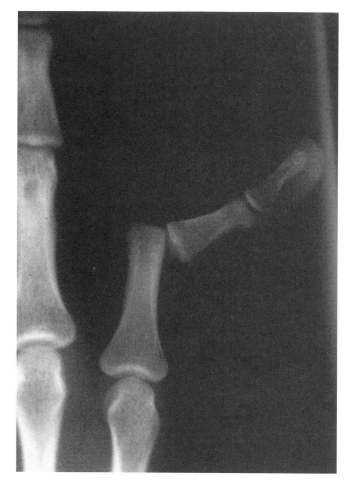

FIGURE 11-10
Proximal interphalangeal joint lateral dislocation.

rule out an extensor tendon tear or volar plate entrapment. The collateral ligaments should then be examined.

PIP joint injuries are usually stable. Range of motion exercises can start almost immediately after the acute swelling has subsided, with buddy taping for 3–4 weeks, which allows early motion of the joint. Patients with soft tissue entrapment (unable to maintain reduction) should be referred.[7, 14]

Volar dislocations are rare. They are frequently difficult to reduce because the proximal phalanx may buttonhole through the extensor mechanism. Also, because of a concomitant tear of the extensor mechanism, a chronic boutonnière deformity may develop (see section on boutonnière deformity). If these conditions exist, appropriate referral should be made.

Phalangeal Fractures

One of the most common phalangeal fractures[7, 16–20] is the bony mallet finger, and management is covered in an earlier section. Distal phalanx fractures can usually be treated by splinting. They are often caused by crush injuries, and ice and elevation are essential to prevent severe swelling. Unless they are severely displaced or angulated, a dorsal splint in extension that immobilizes the DIP joint for 2–3 weeks is usually sufficient. Buddy taping may be used in conjunction with a splint or as a protective measure when the patient is sent back to competition.

Fractures involving the middle phalanx are usually transverse and angulated volarly. If they can be reduced and held in good alignment with the adjacent joints in slight flexion, closed management may be attempted. Maintaining reduction may be difficult because of the deform-

ing forces of the flexor digitorum or extensor mechanism. The dense cortical bone of the middle phalanx takes at least 12 weeks to heal, but range of motion exercises should begin at 4–6 weeks. The fracture should be protected during competition for at least 3–4 months or the rest of that season, whichever is longer. If reduction cannot be maintained, referral should be made to a surgeon for closed reduction and percutaneous pinning.

Fractures of the proximal phalanx are the most disabling and challenging of finger fractures. These fractures are usually oblique or spiral fractures, which cause shortening and malrotation of the fragments. The reduction is difficult to maintain, even if the initial reduction is successful. Also, prolonged immobilization of this fracture often leads to stiffness and adherence of the flexor or extensor tendons, which travel close by it. Therefore, splinting, ice, and elevation with consultation within 24–48 hours are usually warranted.

Articular fractures of the phalanges almost always should be referred to an orthopedic or hand surgeon. Anatomic reduction is desired, so only the perfectly nondisplaced fracture should be managed without some internal stabilization. Small bony avulsions without subluxation of the joint may be managed as outlined in the section on tendon injuries.

METACARPAL AND METACARPOPHALANGEAL JOINT INJURIES

Metacarpophalangeal Joint Sprains

Injuries at the distal ends of the metacarpal are usually a result of a severe abduction or adduction force. The small and index fingers are the ones most commonly injured in athletes, as the fingers are forcibly abducted away by another player or a ball. In addition to tearing the collateral ligaments, the transverse metacarpal ligaments may be injured as well. This injury may be diagnosed by severe pain with separation of the metacarpal heads (see section on ligamentous injuries for grading of injuries).

Treatment. For injuries of grades I and II, usually buddy taping or splinting the fingers with the MCP joints at 45 degrees for 3–4 weeks is sufficient. Another effective treatment, especially in athletes who need to return to competition quickly, is wrapping the patient's hand in a compressive dressing holding the fingers together. This allows the player free use of his or her fingers in flexion and extension.

Grade III injuries may lead to subluxation of the joint and carry risk of chronic instability and pain. If the radiographs reveal normal anatomic position of the joint, immobilization with the MCPs flexed 45 degrees for about 3 weeks is sufficient. Again, the PIP joint does not need to be immobilized. If the joint is not reduced or if there is gross instability, a primary repair should be considered and referral made to the appropriate surgeon.[7, 14, 21, 22]

Metacarpophalangeal Dislocations

Dislocation injuries at the MCP joint are high-energy injuries and are unusual. The classically described and most common injury occurs in the index finger. A hyperextension injury causes a disruption of the volar plate, and the metacarpal head goes through a buttonhole defect in the volar plate. The head rides within the flexor tendons and the lumbricals, and closed reduction by traction is impossible. When present, sesamoid bones may become entrapped with the volar plate between the metacarpal and proximal phalanx.[23]

Treatment. This has been referred to as the "irreducible dislocation." If one attempts a reduction early, however, before significant swelling occurs, a reduction can be performed if the buttonhole defect is reduced first. The correct reduction maneuver is further hyperextension followed by flexion, avoiding any traction. Once someone tugs on the finger, or significant swelling has developed, open reduction is required.

Once a reduction is obtained, the finger should be splinted with a 30-degree extension block for 4–6 weeks and maintained for the duration of the competitive season.[7, 14, 21, 22]

METACARPAL FRACTURES

Boxer's Fractures

The most common fracture of the metacarpal is the boxer's fracture. This is a fracture of the fifth metacarpal neck, which usually occurs after the patient strikes a hard object with a closed fist. Fractures of the metacarpal necks of the other fingers do occur but with less frequency. These fractures angulate volarly, leaving a prominence in the palm if allowed to heal without reduction. Fractures of the fourth and fifth metacarpal necks can functionally tolerate much more flexion than can the radial two rays. Up to 70 degrees of flexion may be acceptable with low morbidity after healing. However, most experts believe that a reduction to less than 30 degrees is more acceptable to the patient. Fractures of the index and long metacarpals tolerate much less volar angulation, because any remaining bony prominence is very tender and functionally limiting on that side of the palm. A reduction to less than 10 degrees of volar angulation should be obtained.[16]

Treatment. Treatment of these fractures can almost always be accomplished with closed reduction and casting. If the proper alignment cannot be maintained, then referral for additional treatment should be made. The reduction maneuver is to put pressure under the metacarpal head with one hand and pressure over the dorsal metacarpal shaft with the other, while maintaining flexion at the MCP joint of approximately 90 degrees. Once the reduction is obtained, the hand is placed in splints with the MCP joints maintaining 50–60 degrees of flexion. This helps maintain the reduction and prevents stiffness of the MCP joint. Radiographic confirmation of the reduction is then made. The fracture should be followed closely with weekly radiographs for 2–3 weeks to assure

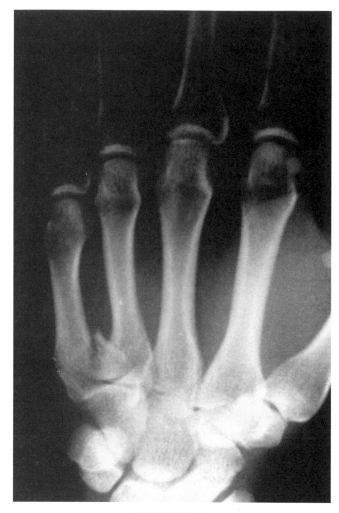

FIGURE 11-11
Fracture at base of fifth metacarpal.

maintenance of the reduction. The athlete should be maintained in a plaster cast for 4–6 weeks.[17] However, a molded orthotic may be made to allow participation in athletics at 3 weeks if adequate callus formation is apparent on an x-ray film.

Metacarpal Shaft Fractures

Metacarpal shaft fractures are often complicated by shortening and malrotation. Maintenance of these fractures is difficult in plaster. Therefore, unless the fracture is essentially nondisplaced, referral should be made to the orthopedic or hand surgeon for treatment and follow-up.[18] A nondisplaced fracture may be treated in a short arm cast for 4–6 weeks. For highly competitive athletes, return to competition may be fairly quick with use of a molded and padded orthosis.[19] Treatment may be variable depending

on the nature of the fracture, and consultation is recommended. Again, splinting, ice, and elevation are extremely important in the acute management of these fractures.

Metacarpal Base Fractures

Metacarpal base fractures usually occur at the base of the thumb metacarpal (Bennett or Rolando fractures), and at the base of the fifth metacarpal (Figure 11-11). These fractures are often intraarticular and involve some subluxation at the carpometacarpal (CMC) joint.[18] Because anatomic reduction is necessary to reduce the long-term morbidity related to these fractures, referral to an orthopedic or hand surgeon is warranted. Again, ice, elevation, and splinting are the mainstays of initial treatment.

THUMB INJURIES

Interphalangeal Joint Sprains

Injury to the thumb CMC or MCP is a much more common occurrence than injury to the interphalangeal joint. When a sprain occurs, however, it is usually low grade and can be managed simply by immobilization until symptoms subside.

Metacarpophalangeal Joint Sprains (Gamekeeper's Thumb or Skier's Thumb)

MCP joint sprains are quite common and occur with forced abduction of the thumb and hyperextension. This results in a complete or partial tear of the ulnar collateral ligament (Figure 11-12). Injuries to the radial collateral ligament are much less frequent but are generally treated in a like manner.

Most injuries are partial tears and will heal with nonoperative treatment. However, complete tears often do not heal well and require operative treatment to gain a satisfactory result. A poor result leads to a very weak and painful thumb, especially with a key or pinch grip. Therefore, distinguishing a complete tear (grade III) is most important. Diagnosis of a complete tear may be made by physical examination after radiographs are obtained. Valgus stress should be applied to the MCP joint while both extended and maximally flexed. A difference of 15 degrees or more of ulnar laxity compared with the unaffected side or an absolute laxity of 35 degrees confirms the diagnosis. Occasionally, it is helpful to examine the thumb under local anesthesia to relax the patient enough to do an examination. The ulnar collateral ligament tear will almost always avulse off its phalangeal insertion. If

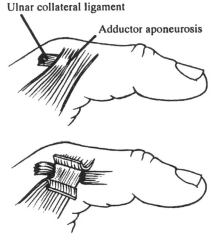

Ulnar collateral ligament

Adductor aponeurosis

FIGURE 11-12

Ulnar collateral ligament complete rupture (Stener lesion). The end of the ruptured ulnar collateral ligament either folds on itself beneath the adductor aponeurosis or becomes trapped outside of it, rendering the ends unapposed and unable to heal.

the ligament pulls itself out from under the adductor aponeurosis where it lies, it will be separated from its insertion and be unable to heal itself without surgical repair. This is referred to as a *Stener lesion.* Confirmation of a Stener lesion can be made with arthrography or at the time of surgery (see Figures 11-12 and 11-13).[24]

Treatment. Grade I and II injuries are treated with immobilization in a thumb spica cast or splint for 2–4 weeks. The patient should be advised that some grade II injuries remain painful, even after appropriate treatment. Figure-eight taping should be continued for competition after cast or splint removal. Treatment of grade III tears is somewhat controversial. Some surgeons attempt treatment in a thumb spica cast in the absence of a Stener lesion. Others think that the most favorable result is obtained on all grade III tears by operative repair. All Stener lesions should be repaired. Either way, the patient should be placed in a thumb spica splint and referred to a hand surgeon for all grade III tears and displaced avulsion fragments.[14, 22, 24]

Fractures

Management of fractures involving the thumb is similar to that of fractures of the fingers (see sections on phalangeal fractures and metacarpal fractures). Because the thumb is often traumatized in sports competition and cannot be buddy taped, early return to competition is usually not possible with phalangeal fractures until the fracture is almost healed and the thumb is nontender. Metacarpal shaft fractures have more inherent stability, and a thumb

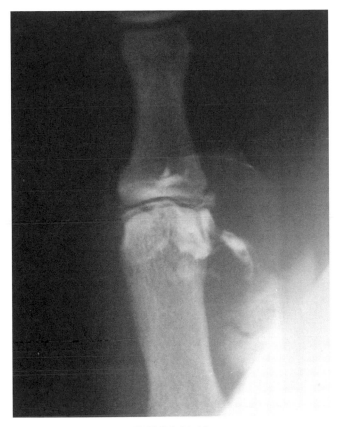

FIGURE 11-13

Arthrogram confirming Stener lesion.

spica orthosis may be worn by athletes in sports that do not require grasping, such as linemen in football.

Fractures at the proximal end of the first metacarpal (Bennett and Rolando fractures) are fairly common fractures. These fractures are intraarticular and usually unstable. Kirschner wire fixation is usually necessary after a closed or open reduction. Referral should be made to an orthopedic surgeon.

LACERATIONS

Lacerations may herald a more significant injury because of the potential involvement of deep structures, including nerve, artery, and tendon. Knowing or reviewing the subcutaneous anatomy of the hand is essential to recognizing potential injury to these structures.

Examination

A thorough examination (see section on physical examination) is needed to assess the neurovascular status before a local anesthetic is used for cleansing, debridement, or further examination. Testing of the superficialis and profundus tendons is particularly important for lacerations on the volar surface of the hand or fingers.

Treatment. A thorough irrigation and debridement of the wound is needed. This is usually most successfully done after a local anesthetic nerve block and with use of a tourniquet. If there is no nerve, artery, joint, or tendon involvement, simple closure with an interrupted 5-0 nonabsorbable suture is performed. (For nerve, artery, joint, or tendon involvement, see subsequent paragraphs.)

Antibiotics are usually not indicated if a thorough irrigation and debridement is performed. If the wound is particularly dirty and concern about infection exists, a first-generation cephalosporin gives good coverage for the usual gram-positive organisms.

For any puncture wound, tetanus immunization status should be determined and tetanus toxoid given if necessary. These wounds must be followed closely for deep-space infections (see section on palmar space infections).

Lacerated Tendons

It is beyond the scope of this book to describe the operative care of lacerated tendons, so the focus will be on their recognition and initial management.

Extensor Tendons

Diagnosis of an extensor tendon laceration is made by physical examination and direct visualization. With a complete laceration, the patient is unable to actively extend the digit at the PIP and DIP joints, but passive range of motion is full. The lumbricals can also extend these joints, so the MCPs must be kept in full extension to block the action of these muscles. Also, if the laceration is proximal to the MCP joints, finger extension may be possible via the extensor juncturae tendinum, which interconnect between adjacent tendons on the dorsum of the hand. When laceration is suspected, the hand should be splinted after initial debridement. The wrist should be placed in extension with a volar splint to relieve tension on the injured tendon. The MCP joints should be flexed 30–45 degrees to prevent contracture of the collateral ligaments. Referral should be made within 48 hours.[12]

Flexor Tendons

The flexor mechanism of the hand is much more complex than the extensor, because flexor tendons run through an intricate system of pulleys and tendon sheaths. These injured tendons should be evaluated by a hand surgeon and repaired in the operating room. These injuries are not emergencies, but referral should be made and the patient seen as soon as reasonably possible (no more than 48 hours).

The most important aspect of the initial treatment of flexor tendon injuries is the initial neural, vascular, and muscular examinations. Because of the proximity of the neurovascular bundle, the appearance of the fingertip, capillary refill, and two-point discrimination must be examined and recorded before treatment. Also, testing and differentiating between a laceration of the flexor superficialis and the flexor profundus will be of great help to the orthopedic surgeon.[25–27]

A thorough irrigation of the wound is indicated in the emergency room. The skin should be closed loosely with interrupted sutures of 5-0 nylon. Actual repair of the lacerated tendon should be performed in the operating room.

A dorsal splint should be applied with the wrist in 45 degrees of flexion, the MCP joints in 60–80 degrees of flexion, and the interphalangeal joints in slight flexion.

Vascular Lacerations

Most vascular injuries of the hand can effectively be managed with direct pressure and elevation. If this appears to be inadequate, a tourniquet may be applied with a blood pressure cuff. If a cuff is used, the hoses must be clamped off with a hemostat to avoid leakage and the development of a venous tourniquet. Most people have a dual blood supply to their hands via the radial and ulnar arteries, and each digit has a dual blood supply through each digital artery. Therefore, even with a complete laceration, collateral flow is usually adequate to provide enough perfusion for the hand to survive.[2]

One should never attempt a blind stab with a hemostat in an attempt to control hemorrhage. Arteries in the hand are almost always accompanied by nerves, and blind stabs often result in nerve damage.

Ischemic fingers—that is, pale, cool fingers with poor capillary refill—should be referred emergently to an orthopedic or hand surgeon for evaluation and treatment.

Nerve Lacerations

Nerve lacerations should be left for repair at a later date by a well-rested hand surgeon in an operating room with good lighting and appropriate instruments. Irrigation and closure appropriate for the laceration are indicated, with prompt referral to a hand surgeon.

Fingertip and Nail Lacerations

Injuries to the fingertip and nail are common in athletes. Usually they are the result of direct trauma and are treated nonoperatively.

Treatment of lacerations to the fingertip pad or pulp is similar to that for other lacerations in the hand. Lacerations resulting in small amputations (<1 cm) may be treated with thorough cleansing and sterile dressing. Larger amputations need more definitive care and should be referred to a hand surgeon immediately. If there is a complete bony amputation, the amputated part should be placed in a waterproof bag and placed in a larger bag with ice water. The amputated part should not be placed in water and allowed to soak.[28, 29]

Badly lacerated nails should be trimmed or removed. If the laceration involves the nailbed, the nail must be removed and the nailbed repaired. The nailbed should be repaired by someone who has had experience with this repair. A 5-0 or 6-0 absorbable suture is ideal.

Contusions beneath the nail are frequent because of its close proximity to bone. A subungual hematoma may develop, which is very painful. This should be relieved by drilling the nail at the center of the hematoma. This may be done with a tip of a knife blade, a large-gauge needle, or a hot paper clip. Many emergency rooms are equipped with disposable electrocautery probes that are effective. Multiple holes (three to five) may be necessary to relieve all of the pain.[28, 29]

Lacerations into a Joint

Lacerations involving a joint should be managed by an orthopedic or hand surgeon to avoid progression to a fulminant septic arthritis. If the laceration has obviously penetrated the joint, irrigation with normal saline and prompt referral are all that is needed. If there is a question as to whether the joint is involved, an injection of dilute methylene blue into the joint and extravasation out through the wound will confirm the diagnosis. This should be done only by someone who has had experience with injecting joints.

INFECTIONS

Serious hand infections are not common in athletes. Minor infections are more common, and if improperly treated may develop into a more serious and devastating problem. Therefore, early recognition and treatment are of paramount importance.

Cellulitis

Cellulitis is the earliest manifestation of a hand infection and the most likely one to occur. There is a local inflammation of the skin, but without localization of pus or involvement of the joint. The treatment follows the basic principles of hand infections, which also apply to more serious infections. They are (1) splinting, (2) elevation, and (3) antibiotics.[30, 31]

Splinting of the hand may be accomplished by a bulky hand dressing, which prohibits any movement of the fingers. A plaster or commercial volar splint also provides adequate immobilization.

The best method of elevation is to place the patient's arm in a stockinette device hanging from an intravenous unit pole. The use of a plaster splint is helpful with this method, because it maintains the proper position of the patient's hand in the stockinette. Other methods may be devised for the home. The use of pillows is less reliable for two reasons: (1) during sleep, the patient's hand is more likely to fall off the pillow and move to a dependent position; (2) it is easier for the patient to be noncompliant and walk around with his or her hand in a dependent position. Warm compresses may be applied and are indeed helpful for minor infections; however, elevation is more important and should be maintained while moist heat is being applied.

Routine use of antibiotics[32] in minor infections is contraindicated and may lead to superinfection. Most hand surgeons maintain that the proper treatment, whether it be splinting and elevation or incision and drainage, is enough to cure most minor hand infections. This is especially true of early, focal cellulitis. More extensive and severe cellulitis may require the use of antibiotics. The most common organism is streptococcus, which responds well to first-generation cephalosporins.

Paronychia

Paronychia is discussed in Chapter 27.

Flexor Tenosynovitis

Flexor tenosynovitis is an infection within the flexor tendon sheath. This sheath provides a tight lubricated path for the tendon to glide within. When infected, this tight space fills with pus and rapidly progresses to a deep palmar space infection or necrosis and destruction of the flexor mechanism. These infections are emergent, and referral to an orthopedic or hand surgeon should be immediate. Treatment is incision and either open or closed irrigation of the tendon sheath.[30, 31]

Recognition of septic flexor tenosynovitis is of primary importance to the primary care person. The two main diagnoses in the differential diagnosis are subcutaneous abscess and cellulitis. In 1912, Kanavael[31] described four "cardinal signs" of flexor sheath infections that still apply today. They are (1) tenderness over the flexor tendon sheath, (2) symmetric swelling of the digit, (3) pain with passive extension of the finger, and (4) flexed posturing of the digit. If these signs are present, prompt referral should be made.[33]

Clenched-Fist Lacerations and Septic Arthritis

Infection involving a joint in the hand should prompt emergent referral to an orthopedic or hand surgeon. Symptoms include swelling and erythema about a joint and severe pain with active or passive motion of the joint. At times, this is difficult to distinguish from a cellulitis overlying a joint, as it will also manifest the same symptoms. The most effective test for distinguishing them is axial compression of the joint. If axial compression produces intense pain, the joint is likely to be infected. Otherwise, the problem is more likely to be a cellulitis but should still be watched closely.

Clenched-fist injuries ("fight bites") almost always overlie the fourth or fifth MCP joint. When they do, it is very likely that the offending tooth entered the joint. These should be considered open, infected joints, and the patient should be referred to the appropriate surgeon. In wounds that involve human bites, one must consider *Eikenella corrodens* as a possible infecting organism. Staphylococcal and streptococcal organisms are still more common, but a first-generation cephalosporin will not be effective against *Eikenella* and other anaerobes. Consequently, either penicillin should be added, or a combination drug with the appropriate coverage should be used (i.e., amoxicillin and clavulanate [875/125 mg twice a day] or ampicillin and sulbactam [1.5 g intravenously every 6 hours]).[30–32] Animal infections are often caused by *Pasteurella multocida*, which also does not respond to a cephalosporin. Again, penicillin should be added to cover this organism or a combination drug (ampicillin and clavulanic acid) used instead.

Palmar Space Infections

Web-space infections or deep-space infections of the thenar space, midpalmar space, or Parona space in the wrist need surgical drainage by a qualified surgeon. These infections are often a result of a puncture wound and can progress rapidly. The patient will need to be admitted and should receive tetanus in the emergency room if needed. Unless a significant delay is expected, antibiotics should not be started until cultures are obtained at irrigation and debridement.[30, 31, 34]

REFERENCES

1. Hollingshead WH. Anatomy for Surgeons: The Back and Limbs (3rd ed). Philadelphia: Harper & Row, 1982;437–562.
2. Green DP (ed). Operative Hand Surgery (2nd ed). New York: Churchill Livingstone, 1982;1–26.
3. Omer G. Management of peripheral nerve problems. Instructional Course Lectures 1984;33:461–498.
4. Chiu DTW, Ishii C. Management of peripheral nerve injuries. Orthop Clin North Am 1986;17:365–373.
5. Recht MP, Burke L, Dalinka MK. Radiology of wrist and hand injuries in athletes. Clin Sports Med 1976;5:741–755.
6. Scott JR, Cobby M, Taggart I. Magnetic resonance imaging of acute tendon injury in the finger. J Hand Surg [Br] 1995;20:286–288.
7. Green DP, Rowland SA. Fractures and Dislocations in the Hand. In CA Rockwood, DP Green (eds), Fractures in Adults (2nd ed). Philadelphia: Lippincott, 1984;313–410.
8. Burton RI, Littler JW. Stenosing tenovaginitis (trigger finger and trigger thumb). Curr Prob Surg 1975;12:29–32.
9. McCue FC, Wooten L. Closed tendon injuries of the hand in athletics. Clin Sports Med 1986;5:741–755.
10. Strickland JW. Management of flexor tendon injuries. Orthop Clin North Am 1983;14:827–846.
11. Leddy JP. Flexor Tendons—Acute Injuries. In DP Green (ed), Operative Hand Surgery (2nd ed). New York: Churchill Livingstone, 1988;1935–1968.
12. Evans RB, Burkhalter WE. A study of the dynamic anatomy of extensor tendons and implications for treatment. J Hand Surg Am 1986;11:774–779.
13. Rooks MD, Johnston RB III, Ensor CD, et al. Injury patterns in recreational rock climbers. Am J Sports Med 1995; 23:683–685.
14. Isani A, Melone C. Ligamentous injuries of the hand in athletes. Clin Sports Med 1986;5:757–771.
15. Abouzahr MK, Poublete JV. Irreducible dorsal dislocation of the distal interphalangeal joint: case report and literature review. J Trauma 1997;42:743–745.
16. O'Brien ET. Fractures of the Metacarpals and Phalanges. In DP Green (ed), Operative Hand Surgery. New York: Churchill Livingstone, 1982;583–636.
17. Belsole R. Physiological fixation of displaced and unstable fractures of the hand. Orthop Clin North Am 1980;11: 393–404.
18. Brunet ME, Haddad RJ. Fractures and dislocations of the metacarpals and phalanges. Clin Sports Med 1986;5:773–776.
19. McCue FC, Mayer V. Rehabilitation of common athletic injuries of the hand and wrist. Clin Sports Med 1989;8: 731–776.
20. Culver JE. Sports-related fractures of the hand and wrist. Clin Sports Med 1990;4:85–109.
21. Eaton RG. Joint Injuries of the Hand. Springfield, IL: Thomas, 1971.
22. Melone CP. Complex Joint Injuries of the Hand. In AAOS Symposium on Upper Extremity Injuries in Athletes. St. Louis: Mosby, 1986;142–169.

23. Hughes LA, Freiberg A. Irreducible MP joint dislocation due to entrapment of the FPL. J Hand Surg [Br] 1993;18:708–709.

24. Stener B. Displacement of the ruptured ulnar collateral ligament of the MCP joint of the thumb. J Bone Joint Surg Br 1962;44:869–879.

25. Keyser JJ. Flexor tendon surgery—retrospective. Clin Plast Surg 1986;13:211–220.

26. Tonkin M, Lister G. Flexor tendon surgery—today and looking ahead. Clin Plast Surg 1986;13:221–242.

27. Lister GD, Kleinert HE, Kutz JE, Atasoy E. Primary flexor tendon repair followed by immediate controlled mobilization. J Hand Surg [Am] 1977;2:441–451.

28. Allen MJ. Conservative management of fingertip injuries in adults. Hand 1980;12:257–265.

29. Louis DS. Amputations. In DP Green (ed), Operative Hand Surgery (2nd ed). New York: Churchill Livingstone, 1988;61–120.

30. Siegal DB, Gelberman RH. Infections of the hand. Orthop Clin North Am 1988;19:779–789.

31. Kanavael AB. Infections of the Hand (7th ed). Philadelphia: Lea & Febiger, 1943.

32. Sandford JP. Guide to Antimicrobial Therapy. Bethesda, MD: Merck, Sharp and Dohme, 1995;18–31.

33. Nevaiser RJ. Infections. In DP Green (ed), Operative Hand Surgery. New York: Churchill Livingstone, 1982;771–792.

34. Spiegel JD, Szabo RM. A protocol for the treatment of severe infections of the hand. J Hand Surg [Am] 1988;13:254–259.

12

Back Pain and Injuries in the Athlete

GREGG W. TAYLOR

Back pain is one of the most common physical complaints in the United States. It is estimated that 80% of the general population will experience at least one temporarily disabling episode of back pain at some time during their lifetime. The vast majority of these episodes resolve over a short period. As a group, 5–8% of athletes are also afflicted with back pain[1] that interferes with their training and performance. One study found that 80% of the injuries occurred during practice, 6% occurred during competition, and 14% occurred during the preseason conditioning program.[2]

At the University of Wisconsin, 4,790 athletes who competed in 17 varsity sports over a 10-year period were noted to have an overall incidence of back injuries of 7%, with the highest incidence in football players at 17% and the lowest incidence in baseball players at 2%.[2] Acute injuries were more common (59%) than overuse injuries (12%) or injuries associated with pre-existing conditions (29%). The most common back injuries were muscle strains (60%), disk injuries (7%), lumbar infraspinous process bursitis (kissing spine) (6%), and spondylolysis (6%). A survey of 143 players on the Men's Professional Tennis Tour revealed that low back problems caused 38% of the players to miss at least one tournament, and 30% of the players experienced chronic low back pain.[3] A study of 143 top Swedish athletes participating in wrestling, gymnastics, soccer, and tennis reported that back pain occurred in 50–85% of these athletes, with the highest percentage in male gymnasts.[4]

This chapter provides a framework for the systematic evaluation and treatment of acute and chronic back pain.

FUNCTIONAL ANATOMY

The thoracic and lumbar spine consists of 12 thoracic vertebrae and five lumbar vertebrae, as well as a sacral unit of five conjoined sacral vertebrae. These vertebrae provide axial skeleton motion in flexion and extension (predominantly in the L4–L5 and L5–S1 interspaces), as well as side bending in the lumbar spine and rotation in the thoracic spine.

In the sagittal plane, the cervical spine and the lumbar spine have a lordotic curve, which is counterbalanced by the thoracic kyphotic curve. These curves provide optimal biomechanical anchoring to the numerous muscle groups that provide both spinal and appendicular motion. These curves also allow optimal load transfer along the spine and abdominal column. Any significant change in these curves structurally or posturally alters the stress transfer across the vertebral units, potentially subjecting them to injury.

The thoracic spine provides for articulation with the ribs, which incidentally provide an additional stabilizing framework with the thoracic vertebrae.

The vertebrae also provide a bony framework for the protection and support of the spinal cord and spinal nerve roots.

STRUCTURAL ANATOMY

Anteriorly, the vertebrae consist of the vertebral bodies, which transmit the greatest part of the axial weight load (Figure 12-1). Between the vertebral bodies are the intervertebral disks. The disk consists of a central nucleus pulposus, which is a reticulated and collagenous substance in mucoid material and is composed of approximately 88% water. The nucleus pulposus is the primary shock absorber for axial loads and acts as a ball bearing for shear loads. Surrounding this is the annulus fibrosus, consisting of concentric lamellae of fibrocartilage fibers arranged obliquely; with each deeper layer, they are arranged in opposite direc-

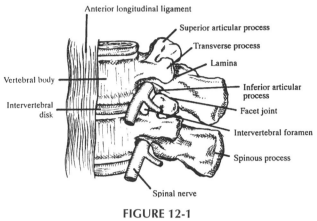

FIGURE 12-1
Lumbar vertebral anatomy.

tions in an alternating pattern to provide excellent resistance to torsional stresses. This arrangement is analogous to the automobile steel-belted radial tire. The major ligamentous structures include the anterior longitudinal ligament, which prevents hyperextension, and the posterior longitudinal ligament, which prevents hyperflexion. Hyperflexion is also resisted by the weaker interspinous ligament, supplemented by the stronger supraspinous ligament linking the spinous processes. Further resistance to hyperflexion of the vertebral unit is provided by the ligamentum flavum; a broad, yellow, elastic, ligamentous band that joins the lamina of adjacent vertebral arches as well as by the lumbodorsal fascia.

The vertebral arch consists of the posterior portion of the vertebrae, which protects the neural tissues and includes the extensions from the vertebral body posteriorly (pedicles). They are joined by the laminae, which extend into four articular processes to make up the facet joints. The facet joints have hyaline cartilage articular surfaces that are oriented toward the coronal plane in the thoracic spine, allowing rotation and limiting flexion and extension of the verte-

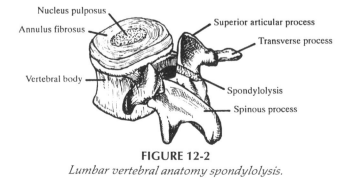

FIGURE 12-2
Lumbar vertebral anatomy spondylolysis.

bral bodies. The orientation in the lumbar spine is toward the sagittal plane, allowing flexion and extension but limiting rotation of those vertebral bodies. These are not weight-bearing joints, but with significant disk space narrowing, they become markedly dysfunctional because of abnormal loading and incongruity. The portion of the lamina that extends to the superior facet joint is called the *pars interarticularis*, which is involved in spondylolysis (Figure 12-2).

Two transverse processes project laterally on each side from the junction of the pedicle and the lamina. Substantial muscle origins are derived from these structures. The apical portions of the two laminae combine to form the spinous process.

The spinal cord extends from the foramen magnum to the L1–L2 disk where the cauda equina is the continuation of the nerve roots to the coccygeal region.

HISTORY

The athlete presenting with symptoms of back pain should be carefully questioned about the following:

- The location of the pain
- The nature of the pain
- When the pain started
- Events surrounding the onset of the pain
- Subsequent events related to the pain (including any self-treatments or medical treatment and the response to those treatments)
- The nature of the pain over time
- What makes the pain worse
- What makes the pain better
- The overall change in the pain with time

Additionally, previous injuries or prior pain events should be noted. Radicular symptoms, sensory changes (such as hypoesthesia, hyperesthesia, tingling, or a pins-and-needles sensation), burning, or numbness should be sought. The athlete should be queried as to how it has affected performance and if any weakness or loss of agility, speed, or endurance has been noted. The athlete should be questioned as to the response to Valsalva maneuvers (pain exacerbated by Valsalva suggests nerve root or dural tension or inflammation), such as coughing, sneezing, or straining at the toilet, and whether there is any urinary or fecal incontinence. Questions concerning the sleeping pattern and sleeping positions should also be asked. A thorough review of systems should be undertaken, including previous surgical and medical history as well as questions regarding smoking, alcohol, and illicit drugs.

PHYSICAL EXAMINATION

The patient is carefully observed walking into the examination room, getting into and out of a chair, and getting onto and off the table. The patient's posture is observed throughout the history taking. How the patient moves when removing shoes, socks, and articles of clothing should also be noted. The examination should be performed with the patient in underwear to note the overall body posture and stance.

With the patient standing, the spinal alignment in both the posterior and lateral aspects is noted. The level of the iliac crests should be noted, looking for ilial rotation, pelvic obliquity, or leg length discrepancy while making sure both of the patient's knees are fully extended. If a discrepancy is present, blocks are placed underfoot to level the iliac crest, and the block thickness necessary to level off the crest is measured. Measurement of the leg lengths may be done on the supine patient from the anterosuperior iliac spine to the medial malleolus; however, studies have shown this to be more variable than the block-leveling technique. The block technique is less reliable when the patient has pelvic obliquity that is due to severe muscle spasm or sacroiliac dysfunction (see the sacroiliac discussion in Chapter 14). The presence of a list, scoliosis, and muscle symmetry or asymmetry should be noted. Asymmetry of iliac crests is more likely due to ilial rotation, pelvic obliquity, or sacroiliac dysfunction than leg length discrepancy. In treatment, a true leg length discrepancy should be one of the last treatment trials.

The patient should indicate where the pain is located, and that area is examined last. Palpation of the back is done in all other areas, such as the spinous processes, posterior superior iliac spines, iliac crests, sacrum and coccyx, and the paraspinous muscles, before examining the painful area. Light axial loading is performed on the shoulders or at the head, a gentle rotational motion as a whole unit is done with the arms at the patient's side (en bloc rotation), and the skin of the back is lightly palpated. These three Waddell procedures should not produce any pain. The patient's reaction during these maneuvers and the severity of pain vocalized indicate the amount of embellishment by the patient. (An exception to this is moving a patient who has marked muscle spasm that produces a significant amount of pain and who is fearful of increasing the pain.)

Muscle spasm is characterized by muscular tightness that does not decrease in any position, whether standing, sitting, or lying. To test for this, palpate the erector spinal muscles with thumbs on each side and rest your hand on the patient's flanks while he or she walks in place. No relaxation occurs in the erector spinae muscle that is in spasm. When no spasm is present, the erector spinae muscle on the weightbearing side relaxes, and the palpating thumb moves anteriorly toward the spine; the contralateral side tightens and pushes the other thumb away. It is important that the patient stand in an upright position and not lean forward or be in extension while performing this test.

An asymmetric muscle spasm is indicated by the presence of a list. The presence or absence of spasm may also be assessed with the patient supine and resting on his or her elbows, holding his or her chest off the table. If no spasm is present and the patient is passively hyperextending his or her back, the erector spinae muscles are relaxed and soft to palpation.

The patient's stance should be observed. If significant nerve root irritation is present, the patient may stand with his or her knee flexed on the painful side in an attempt to take tension off the nerve root. The patient's gait is observed for the presence or absence of a limp. If present, the type of limp is noted: an antalgic limp favoring the painful side; a leg length discrepancy limp; an abductor muscle weakness limp (Trendelenburg gait) with the pelvis dropping down toward the side opposite the weak side; or a hip limp, leaning the body over the side of the painful hip. The patient is asked to toe walk (S1) and then heel walk, while particular attention is paid to the degree of great toe extension (L5) as well as to the ankle dorsiflexion (L4 and L5). The patient is asked to go into a full squat and arise (L3 and L4). (The parentheses indicate the predominant nerve root[s] involved in performing the indicated test.) S1 nerve root weakness may be subtle, and 10 repetitions of single-leg stance toe raises (done to fatigue the gastrocnemius and soleus muscle groups) may be necessary to detect this weakness. The patient's lumbosacral range of motion is measured with a goniometer or inclinometer. Side bending is noted by having the patient slide his or her hand down the side of his or her leg as far as possible then repeating this on the other side (normal is 40 degrees tilt to each side). Backward extension is measured (normally 35 degrees). Last to be measured is forward flexion without bending the knees (normally 80 degrees). The examiner places his or her thumb and middle fingertip on the spinous processes of L5 and L3 and notes the separation between the digits increases when the patient flexes and decreases when the patient returns to the upright stance. If significant muscle spasm is present, then the distance between the digits remains unchanged as the forward flexion is through the pelvis and hips and not the lumbar spine. The patient is now asked to be seated. Rotation of the thoracic spine is measured with maximal upper torso rotation to each side. The seated position helps to prevent pelvic rotation and thus allows a more accurate measurement.

Sensation in the lower extremities is tested with light touch and pinprick (paper clip sharp end) as well as with a cold object. The area of decreased sensation is noted, as well as the presence or absence of a dermatomal pattern and any inconsistencies between the different modalities.

The patient's maximal strength is tested in both lower extremities simultaneously using resistance to toe flexion (S1) and extension (L5); ankle plantar flexion (S1) and extension (L4), inversion (L5), and eversion (S1); knee flexion (L5 and S1) and extension (L3 and L4); hip flexion (L2 and L3) and extension (S1 and S2), abduction (L5 and S1), and adduction (L1 and L2). The reflexes at the Achilles tendons (S1) and the patellar tendons (L3 and L4) are assessed at rest. If asymmetric or decreased, augmentation is used (i.e., pushing or pulling the hands while simultaneously tapping the tendon), and the response is noted. If the Achilles reflex is difficult to determine, it may be repeated with the patient kneeling in a chair and augmenting if necessary. Check for clonus by rapidly dorsiflexing the foot. A normal response is three beats downward or less. Four beats or more is abnormal. While the seated patient is distracted with the pretense of examining the foot, the knee is fully extended, then the foot is dorsiflexed, and the patient's response is noted. With significant radicular symptoms, the patient leans backward and reports discomfort in the leg. The patient's dorsalis pedis and posterior tibial arterial pulses are noted.

Measurements of the maximum girth of the calf and at a fixed reproducible point on the thigh are made to document atrophy. A convenient method for thigh girth measurements is 20 cm proximal to the anteromedial tibial plateau, owing to the difficulty in noting the superior pole of the patella level. If the measurements are asymmetric, the marks are again checked, and the examiner makes sure that the tape measure is perpendicular to the long axis of the limb.

The patient is then asked to lie supine and do an active straight leg raise (SLR). If significant hip pathology is present or the iliopsoas or rectus muscles are injured, the patient will have groin pain on elevating the leg. The hip range of motion is determined with flexion and internal and external rotation and then brought down into an abduction external rotation position, which stresses the hip and the sacroiliac joint. (Examination for sacroiliac joint problems is described in Chapter 14.) If significant hip arthritis is present, internal rotation is the first to decrease. Maneuvers to assess for nerve root irritation are then performed. The knee is extended and the hip flexed, noting the degree of hamstring tightness and if leg pain radiating distally is produced (positive SLR) or exacer-

bated by ankle dorsiflexion (positive Lasègue sign) or ankle plantar flexion (functional sign). Record the degree of hip flexion when the leg pain was produced. Nerve root inflammation typically causes pain with the hip flexed 70 degrees or less. At the level of supine hip flexion that produces the leg pain, the knee is flexed slightly, and the symptoms should be relieved if symptoms are due to nerve root tension. With thumb compression into the popliteal space, tension is again placed onto the sciatic nerve, and the radiating leg pain may be reproduced if nerve root irritation and tension is present (positive bowstring sign). Reproduction of back pain only during SLR is not a positive SLR. The contralateral SLR test is positive when the patient's asymptomatic leg is elevated from the table by the examiner and radicular pain is reproduced down the patient's opposite leg. This is a significant finding when present, because it indicates the presence of a large disk fragment that lies near the axilla of the nerve root and the thecal sac.

Palpation of the abdomen is done to note if any abdominal pathology is present. The patient is asked to assume a prone position, and the musculature of his or her back is observed. The sciatic notch, piriformis and gluteal muscles, and greater trochauteric bursa are palpated for excess tenderness. The anterior thigh (L4), anterolateral lower leg (L5), and posterior calf (S1) are then palpated, as nerve root irritation often results in localized tenderness of the innervated muscles. The reverse SLR test is done with the patient prone and flexing his or her knee 90 degrees and extending his or her hip. If the femoral nerve or nerve roots L2, L3, and L4 are irritated, this test will reproduce the patient's anterior thigh pain. For a complete examination, a rectal examination is also carried out, with a Hemoccult (SmithKline Diagnostics, Sunnyvale, CA) test for occult blood.

Throughout this history and examination, the appropriateness of the patient's responses is noted. It must be remembered that even in the patient with many nonorganic signs, meticulous attention must be given to thoroughly searching for any underlying organic findings. The nonorganic signs indicate the degree of pain behavior the patient demonstrates. Waddell developed the following standardized group of five types of physical signs:

1. Nonanatomic superficial tenderness
2. Simulation tests, as noted earlier in this section, with axial loading and en bloc rotation producing pain
3. Distraction test or flip test in which the patient has no pain with full extension of the knee while seated, but the supine SLR is markedly positive
4. Nonanatomic weakness or sensory loss
5. Overreaction verbally or exaggerated body language

When three or more of these signs are present, the patient is likely exaggerating.[5] However, a complete examination must be done to uncover any potential underlying organic pathology.

DIAGNOSTIC IMAGING

Diagnostic imaging is rarely indicated in acute episodes of back pain unless there has been significant trauma; significant or progressive neurologic deficits; or atypical pain, such as pain at rest; at night; or associated with fever, chills, or sweats (suspicion of infection or neoplasm). The natural history of low back pain without radiculopathy is 50% recovery expected in a week and 95% recovery in 3 months. At 3 months, plain spine radiographs may be taken if the symptoms are still significant.

Magnetic resonance imaging (MRI) is the diagnostic imaging modality of choice for patients with neurologic findings because it is noninvasive, does not expose the patient to radiation, has a large field of view, and produces excellent sagittal images. Computed tomography (CT) myelography is helpful in the rare patient with a lateral recess and foraminal disk herniation. CT is best for assessment of spinal fractures when spinal canal compromise is present or suspected. Many studies of normal asymptomatic patients with these modalities reveal a 40% false-positive abnormal finding rate that increases with age. It is important to order and interpret the findings in light of the patient's history and physical examination.

A bone scan and single photon emission CT is helpful with detecting occult fractures, arthritic processes, tumor, or infection and with distinguishing between old versus new pars fractures.

Electrodiagnostic testing is useful when determining the level of nerve root involvement to eliminate peripheral neuropathy or other neurologic disorders. Electrodiagnostic testing can be done after an injury to prove that there was no nerve root problem before injury. A positive electromyogram for radiculopathy 6 weeks postinjury correlates radiculopathy and injury.

DIFFERENTIAL DIAGNOSIS

When the patient presents with chronic as well as acute back pain, it must be kept in mind that conditions other than those related to the vertebral and surrounding structures may produce back pain, including viscerogenic sources that originate from disorders of the kidney, the urinary tract, the female reproductive tract, or the gastrointestinal tract. Vascular causes include an abdominal

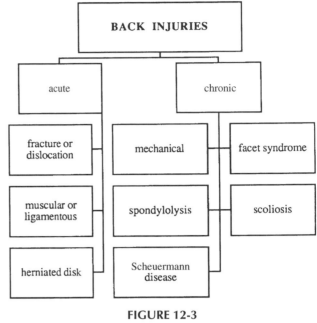

FIGURE 12-3
Evaluation of back injuries.

aortic aneurysm, which may produce excruciatingly severe low back pain. Neoplastic diseases (both primary and metastatic), as well as intra- and extradural spinal cord tumors, may produce back and leg pain. Infectious processes—including vertebral body osteomyelitis and disk space infection (with or without abscess formation) and sacroiliac joint infection—may also produce back or leg pain. Inflammatory diseases, such as ankylosing spondylitis or inflammatory bowel disease, should also be considered. The sacroiliac joint can also produce low back pain and may exacerbate an underlying lumbar condition. Sacroiliac strain is frequently seen in throwing athletes secondary to rotation through the pelvis.[6] (See Chapter 14 for evaluation of sacroiliac dysfunction.) Psychogenic causes may also significantly affect the patient, especially if there is a medicolegal aspect to the injury.

SPECIFIC INJURIES

See Figure 12-3.

Traumatic Back Injuries

Fractures and Dislocations
Fractures and fracture dislocations of the thoracic and lumbar spines are rarely produced by athletic pursuits. In the younger athlete in the second decade of life, however,

almost half of the thoracic and lumbar spine fractures are attributable to sports injuries such as tobogganing and bicycling. The force is transmitted over many segments, usually resulting in multiple vertebral fractures. In these patients, there is also a high incidence of associated injuries, both abdominal and thoracic, especially when transverse process fractures are present.

Fracture dislocations of the spine, particularly of the thoracolumbar junction, can produce neurologic deficits. In young patients, careful follow-up must be made over the years until maturity, because a progressive spinal deformity can occur with asymmetric spinal growth resulting from growth plate damage.

History

The examiner must take the time to obtain an accurate history, because this helps provide an understanding of the mechanism of injury and severity of symptoms. Many of these injuries are due to hyperflexion and produce compression fractures. It is important to determine if any neurologic abnormality is present, if any other associated symptoms are present to indicate injuries to other structures, and if a cervical or cranial injury has also occurred. In general, the force involved and the symptoms are significant enough that the patient will present within a short period for evaluation and treatment.

Physical Examination

A complete examination should be carried out, noting carefully areas of pain, degree of pain, soft tissue disruption, soft tissue swelling, and distortion of spinal alignment. The sensory status to light touch, pinprick, and temperature is determined. The motor examination of the extremities, reflexes, and Babinski reflex should also be noted. If any neurologic deficit is noted, the presence of the bulbocavernosus reflex must be checked (stimulation to the glans of the penis and noting that the anal wink is present). If this reflex is absent, the patient is in spinal shock, and no determination can be made concerning long-term prognosis of the neurologic deficit.

Radiography

Radiographic examination is essential to determine the extent of the injury. In the thoracic spine, this includes anteroposterior and lateral views. In the lumbosacral spine, this includes anteroposterior, lateral, and lumbosacral spot views, as well as oblique x-ray films if a questionable appearance suggesting spondylolysis is present in the pars interarticularis region.

If a question arises as to the presence of a fracture or the acuity of a radiographic appearance, a technetium bone scan should obtained. If a neurologic deficit is present or a question of posterior displacement of fragments into the spinal canal occurs, then CT is helpful in delineating the extent of the injury, especially assessing the bony fragments and the narrowing of the spinal canal, and detecting posterior arch fractures. MRI is used to define injuries to the soft tissues, such as the spinal cord, the intervertebral disks, the ligaments, and the muscles.

Treatment. The majority of vertebral fractures that result from athletic injuries are compression injuries and involve less than 50% compression of the vertebral body. These may be treated symptomatically with a hyperextension brace or a corset for very mild wedging for a period of 2–3 months, or until asymptomatic. As the vertebral compression approaches 50%, care must be taken to watch for progression of the flexion deformity. Transverse process fractures should warn of associated intraabdominal or thoracic injuries. Patients are treated symptomatically with analgesics and restriction of activity and are observed closely for the development of a paralytic ileus (secondary to the hematoma in the initial few days after the trauma). The patient may continue with activity to the point at which he or she begins to note increasing discomfort. When painless full mobility and agility have resumed, the athlete may return to competitive sports, taking great care to prevent reinjury. With injuries requiring surgical treatment, it may not be prudent to return to rigorous sports activities because of the severity of injury and extensive mechanical changes. Case-by-case determination can be made by the operating physician.

A fracture dislocation or unstable spinal fracture is extremely unusual and requires immediate surgical consultation.

In skeletally immature children, care must be taken to observe for the development of posttraumatic scoliosis. The treatment is identical to that for idiopathic scoliosis, with bracing being used for progressive curves between 25 and 45 degrees and surgical stabilization for curves that exceed 45–50 degrees.

Musculoligamentous Injuries

The most common acute injury sustained by the athlete in both contact and noncontact sports at all levels of competition is to the musculoligamentous structures in the spine. These are soft tissue injuries and are self-limiting.[7] The pain can be quite debilitating and can prevent the athlete from standing erect. Significant muscle spasm can be present and can make sitting very painful or impossible to tolerate. This leads to rapid deconditioning that must be overcome with a rehabilitation program or the symptoms will persist.

Lumbosacral spine radiographs are taken to rule out the presence of a fracture if there is a history of significant trauma.

Treatment. Initial treatment consists of relative rest of the back while encouraging as much activity as possible.[8] The efficacy of bed rest in the acute management of low back pain has been questioned and indeed may actually delay recovery and negatively affect long-term outcome.[9] During the acute phase, the patient performs frequent sessions of gentle stretching exercises. Examples of these exercises include lying supine and bringing one knee at a time toward the chest, bringing both knees to the chest, tilting the knees from side to side with the feet flat on the floor, tightening the abdomen while tilting the pelvis, and gently hyperextending the back by assuming a prone position and raising up on the elbows. Analgesics and nonsteroidal anti-inflammatory drugs (NSAIDs) may help during the initial recovery phase. This may be augmented by physical modalities, including heat, cold, ultrasound, and electrical current therapy. In addition, manual therapies—including mobilization, osteopathic manipulation, and chiropractic adjustment—may be useful in providing pain relief. The patient may increase activity level as the symptoms subside and begin a program of low back and hamstring stretching, and back and abdominal musculature strengthening. These exercises should not be pushed to the point of increasing back pain. The athlete may return to sports activities as soon as is comfortable, beginning with basic activities and gradually increasing activity until normal range of motion and agility are obtained. Return to full competition is allowed only after full range of motion and sport-specific agility exercises can be performed without pain. The patient must pay great attention to proper body mechanics with all activities to prevent reinjury.

Herniated Nucleus Pulposus

Herniated nucleus pulposus is present in as many as 10% of young athletes who have persistent pain more than 3 weeks after an injury (Figure 12-4).[7] The classic history associated with a symptomatic lumbar disk is pain radiating into the lower extremity in a near dermatomal pattern that is brought on with any position that produces nerve root stretching or disk compression, such as forward flexion of the back with the knees extended. This pain is usually a sharp shooting pain, but it may later become a deep aching pain in the dermatomal distribution. These radiating symptoms are due to both the inflammatory response to the herniated disk and the mechanical pressure on the nerve root. Low back pain alone without radiating symptoms into the leg may be due to a small

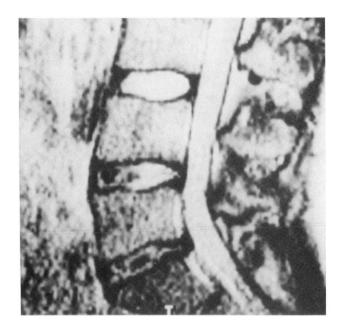

FIGURE 12-4

Magnetic resonance imaging of the lumbosacral spine. The top disk is normal. The middle disk is degenerated. The lowest disk is herniated.

disk herniation without nerve root irritation or to disk herniation through the end plates of the vertebral bodies (commonly in the thoracolumbar region), producing what are called *Schmorl nodes*. This may result in subsequent narrowing of the disk space and altered disk and facet joint mechanics, which produces the low back pain. However, there is no correlation between the finding of Schmorl nodes radiographically and the report of low back pain.

The herniated intervertebral disk is commonly noted in athletes in vigorous training programs such as gymnastics[10] and wrestling. More than 90% of herniated lumbar disks occur at the L4–L5 or L5–S1 levels, which are the levels through which the majority of flexion and extension occurs in the back. The athlete usually starts with back pain, which later radiates into the posterior to posterolateral aspect of lower extremity, to any level from the buttock to the toes (sciatica). Some athletes may experience leg pain as the only symptom. Most have varying degrees of back and leg pain.

The L4–L5 herniated disk most commonly impinges on the L5 nerve root, producing paresthesias or numbness in the dorsum of the foot, particularly the first web space (Table 12-1). L5 nerve root weakness is manifested by decreased great toe extensor power and, to a less pronounced degree, by loss of ankle dorsiflexion power (as this is also predominately innervated by L4). There may be tenderness to palpation of the anterior compartment musculature.

TABLE 12-1
Neuromotor Evaluation of Lower Lumbosacral Segment

Level of Disk Injury	Motor Testing	Reflex Testing	Sensory Distribution
L4	Tibialis anterior Quadriceps	Patellar tendon (knee jerk)	Medial arch
L5	Extensor hallucis longus	None	Dorsal foot (first web space)
S1	Peroneus longus/ brevis Gastrocnemius- soleus	Achilles tendon (ankle jerk)	Lateral and plantar foot

The L5–S1 herniated disk most commonly impinges on the S1 nerve root, producing paresthesias or numbness characteristically located at the posterolateral calf and foot. The weakness is noted with great toe flexion and ankle plantarflexion. The Achilles (ankle jerk) reflex may be diminished or absent. There may be tenderness to palpation of the calf musculature.

L4 nerve root irritation is much less frequent and is produced by a herniated L3–L4 disk or by an L4–L5 herniated disk that encroaches on the nerve root as it exits the neural foramen. The radicular pain may be present in the anterior thigh. The paresthesias and numbness may be found at the medial border of the thigh and calf. Weakness of knee extension may be present, and the patellar reflex may be diminished. The reverse SLR test may be positive.

Treatment. Treatment consists of decreasing the activity to a level at which symptoms are minimal (relative rest) while initiating a program of stretching and strengthening of the back, abdomen, and hamstrings. Positions with increased pressure on the disk, such as prolonged sitting and standing, should be avoided. Sitting and leaning forward create greater pressure on the disk. If symptoms are severe, limited bed rest for 24–48 hours may be prescribed, although the efficacy of this treatment is questionable.[8, 9]

NSAIDs and analgesics (in the most acute phase) help to decrease symptoms. A short 4- to 6-day course of oral steroids may help calm perineural inflammation and symptoms quickly; however, longer courses of 7 days or more have been implicated in the development of femoral and humeral osteonecrosis. Epidural steroids have not produced significant improvement in symptoms, but they may be useful in providing pain relief in some patients.

A structured and supervised physical therapy program is essential. This should initially involve gentle stretching and physical modalities, followed by a back stabilization program. An important but frequently overlooked issue is allowing adequate time for the injury to heal. Often, the pain symptoms are extreme, causing the patient to repeatedly seek care from several providers. Time must be taken to explain the anticipated course and outcome to the patient.

As radicular symptoms decrease, the athlete may progress activity with a gradual return to competition, taking care to maintain proper stretching, strengthening, fitness, and body mechanics. The majority of patients with documented ruptured disks, with or without radicular symptoms, do not require surgery and will improve significantly with nonoperative care. If, however, there is no significant improvement after 2–3 months of treatment, or in patients with focal neurologic findings, further evaluation with MRI, CT, intrathecal contrast, technetium bone scan (to rule out acute bony injury), and electromyography should be considered. Caution must be given to attributing the imaging abnormalities seen, because 30–40% of asymptomatic individuals demonstrate at least one abnormality. Clinical correlation is mandatory before concluding the abnormality noted on the study is the etiology of the patient's symptoms. At this time, consideration should be given to orthopedic or neurosurgical referral for further evaluation and possible surgical treatment.

A review of relevant studies by Young and colleagues highlighted several important issues regarding surgical and nonsurgical treatment of discogenic back pain.[11] First and foremost, although surgical treatment may lead to more rapid resolution of symptoms, there is no long-term difference in outcome in those treated surgically or with conservative measures. The decision to undergo surgical treatment depends on several factors, including the level of athletic competition, the length of time the athlete can allow for conservative treatment (6–9 months are typically required), and the desired level of continued participation.[11]

The existence of concomitant lumbar pathology, such as spondylolysis or spinal stenosis, deserves special consideration and should be referred to a spine specialist.[11] Similarly, a fractured disk with loose bodies in the spinal canal requires surgical evaluation. Immediate referral is warranted in the athlete with loss of bowel or bladder control or rapidly progressing lower extremity motor weakness.

Although many athletes are able to return to their former competitive level after surgical treatment, some will never return to their performance level and may have to select a less demanding position in their sport, select other less demanding sports, or possibly be unable to participate in any sport.

The unusual herniated disk is located in the thoracic spine, and the majority of these disks are asymptomatic.

Symptomatic thoracic disks cause radicular pain radiating to the rib at the level of the herniation, or myelopathy with numbness, weakness, bladder and bowel dysfunction, spasticity, or ataxia. Usually, surgery is not required unless progressive neurologic abnormalities are present or the radicular pain is severe after 6 months of treatment.

It is very rare for a patient to develop a cauda equina syndrome. The symptoms are produced by a very large central disk herniation pressing the thecal sac and the contained sacral nerve roots. The clinical presentation is a dramatic one of loss of bladder and bowel control, perianal numbness, anal sphincter weakness, pain radiating down both legs, and weakness in the legs. This is a true surgical emergency to decompress the sacral nerve roots before establishment of permanent damage.

Chronic Back Pain: Mechanical Low Back Pain

Mechanical low back pain is common in both the general population and athletes and is likely due to chronic muscular strain or ligamentous injuries of the spine. Factors that predispose athletes to this include tight hamstrings, lumbodorsal fascia posteriorly, and weak abdominal musculature anteriorly. This results in increased lumbar lordosis, which increases muscular and ligamentous stresses and overloads the posterior elements. In younger athletes, the adolescent growth spurt (with the inability of the musculotendinous units and ligaments to keep up with the growth of the bony elements) produces significant imbalances, resulting in susceptibility to recurrent injuries and pain (hyperlordotic low back pain syndrome).

In the majority of cases of mechanical low back pain, diagnostic examination and testing fails to reveal a specific mechanism or a precise anatomic site of the disorder, suggesting that it is a chronic intrinsic process rather than an acute and traumatic process.

Treatment. The treatment for mechanical low back pain (as well as most chronic back injuries) revolves around the basic program of careful education and explanation of the condition, with reassurance that with proper treatment, the symptoms can be resolved and the athlete returned to his or her former level of performance.

Instruction in proper body biomechanics is essential. Particularly when sitting for long periods, the athlete should make sure that his or her knees are slightly higher than his or her hips and that good erect sitting posture is maintained, with the possible addition of a small lumbar support. When standing for long periods, the athlete should attempt to place one foot on a step, thus tilting his or her pelvis forward.

The athlete is to maintain a rigorous twice-a-day program of stretching and strengthening until several asymptomatic months have passed. Flexibility of the hamstrings and lumbodorsal fascia is particularly important. Initial gentle stretching can be done in a supine position, bringing one knee at a time to the chest and progressing to both knees to the chest into a curled position, using the arms to pull the flexed knees toward the chest. This position is held for 30–60 seconds and repeated five times.

Hamstring stretching can be done one leg at a time with the heel on an elevated structure, such as a desk or table, and bending forward. It is essential that this is done slowly with the spine relatively straight and without bouncing. Another method, less stressful to the back, can be done before going to sleep and again on awakening. With this method, the athlete sits in bed with his or her legs outstretched in front, then flexes, abducts, and externally rotates one leg, placing the plantar foot adjacent to the contralateral knee. The athlete slowly bends at the waist and holds onto his or her outstretched leg as far distally as possible without bending his or her knee, for a count of 10. The maneuver is reversed for the contralateral leg. Four repetitions are done three to five times a day. If there is significant back pain with these stretches, a towel roll is placed behind the lumbar spine and the athlete lies supine. One leg at a time is pulled toward the ceiling with a towel behind the knee or calf, keeping the knee extended.

Anterior hip structures should be stretched by hyperextending the hip with the knee flexed, grasping the ankle, and pulling backward while in a standing position.

Pelvic tilting exercises in both the standing and supine position are done. The supine pelvic tilt is done with the knees bent and the feet flat on the floor. The buttocks are squeezed together and the stomach pulled inward, flattening the low back against the floor. The standing pelvic tilt is done with the back to the wall, pressing the small of the back to the wall by tucking the buttocks in and tightening the stomach muscles. Abdominal strengthening exercises are done during slow sit-ups or curl-ups with the knees and hips flexed at a 90-degree angle. The sit-ups are done in both a straight-up and oblique fashion. Extension exercises are done by lying in the prone position and pushing the torso upward with the arms until the arms are straight. Later, this extension exercise may be done actively by clasping the hands behind the back and then lifting the chest and legs off the ground. This may aggravate pain that is due to posterior element disease and should be avoided if painful.

Later, a weight-training program specific to the sport involved may be instituted, with attention to assure symmetric training of the agonist (paraspinous, rotatory muscles, gluteus, hamstrings) and antagonist (abdominals

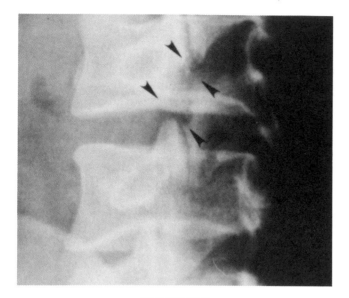

FIGURE 12-5
Oblique lumbar spine radiograph with arrows indicating bony edges of the pars interarticularis defect (spondylolysis).

[including obliques], quadriceps, iliopsoas) muscle groups. It is essential that the athlete gradually increase the rehabilitation program and training within the pain-free boundaries and prevent sudden changes in activity level.

Leg length discrepancy exceeding one-fourth inch may be addressed by placing a shoe lift amounting to one-half the discrepancy and gradually increasing it to one-eighth inch under the amount of the discrepancy over a 3-month period as the patient tolerates it. If the patient tends to catch the shoe while walking on a level surface, the lift is too thick and should be decreased in thickness.

A lumbosacral corset or a thoracolumbosacral orthosis is frequently used to prevent the hyperlordotic position of the back and to allow the patient to gradually increase the level of activity. It is essential that the support be used only for 2–3 months as a "crutch" while the patient is improving with the rehabilitation program. Ice massage to the painful area for approximately 10–12 minutes helps decrease pain. The patient may also benefit from physical therapy modalities, such as ultrasound, massage, and transcutaneous electrical nerve stimulation, as well as "back school" instruction and supervision of the exercise program. Referral to a spine specialist is recommended when no significant progress is made after 3 months or when symptoms appear confusing.

Differential Diagnosis

When the patient presents with low back pain, nonmusculoskeletal sources for this condition must be considered. Examples include viscerogenic sources that originate from disorders of the kidney, the urinary tract, the female reproductive tract, or the gastrointestinal tract; vascular causes, such as an abdominal aortic aneurysm; neoplastic diseases of the vertebral column itself, as well as intra- and extradural spinal cord tumors; and infectious processes, including vertebral body osteomyelitis, disk space infection, and sacroiliac joint infection.

The sacroiliac joint can produce pain in the very low back in the region of the sacroiliac joint without any symptoms in the lumbar musculature, unless the sacroiliac symptoms have exacerbated an underlying lumbar condition. There is only a small amount of rotational motion at the sacroiliac joint, but when this motion is asymmetric, pain commonly occurs. Sacroiliac strain is frequently seen in throwing athletes secondary to rotation through the pelvis.[6] (See Chapter 14 for evaluation of sacroiliac dysfunction.)

Facet Joint Syndrome

Facet joint injuries most commonly affect middle-aged athletes. Younger athletes also develop this problem when minor congenital anomalies—such as facet asymmetry or sacralization of the transverse processes—are present, placing unusual stresses on the facet joint. Other factors that contribute to facet joint syndrome include leg-length discrepancies and degenerative joint disease.

Patients generally report central or unilateral low back pain precipitated by extending from a flexed position or hyperextending the back. Pain may be referred to the buttock or posterior thigh. The diagnosis is often one of exclusion, but CT or MRI may demonstrate facet hypertrophy or degeneration. Selective fluoroscopic-guided facet injections help to confirm the diagnosis but offer little in the way of lasting relief.

Treatment. The treatment consists of avoiding hyperextension activities and otherwise following the mechanical low back pain program of treatment. Consideration may be given for corticosteroid injection into the facet joint.

Spondylolysis and Spondylolisthesis

Wiltse[12] reported that the incidence of spondylolysis (Figure 12-5) in the United States is 5.8% in the white population, with only one-third of this incidence in the black population. In the Eskimo population, the incidence may be as high as 60%. This indicates that there is a genetic predilection to this disorder. This condition is very rarely found before the age of 5 years and most frequently occurs between the ages of 5 and 8 years, with a lesser incidence after 8 years of age.

A prospective study of University of Indiana football players showed that 13.1% had a pars interarticularis defect at the start of their football program—more than twice the incidence in the general population.[13] A further 2.4% of the football players developed a defect in the pars interarticularis during their 4 years in college football.

Wiltse, in addition to many other authors, believed that a spondylolysis is a fatigue fracture from multiple repetitive stresses at the pars interarticularis.[12] In the general population, it is much more frequent in males than in females. This is thought to be due to the more vigorous activities traditionally pursued by males. In the realm of sports injuries to the low back, however, the predisposition is more sport-specific. Goldstein[14] used MRI evaluation of top-level female gymnasts and swimmers and found that spinal abnormalities increased dramatically as the level of competition and expertise increased. Spinal abnormalities were demonstrated in 9% of the pre-elite and 63% of the Olympic-level gymnasts, compared with 16% of all-level swimmers. It was thought that the female gymnast was prone to spinal injuries, because she often placed nonphysiologic, extreme stresses on her back during the maneuvers characteristic of that sport.

In spondylolysis itself, the incidence was found to be 11% in competitive female gymnasts versus 2–3% in the general female population.[15] The pain initially may be elicited only with back hyperextension maneuvers, but later may become progressively more severe and interfere with the activities of daily living, including sitting or sleeping. It is relieved by the supine position. The pain may radiate from the back into the buttocks and thighs. More leg pain may be noted with higher-grade slips. Most patients are entirely symptom free.

For further discussion on spondylolysis, see Chapter 13.

Physical Examination

The classic presentation is an adolescent athlete who has a hyperlordotic posture with tight hamstrings and restricted forward bending that is usually painless; however, when returning to the position standing upright, the athlete notes pain. The provocative test is a single-leg stance while hyperextending the back (to stress the posterior elements) and then standing on the other leg while continuing to hyperextend the back. If the pars fracture is unilateral, the pain will be greatest on the single-leg stance on the ipsilateral weightbearing leg that is on the same side as the spondylolysis. High-grade slips may produce a palpable spinous process step-off.

Radiography

Lumbosacral spot x-ray films will reveal the lesion to be most commonly at L5 on S1 and followed by L4 on L5.

There may be a grade I spondylolisthesis, but it is extremely rare to find a higher-grade slip. A slippage usually occurs between the ages of 9 and 14 years, and seldom does any progression occur after 14 years of age. A bone scan is done if initial x-ray films are normal but suspicion remains. A positive scan usually means that either a spondylolysis or an exacerbation of a previously spondylolytic area has occurred in the previous 6–12 months. Flexion and extension lateral views—both translational and angular aspects—are done to note if the segment is unstable in the sagittal plane.

Treatment. The patient usually responds to the treatment described in the section on mechanical low back pain, with more rigorous emphasis on bracing, avoiding back extension, and avoiding sport activity until the symptoms resolve. Usually, the resolution of pain corresponds to resolution of activity on the bone scan, and once the pain has been eliminated and agility has increased, the patient may return to the sports activity. Resolution of the hamstring spasm mirrors the success of the treatment program.[16]

Many patients are competing without awareness that they have spondylolysis or a grade I spondylolisthesis. Once the spondylolisthesis is 50% or greater, however, the patient has increasingly marked structural changes that interfere with the ability to participate in competitive sports.

In patients whose symptoms persist longer than 6–12 months in spite of the aggressive nonoperative program, care should be taken to make sure that none of the other conditions noted in the differential diagnosis section are present. Consideration may be given to fusion of the involved segment to the adjacent level. Fusion is done in very few patients, because the majority respond to the nonoperative treatment program. Some athletes have been able to return to successful levels of competition after a fusion.[17]

Spinal Stenosis

Older athletes with lumbar degenerative spondylosis may develop symptoms related to the narrowed spinal canal. Significant spinal stenosis produces neurogenic claudication that presents as bilateral leg pain produced by prolonged standing, walking upright, or with spine extension. The narrowing of the spinal canal is worsened with the extended position, and further pressure and ischemia occurs in the neural tissues. Flexion typically relieves the symptoms as the canal is widened.

The symptoms start proximally and progress distally. Relief with stopping or forward flexing at the waist comes very slowly and may take longer than 30 minutes. Spinal stenosis must be differentiated from vascular claudication, in which the pain starts in the calf and progresses proximally. Pain from vascular claudication differs from spinal stenosis in that it is relieved by stopping for less than 1 minute, bending forward does not relieve the pain, and peripheral pulses are often decreased.[18]

Diagnosis is made by the characteristic history and an MRI, which confirms the narrow spinal canal. Physical examination is generally unremarkable except for possibly brisk lower extremity reflexes.

Treatment. Treatment initially consists of activity limitation below the pain threshold, NSAIDs, low back stretching and strengthening, and hamstring stretches. Epidural steroids are generally more effective in this condition than with a herniated disk, but the duration of relief is quite variable. Decompressive laminectomy should be considered in progressive or more severe cases.

SUMMARY

The etiology of the athlete's back pain is often very difficult to diagnose and thus properly treat. The vast majority of patients have resolution of their pain in a short period, especially with the rehabilitation program. The physician should rule out the more serious spine disorders, which are experienced by only the minority of patients.[1] A meticulous history and physical examination accomplishes this goal without having to pursue expensive diagnostic testing that has a high false-positive rate.

REFERENCES

1. Harvey J, Tanner S. Low back pain in young athletes. Sports Med 1991;12:394–406.
2. Keene JS, Albert MJ, Springer SL, et al. Back injuries in college athletes. J Spinal Disord 1989;2:190–195.
3. Marks MR, Haas SS, Wiesel SW. Low back pain in the competitive tennis player. Clin Sports Med 1988;7:277–287.
4. Sward L, Hellstrom M, Jacobsson B. Back pain and radiologic changes in the thoracolumbar spine of athletes. Spine 1990;15:124–129.
5. Waddell G, McCulloch JA, Kummel E, Venner RM. Nonorganic physical signs in low-back pain. Spine 1980;5:117–125.
6. Stanish W. Low back pain in middle-aged athletes. Am J Sports Med 1979;7:367–369.
7. Tall RL, DeVault W. Spinal injury in sport: epidemiological considerations. Clin Sports Med 1993;12:441–448.
8. Malmivaara A, Hakkinen U, Aro T, et al. The treatment of acute low back pain—bed rest, exercises, or ordinary activity. N Engl J Med 1995;332:351–355.
9. Wilkinson MJ. Does 48 hours' bed rest influence the outcome of acute low back pain? Br J Gen Prac 1995;45:481–484.
10. Jackson DW. Low back pain in young athletes: evaluation of stress reaction and discogenic problems. Am J Sports Med 1979;7:364–366.
11. Young JL, Press JM, Herring S. The disk at risk in athletes: perspectives on operative and nonoperative care. Med Sci Sports Exerc 1997;29(suppl):222–232.
12. Wiltse LL, Widell EH, Jackson DW. Fatigue fracture: the basic lesion in isthmic spondylolisthesis. J Bone Joint Surg Am 1975;57:17–22.
13. McCarroll JR, Miller JM, Ritter MA. Lumbar spondylolysis and spondylolisthesis in college football players: a prospective study. Am J Sports Med 1986;14:404–406.
14. Goldstein JD, Berger PE, Windler GE, Jackson DW. Spine injuries in gymnasts and swimmers: an epidemiologic investigation. Am J Sports Med 1991;19:463–468.
15. Ciullo JV, Jackson DW. Pars interarticularis stress reaction, spondylolysis and spondylolisthesis in gymnasts. Clin Sports Med 1985;4:95–110.
16. Stinson JT. Spondylolysis and spondylolisthesis in the athlete. Clin Sports Med 1993;12:517–528.
17. Micheli LJ. Back injuries in gymnastics. Clin Sports Med 1985;4:85–93.
18. Watkins RG, Campbell DR. The older athlete after lumbar spine surgery. Clin Sports Med 1991;10:391–399.

13

Back Pain in the Young Athlete

Laura Jean Trombino

The evaluation of back pain in children generally requires a more aggressive approach than in the adult. Approximately 60–80% of adults experience back pain[1] that is generally mechanical or related to disk degeneration or musculotendinous strain.[2, 3] Unlike adults, children more commonly have an organic and demonstrable etiology of their pain.[4-7] Indeed, Hensinger[8] reported that 84 out of 100 skeletally immature patients with back pain had an identifiable cause; these included 33 with occult fractures, spondylolysis, or spondylolisthesis; 33 with scoliosis or kyphosis; and 18 with tumors or infection.

In school-based surveys, 20–36% of adolescents report low back pain[9, 10] with the prevalence increasing from 11.6% at age 11 years to 50.4% by age 15 years.[9] Both inactivity and participation in strenuous sports have been associated with recurrent back pain in children.[1, 9-12] Although back pain is frequently a result of macrotrauma or repetitive microtrauma, underlying neoplasm, developmental anomaly, or infection should always be considered in younger athletes. An occult neoplasm or infection is not infrequently discovered while evaluating back pain presumed to be from an injury.[4, 5, 10]

EVALUATING THE CHILD WITH BACK PAIN

Figure 13-1 is an algorithm for evaluating low back pain in children.

History

The primary distinction to be made is whether the back pain was caused by trauma or activity or whether the back pain coincidentally developed in an active child.

The young athlete and parents should be carefully queried regarding characteristics of the back pain, including onset, quality (burning, aching, sharp, dull), radiation, duration, precipitating activities, and positions of relief. Systemic symptoms, such as weight loss, anorexia, bruising, fatigue, fever, chills, night sweats, or night pain, suggest underlying infection or neoplasm.[5, 7] Pain provoked by specific activities or positions strongly favors a structural etiology. Lesions of the posterior elements (e.g., pars interarticularis stress reactions) are aggravated by back extension and relieved by flexion. Conversely, disk problems are aggravated by flexion and often relieved by extension. A family history can be useful if there is a suspicion of spondyloarthropathy or a developmental anomaly.

Historic features that concern and should prompt an expedient workup include progressively increasing pain, systemic symptoms, neurologic symptoms, bowel or bladder dysfunction, and age younger than 4 years.[5, 8]

Physical Examination

The examination should begin by observing the child's posture and gait. The back is then inspected for midline dermatologic signs of spinal cord abnormalities, such as deep dimpling, hemangiomas, or hairy patches.[6] The patient is next examined for spinal curvatures, muscle spasm, lumbosacral and hamstring flexibility, and leg length discrepancy. Hamstring tightness is common in many back pain syndromes, especially spondylolisthesis.[6, 7, 10, 13-16]

The neurologic examination includes gait analysis, deep tendon reflexes, abdominal reflexes, Babinski test, sensory examination, motor strength, and straight leg raise. Findings of concern include a left thoracic scoliosis curve or neurologic abnormalities. Significant loss of spinal

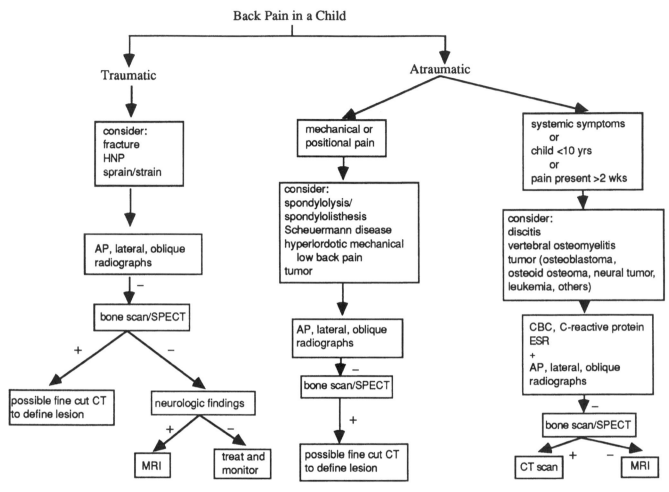

FIGURE 13-1

Algorithm for evaluating low back pain in children. (AP = anteroposterior; CBC = complete blood count; CT = computed tomography; ESR = erythrocyte sedimentation rate; HNP = herniated nucleus pulposus; MRI = magnetic resonance imaging; SPECT = single photon emission computed tomography.)

motion and inability to bear weight are particularly worrisome for underlying pathology.[5, 6]

Imaging

Plain radiographs (anteroposterior and lateral views) are indicated in children with acute or persistent back pain[6, 7, 10] and pain associated with systemic symptoms. Oblique views are useful to evaluate pars interarticularis defects (spondylolysis), and standing full-length views are necessary to adequately evaluate scoliosis or Scheuermann disease.

More sophisticated imaging techniques are frequently required to diagnose occult spinal problems. Technetium nuclear imaging (bone scan) is generally the best test after plain radiographs and is helpful to rule out infection, most

neoplasms, and occult stress fractures.[6, 7] Single photon emission computed tomography (SPECT) is more sensitive and is particularly helpful in identifying stress reactions of the pars interarticularis.[6,7] Computed tomography (CT) scans give excellent resolution of bone and are helpful in delineating bony lesions identified on bone scan. Magnetic resonance imaging (MRI) is used to delineate soft tissue abnormalities of the neural or perineural elements. MRI is particularly useful to identify herniated nucleus pulposus (HNP), spinal cord anomalies, tumors, discitis, and vertebral osteomyelitis.[17, 18]

Laboratory Tests

The need for laboratory evaluation is determined by the clinical presentation but should be considered in children with atypical back pain, night pain, fever, or other systemic symptoms. A complete blood count with differential, erythrocyte sedimentation rate, and C-reactive protein is helpful in evaluating back pain that may be due to infection or neoplasia.[6, 7, 10] Back pain is the presenting symptom in 6% of children with leukemia. A number of spondyloarthropathies can be associated with a positive HLA-B27 assay.[5]

ACQUIRED CONDITIONS CAUSING LOW BACK PAIN

Spondylolysis and Spondylolisthesis

Spondylolysis is an acquired defect (stress fracture) through one or both pars interarticularis, predominately at the L5–S1 level (see Figure 12-2). Spondylolisthesis is slippage of one vertebral body on another due to bilateral pars defects at a given vertebral level. Spondylolysis typically occurs between 5 and 10 years of age and is present in 5–10% of North Americans.[5, 13] Symptoms often do not develop until the teenage years when the child becomes more active. There is a genetic predisposition with a 27% incidence in first order relatives[10] and a 50% prevalence in the Eskimo population.[13]

Involvement in certain sports appears to predispose an athlete to spondylolysis. Repetitive cycles of spine flexion and extension presumably lead to microfractures and attempted repair of the posterior elements (pars interarticularis).[5, 10, 19–21] Additionally, some individuals have hip flexion contractures and accentuated lumbar lordosis, which transfer more stress to the posterior elements.[13] Virtually any athlete can develop spondylolysis, but higher-risk sports (that require repetitive back extension) include down linemen in football, dancers, figure skaters, and gymnasts. Female gymnasts, for example, have a fourfold higher prevalence than the general population,[22] and increased training is associated with a higher incidence.[19] Pars defects are present in 15.2% of college football players, but only 2.4% develop the defect while in college.[23] Acute fractures of the pars interarticularis are more commonly being recognized and should be considered in any athlete with traumatic low back pain.[10, 13, 19, 20, 22, 24, 25]

History

Affected athletes generally report recurrent lower back pain or a chronic ache that is aggravated by extension or rotation.[7, 13, 14, 25] Rest or discontinuing the inciting activity often relieves the pain. Occasionally, a specific traumatic event is identified, but generally months go by before athletes seek medical attention.[14, 25] Younger children with minimal symptoms are sometimes brought in by the parents when they notice a hyperlordotic posture or waddling gait.[14, 15, 21]

Physical Examination

A waddling gait may be observed that is due to hyperlordosis and tight hamstrings. The patient should be observed from behind while standing in his or her shorts with attention to leg length discrepancy, increased lumbar lordosis, and any spinal curvature. Individuals with spondylolisthesis may have a visible lumbar step-off posteriorly and a transverse abdominal crease anteriorly.[21]

Next, the patient is asked to flex and extend at the waist. Flexion may be limited due to tight hamstrings, but extension is generally full or excessive. Extension while standing loads the posterior elements and may be painful.

The single-leg hyperextension test loads the ipsilateral pars even more and is considered the best clinical test for spondylolysis. In this test, the patient stands on one leg while holding the contralateral flexed knee toward the chest. He or she is balanced by the examiner and asked to hyperextend his or her low back, thereby loading the ipsilateral pars interarticularis. Reproduction of pain is consistent with posterior element injury.[21, 24]

Motor strength, deep tendon reflexes, and straight leg raise should be performed to assess for associated neurologic deficit. Neurologic deficits are unusual but are seen in as many as 35% of spondylolisthesis cases when slippage is more than 50%.[21]

Imaging Studies

Standing anterior-posterior and lateral radiographs are adequate in diagnosing spondylolisthesis (Figure 13-2). Spondylolysis is best visualized on the oblique projections showing abnormalities of the pars interarticularis (the neck of the "scotty dog," Figures 12-2 and 13-3). The most common level involved is L5–S1 in spondylolysis and isthmic spondylolisthesis followed by L4–L5.[7, 21]

If the clinical picture strongly suggests spondylolysis and plain radiographs are normal, the patient should be evaluated with a technetium bone scan or SPECT (Figure 13-4). Additionally, these scans are useful to determine whether visualized pars defects are active or acute.[10] The SPECT scan is the most sensitive test to demonstrate stress reactions that occurred before plain radiograph abnormalities.[13, 24, 26, 27] CT scans are not always necessary but can be useful to delineate the extent of a fracture and plan treatment.

Radiographic classification of spondylolisthesis can be described through percentage of slipping or determination of slip angle[21] (Figure 13-5). MRI may also be useful in diagnosing early spondylolysis.[26]

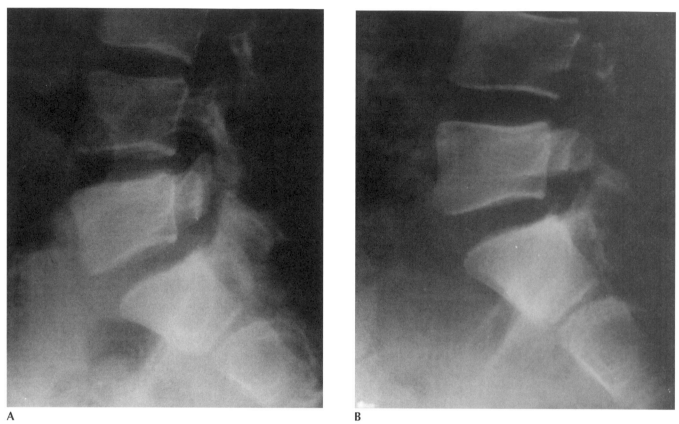

FIGURE 13-2

Radiographs of an 11-year-old boy with painful spondylolisthesis. A. Standing lateral radiograph demonstrates the L5 vertebral body slipped forward on S1. B. The unstable nature of this lesion is evident with this supine view of the same patient, which shows reduction of the spondylolisthesis.

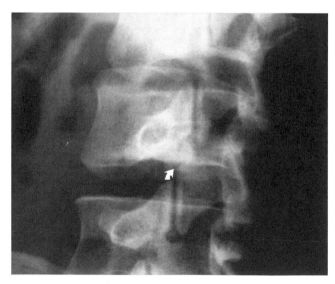

FIGURE 13-3

Spondylolysis in a 20-year-old baseball player. This oblique projection demonstrates a fracture line through the pars inter-articularis (arrow). These fractures resemble a collar on the neck of the "scotty dog" (see also Figure 12-2).

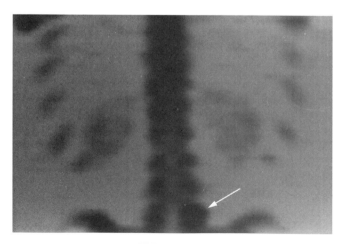

FIGURE 13-4

Single photon emission computed tomography image demonstrating early stress reaction of the pars interarticularis (arrow).

Treatment. Symptomatic spondylolysis often responds to restriction of activities, hamstring and lumbosacral fascia stretching, and abdominal strengthening exercises.[5, 7, 22] Many authors think that simply removing the patient from the exacerbating activity is adequate treatment.[5, 7, 22] Most think a period of limited activity for 3–6 months is necessary to improve symptoms and, at times, allow full healing of these fractures. Complete healing of pars interarticularis lesions is possible and has been demonstrated by bone scan.[13, 25] If relative rest fails to improve symptoms, bracing in a lumbar jacket from 6 weeks to 6 months or longer may be necessary.[7, 10, 14] Other indications for bracing are traumatic injuries or sudden-onset atraumatic injuries.

Spondylolysis that fails to respond to conservative therapy may require surgery. Surgical treatments include bone grafting of the pars defect with wire or screw fixation[20, 24, 27, 28] or posterior lateral fusion of the two involved levels.[7]

Indications for spinal fusion in spondylolisthesis include the following: (1) slips greater than 50% in the immature skeleton, (2) slip progression, (3) persistent deformity and abnormal gait, (4) refractory pain, and (5) neurologic deficit and high-angle slip.[10, 21] Virtually every degree of slip has been successfully treated with in situ fusion. The higher grade slips (50% or greater) require a three-level fusion (e.g., L4–S1).[16, 21, 29-32]

Scheuermann Disease

Scheuermann disease (juvenile kyphosis) is the second most common cause of back pain in children and adolescents[6] and is radiographically evident in 20–30% of the adult population.[5] There is a strong genetic predisposition.[7] The usual presentation of an adolescent with Scheuermann disease is back pain (50%) or painless thoracic kyphosis.[5] Scheuermann disease should be distinguished from postural round back, which is more flexible and lacks radiographic changes in the vertebrae (Figure 13-6). The pain associated with Scheuermann disease usually starts later in the day after activity and is typically aggravating but not activity limiting.[5, 7] These patients are also predisposed to spondylolysis at L5–S1 because of excessive lumbar lordosis.

Physical Examination

Two main forms of kyphosis are seen: the thoracic form (apex at T7–T9) and the thoracolumbar form (apex at T11–T12), with the latter associated with more persistent back pain. Physical examination demonstrates excessive thoracic or thoracolumbar kyphosis with a compensatory lumbar lordosis. Forward bending in both forms accentuates the apical kyphosis[33] (see Figure 13-6), and back extension may cause low back pain if there is associated

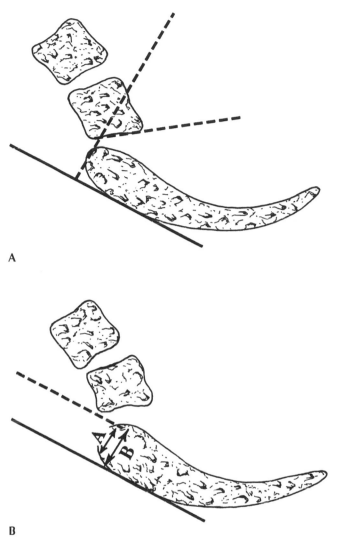

FIGURE 13-5
Two methods of radiographic evaluation of retrolisthesis to objectively measure progression of a slip. A. The slip angle is used to monitor progression of deformity. Angles greater than 40–50 degrees are at high risk of progression. B. Percentage slip of one vertebral body on the lower one. A is the distance from the anterior aspect of the L5 vertebral body to the anterior aspect of the sacrum, and B is the width of the sacrum. Percent slip = [1 − (B − A)/B] × 100.

spondylolysis. Concomitant scoliosis is present in 32–50% of patients with Scheuermann kyphosis.[6, 7] The neurologic examination is generally normal but should be done in all patients.

Radiographs

Standing lateral radiographs will show 5 degrees or more of anterior wedging of three or more consecutive verte-

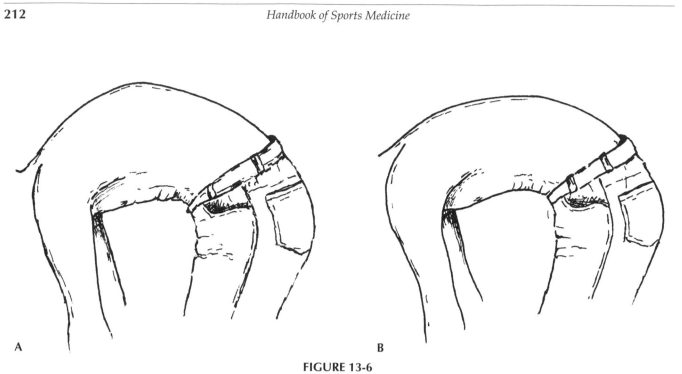

FIGURE 13-6
The clinical evaluation of Scheuermann disease includes a forward bending test. A. An apical kyphosis typical of Scheuermann disease. B. Smooth round back posture seen in postural kyphosis.

brae in the thoracic form, or one or two vertebral bodies in the thoracolumbar form (Figure 13-7). Lateral hyperextension views help determine the flexibility of the deformity. Normal kyphosis in the thoracic spine is 25–40 degrees, and measurements greater than 45 degrees are generally considered significant. Additional abnormalities associated with Scheuermann disease include end plate irregularities and Schmorl nodes.[33]

Natural History
Murray and colleagues[34] assessed the functional level of patients over an average of 32 years after their diagnosis of Scheuermann kyphosis. Patients with Scheuermann were found to have more intense back pain than the general population and to have jobs with lower physical demands. No differences, however, were found in level of education, extent that pain interfered with daily living, level of recreational activities, self-consciousness, self-esteem, or social limitations.

Treatment. Treatment is determined by the degree of kyphosis, skeletal maturity, and symptoms. Mild symptoms and deformities are treated with postural exercises and mild analgesics as needed. Follow-up should be done every 3–4 months during periods of rapid growth. Bracing with a Milwaukee brace or antigravity thoracolumbar sacral orthosis should be considered in the skeletally immature spine with angles greater than 55 degrees.[33] Thoracolumbar and lumbar Scheuermann disease may be treated with an underarm brace that is well molded and padded

properly to correct kyphosis. Because bracing is cumbersome and often needs to be continued for 12–18 months, referral to a pediatric spine specialist should be considered. Surgical treatment is generally reserved for patients with symptoms and curves greater than 75 degrees or with rapidly increasing kyphosis despite conservative care.[33]

DISK INJURIES AND FRACTURES

Herniated Nucleus Pulposus

HNP is relatively uncommon in children, accounting for only 1–4% of all patients with herniated disks.[10] Herniated disks in children differ from adults in that they are often atraumatic and may not cause classic sciatica.[35] In later adolescence, there is a preponderance of males to females with this condition, but the gender difference is reversed in younger patients.[36]

Physical Examination
Patients typically have signs of significant back discomfort with or without leg pain. Sciatic scoliosis, gait abnormalities, limitation of spinal flexion, loss of lordosis, and spinal deformities are more common than in adults.[35, 36] Neurologic findings, however, are less frequent, although motor changes, sensory dermatomal findings, and decreased ankle jerks have all been described. Most patients have a positive straight leg raise.[4–6, 10]

Imaging

Imaging should begin with plain radiographs to assess for other causes of back pain or associated spinal deformity. MRI is the study of choice for suspected herniated disks because it is less invasive than myelogram (Figure 13-8).

Treatment. Approximately 40% of children and adolescents with HNP respond to conservative care.[36] Initial treatment includes relative rest (with particular attention to avoid twisting and flexing of the waist) and nonsteroidal anti-inflammatory medications to decrease inflammation around the nerve root. Physical therapy is useful to maintain flexibility and muscle tone around the spine. Epidural steroid injections have been found to hasten the recovery in 50% of athletes with HNP. Activity is increased as symptoms resolve, progressing from low impact to jogging or running to cutting to contact.

Surgical treatment should be considered in patients with neurologic findings or persistent pain.[37] Herniated disks are generally posterior or posterolateral and best treated with laminotomy and removal of the herniated portion of the disk. There are generally few sequelae after surgery.[35]

Fractured Vertebral Apophysis

A variation of HNP unique to children is the fractured vertebral apophysis. Apophysis fractures occur when fusion between the vertebral rim apophysis and central cartilage is incomplete or delayed.[37] The usual mechanism is traumatic flexion causing posterior disk rupture where the annulus pulls (avulses) the ring apophysis portion of the vertebral body into the spinal canal.[38] It is frequently related to falls, motor vehicle accidents, weight lifting, and gymnastics. Four types of injuries have been described, ranging from a localized injury that includes small posterior irregularities of the cartilaginous end plates to a fracture spanning the entire length of the vertebrae.

Presentation

The presentation of a fractured vertebral apophysis is similar to a herniated disk. Neurologic symptoms however, are far more common and include both sensory and motor deficits. Electromyogram findings were found to be positive in 10 of 27 patients studied by Epstein and Epstein.[37]

Imaging

Radiographs may be negative, but the lateral view often shows a small vertebral chip posterior to the vertebral body (Figure 13-9A). CT or MRI scans should be used to

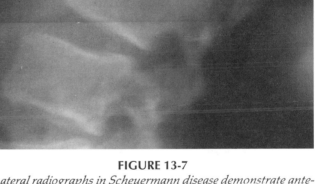

FIGURE 13-7

Lateral radiographs in Scheuermann disease demonstrate anterior wedging of 5 degrees or more in three contiguous thoracic vertebrae.

assess the cartilaginous extent of this injury and degree of displacement into the spinal canal (Figure 13-9B).

Treatment. Treatment generally requires surgery, and these patients should be referred to a spine specialist.[35]

Other Spine Fractures

Spinal column trauma is relatively uncommon in children, accounting for only 2–3% of all spinal trauma cases. Although these rarely occur in athletes, more violent trauma in sport can lead to compression fractures of the vertebral bodies (Figure 13-10). Burst fractures involve the anterior and posterior aspects of the vertebral body and can lead to neurologic problems that are due to extruded fragments into the spinal canal.[38] Seat belt (or Chance) fractures are caused by flexion of the anterior aspect of the spine with distraction of the middle and posterior elements.

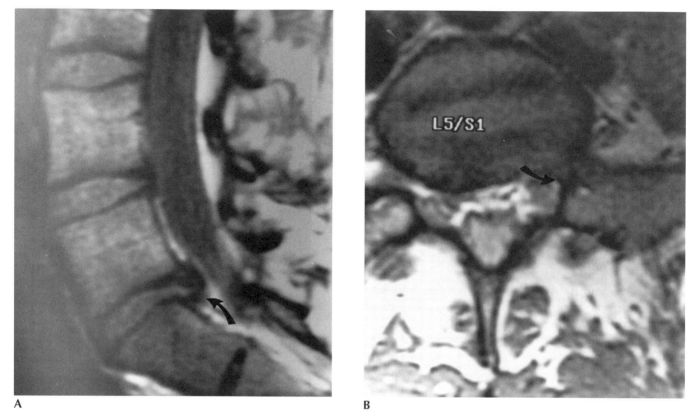

A   B

FIGURE 13-8

Magnetic resonance imaging demonstrating a posterolateral disk herniation in a teenage patient. A. Sagittal view demonstrating posterior prolapse of an L5–S1 disk (arrow). B. Axial section demonstrating the eccentric posterolateral prolapse and nerve root compression (arrow).

This can be identified on plain radiographs by an increased intraspinous distance on the lateral view.[38] Patients with these fractures should be referred for definitive care.

INFECTIONS

Discitis and vertebral osteomyelitis must be considered in all children and adolescents with back pain. In vertebral osteomyelitis, 21% of patients have back trauma that precedes symptoms.[39]

Discitis

Discitis is osteomyelitis of the end plate that invades the disk. It occurs in younger children (often younger than 4 years old) and rarely occurs in those older than 10 years.[5, 7] Children generally present with a stiff back or abdominal pain, and younger children will often refuse to walk.[7, 10] Children with discitis rarely

have severe systemic signs, although they may have a fever.[7, 10, 18]

Physical Examination

Physical examination demonstrates tenderness in the spine and loss of motion. Neurologic findings are rarely present.[7, 10, 18]

Laboratory

Laboratory evaluation should included a complete blood count with differential, erythrocyte sedimentation rate, and C-reactive protein. The white blood cell count is often normal, but the sedimentation rate is almost always elevated.[5, 7, 10, 18] C-reactive protein levels are also elevated to varying degrees.

Imaging

Radiographs show narrowing of the disk space and erosion of the end plate but are often not positive for 10 days to 2 weeks. Technetium bone scans and MRI scans can be

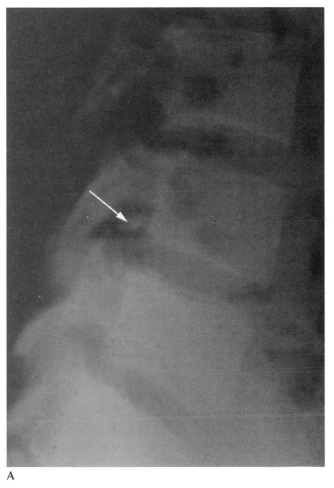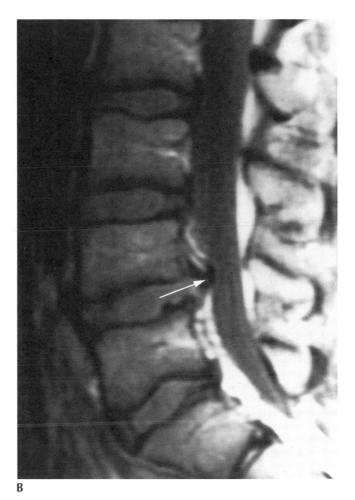

A   B

FIGURE 13-9

Ruptured vertebral ring apophysis in a 14-year-old gymnast from a hard landing with the waist flexed. A. Displaced bony avulsion fragment in the spinal canal (arrow). B. Magnetic resonance imaging demonstrates associated herniated disk and nucleus pulposus (arrow).

predictive early and should be obtained in suspected cases.[10, 17, 18]

Treatment. The majority of cases are secondary to *Staphylococcus aureus* and respond to intravenous antibiotics.[7, 18] Aspiration of the disk space is generally not necessary and should be reserved for patients who do not respond to antibiotics. Bed rest and immobilization with casts or braces have also been advocated.[5, 7]

Vertebral Osteomyelitis

Vertebral osteomyelitis is a more severe infection than discitis and most commonly involves the vertebral bodies of the lumbar spine.[39] It accounts for 1–4% of all cases of pyogenic osteomyelitis and is preceded by blunt trauma in approximately one-third of all cases. Ninety-two percent of these patients have back pain, and fever is common (58%).[39] Neurologic complications are far more common than in discitis and include nerve root compression, paraparesis, neurogenic bladder, meningitis, and torticollis.[39, 40]

Seventy-three percent of patients with vertebral osteomyelitis have an elevated sedimentation rate, and white blood cell counts are elevated in 35%. Erosive changes on plain radiographs will not be evident until 4–8 weeks, so MRI or technetium 99 bone scan should be used to detect early infections.[39, 40]

Treatment. Aspiration for culture and sensitivity may be necessary in these patients. *Staphylococcus aureus* is the most common causative organism, but infection can also be due to coagulase negative staphylococcus, streptococcus, and *Escherichia coli*. Abscesses can form and require surgical drainage.[39, 40]

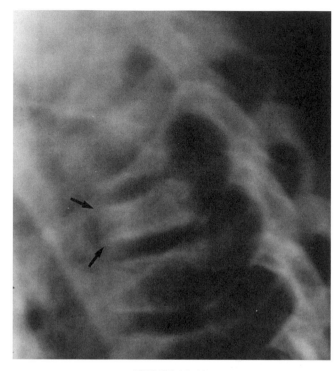

FIGURE 13-10

Anterior thoracic compression fracture demonstrated on lateral radiograph (arrows). Follow-up films should be repeated throughout growth, especially if vertebral end-plate damage is suspected.

SPINAL TUMORS AND PAINFUL SCOLIOSIS

Idiopathic scoliosis is rarely a painful condition, even in advanced curves. For this reason, any painful scoliosis should be viewed with suspicion. Stress fracture, infection, HNP, and neoplasia can all be responsible for a painful scoliosis.

Osteoid osteoma and osteoblastoma are common childhood tumors that can cause both pain and scoliosis and have a predilection for the posterior elements of the spine.[41, 42] The main differentiation between these two benign neoplasms is size. Some authors think that in fact these are the same lesion because of the similar histologic appearance.[41] Osteoid osteomas are painful, small lesions—less than 1.5–2.0 cm—with a small nidus surrounded by sclerosis. Osteoblastomas are larger than 1.5–2.0 cm with mixed osteosclerotic and osteoblastic characteristics. Osteoid osteomas occur 10 times more frequently than osteoblastomas.[41] The predominate symptom with both of these lesions is back pain that is more intense at night and relieved with aspirin.[41, 42]

Plain radiographs are usually sufficient to make a diagnosis of osteoblastoma,[43] and bone scans are useful to screen for an osteoid osteoma. A fine-cut CT scan is then

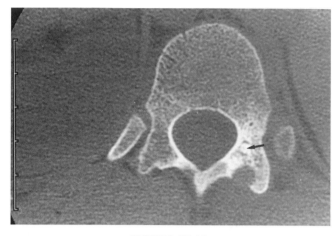

FIGURE 13-11

Osteoid osteoma. This teenage athlete had back pain initially aggravated by activity, but which later became constant, especially at night. This computed tomography scan demonstrates sclerosis in the posterior elements of the thoracic spine and a central round nidus (arrow), which is typical of an osteoid osteoma.

used to better define the lesion (Figure 13-11). Although the spontaneous resolution of an osteoid osteoma is possible, excision is often necessary for both types of lesions.[41–43]

An aneurysmal bone cyst is another benign neoplasm that commonly affects the spine. Most cases involve the posterior elements but, unlike osteoid osteomas, these tumors tend to be expansile and may involve the pedicles and vertebral bodies. Symptoms include back pain, a decrease in range of motion, and neurologic deficits that are due to the mass effect of the expansile lesion. Treatment requires resection or curettage and bone grafting.[44, 45]

Malignant tumors that affect the child's spine include Ewing sarcoma, osteosarcoma, and leukemia.[5, 10] Spinal cord abnormalities, such as syrinx and neoplasms (e.g., neuroectodermal tumors), should also be considered in persistent back pain.[5, 46]

REFERENCES

1. Salimen J, Erkintalo M, Laine M, Pentti J. Low back pain in the young: a prospective three-year follow-up study of subjects with and without low back pain. Spine 1995;20: 2101–2107.
2. Burton AK. Low back pain in children and adolescents: to treat or not. Bull Hosp Jt Dis 1993;55:127–129.
3. Micheli LJ, Wood R. Back pain in young athletes: significant differences from adults in causes and patterns. Arch Pediatr Adolesc Med 1995;149:15–18.

4. Combs JA, Caskey PM. Back pain in children and adolescents: a retrospective review of 648 patients. South Med J 1997;90:789–792.

5. Hollinsworth P. Back pain in children. Br J Rheumatol 1996;35:1022–1028.

6. King H. Back Pain in Children. In SL Weinstein (ed), The Pediatric Spine, Principles and Practice. New York: Raven, 1994;173–183.

7. Thompson G. Back pain in children. J Bone Joint Surg Am 1993;75:928–938.

8. Hensinger R. Back Pain in Children. In DS Bradford, R Hensinger (eds), The Pediatric Spine. New York: Thieme, 1985;41–60.

9. Burton KA, Clarke RD, McClune TD, Tillotson KM. The natural history of low back pain in adolescents. Spine 1996;21:2323–2328.

10. Payne WK, Ogilvie JW. Back pain in children and adolescents. Pediatr Clin North Am 1996;43:899–917.

11. Kujula UM, Taimela S, Erkintalo M, et al. Low back pain in adolescent athletes. Official J Am Coll Sports Med 1996; 28:165–170.

12. Sward L, Hellstrom M, Jacobsson B, et al. Disc degeneration and associated abnormalities of the spine in elite gymnasts, a magnetic resonance imaging study. Spine 1991;16:437–443.

13. Stinson J. Spondylolysis and spondylolisthesis in the athlete. Clin Sports Med 1993;112:517–528.

14. Turner R, Bianco A. Spondylolysis and spondylolisthesis in children and teenagers. J Bone Joint Surg Am 1971;53:1298–1306.

15. Saraste H. Long-term clinical and radiological follow-up of spondylolysis and spondylolisthesis. J Pediatr Orthop 1987;7:631–638.

16. Seitsalo S, Osterman K, Poussa M, Laurent L. Spondylolisthesis in children under 12 years of age: long-term results of 56 patients treated conservatively or operatively. J Pediatr Orthop 1988;8:516–521.

17. Szalay EA, Green NE, Heller RM, et al. Magnetic resonance imaging in the diagnosis of childhood discitis. J Pediatr Orthop 1987;7:164–167.

18. Ring D, Wenger D. Magnetic resonance imaging scans in discitis. J Bone Joint Surg Am 1994;76:596–601.

19. Goldstein J, Berger PE, Windler G, Jackson D. Spine injuries in gymnasts and swimmers: an epidemiological investigation. Am J Sports Med 1991;19:463–468.

20. Hardcastle PH. Repair of spondylolysis in young fast bowlers. J Bone Joint Surg Br 1993;75:398–402.

21. Hensinger RN. Spondylolysis and spondylolisthesis in children and adolescents. J Bone Joint Surg Am 1989;71:1098–1107.

22. Jackson D, Wiltse L, Cirincione R. Spondylolysis in the female gymnast. Clin Orthop 1976;117:68–73.

23. McCarroll J, Miller JM, Ritter MA. Lumbar spondylolysis and spondylolisthesis in college football players: a prospective study. Am J Sports Med 1986;14:404–406.

24. Jackson D, Wiltse L, Dingeman R, Hayes M. Stress reactions involving the pars interarticularis in young athletes. Am J Sports Med 1981;9:304–312.

25. Jackson D. Low back pain in young athletes: evaluation of stress reaction and discogenic problems. Am J Sports Med 1979;7:364–366.

26. Yamane T, Yoshida T, Mimatsu K. Early diagnosis of lumbar spondylolysis by MRI. J Bone Joint Surg Br 1993;75:764–768.

27. Collier BD, Johnson RP, Carrera GF, et al. Painful spondylolysis or spondylolisthesis studied by radiography and single photon emission computed tomography. Radiology 1985;154:207–211.

28. Nicol RO, Scott JHS. Lytic spondylolysis repair by wiring. Spine 1986;11:1027–1030.

29. Seitsalo SW, Osterman K, Hyvarinen H, et al. Progression of spondylolisthesis in children and adolescents: a long-term follow-up of 272 patients. Spine 1991;16:417–421.

30. Pizzutillo PD, Hummer CD. Nonoperative treatment for painful adolescent spondylolysis or spondylolisthesis. J Pediatr Orthop 1989;9:538–540.

31. Velikas EP, Blackburne JS. Surgical treatment of spondylolisthesis in children and adolescents. J Bone Joint Surg Br 1981;63:67–70.

32. Boxall D, Bradford D, Winter R, Moe J. Management of severe spondylolisthesis in children and adolescents. J Bone Joint Surg Am 1979;61:479–495.

33. Ascani E, La Rosa G. Scheuermann's Kyphosis. In SL Weinstein (ed), The Pediatric Spine: Principles and Practice. New York: Raven, 1994;557–584.

34. Murray PM, Weinstein SL, Spratt KF. The natural history and long-term follow-up of Scheuermann's kyphosis. J Bone Joint Surg Am 1993;75:236–248.

35. Bradford DS, Garcia A. Herniations of the lumbar intervertebral disk in children and adolescents: a review of 30 surgically treated cases. JAMA 1969;210:2045–2051.

36. Clarke NMP, Cleak DK. Intervertebral lumbar disc prolapse in children and adolescents. J Pediatr Orthop 1983;3:202–206.

37. Epstein N, Epstein J. Limbus lumbar vertebral fractures in 27 adolescents and adults. Spine 1991;16:962–966.

38. Crawford A. Operative treatment of spine fractures in children. Orthop Clin North Am 1990;21:325–339.

39. Correa AG, Edwards MS, Baker CJ. Vertebral osteomyelitis in children. Pediatr Infect Dis J 1993;12:228–233.

40. Schwartz ST, Spiegel M, Ho G. Bacterial vertebral osteomyelitis and epidural abscess. Seminars in Spine Surgery 1990;2:95–105.

41. Azouz EM, Kozlowski K, Marton D, et al. Osteoid osteoma and osteoblastoma of the spine in children. Pediatr Radiol 1986;16:25–31.

42. Pettine KA, Klassen RA. Osteoid osteoma and osteoblastoma of the spine. J Bone Joint Surg Am 1986;68:354–361.

43. Akbarnia BA, Rooholamini SA. Scoliosis caused by benign osteoblastoma of the thoracic or lumbar spine. J Bone Joint Surg Am 1981;63:1146–1155.

44. Hay MC, Paterson D, Taylor TKF. Aneurysmal bone cysts of the spine. J Bone Joint Surg Br 1978;60:406–411.

45. Capanna R, Albissini U, Picci P, et al. Aneurysmal bone cyst of the spine. J Bone Joint Surg Am 1985;67:527–531.

46. Svenson J, Stapczynsi JS. Childhood back pain: diagnostic evaluation of an unusual case. Am J Emerg Med 1994;12: 334–336.

14

Pelvis, Hip, and Thigh Injuries

TIMOTHY W. FLYNN

The pelvis is the transfer point for forces generated in both the upper and lower extremities. Although motion of the pelvic joints is relatively small in comparison to that of the extremities, it is extremely important in providing a smooth dissipation of energy between the lower extremities and spine. The pelvis and thigh are commonly injured regions, but pain arising from this area is often difficult to diagnose. The examiner must always perform a screening examination of the spine to rule out pain of a radicular nature. This chapter reviews the functional anatomy and arthrology of the pelvis and hip and follows with the identification and treatment of common injuries.

FUNCTIONAL ANATOMY

Osseous Anatomy

The pelvic girdle consists of the following bony units: (1) the sacrum, which is composed of fused elements of the five sacral vertebrae; (2) the coccyx, which is composed of fused elements of the four coccygeal vertebrae; and (3) the paired (right and left) innominate bones, which are formed by the fused elements of the ilium, ischium, and pubis (fusion is usually complete by age 15 years). The examiner should be proficient in palpation of the following pelvic girdle bony landmarks: anterosuperior iliac spine (ASIS), anteroinferior iliac spine (AIIS), iliac crest, pubic tubercle, posterosuperior iliac spine (PSIS), and the ischial tuberosity (Figure 14-1).

The femur attaches the lower extremity to the pelvic girdle. The acetabulum of the innominate provides a deep and stable cavity to accept the femoral head. The examiner should readily identify the greater and lesser trochanter of the femur.

The femoral neck is approximately 5 cm in length and attaches the head to the shaft. Blood supply to the femoral head comes primarily from the neck of the femur with an additional supply from the artery that travels through the ligament of the head of the femur. Blood supply to the head is jeopardized in femoral neck fractures and hip dislocations.

Muscular Anatomy

The muscles of the pelvis and thigh are capable of generating huge forces. The scope of this text does not allow for a thorough review of the numerous muscles in this region, but several bear mentioning. The psoas major arises on the transverse processes of the lumbar spine and inserts on the lesser trochanter of the femur, thereby acting on the lumbar spine, pelvis, and femur. The biceps femoris and the rectus femoris actions affect the pelvis, hip, and knee joints. Other musculature is addressed later in the chapter.

LEG LENGTH DISCREPANCY

An inequality of limb length has been implicated as a causative factor in pain arising in the low back, pelvis, and hip region.[1] Gofton[2] stated that unilateral osteoarthritis of the hip regularly occurs in patients with leg length disparity on the side of the longer leg. Greenman[3] reported that two-thirds of the cases of low back pain with leg length discrepancy were improved with heel-lift therapy.

The athlete reporting nontraumatic pelvis and hip pain should always be screened for leg length discrepancy. The screen is performed by having the athlete stand with equal weight on each leg and with feet shoulder width apart. The

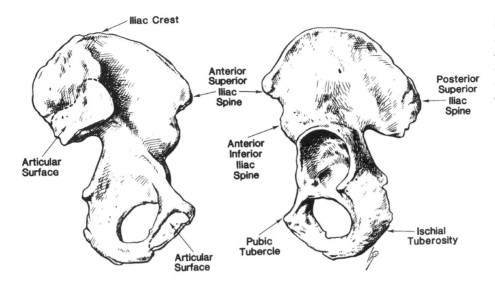

examiner's hands are then placed on each iliac crest to assess for differences in vertical height from right to left. This is repeated with the examiner's hands on the patient's ASIS and finally on the superior aspect of each greater trochanter. The standing examination ensures a dynamic measurement, which simulates functional weightbearing activities. Unleveling of the iliac crest and ASIS may be caused by ilia rotations, sacral torsion, scoliosis, or a leg length discrepancy. An unleveling of the greater trochanters indicates a closed-chain leg length discrepancy. Causes include unilateral pes planus or overpronation; unilateral joint asymmetries of the lower extremity, such as genu valgum; or bony segmental shortening.

Several methods are available for performing leg length measurements. One method is done with the athlete standing against a wall. The examiner places full-length shims of one-eighth–in. or 2-mm thickness under the short side and adds additional shims until the trochanters are level. A second method is the supine tape measure examination, whereby the examiner measures the distance from the athlete's ASIS to the ipsilateral medial malleolus. This is repeated three times, and the distances are averaged and compared with the other limbs' measurements.

The gold-standard measurement for leg length discrepancy and pelvic unleveling is the standing anteroposterior x-ray film of the pelvis. This view should be taken from the upper lumbar spine and distally to include the femoral heads.[4] While the radiograph is being taken, the athlete must stand with his or her feet shoulder width apart and with equal weightbearing. Lines are drawn on the radiograph at the superior sacral ala bilaterally to form a sacral base plane and at the superior margin of each femoral head. The examiner then measures from the sacral base plane and femoral heads to the base of film

(Figure 14-2). Because of the often inappropriate and excessive use of radiography, the examiner is strongly cautioned to use this method only on the athlete for whom precision is needed and for whom the standing measurements have not achieved the desired accuracy. In the evaluation and treatment process of spine and pelvic pain, treatment of leg length discrepancies should generally not be the first intervention. Often, leg length discrepancies are not the cause of the problem, and intervention with a heel lift will complicate the diagnosis and treatment. Leg length discrepancies may be a contributing factor and should always be evaluated and addressed before discharge from therapy.

If a discrepancy is found, the examiner should lift the short side by using a heel lift or full orthotic device. If the athlete is experiencing hip pain, the amount of lift should equalize the femoral head height. If the pain is at the sacroiliac (SI) joint, the goal is to level the sacral base. In a discrepancy of greater than one-fourth in., the initial correction should be only one-half of the total discrepancy and, after an accommodation period, increased to the appropriate height.

PELVIS AND HIP PAIN

Pelvis and hip injuries are divided into three regions: anterior, lateral, and posterior. See the algorithm (Figure 14-3) for quick reference.

Anterior Pelvis, Hip, and Groin Pain

Groin injury in athletes is recognized as one of the most difficult problems in sports. Symptoms associated with chronic groin injury are often diffuse and uncharacteristic.[5] Typically, the injury is in a chronic or subchronic state when the athlete is examined by the practitioner. This results in major diagnostic and therapeutic challenges. Hernias should be suspected in athletes with persistent groin pain despite adequate treatment and physical therapy. In particular, athletes that have incipient groin hernias (i.e., symptoms that worsen after strenuous activities) should be evaluated using herniography.[6]

Pubic Symphysis Dysfunction

A common yet underappreciated source of pubic pain is pubic symphysis dysfunction. This injury occurs frequently during a high-speed cutting activity and is often present concurrently with a groin pull. If it is suspected, the examiner should evaluate the position of the pubic tubercles bilaterally by palpating the superior border of the pubic tubercles to assess right-to-left variation in the frontal plane. If the pubic bones are not level and tension of the two inguinal ligaments is asymmetric, a pubic symphysis dysfunction is present.[7] Differential diagnoses include osteitis pubis or pubic rami stress fracture.

A quick approach to reduction of an elevated or depressed pubic bone is the "adductor squeeze." The athlete should be in the supine position while the knees and hips are flexed and abducted (Figure 14-4). The examiner's forearm is then placed between the athlete's knees and the opposite knee grabbed with the free hand. The athlete is asked to abduct the knees for 5 seconds and to repeat this three times. This is followed by three maximal adduction contractions for 5 seconds. An audible "pop" signals reduction.

Recurrent dysfunction of the pubis can be attributable to mechanical dysfunction of the lumbar spine, pelvis, or lower extremity. Exercises should include a stabilization program, avoidance of positions that cause the dysfunction, and occasional use of an SI belt. Recurrent dysfunctions are optimally managed under the supervision of a practitioner skilled in manual medicine techniques (physical therapist, osteopath, physical medicine and rehabilitation physician).

Osteitis Pubis

Osteitis pubis is a chronic inflammatory condition of the pubic symphyseal joint that is more commonly reported in sports requiring twisting and cutting—notably soccer, rugby, ice hockey, tennis, football, basketball, cycling, and running.[6] A number of etiologic factors have been proposed for the development of osteitis pubis, including overuse and microtrauma of the muscles associated with running and kicking, instability of the SI joint, repetitive adductor muscle pull at the origins of the pubic rami,

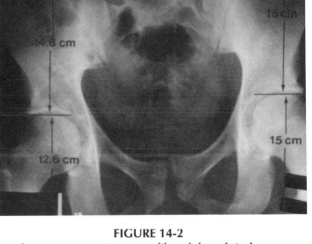

FIGURE 14-2

Standing anteroposterior x-ray film of the pelvis demonstrating a long left lower extremity with an unleveling of the sacral base.

excessive frontal or up-and-down pelvic motion, and limitations of hip joint movement.[8] On physical examination, there is marked tenderness over the superior aspect of the pubic symphysis and the adductor origins of the inferior pubic ramus. Symptoms are often exaggerated by active hip flexion and adduction.

Differential diagnoses include pubic rami stress fracture, pubic symphyseal dysfunction, and hernias (inguinal and femoral). Radiographs of the pelvis often demonstrate sclerosis, irregularity, and widening of the symphysis pubis (Figure 14-5). If the pain is long-standing, a bone scan should be performed. If instability is suspected, Flamingo view roentgenograms are warranted. Appropriate screening measurement for leg length discrepancy is indicated.

Treatment consists of nonsteroidal anti-inflammatory drugs (NSAIDs) for symptom reduction. Training mod-

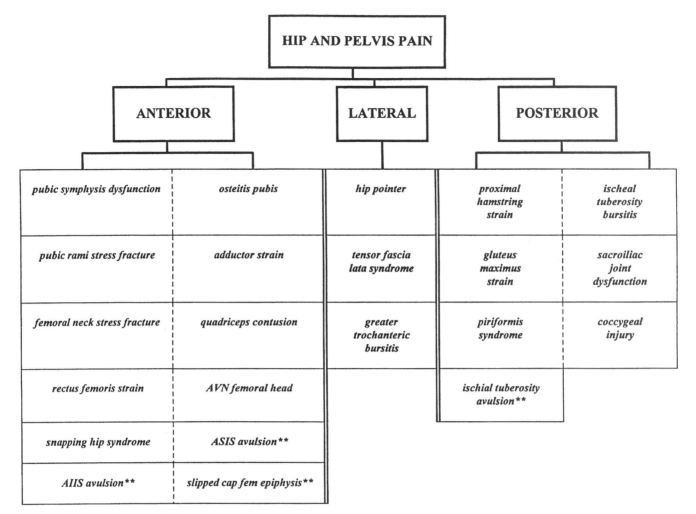

FIGURE 14-3

Algorithm of common pelvis and thigh injuries presented in this chapter. (** Designates pediatric athlete concern.) (AIIS = anteroinferior iliac spine; ASIS = anterosuperior iliac spine; AVN = avascular necrosis.)

ifications should include reduction of mileage, prevention of overstriding, and elimination of downhill running. Leg length inequality should be corrected by using a heel lift and orthotic devices (if excessive pronation is noted). Additionally, the hip joint capsules should be thoroughly evaluated for abnormal tightness. In my experience, mobilization of the hip joint capsule has greatly reduced the symptoms associated with osteitis pubis (Figure 14-6 demonstrates a mobilization of the anterior hip joint capsule). In athletes with recalcitrant symptoms, corticosteroid injection into and around the symphysis may be considered.[8]

Pubic Rami Stress Fracture

This condition often starts as a periosteal reaction at the adductor muscle origin on the pubis. The stress fracture has an insidious onset, usually incurred by runners undergoing a too-rapid change in distance or speed. On physical examination, tenderness is noted on the inferior aspect of the pubic rim.

The bone scan is the most sensitive test in the early diagnosis of stress fractures. If symptoms have existed for longer than 3 weeks, an x-ray study can be performed, but if it is negative and a stress fracture is still suspected, a bone scan is indicated.

Treatment consists of avoidance of pain-inducing activity for 4–6 weeks. During this time, the athlete should concentrate on nonweightbearing activities (swimming or biking) and stretching the adductor muscle group and hip joint capsule. Furthermore, a careful evaluation of the athlete's nutritional intake, estrogen status, and training program is warranted.

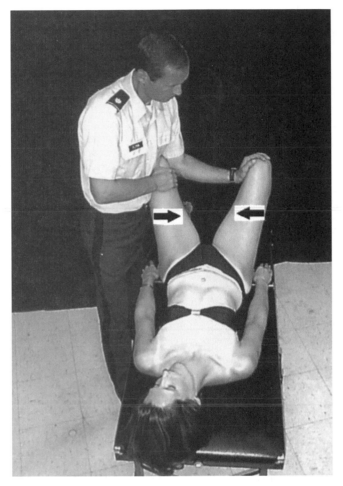

FIGURE 14-4

Adductor squeeze technique for the treatment of pubic symphysis dysfunction. The athlete is asked to maximally adduct his or her legs from the above position against the practitioner's resistance.

Adductor Strain ("Groin Pull")

Adductor strain is a debilitating injury usually caused by sprinting or a sudden change in direction. Physical examination reveals pain and swelling in the groin region, and in severe cases, a muscle herniation or defect may be present. If onset is insidious, one should consider proximal-medial femoral shaft stress fracture or periostitis.

Treatment consists of intermittent application of ice massage or an ice pack under a compression wrap until swelling subsides. This is followed with a contrast of heat and ice (3–5 minutes each) and pulsed ultrasound in conjunction with adductor stretching. The strengthening phase should emphasize eccentric loading and a gradual progression of lateral functional activities. Return to competition must proceed carefully to avoid reinjury.

Femoral Neck Stress Fracture

Femoral neck stress fracture is a potentially career-ending injury if the diagnosis is delayed or missed (Figure 14-7). The examiner should be highly suspicious of any hip, groin, or vague medial knee pain in the athlete. Physical examination reveals pain on a single-leg stance on the affected side, pain with a Patrick or quadrant test, and frequently a painful Trendelenburg gait. Differential diagnoses include avascular necrosis, slipped femoral capital epiphysis, hip flexor tendinitis or bursitis, hernia, and osteitis pubis.

The bone scan is the most sensitive test in the early diagnosis of stress fractures and is indicated if pain has been present for less than 3 weeks. If pain has existed for longer than 3 weeks, plain radiographs are indicated. If radiographs are negative and the examiner is still suspicious of a stress fracture, then a bone scan or magnetic resonance imaging (MRI) is performed. If suspected, these patients should not bear weight on the involved leg until a stress fracture is ruled out.

All stress fractures on the tension (superolateral) side should be referred immediately to an orthopedic surgeon for surgical fixation. Compression side fractures can heal with prolonged nonweightbearing (more than 6 weeks) followed by gradual resumption of activities. Because of the prolonged recovery, referral should be considered. A careful evaluation of the athlete's nutritional intake, estrogen status, and training program is especially warranted in the female athlete, because this injury may be the result of athletic amenorrhea.

Quadriceps Contusion

Quadriceps contusion is a common injury in contact sports and is caused by a direct blow to the thigh, which compresses the quadriceps into the femur. Examination reveals tenderness, swelling, and often a large hematoma on the anterior thigh. A loss of knee range of motion is present. The incidence of myositis ossificans as a sequela is 4–20% and directly proportional to the severity of injury.[9] A loss of full knee flexion can also occur. Complications can be reduced by immediate treatment intervention.

Radiographs should be taken to rule out femur fracture. A bone scan is often used to track myositis ossificans formation. These injuries are optimally managed by a qualified physical therapist or athletic trainer.

Treatment begins immediately with application of ice packs with compression wrap for 10 minutes per waking hour for 3–5 days. In between ice treatments, a compression wrap with a thin layer of felt padding over the effused area should be worn. Pillows should be placed under the knee to achieve knee flexion to the pain barrier. Ambulation is by means of crutches with weightbearing

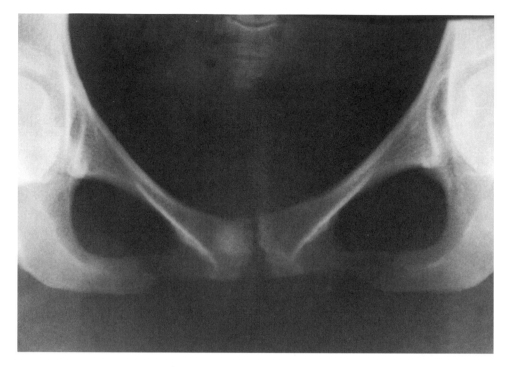

FIGURE 14-5
Anterior-posterior x-ray film of the pelvis demonstrating osteitis pubis with irregularity and sclerosing of the symphysis pubis.

to tolerance. Active range of motion is to be performed within the pain-free range. Passive stretching, deep massage, and ultrasound should be avoided because these can increase muscle bleeding. Active flexion should be encouraged. After the swelling begins to decrease, heat and cold contrasts are initiated with quadriceps-strengthening exercises. Active range of motion should be continued frequently. The athlete may return to play after gaining quadriceps length and strength equal to 90% of the unin-

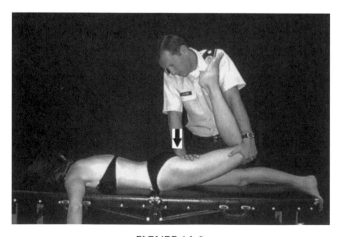

FIGURE 14-6
Position of practitioner and athlete for mobilization or stretching of the anterior hip joint capsule.

jured side. Length can be measured with the athlete prone and actively flexing both knees.

Rectus Femoris Strain

This injury commonly occurs in the sprinting athlete. The athlete reports feeling a "pulling" sensation and pain in the anterior thigh. Examination finds tenderness to palpation, which increases during resisted knee extension. An avulsion of the ASIS or AIIS should be considered.

Radiographs are indicated if an avulsion is suspected. Moderate to severe cases may require physical therapy.

Treatment begins with ice massage progressing to ultrasound and ice contrast. Range of motion and quadriceps setting exercises should be done immediately. A compression wrap with a felt pad placed over the effused area is used to control swelling. Strengthening exercises are initially concentric and progress to eccentric. Cycling may be initiated early if it is not painful. The athlete returns to running when his or her knee's range of motion is 80% that of the uninvolved side. Start the athlete with backward walking and running, which is a good concentric strengthening exercise for the quadriceps, and then progress to forward running.

Avascular Necrosis of the Femoral Head

Avascular necrosis (AVN) is a relatively rare but serious condition caused by the disruption of blood supply to the femoral head, resulting in bone cell death. AVN

FIGURE 14-7

Anteroposterior x-ray film of the left hip in a female with a severe femoral neck stress fracture requiring orthopedic fixation. Arrow shows complete fracture through the cortex.

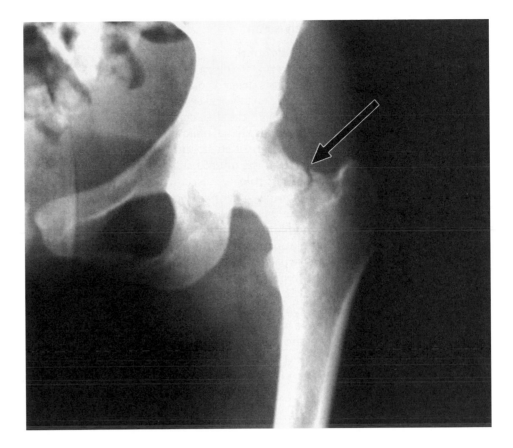

should be suspected when there has been trauma to the hip joint resulting in limited range of motion and persistent pain on weightbearing. An athlete with a history of high-dose steroid use is also at greater risk. X-ray films taken at the time of injury are normal unless a fracture is present (flattening of the femoral head may be seen in long-standing cases). The bone scan and MRI are the standard diagnostic studies if AVN of the femoral head is suspected. These injuries should be managed by an orthopedic surgeon.

Snapping Hip Syndrome

The snapping hip syndrome is characterized by hip pain and an audible "pop" during hip range of motion and physical activity. The exact etiology is difficult to ascertain, but the syndrome is typically caused laterally by friction on the greater trochanter from either the iliotibial band (ITB) or the anterior border of the gluteus maximus. In addition, Schaberg and colleagues[10] found that the iliopsoas tendon slipping over an osseous ridge on the lesser trochanter or the iliopectineal eminence can cause the snapping hip. The examiner attempts to localize the snapping either to the greater trochanter (which implicates the ITB or the gluteus maximus) or antero-

medially (which implicates the iliopsoas). This is done by careful palpation during active and passive manipulation of the hip. Iliopsoas snapping can often be elicited by asking the supine patient to actively flex his or her hip and knee, abduct and externally rotate his or her hip, and then extend his or her leg. Hip flexor tightness is commonly associated with snapping hip. Differential diagnosis includes recurrent hip instability or subluxation (which is quite uncommon in the absence of significant trauma).

Conservative treatment consists of ice and phonophoresis to the affected structures (gluteus maximus tendon, ITB, or iliopsoas tendon) to decrease inflammation. After the acute phase, one should initiate 10 minutes of moist heat and specific prolonged stretching of the involved structures (anterior or posterior muscle group). Additionally, joint mobilization to the hip capsule should be performed. The athlete should then perform strengthening exercises of the antagonist muscle group. The athlete should respond to treatment in 3–6 weeks and then begin the return to a full sports program.

Athletes failing conservative treatment are referred to an orthopedic specialist for evaluation and possible steroid injection and surgical consideration.

Lateral Hip and Pelvis Pain

Contusion of the Iliac Crest (Hip Pointer)

The hip pointer occurs in contact sports from a direct blow to an unprotected iliac crest. Diagnosis depends on the history of a direct blow with the finding on physical examination of tenderness on and superior to the iliac crest extending superiorly into the internal and external oblique musculature. Swelling and ecchymosis are often present. Side-bending of the trunk away from the injured side increases the pain. The examiner must rule out visceral injury. Often, the T12–L3 lateral cutaneous nerve branches can be injured, which will cause numbness and decreased sensation in the lateral buttock and hip region.

Radiographs are indicated to rule out iliac fracture. Initially, the injury is treated with ice packs for 10 minutes on and 20 minutes off; this is done frequently until swelling subsides. Adhesive tape support is used to limit trunk motion and for comfort. After 3–4 days, moist heat should be applied for 10 minutes, followed by ice packs. Abdominal muscle stretching and strengthening are done as tolerated. Before returning to contact sports, trunk range of motion must be pain free, and the athlete should be adequately padded.

Tensor Fascia Lata Syndrome

Inflammation of the tensor fascia lata (TFL) as it passes over the greater trochanter of the femur is common in runners and cyclists. The history is usually of a gradual onset of lateral hip pain coinciding with a change in a training program. Other causative factors include a leg length discrepancy (with the long side being most often affected) and improperly adjusted seating and shoe systems in cyclists. Physical examination reveals tenderness along the TFL and often a "snapping" during hip flexion and extension between the TFL and greater trochanter. An Ober test (tight ITB) is usually positive. The Ober test is performed with the athlete on one side, with the painful side up. The leg is passively abducted and extended while the pelvis is stabilized, and it is then allowed to drop. If the leg cannot return to midline, a tight ITB is present. Differential diagnoses include femoral neck stress fracture and trochanteric bursitis.

Radiograph or a bone scan is indicated if a femoral neck stress fracture is suspected. Treatment should begin with a modification of training (decrease mileage, speed, or hills). Short-term NSAIDs may be helpful. Ice and heat contrast with phonophoresis treatment can reduce inflammation. A stretching program for the TFL followed by adductor muscle strengthening should be implemented. Correction of leg length or other biomechanical discrepancy will prevent recurrence.

Greater Trochanteric Bursitis

Greater trochanteric bursitis is often difficult to differentiate from TFL syndrome, except the pain is usually more posterior to the greater trochanter and can often radiate into the buttock. Differential diagnoses should include radicular symptoms of lumbar origin and radiation from the SI joint.

Initial treatment begins with ice massage and heat contrasts. This is followed by stretching of the hamstrings and TFL with joint mobilization of the hip. Strengthening of hip adductors (antagonists) is often effective. Certain cases respond well to phonophoresis; others require steroid injection. Stretching and strengthening should continue.

Corticosteroid injection may provide several weeks of pain relief and allow the patient to achieve his or her rehabilitation goals. To accomplish this, the patient is positioned lying on the uninjured side. The injection area is prepared with povidone-iodine (Betadine) or alcohol and the tender bursa is palpated to identify the injection site. The corticosteroid (betamethasone 6 mg or triamcinolone 40 mg) is injected using a 2-in., 25-gauge needle. To aid in delivery of the medication and to assure the proper positioning of the injection, 10 ml of lidocaine is usually added to the syringe. The bursa lies deep to the iliotibial band. Often, there are substantial overlying soft tissues, so the needle is inserted relatively deep. To assure accurate depth of injection, the patient is asked if he or she feels the discomfort from the initial contact with the lidocaine. The needle depth is adjusted until the "burn" is felt in the target tissue, at which time the remainder of the solution is delivered.

Posterior Hip and Pelvis Pain

Proximal Hamstring Strain

The hamstring group is made up of the semitendinosus, semimembranosus, and the long head of the biceps femoris. These three muscles have a common origin on the ischial tuberosity. The "pulled" hamstring frequently occurs during the last half of the swing phase, when the hamstrings are working eccentrically, or during early stance phase, when there is a large concentric burst.[11] The injury usually extends longitudinally within the muscle rather than in a single cross-sectional area. The athlete generally self-diagnoses the problem at the time of injury. Reports of "I felt a pull" or "pop" are common. During palpation, the examiner should locate the ischial tuberosity and follow the muscles inferiorly to locate the area of maximum tenderness. If the ischial tuberosity is exquisitely tender, then an avulsion fracture is suspected and should be referred to an orthopedic specialist. In the hamstring strain, swelling usually occurs within 2 hours, and ecchymosis within 48 hours. Resisted knee flexion increases symptoms. The athlete is often unable to straighten his or her knee during the terminal swing phase of gait.

The differential diagnoses include radicular pain of a lumbar origin, referred pain from the SI joint, and avulsion fracture of the ischial tuberosity. Radiographs are indicated if an ischial tuberosity avulsion is suspected. Patients who have a large amount of swelling and ecchymosis associated with clear weakness in knee flexion may have completely ruptured the hamstring origin. MRI and referral for surgical repair should be considered.

Initial treatment consists of ice packs or ice massage, compression wraps, and possibly crutches. After 72 hours or when swelling begins to subside, a program of ice and heat contrasts and pulsed ultrasound over the affected area is instituted. This is followed by 30-second passive hamstring stretches in the pain-free range. The treatment session ends with ice massage. The athlete progresses to active hip and knee range of motion exercises and contract-relax techniques to the hamstrings, followed by hamstring isometrics at varying angles.

The final phase is the active strengthening phase, which emphasizes eccentric (negative) exercise. Speed and resistance are gradually increased (Figure 14-8). The athlete assumes the position shown and lowers the ankle weight at successively faster speeds. Eventually, the athlete should drop his or her ankle and then "catch" the weight before his or her knee reaches full extension.[9]

Running should begin with backward running, which helps to stretch the hamstrings. Forward running should begin at 60% speed with frequent hamstring stretch breaks during the workout.

The athlete may develop TFL syndrome, which may require steroid injection; caution is always advised in considering an injection into a major weightbearing tendon.

Gluteus Maximus Strain

An isolated strain of gluteus maximus is uncommon but can occur in sprinters. Often, there is associated SI joint involvement. The examiner must evaluate the lumbar spine, SI joint, and the hip in athletes reporting buttock pain. Piriformis muscle involvement can be ruled out by palpation in the area of the sciatic notch while the examiner resists the athlete's hip external rotation. If the examiner cannot elicit symptoms in these areas, but palpation finds tenderness in the muscle bulk of the gluteus maximus, a strain is suspected. The history should confirm a sudden sharp pain in the buttock during a burst of speed or sudden direction change.

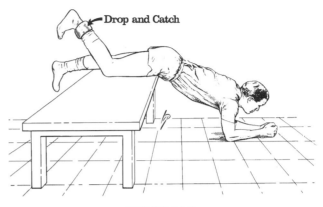

FIGURE 14-8
Eccentric "catch" exercise for strengthening the hamstrings. The athlete is lying prone over the edge of the table to approximate the hip and knee angles during late stance phase. (Adapted from D Stanton, C Purdham. Hamstring injuries in sprinting—the role of eccentric exercise. J Orthop Sports Phys Ther 1989;10:347. © The Orthopaedic and Sports Physical Therapy Sections of the American Physical Therapy Association.)

If the lumbar spine or SI joint is involved, then a rehabilitation program that is specific to these areas should be implemented. Further diagnostic studies may be indicated.

Initially, gluteus maximus strain is treated with ice massage. After 72 hours, ultrasound is begun to attain deep heating of the muscle belly and followed by knee-to-chest exercises. A strengthening program should use leg-press machines and stair-climbing exercises.

Sacroiliac Joint Dysfunction

Injury to and pain arising from the SI joint is a common and often overlooked injury in athletes. Movements between the sacrum and the ilia are rotatory or translatory, or a combination of the two.[12] It is possible that minor loss of motion in the joint leads to pain. It is also postulated that the pain results from sustained contraction of the muscles overlying the joint.[13] The athlete typically presents with pain over one SI joint, which may have resulted from trauma or may have been insidious in nature. SI dysfunction can cause low back pain and other spine pain—including thoracic and cervical—and even muscle contraction headaches.

Physical examination finds unilateral tenderness to palpation over the affected PSIS and along the sacral sulcus. The athlete often has referred pain radiating into the buttocks, groin, and posterolateral thigh on the side of dysfunction. The pain pattern may mimic radicular pain from a herniated nucleus pulposus or lateral spinal stenosis. The lack of nerve root tension signs and absence of motor, reflex, or sensory deficits helps to distinguish SI joint dys-

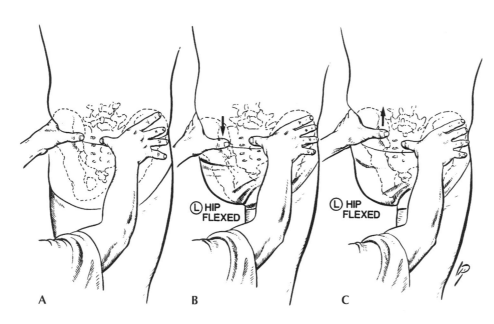

FIGURE 14-9
Sacroiliac fixation test. A. The examiner's thumbs are placed on the inferior slope of the posterosuperior iliac spine and medially on the spinous process of S2. The athlete then flexes the involved hip. B. A negative test occurs when the examiner's thumb swings downward and laterally. C. A positive test occurs when the examiner's thumb swings upward or does not move relative to the other side. (L = left.) (Adapted from WH Kirkaldy-Willis. Managing Low Back Pain [2nd ed]. New York: Churchill Livingstone, 1988.)

function from nerve root compression lesions.[11] Motion in the joint is restricted and can be detected by a positive SI fixation test, also called the "one-legged stork test" or Gillet test (Figure 14-9). When performing this test, one should compare movement from side to side and assess for a lack of mobility. A positive test is always on the hypomobile side. Bilateral SI involvement can be present, and there will be a general lack of movement in both SI

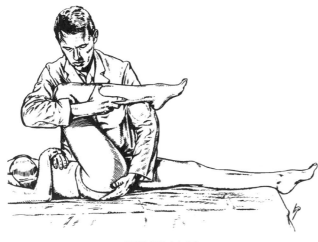

FIGURE 14-10
Treatment of a right anterior innominate dysfunction using the athlete's hip extensor muscles as the correcting force. The examiner flexes the athlete's hip and knee while attempting to rotate the innominate posterior. The athlete then attempts to extend his or her hip against the examiner's unyielding resistance. This is held for 5 seconds and repeated three times.

joints. Compression on the sacrum just medial to the PSIS often causes localized pain.

The SI joints are common lesion sites in ankylosing spondylitis and Reiter syndrome. In these conditions, both SI joints are affected and painful. In athletes who do not benefit from appropriate conservative treatment, systemic disease affecting the SI joints should be considered. A radiographic series often demonstrates bilateral symmetric sacroiliitis.[14]

Initial treatment is designed to reduce inflammation and consists of ice packs or ice massage to the area overlying the SI joint. The goal of treatment is restoration of normal movement. Multiple dysfunctions of the SI joint have been identified, but two common dysfunctions and treatments are described.[7]

The *anterior innominate dysfunction* is diagnosed when the athlete has a positive SI fixation test and an ASIS that is relatively inferior in relation to the contralateral ASIS. Treatment requires the examiner to resist hip extension with the hip and knee flexed on the athlete's affected side (Figure 14-10). The athlete holds this position for 5 seconds, then relaxes; this is repeated three times. If correction is not achieved using this method, an alternate technique is required.

The alternate technique is demonstrated in Figures 14-11 and 14-12 and uses the practitioner's left arm as the corrective mobilizing force. The starting position requires the athlete to be supine on the treatment table with maximum right side-bending of his or her lumbar spine. The practitioner engages the barrier by left rotation of the patient's trunk without losing the right side-bending until the patient's right ilium comes off the table. A very quick

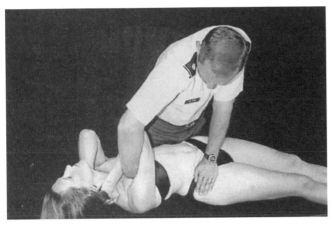

FIGURE 14-11
Starting position for treatment of a right anterior innominate dysfunction using a high-velocity, low-amplitude manipulative technique.

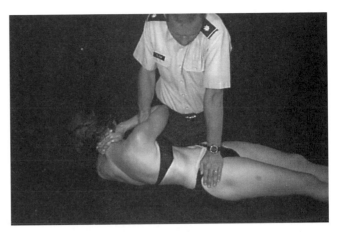

FIGURE 14-12
End position for treatment of a right anterior innominate dysfunction using a high-velocity, low-amplitude manipulative technique.

low-amplitude thrust is given by the practitioner's left hand, which rotates the patient's ilium posteriorly.

A second common dysfunction of the SI joint is the *posterior innominate dysfunction*. This is diagnosed by a positive SI fixation test and a superior ASIS on the same side. Treatment requires the examiner to resist the athlete's isometric hip flexor contraction while the athlete's affected hip is extended (Figure 14-13). The athlete holds this position for 5 seconds, then relaxes and repeats.

In athletes with SI dysfunction, evaluation of a leg length discrepancy should be performed on initial evaluation. Management may require a physical therapist or physician skilled in manual medicine techniques. Further treatment should consist of pelvic stabilization exercises and often stretching and strengthening of the piriformis muscle.

Piriformis Syndrome

The piriformis muscle lies deep to the gluteus maximus, originating on the anterolateral aspect of the sacrum and inserting on the upper border of the greater trochanter of the femur. A prolonged spasm in this muscle can be caused by a twisting injury sustained during a single-leg stance.

Physical examination reveals exquisite point tenderness in the midsubstance of the piriformis. Referred pain (sciatic in nature) down the posterior thigh and calf is common. The sciatic nerve lies in close proximity to the piriformis, and it can pierce the muscle belly, making it susceptible to compression. Resisted hip abduction and hip external rotation increase the symptoms. A loss of hip internal rotation is often present. Passive hip extension should relieve symptoms.

The examiner must evaluate the lumbar spine and SI joints to rule out underlying or coexisting lesions. Differential diagnoses include lumbar herniated nucleus pulposus, lateral stenosis, nerve root irritation, and SI joint dysfunction. Occasionally, evaluation and treatment by a manual or manipulative medicine specialist are indicated.

The goal of treatment is spasm reduction. Local treatment with ice massage and ultrasound–electrical stimulation combination may be effective. The therapeutic effect

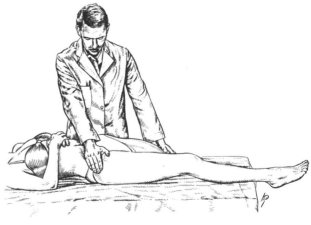

FIGURE 14-13
Treatment of a left posterior innominate dysfunction using the athlete's hip flexor muscles as the correcting force. The examiner extends the athlete's hip while stabilizing the contralateral ilium. The athlete attempts to raise his or her left knee to the ceiling against the examiner's unyielding resistance. The position is held for 5 seconds and repeated three times.

can be enhanced by applying a low-load passive stretch to the piriformis (achieved by internal hip rotation). Spraying ethyl chloride on the buttock overlying the piriformis followed by stretching may also be effective (spray and stretch). To prevent recurrence, any imbalance in the surrounding musculature must be treated (for example, tight or weak hamstrings). Self-stretching of the piriformis is performed by having the athlete lie on his or her back and pull his or her knee on the affected side toward the opposite shoulder. A sustained 30-second stretch is repeated several times. Dysfunction of the lumbosacral region can lead to chronic piriformis tension and spasm and should be addressed.

Coccygeal Injuries

The coccyx is joined to the sacrum via cartilage, forming a synchondrosis.[15] Because of its location, it is susceptible to injury during a fall on the buttocks or when struck from behind by a football helmet.

Physical examination finds localized tenderness and reports of pain in the coccygeal region (coccydynia), which is exacerbated with sitting. There may be localized swelling or ecchymosis.

Radiographs are required to rule out fracture of the inferior sacrum and to determine whether the coccyx is dislocated or displaced. If there is no history of trauma, rectal examination and lower gastrointestinal evaluation are indicated.

The dislocated or displaced coccyx can be reduced by the examiner.[16] The examiner's surgically gloved and lubricated index finger is inserted into the rectum. The index finger is then rotated so the palmar surface rests against the anterior aspect of the coccyx. The examiner then palpates the posterior aspect of the coccyx externally, applies gentle traction on the coccyx, and glides the coccyx into its normal (reduced) position. Pain relief is usually immediate.

SPECIAL CONSIDERATIONS IN THE PEDIATRIC ATHLETE

Slipped Capital Femoral Epiphysis

A slipped capital femoral epiphysis (SCFE) is a serious condition in children and adolescents in which the femoral head shears off the femoral neck along the growth plate. It typically occurs in boys aged 10–17 years and girls aged 8–15 years. The incidence is greater in blacks than in whites and is especially high in overweight children.[17] A variety of factors can contribute to SCFE: trauma, adolescent growth spurt, hormonal influences, increased body weight, and increased physical activity. AVN of the femoral head

can occur. SCFE should be considered in any child or adolescent presenting with hip, groin, thigh, or traumatic medial knee pain. Bilateral, anteroposterior, and lateral or frog-leg radiographs are indicated in any adolescent with these symptoms. Radiographic evidence of slips are often subtle and in preslips are normal. When the diagnosis is entertained, patients should be put on crutches immediately with no weightbearing pending further evaluation. Any degree of slip should be referred immediately to an orthopedic surgeon for possible pinning. Preslips can be diagnosed with either MRI or bone scan and when diagnosed should also be referred.

Avulsion Fractures

Avulsion fractures of the pelvis primarily occur in young athletes between the ages of 14 and 25 years. In general, these fractures occur through secondary centers of ossification before the center is fused with the pelvis.[18] For this reason, comparison x-rays of the contralateral apophysis should be taken to ascertain that an avulsion fracture is not, in reality, a normal adolescent anatomic variant.

Avulsion of the Anterosuperior Iliac Spine

When there is overpull of the sartorius muscle, usually with the hip in extension and the knee flexed while the foot is planted, an avulsion fracture can occur. Physical examination demonstrates pain, swelling, and exquisite tenderness over the ASIS. Resisted hip flexion with external rotation aggravates the symptoms. In addition, local swelling is often appreciated.

Avulsion of the Anteroinferior Iliac Spine

When there is overpull of the rectus femoris muscle, usually with the hip in extension and knee flexed while kicking, an avulsion fracture can occur. Physical examination demonstrates pain, swelling, and exquisite tenderness over the AIIS. Resisted straight leg raise aggravates the symptoms, and local swelling is often present. This injury is most frequently seen in soccer, rugby, and football.

Avulsion of the Ischial Tuberosity

Avulsion fractures of the ischial tuberosity can occur after maximum contraction of the hamstring muscles. Physical examination demonstrates pain, swelling, and exquisite tenderness over the ischial tuberosity. Both passive hamstring stretching and resisted knee flexion aggravate the symptoms. Local swelling is often present.

Treatment of Avulsion Fractures

Treatment depends on the size of the fragment; however, conservative nonsurgical treatment is nearly always successful.[18] It should include the avoidance of active muscle contraction of the involved segment and the use of crutches with partial weightbearing until the athlete is pain free. A range of motion and strengthening program is implemented when the athlete is pain free. Patients with significant apophyseal displacement should possibly be managed by an orthopedic surgeon. Return to athletics can typically be resumed at 6–10 weeks.

SUMMARY

The pelvis and hip region is a complex anatomic system that is the transitional point for forces entering the upper and lower limbs. The examiner should be aware that the lower extremity includes the paired innominate complex and that the SI joints are the beginning of the torso. The extreme forces that enter this region and that must be dissipated and redirected are often the reason for recurrent pelvic problems. Athletes who do not respond to initial treatment often may warrant referral to a clinician skilled in mechanical diagnosis and manual medicine.

REFERENCES

1. Wallace LA. Limb Length Difference and Back Pain. In GP Grieve (ed), Modern Manual Therapy of the Vertebral Column. New York: Churchill Livingstone, 1986; 463–472.
2. Gofton JP. Studies in osteoarthritis, part IV: bio-mechanics and clinical considerations. Can Med Assoc J 1971;104: 1007–1011.
3. Greenman PE. Lift therapy: use and abuse. J Am Osteopath Assoc 1979;79:238–250.
4. Giles LGF, Taylor JR. Low back pain associated with leg length inequality. Spine 1981;6:510–521.
5. Renstrom AFH. Tendon and muscle injuries in the groin area. Clin Sports Med 1992;11:815–831.
6. Batt ME, McShane JM, Dillingham MF. Osteitis pubis in collegiate football players. Med Sci Sports Exerc 1997;27:629–633.
7. Greenman PE. Principles of Manual Medicine (2nd ed). Baltimore: Williams & Wilkins, 1996;305–368.
8. Holt MA, Keene JS, Graf BK, Helwig DC. Treatment of osteitis pubis in athletes: results of corticosteroid injections. Am J Sports Med 1995;23:601–606.
9. Ryan JB, Wheeler JH, Hopkinson WJ, et al. Quadriceps contusions—West Point update. Am J Sports Med 1991;19:299–304.
10. Schaberg JE, Harper MC, Allen WC. The snapping hip syndrome. Am J Sports Med 1984;12:361–365.
11. Stanton D, Purdam C. Hamstring injuries in sprinting—the role of eccentric exercise. J Orthop Sports Phys Ther 1989;10:343–348.
12. Beal MC. The sacroiliac problem: review of anatomy, mechanics, and diagnosis. J Am Osteopath Assoc 1982;81:667–674.
13. Kirkaldy-Willis WH. Managing Low Back Pain (2nd ed). New York: Churchill Livingstone, 1988;135–137.
14. Borenstein DG, Wiesel SW. Low Back Pain: Medical Diagnosis and Comprehensive Management. Philadelphia: Saunders, 1989;175–239.
15. Moore KL. Clinically Oriented Anatomy. Baltimore: Williams & Wilkins, 1980;145–336.
16. Hoppenfeld S. Physical Examination of the Spine and Extremities. New York: Appleton-Century-Crofts, 1976;169.
17. Resnick D, Niwayama G. Diagnosis of Bone and Joint Disorders. Philadelphia: Saunders, 1988;2962–2965.
18. Canale ST. Pelvis and Hip Fractures. In CA Rockwood, KE Wilkins, JH Beaty (eds), Fractures in Children (4th ed). Philadelphia: Lippincott, 1996;1109–1193.

15

Evaluation of Knee Injuries

RICHARD W. KRUSE

ANATOMY OF THE KNEE

The anatomy of the knee is illustrated in Figures 15-1 through 15-8.

HISTORY

Questioning should focus on the nature of injury, positioning, and weightbearing status of the leg as well as the direction of any blow or contact. A popping sensation may occur with ligamentous disruption, patellar dislocation or subluxation, meniscal tear, or fracture. The sensation of the knee popping out may be patellar subluxation or dislocation, or ligamentous injury. Hyperextension injuries may cause injuries to both the posterior and the anterior cruciate ligaments (ACLs).

Swelling of the knee within 4–6 hours after acute injury most likely represents hemarthrosis and significant ligamentous disruption[1] or fracture. If the knee capsule is torn, however, swelling may not occur despite severe injury. Inability to extend the knee after acute injury may represent joint locking due to meniscal tear, disruption of the extensor mechanism, patellar dislocation, intraarticular fracture, or loose body.

Questions about sensory and motor function can elicit important clues to neurovascular injury, particularly with a knee dislocation, in the severely traumatized knee. Referred pain from other sources, such as radicular pain or hip pain, may cause knee pain. Similarly, a slipped capital femoral epiphysis may present as knee pain in the adolescent.

ACUTE KNEE INJURY

Figure 15-9 illustrates evaluation of acute knee injury.

Physical Examination

Pedal pulses, sensory function, and motor function of the lower extremity should initially be checked. Any visible deformity or nonphysiologic positioning is noted. Severe trauma may cause complete knee dislocation with interruption of the popliteal artery, which is a limb-threatening emergency. A knee dislocation may spontaneously reduce, and because of capsular disruption, swelling may not be seen. In this injury, the knee is unstable in multiple planes. Fractures about the knee may present similarly; once they are suspected, splinting, reevaluation of pulses, and emergent referral are indicated.

Palpation should localize any tenderness anatomically. Joint laxity is assessed in anterior, posterior, medial, and lateral planes to test, respectively, the anterior and posterior cruciate ligaments and the medial and lateral collateral ligaments. Any perceived laxity should be compared with the opposite normal knee.

Anterior Cruciate Ligament Injury

Mechanism of ACL injury may be a sudden direction change during running, pivoting, hyperflexion or extension, or initiating or landing a jump. A "pop" may be noted at the time of injury.[2]

Knee swelling is common within 6 hours. X-ray films of the knee should be obtained. Bony avulsion of the tibial spine (most evident on lateral view) may be seen, particularly in the pediatric population. Femoral avulsions are best seen on anteroposterior (AP) tunnel view. Most adult tears are midsubstance.[1] A small lateral capsular bony avulsion may also be seen lateral to the tibia at the level of the joint (lateral capsular or Segond sign). This suggests an associated ACL rupture.[2] Examination by means of the Lachman test (Figure 15-10) is most accu-

233

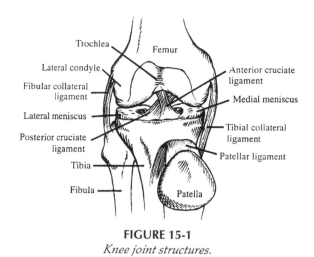

FIGURE 15-1
Knee joint structures.

rate at the acute stage. The patient is supine with his or her head resting on the table, and his or her knee is held flexed at 30 degrees.[3] The examiner holds the patient's distal femur with one hand while grasping the patient's proximal tibia with the other hand and applies a slow anterior directed force to the patient's proximal tibia just below his or her knee. Care must be taken to make sure that the hamstrings are relaxed to avoid a false-negative examination. Increased laxity or absence of a firm end point compared with the normal side is indicative of ACL injury.

Anterior drawer testing (Figure 15-11) is less accurate.[3] The patient is supine with his or her knee flexed 90 degrees and feet resting on the table. The examiner grasps the patient's proximal tibia with thumbs on the tibial condyles. The patient's foot is stabilized in neutral rotation by another examiner or by sitting on it. A slow anterior force on the proximal tibia may reveal any laxity or rotational instability.

The pivot shift test (Figure 15-12)[4] and variants of it have also been described.[5] It requires patient relaxation and cannot usually be performed in acute injury. This test should be performed last, because it can be painful. The patient is supine. The patient's foot of the affected side is lifted with his or her knee extended and leg internally rotated. The examiner applies a valgus stress with one hand in the area of the patient's fibular head while the patient's knee is slowly flexed and the tibia internally rotated. If the ACL is deficient, a subluxation (pivot-shift) of the tibia is noted at 30–40 degrees of knee flexion.[2]

Initial management of the suspected ACL injury includes splinting (e.g., knee immobilizer or bulky Jones dressing), ice, elevation, and orthopedic evaluation. Magnetic resonance imaging (MRI) is generally indicated to assess for associated meniscal tears, bone bruising, and confirmation of ACL disruption. Subsequent orthopedic management is somewhat controversial, depending on the patient's age, activity, motivation, and associated injuries.

Posterior Cruciate Ligament Injury

The posterior ligament is usually injured by hyperextension or a direct anterior blow to the proximal tibia of the flexed knee.[6] Examination may show swelling and tenderness in the popliteal fossa. Posterior sag of the tibia on the femur may be visible when the patient's knee is flexed to 90 degrees in preparation for performing the drawer test. The tibial plateau is not as prominent to palpation compared with that of the noninjured knee. Posterior laxity may be noted on the posterior drawer test.[7] Because the tibia is dropped back,[8] a careful distinction must be made not to misinterpret this as excessive anterior laxity on the Lachman or drawer test. When the patient is in the position of drawer testing, attempts to actively extend the

FIGURE 15-2
Bursae of knee.

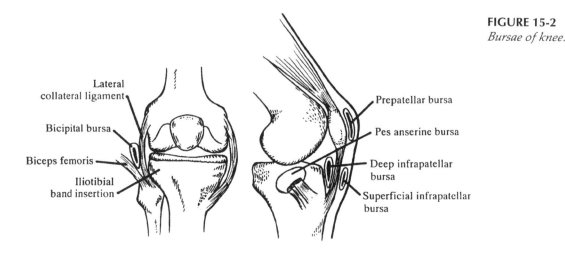

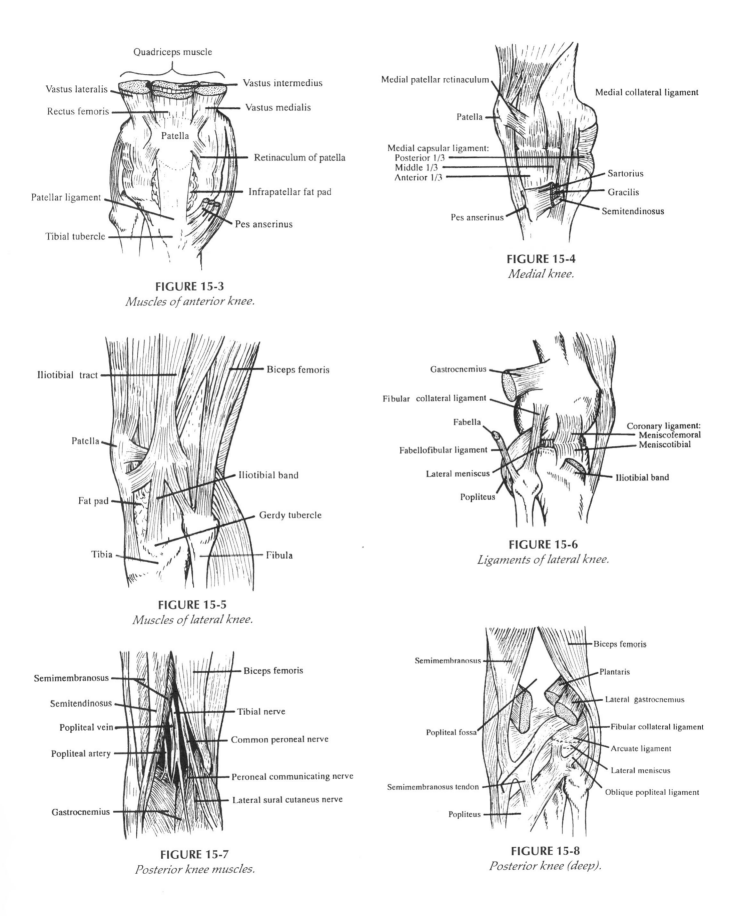

FIGURE 15-3
Muscles of anterior knee.

FIGURE 15-4
Medial knee.

FIGURE 15-5
Muscles of lateral knee.

FIGURE 15-6
Ligaments of lateral knee.

FIGURE 15-7
Posterior knee muscles.

FIGURE 15-8
Posterior knee (deep).

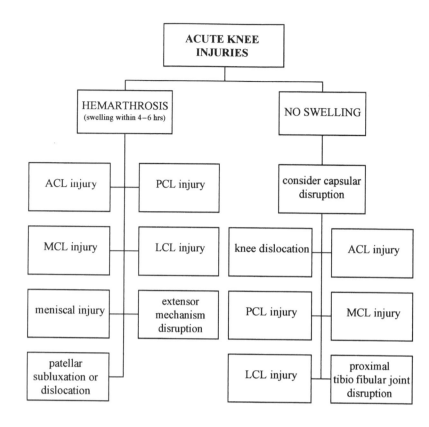

FIGURE 15-9
Evaluation of acute knee injuries. (ACL = anterior cruciate ligament; LCL = lateral collateral ligament; MCL = medial collateral ligament; PCL = posterior cruciate ligament.)

patient's knee against resistance may cause the proximal tibia visibly to move anteriorly (quadriceps active drawer test).[9] Hyperextension of the knee may also be noted by holding the patient's foot and lifting his or her leg off the table while the patient is supine.[10]

X-ray films may show bony avulsion from the proximal tibia. Children should be checked for distal femoral or proximal tibial physeal fractures. Initial treatment should consist of a knee immobilizer, crutches until the athlete is no longer limping, and routine orthopedic referral, because treatment is somewhat controversial.

Medial Collateral Ligament Injury

The medial collateral ligament (MCL) is usually injured by valgus stress through a direct blow from the lateral side.

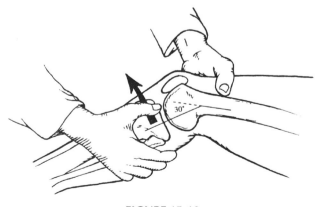

FIGURE 15-10
Lachman test.

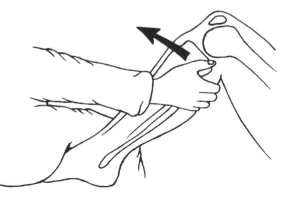

FIGURE 15-11
Drawer test.

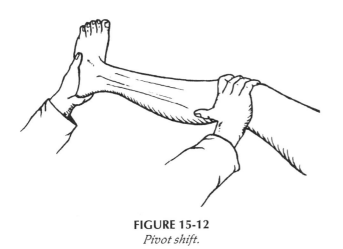

FIGURE 15-12
Pivot shift.

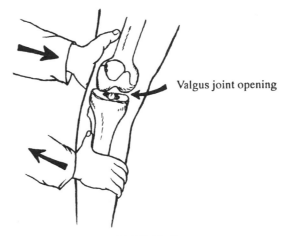

Valgus joint opening

FIGURE 15-13
Medial collateral ligament test.

In the pediatric population, this mechanism of injury may produce physeal separation. Tenderness is noted along or adjacent to the medial joint line, and swelling may be present. The MCL is best tested with the patient supine and his or her knee flexed 25 degrees to take away the stabilizing effect of the posterior cruciate ligament.[11] With one hand, the examiner stabilizes the joint, and his or her thumb palpates the patient's medial joint line while the examiner's other hand grasps the patient's ankle to hold his or her foot in neutral rotation. A valgus stress is applied, and the amount of opening of the medial joint line is noted (Figure 15-13). No joint laxity is a grade I stretch, laxity with a firm end point is a grade II partial tear, and no firm end point on stress is a grade III or complete tear.[12] The test is repeated with the knee in full extension. Excessive varus or valgus laxity in knee extension may indicate associated injury to the posterior cruciate ligament.[13]

Treatment of grade I and II injuries is ice, a hinged knee brace with full range of motion, and limited weightbearing until the pain subsides. Rehabilitation exercises—including straight leg raising, quadriceps setting, active range of motion, and hamstring isometrics—may begin immediately for patients with grade I injuries and within a week for those with grade II injuries. A knee immobilizer is used symptomatically and may be needed for 3–4 weeks with grade II injuries. In general, early active motion as soon as possible is reasonable for grades I and II injuries. The patient can return to sports when full range of motion is achieved and when knee strength is within 10% that of the opposite knee. This may take 3 months with a grade II injury.[2]

Although grade III injuries may be treated nonoperatively, splinting and orthopedic referral are recommended because of potential associated injuries. One nonoperative protocol for treating isolated grade III MCL injuries involves knee immobilization in 30 degrees of flexion for 2 weeks in a locked, hinged knee brace and with the knee nonweightbearing. For the next month, range of motion from 30 to 80 degrees is allowed, but the athlete remains nonweightbearing. This is followed by weightbearing as tolerated, until motion and strength are near normal.[14]

Lateral Collateral Ligament Injury

The lateral collateral ligament (LCL) is most commonly injured by varus stress to the knee. Localized lateral tenderness may be noted. The LCL is most effectively tested by varus stress at 25 degrees of flexion (similar to MCL testing).[11] Laxity is graded as for MCL injuries. X-ray findings may reveal a lateral capsular avulsion fracture indicative of associated cruciate injury. Avulsion of the biceps femoris from the proximal fibula may be seen in severe injury.

Treatment is as for MCL injuries. Orthopedic referral is recommended for grade III injuries and those with associated bony avulsions.

Meniscal Injury

Twisting or hyperflexion injuries are the common mechanisms of meniscal injuries. A popping sensation may be noted. A firm block to passive extension or inability to fully extend the knee may occur with displaced meniscal tears. Effusion may be noted if the meniscus is torn near its vascular connection to the capsule. Joint line tenderness is generally present. Other injuries may cause apparent locking of the knee and are often confused with meniscal tears: (1) patellar dislocation or osteochondral

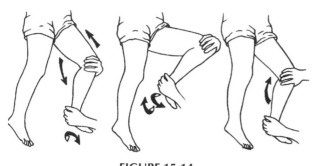

FIGURE 15-14
McMurray test.

fracture, (2) intraarticular fracture or loose body, and (3) severe hamstring spasm.

Examination should include McMurray test (Figure 15-14). This is done with the patient supine. The heel of the patient's injured leg is held in one hand by the examiner while the patient's knee is fully flexed. The fingers of the examiner's other hand palpate the patient's medial joint line while the examiner's thumb and thenar eminence are on the lateral aspect of the joint. A valgus stress is applied by the examiner, and the patient's knee is extended with the tibia held externally rotated. Pain or a palpable click over the medial joint line indicates medial meniscal tear.[2]

Apley compression test is performed with the patient prone and his or her injured knee flexed to 90 degrees. The examiner grasps the patient's foot with both hands. The examiner's knee and leg may be used to stabilize the patient's thigh. The patient's foot is laterally rotated while a downward force is applied to the foot. Pain at the medial joint line may indicate medial meniscal tear. The lateral meniscus may similarly be tested by medially rotating the patient's foot.

X-ray films should be obtained to evaluate for fracture or loose osseous bodies. Treatment consists of protection from full weightbearing, a knee immobilizer, nonsteroidal anti-inflammatory drugs (NSAIDs), and weightbearing as tolerated. Range of motion, isometric, and straight leg raising exercises are begun as soon as symptoms permit. Orthopedic referral is indicated for joint locking, frequent catching or giving-way sensations, associated ligamentous or osseous injury, or failure of any other symptoms to resolve fully within 3 months.[2]

Proximal Tibiofibular Joint Disruption

Dislocation of the proximal tibiofibular joint is a very uncommon injury. If dislocation is suspected, splinting and immediate orthopedic referral is recommended. The most common mechanism of injury resulting in anterolateral instability is

falling on a flexed, adducted leg with the ankle inverted.[15] Posteromedial dislocation is caused by direct trauma to the flexed knee. Superior dislocation is associated with displaced tibia fractures, ankle injuries (including diastasis), or congenital knee dislocation.

Anterolateral dislocation is the most common dislocation, occurring in approximately 90% of the patients, and it is especially common in athletes.[16] These usually present after some significant injury to the knee. Many will describe falling into so-called *hurdler's position*, with the knee flexed, foot adducted, and ankle everted. Patients will report lateral knee pain.

Physical examination reveals a prominent, tender, and mobile fibular head. Occasionally, peroneal nerve injury may be seen in this injury. AP and lateral radiographs of both knees must be obtained. AP x-ray films will usually reveal a laterally displaced fibular head, with widening of the proximal interosseous space. A bone scan may also be of benefit.

Orthopedic treatment options include closed reduction with or without immobilization, biceps femoris strengthening, open reduction, reconstruction, arthrodesis of the tibiofibular joint, and fibular head resection.[16]

Other Causes of Inability to Extend the Knee

Disruption of the Extensor Mechanism

Disruption of the extensor mechanism[2, 10] may be caused by sudden forceful contraction of the quadriceps during jumping or deceleration, or by a direct blow to the knee. Disruption may occur by means of the following:

- Quadriceps tendon rupture (proximal to patella)
- Patellar fracture
- Patellar tendon rupture (just distal to patella)
- Tibial tubercle avulsion (in the pediatric population)

Examination may show effusion and a palpable gap at the site of rupture. Affected individuals are unable to hold the knee straight against gravity once it has been passively extended. X-ray films reveal any fracture or bony avulsion. In the pediatric population, a displaced patellar fracture may appear only as a small fleck of bone because of the cartilaginous nature of the immature patella. Tibial tubercle avulsions may also be seen in the pediatric population. Treatment of all these injuries is immobilization of the knee in extension and immediate orthopedic referral.

Acute Patellar Dislocation or Subluxation

Acute patellar dislocation or subluxation may occur by a mechanism similar to that causing extensor disruptions

FIGURE 15-15
Evaluation of chronic knee pain. (ITB = iliotibial band.)

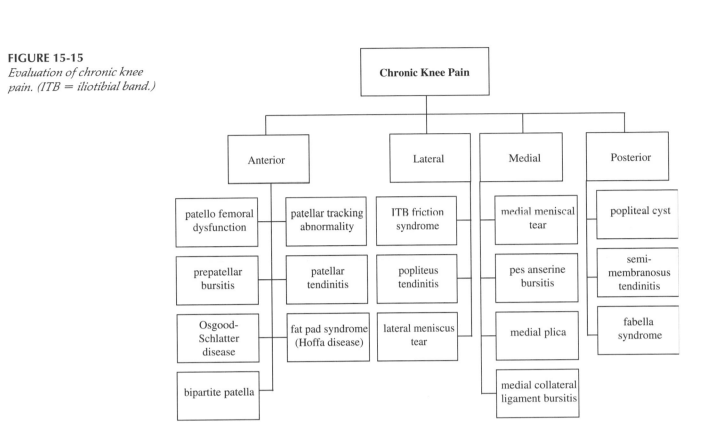

or by sudden cutting movements. Dislocations are usually lateral and may spontaneously reduce, making diagnosis difficult. Knee swelling and medial retinacular tenderness above the joint line and at the adductor tubercle may be noted, and the patella may be hypermobile to medial and lateral pressure. Affected patients demonstrate significant apprehension and pain when the patella is pushed laterally while the knee is passively flexed to 20–30 degrees (patellar apprehension text). X-ray films (AP, lateral, and sunrise) should be taken to rule out any associated osteochondral fractures of the patella or femoral condyle.

Initial treatment consists of a knee immobilizer or cylinder cast in near full extension for approximately 3 weeks, followed by gentle active range of motion exercises. The athlete may begin quadriceps setting and straight leg raising immediately, but dynamic resistance exercises are avoided until full range of motion is achieved.[2] Orthopedic referral is recommended for osteochondral fracture, joint locking, or recurrent dislocation indicating severe hypermobility of the patella.

CHRONIC KNEE PAIN OR SWELLING

Figure 15-15 illustrates evaluation of chronic knee pain.

Anterior Knee Pain

History
Attention must be given to age at onset and associated trauma. Sudden traumatic onset may indicate patellofemoral dislocation or subluxation, or osteochondral fracture. Gradual onset may be seen with patellar tendinitis, synovial plica, patellofemoral tracking disorder, tibial tubercle apophysitis (Osgood-Schlatter disease), osteochondrosis of the inferior pole of the patella (Sinding-Larsen-Johansson disease), retropatellar pain syndrome, or patellar chondrosis. Associated catching or popping is seen with synovial plica or patellar subluxation. Pain that is worse with knee flexion is usually retropatellar in origin. Persistent night pain that wakes the patient from sleep should be evaluated by x-ray examination for osteonecrosis, tumors, or tumorlike conditions. Persistent joint effusions or polyarticular involvement may be the result of arthritides or connective tissue disorders. Acute atraumatic effusions with pain on joint motion may represent joint infection or crystalline synovitis,[2] as in gout or pseudogout. A large, painless effusion may represent pigmented villonodular synovitis.

Physical examination should include overall extremity alignment for increased hip internal rotation (increased femoral anteversion), excessive knee varus or valgus, internal or external tibial torsion, leg length discrepancy, calcaneal valgus and varus, and pes planus and cavus. Thigh circumference is measured to check for atrophy. The quadriceps angle (Q-angle) is measured as the angle from the anterior superior iliac spine to the center of the patella to the center of the tibial tubercle.[17] A normal Q-angle is usually up to approximately 10 degrees for males and 15 degrees for females.[18] An increased Q-angle suggests patellofemoral malalignment.

Patellar tracking is assessed by having the patient sit on the edge of the examining table with his or her knees hanging over the edge. The examiner places his or her index finger on one side of the patient's patella and his or her thumbs on the other. The patient then actively raises and lowers his or her leg. Normally, the patella will track straight in the femoral groove. With maltracking, the patella can be felt gliding or tilting laterally, especially as the leg is fully extended (J-shift sign).

Palpation determines any localized tenderness. The infrapatellar fat pad behind the patellar tendon is palpated for tenderness and any hypertrophy indicating inflammation. The knee is then moved through a passive range of motion, and any patellofemoral crepitus or tracking difference from the contralateral knee is noted.

Patellofemoral stability is tested by pushing medially and laterally on the patella while the patient is supine and relaxed and his or her knee is passively flexed 30 degrees.[2] The amount of displacement is compared with that on the opposite side. With excessive instability, the patient may sense impending dislocation and grab at the examiner's hand (apprehension sign). Pain on compression of the patella while the patient actively contracts the quadriceps with his or her knee extended suggests a retropatellar origin.[2]

A detailed examination should also include evaluation of strength and flexibility of the hip flexors, quadriceps, hamstrings, and gastrocnemius-soleus complex.

Patellofemoral Dysfunction

Patellofemoral dysfunction refers to anterior knee pain emanating from the patellofemoral joint and its supporting soft tissue structures. It is also referred to as *retropatellar pain syndrome, chondromalacia patella, anterior knee pain,* or *lateral facet compression syndrome.* Patients generally report anterior, anterolateral, or anteromedial knee pain that is worsened when the patellofemoral joint is loaded (e.g., climbing or descending stairs, prolonged sitting, or squatting). The knee may occasionally give out as a result of pain-induced reflex inhibition of the quadriceps. Swelling is generally minimal to absent, and symptoms are frequently bilateral.

The physical examination is directed toward both confirming the diagnosis and evaluating for predisposing bio-

mechanical factors. Knee range of motion is full, and there is generally trace to no effusion and no ligamentous instability. Pain is reproduced with direct pressure over the patella and "rocking" it in the femoral groove (patellar grind test). The patella should ideally track in a straight line from distal to proximal as the knee is actively extended. Numerous factors can cause the patella to track "off course," leading to painful increased intraosseous pressure within the patella or excessive stress of the peripatellar structures (particularly the medial and lateral retinaculum). The anatomic factors include excessive femoral anteversion, external tibial torsion, genu valgum, calcaneovalgus, and pes planus. Functional factors include tightness of the lateral retinaculum, iliotibial band, quadriceps, and hamstrings and relative weakness of the vastus medialis obliques. Radiographs are not necessary on initial evaluation but should be procured if patients fail to respond to treatment. AP views assess for a bi- or tripartite patella, the lateral view assesses for evidence of a high-riding patella (patella alta), and sunrise views should be evaluated for lateral patellar tilt or subluxation.

Treatment is generally conservative with the goal of decreasing the patellofemoral forces. Patients should be instructed to avoid squatting, deep knee bends, hill running, and excessive stair climbing. Physical therapy is directed toward loosening the lateral structures and functionally strengthening the medial structures, with particular attention to the vastus medialis. A qualified therapist can instruct the patient in McConnell taping techniques, which facilitate proper patellar tracking. This is done in conjunction with a program of lateral retinacular, hamstring, iliotibial band, and quadriceps stretching and quadriceps and vastus medialis strengthening exercises. Exercises that involve flexing the knee more than 30–40 degrees or that are painful should be avoided. Ice massage after exercise and NSAIDs are useful adjuncts.

Patellar support braces may be useful in patients when McConnell taping is ineffective, and orthotics may benefit patients with associated flatfoot. The evaluation of gait—observing for overpronation, prolonged pronation, and loss of the arch (flatfoot)—should always be done in patellofemoral dysfunction resistant to other treatment. Watching the patient walk barefoot in an office hallway may be all that is needed to identify these contributing conditions. LowDye strapping, over-the-counter arch supports, or custom-made in-shoe orthotics are often very effective. Custom-made in-shoe orthotics can be obtained from several sources. Measurements and plaster casts of the feet are sent to an orthotics company or occasionally made in the office of a physical therapist, podiatrist, or orthotist.

Referral to an orthopedic surgeon is indicated if conservative measures fail after 6–12 months. Surgical options include lateral retinacular release, tibial tuberosity transfer, advancement of the vastus medialis, or derotational osteotomy.

Patellar Tracking Abnormalities

Recurrent patellar subluxation or dislocation or extensor mechanism malalignment may present as chronic knee pain or swelling. Thigh atrophy may be noted. Management is as outlined for patellofemoral disorders. In addition, correction of any foot overpronation with temporary orthotics may be helpful. A variety of bracings (such as a knee sleeve with patellar cutout) may be helpful.

Prepatellar Bursitis

Repeated minor trauma or kneeling may incite inflammation of the subcutaneous bursa over the patella or patellar tendon. Pain and superficial swelling are noted on palpation. Knee padding, avoidance of kneeling, and NSAIDs may be tried. Knee rehabilitation exercises are also prescribed. The bursae should be watched, because infection may develop. The natural history of bursitis is slow resolution, regardless of treatment.

Patellar Tendinitis

Inflammation and pain in the patellar tendon is often seen in jumping sports (jumper's knee). Localized pain on palpation may be worsened by resisted active knee extension. In the pediatric athlete, pain may be localized to the inferior pole of the patella, and fragmentation of the inferior pole may be noted on lateral x-ray films (Sinding-Larsen-Johannson disease). Treatment includes NSAIDs and focuses on reduction of activity and on strengthening and flexibility of quadriceps and hamstring as symptoms subside. Jumpers should use eccentric exercises to recondition the extensor mechanism. A compression strap similar to that used in tennis elbow may be useful to decrease symptoms.

Hoffa Syndrome

Hoffa syndrome, also known as *infrapatellar fat pad syndrome*, is hypertrophy and inflammation of the infrapatellar fat pad. Although the etiology is not completely understood, most authors believe that the primary cause may be repeated trauma of the infrapatellar fat pad during activities requiring constant repetition of maximal extension of the knee.[16, 19] The fat pad can become inflamed as a result of direct trauma as well.

Diagnosis is usually one of exclusion. Patients usually report pain below the inferior pole of the patella, exacerbated by physical activity or knee extension. Examination reveals swelling on either side of the patellar ligament and pain on palpation of the fat pad deep to and along the edge of the patellar ligament.

The bounce test, as described by Hoffa, is performed by applying fingertip pressure to the fat pad while the knee is passively extended. If pain is elicited near terminal extension, the result is considered positive. However, this test is not specific. Radiographs typically are negative.

In most cases, treatment is nonoperative.[16] Treatment involves rest, ice, NSAIDs, and a sequential exercise program (see section on knee rehabilitation guidelines). Exercise range of motion should be modified to avoid terminal extension. Physical therapy modalities, including high-voltage galvanic stimulation and phonophoresis with hydrocortisone, may be helpful. Resistant cases may benefit from judicious placement of a steroid injection deep in the fat pad. If pain does not resolve after 6 months, surgical treatment for resection of the fat pad may be considered but is rarely necessary.

Bipartite or Multipartite Patella (Patella Partita)

Patella partita (Figure 15-16) is a malformation of the patella. It is characterized by one or multiple vertical lines of discontinuity secondary to incomplete ossification, most commonly in the anterolateral portion of the patella.[20]

Most bipartite patellas are asymptomatic, and the diagnosis often is made as a coincidental finding on a radiograph obtained for another reason. However, pain may be present after direct trauma to the knee or secondary to repetitive athletic activities.

If tenderness exists and x-rays show a bipartite patella at the point of tenderness, a short period of immobilization may be tried to decrease inflammation and pain. If conservative treatment fails, referral to an orthopedist for possible excision of the fragment is considered but is rarely necessary.

Lateral Knee Pain

Iliotibial Band Friction Syndrome

Pain over the posterolateral knee (Figure 15-17) is often associated with running on hills or banked surfaces.[1] Localized tenderness is located over the lateral femoral condyle just above the joint line. Ober test is useful to document iliotibial band tightness. The patient lies in the lateral decubitus position with his or her affected side up. The unaffected hip and knee are flexed to eliminate the lumbar lordosis. The examiner stands behind the patient and grasps the ankle of the patient's affected leg while the other hand stabilizes the pelvis. The patient's affected knee is flexed 90 degrees while his or her hip is abducted and extended to align the patient's thigh with his or her body. The patient's thigh is then allowed to adduct passively. If the iliotibial band is tight, the patient's hip may

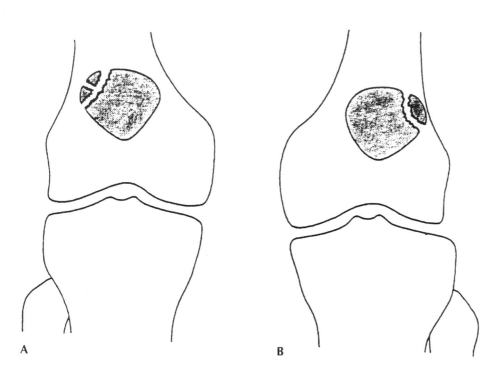

FIGURE 15-16
A. Tripartite patella. B. Bipartite patella. (Reprinted with permission from H Schmidt, J Freyschmidt, W Holthusen. Knee. In P Winter [ed], Borderlands of Normal and Pathologic Findings in Skeletal Radiography. New York: Thieme Medical Publishers, 1993;730.)

remain passively abducted. Tenderness over the posterolateral knee near the insertion of the iliotibial band may be noted.

Treatment includes reduction of mileage run and avoidance of banked surfaces and hill running. Ice massage, NSAIDs, and iontophoresis may be beneficial. The iliotibial band may be stretched by standing with both knees fully extended and adducting and extending the hip of the affected side as far as possible. The trunk is simultaneously flexed toward the unaffected side. This position is held for 10 seconds, and the exercise is repeated 10–20

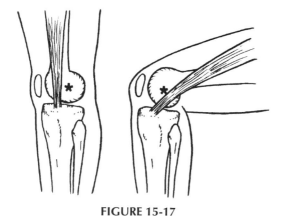

FIGURE 15-17
Iliotibial band friction syndrome. (∗ = point of tenderness.)

times three times daily. Correction of any forefoot pronation with a medial longitudinal arch support or correcting of leg length discrepancy may be helpful. Pain may persist for approximately 6 weeks. Steroid injection between the iliotibial band and lateral femoral condyle (the area of maximal tenderness) is indicated when more conservative measures fail. The return to running must be gradual after symptoms subside. A good return-to-running program, which may be applied safely during most knee rehabilitation programs, follows.[8]

1. Jog 15 minutes per day for 1 week.
2. Add 5 minutes to daily time per week if no symptoms appear.
3. Progress to 40 minutes daily (or, if <40 minutes, to prior level of training).
4. Return to prior training if no symptoms appear at this duration of the run.

Popliteus Tendinitis
Popliteus tendinitis is often seen with downhill running. Pain is felt over the posterolateral knee during running or sitting cross-legged. X-ray films are not needed unless symptoms persist. This may be confused with biceps femoris tendinitis, in which tenderness is over the biceps tendon and its insertion. Treatment is ice, activity limitation, NSAIDs, physical therapy modalities, hamstring

stretching, and a gradual return to activity when the patient is symptom free.

Lateral Meniscus Tear

Lateral meniscus tear may cause lateral joint line pain, locking, or catching. Treatment is addressed in the discussion of acute knee injury.

Medial Knee Pain

Medial Meniscus Tear

Presentation and treatment of medial meniscal tear are addressed in the discussion of acute knee injury.

Pes Anserine Bursitis

Pes anserine bursitis presents as insidious-onset pain over the medial proximal tibial metaphysis approximately 2–4 cm below the joint line. Pain in this area must be distinguished from the following:

- Meniscal injury (meniscal pain is usually a joint line)
- Degenerative joint disease in the mature athlete
- Tumors and tumorlike conditions
- Tibial stress fracture
- Hamstring tendinitis

In pes anserine bursitis, localized swelling may be noted in the bursa underlying the tendons. X-ray films of the knee should be reviewed carefully for any bony lesion or fracture. A bone scan may be indicated if pain is diffuse or persistent. Treatment includes rest, local ice application for 10–15 minutes, NSAIDs, iontophoresis, and possibly a trial of local anesthetic and steroid injection. Hamstring stretching and strengthening should be emphasized as symptoms subside. Medial longitudinal arch supports and heel wedges may be helpful for any excessive knee valgus or hindfoot pronation. Runners should reduce the distance run, shorten the stride, and gradually return to prior training.

Mediopatellar Plica Syndrome

The mediopatellar plica runs from the medial lining of the suprapatellar pouch distally to the synovium over the infrapatellar fat pad (Figure 15-18). It may impinge on the femoral condyle during knee flexion. Inflammation and hypertrophy may ensue.[16] Pain is noted in this area of the medial retinaculum. X-ray films should be obtained if pain is persistent. Treatment is as for patellofemoral disorders. A local anesthetic and steroid agent may be injected directly into the plica to give temporary relief. Orthope-

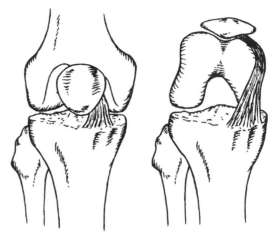

FIGURE 15-18
Mediopatellar plica.

dic referral should be made after 6 months of unresponsiveness to treatment.

Medial Collateral Ligament Bursitis (Bursa of Stuttle)

Patients with MCL bursitis report medial joint line pain; however, they deny any history of locking or giving way.

Physical examination reveals a palpable, tender enlargement under the MCL at the level of the medial joint line. This pain is exacerbated by valgus stress, extension or hyperextension of the knee, or with external rotation of the leg. X-ray films should be obtained to rule out bony avulsion or other bone pathology.

Treatment should include rest, rehabilitation emphasizing quadriceps strengthening, NSAIDs, and occasional steroid injection. If there is no improvement in 2–4 weeks, then referral to an orthopedic surgeon should be considered.

Posterior Knee Pain

Popliteal Cyst (Baker Cyst)

A popliteal cyst may present as aching posterior knee pain with a palpable cystic mass, which is usually the result of distention of the gastrocnemius or semimembranosus bursa. If no mass is noted, pain may be due to semimembranosus tendinitis. The cyst may communicate with the joint and change in size.

The examination should rule out a palpable pulsatile mass of popliteal artery aneurysm. X-ray films should be obtained to rule out tumor. Normal x-ray findings in the face of a mass in the popliteal area do not rule out tumor. In the absence of a good explanation for Baker cyst and

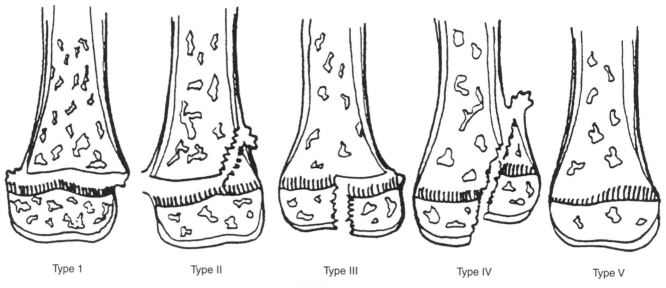

| Type 1 | Type II | Type III | Type IV | Type V |

FIGURE 15-19

Salter-Harris classification of injuries to the physis. (Reprinted with permission from WB Kleinman, WH Bowers. Fractures, Ligamentous Injuries to the hand. In FW Bora [ed], The Pediatric Upper Extremity. Philadelphia: Saunders, 1986;154.)

in the absence of transillumination or ability to aspirate fluid, masses in the popliteal area should be evaluated by MRI. Treatment is primarily by activity modification.

Orthopedic referral is recommended for large or painful cysts or cysts in the young child because of the possible association with meniscal tears or rare cystic tumors. Any cyst with calcifications seen on x-ray films should be referred for orthopedic evaluation. Aspiration of the cyst is not initially recommended.

Fabella Syndrome

The fabella is a sesamoid bone that, when present, is located in the tendinous portion of the lateral gastrocnemius muscle directly posterior to the lateral femoral condyle. The fabella serves as an attachment site for strands from the popliteus, arcuate complex, and the fabellofibular ligament. The fabella is present in 10–18% of the normal population and is bilateral in approximately half of these patients.[21]

Fabella syndrome is characterized by gradual onset of sharp, intermittent pain localized to the posterolateral aspect of the knee.[16] Examination reveals localized tenderness over the fabella, accentuated with knee extension. This condition occurs most frequently in late adolescence but can be seen in older patients as well.

Treatment should consist of restricted activity, relative rest, and NSAIDs to control the inflammation. Heel lifts are occasionally useful to functionally shorten the gastrocnemius muscle. Conservative management should be continued for 6 months. If pain continues, then surgical excision of the fabella is indicated.

SPECIAL CONSIDERATIONS IN THE PEDIATRIC ATHLETE

Knees are a frequent site of injury in childhood sports. Increasing participation in cutting sports, such as football, soccer, and basketball, has increased the potential for knee injuries. The young athlete's knee anatomically resembles that of an adult; however, because of the presence of open epiphyses, they are biomechanically prone to different patterns of injury. This section addresses some of these unique injuries.

Fractures About the Knee (Salter-Harris Classification)

The Salter-Harris classification of fractures describes five types (Figure 15-19).

Fracture Separations of the Distal Femoral Physis

Fracture separations of the distal femoral physis are relatively uncommon fractures, accounting for approximately 7% of all lower extremity physeal injuries. A hyperextension force is the most common mechanism of injury. Salter-Harris type II fractures are the most common pattern seen in the distal femoral physis.

Epiphyseal fracture

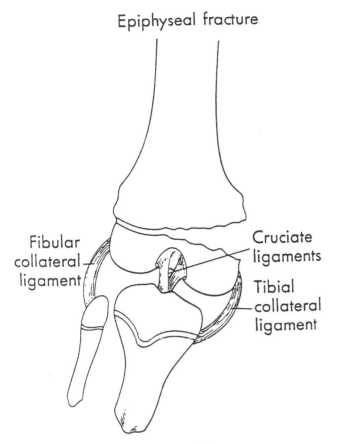

Fibular collateral ligament

Cruciate ligaments

Tibial collateral ligament

FIGURE 15-20
Major ligamentous attachments of distal femoral and proximal tibial epiphysis. (Reprinted with permission from ST Canale. Fractures and Dislocations in Children. In AH Crenshaw [ed], Campbell's Operative Orthopaedics [8th ed]. St. Louis: Mosby–Year Book, 1992;1197.)

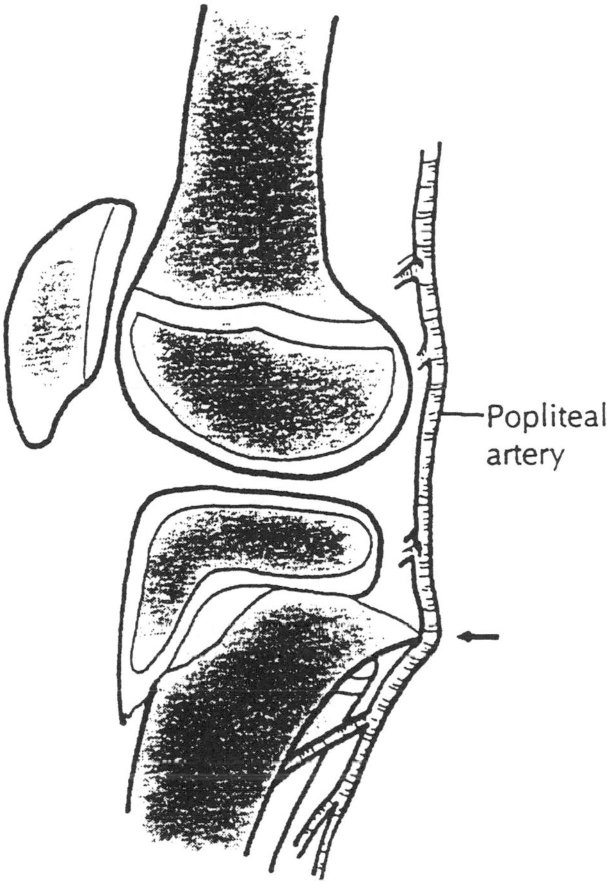

Popliteal artery

FIGURE 15-21
Medial view of the right knee with fracture-separation of the proximal tibial epiphysis resulting from hyperextension. Posteriorly displaced proximal tibial metaphysis impinges on the adjacent popliteal artery (arrow). (Reprinted with permission from JM Roberts. Fractures and Dislocations of the Knee. Part I: Fractures and Separations of the Knee. In CA Rockwood Jr, KE Wilkins, R King [eds], Fractures in Children [3rd ed]. Philadelphia: Lippincott, 1991;1196.)

Pain over the distal femur and knee effusion is suspicious for a Salter-Harris fracture of the distal femoral physis until proved otherwise. If displaced, then shortening and angulation of the thigh may be seen.[22]

X-rays of the knee should be obtained to evaluate the fracture (Figure 15-20). However, the x-ray findings must be correlated with the physical examination, especially in the case of a nondisplaced Salter-Harris type I fracture, in which no x-ray abnormalities may be present. Stress x-rays may be required by an orthopedic surgeon to detect this fracture.

Initial treatment should include a careful neurovascular examination, checking for dorsalis pedis and posterior tibialis pulses, evaluating capillary refill, and carefully examining both sensory and motor function. The next step in management should involve long leg splint to immobilize the entire leg, followed by imme-

diate referral to an orthopedic surgeon for definitive treatment.

Fractures of the Proximal Tibial Epiphysis
Injuries of the proximal tibial epiphysis are also rare. Mechanism of injury usually is a hyperextension force that displaces the tibial metaphysis posteriorly (Figure 15-21). It is usually seen in older children and adolescents. Salter-Harris type II fractures are the most common pattern of fracture seen in proximal tibial epiphyseal injuries.[22]

Physical findings include severe pain and swelling and limitation of motion of the knee. Pain is present over the

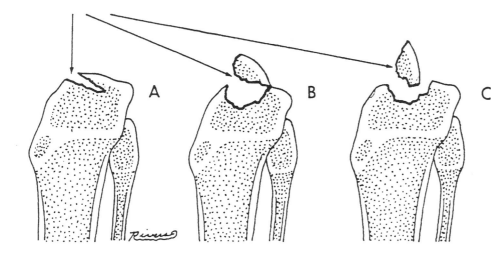

FIGURE 15-22

Fractures of intercondylar eminence of the tibia. A. Type I, avulsion fracture, nondisplaced. B. Type II, hinged fracture, displaced but posterior rim remains intact. C. Type III, completely displaced fracture. (Reprinted with permission from ST Canale. Fractures and Dislocations in Children. In AH Crenshaw [ed], Campbell's Operative Orthopaedics [8th ed]. St. Louis: Mosby–Year Book, 1992;1193.)

proximal tibial physis distal to the joint line; however, soft tissue swelling may make localization of pain difficult. Posterior displacement may produce a visible and palpable concavity anteriorly at the level of the tibial tuberosity.

As discussed in the preceding section, x-rays of the knee must be obtained to evaluate the nature of the injury, correlating any findings with the physical examination.

Treatment of this injury should include immediate assessment of the neurovascular status, followed by immobilization of the entire leg and emergent referral to an orthopedic surgeon because of the high potential for vascular complications associated with this type of injury.

Fractures of the Tibial Eminence

Fractures of the tibial (intercondylar) eminence in children are frequently caused by a fall that results in forceful hyperextension of the knee, or by a direct blow to the distal end of the femur with the knee flexed (Figure 15-22). They are most commonly seen in children between the ages of 8 and 14 years. These injuries are usually an avulsion fracture of the anterior intercondylar eminence from the pull of the ACL.

Physical examination reveals pain and effusion around the knee, hemarthrosis, and reluctance to bear weight. There may be a positive anterior drawer sign and associated collateral ligament injury present; however, a thorough physical examination may not be possible secondary to pain. X-rays of the knee must be obtained.

Treatment should include immobilization with a knee immobilizer or long leg posterior splint, no weightbearing on the leg, ice, and elevation, followed by urgent referral to an orthopedic surgeon.

Fractures of the Tibial Tuberosity

Avulsion fractures of the tibial tuberosity are uncommon Salter-Harris type III fractures of the proximal tibial physis (Figure 15-23). Mechanism of injury is usually a violent flexion of the knee against a contracted quadri-

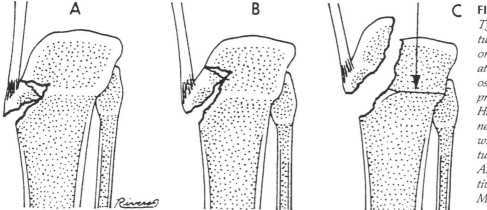

FIGURE 15-23

Types of avulsion fracture of tibial tuberosity. A. Type I, through secondary ossification center. B. Type II, at junction of primary and secondary ossification centers. C. Type III, across primary ossification center (Salter-Harris type III) with epiphyseal plate near closing posteriorly. (Reprinted with permission from ST Canale. Fractures and Dislocations in Children. In AH Crenshaw [ed], Campbell's Operative Orthopaedics [8th ed]. St. Louis: Mosby–Year Book, 1992;1194.)

FIGURE 15-24
Osteochondral fractures associated with dislocation of the patella. A. Medial facet. B. Lateral femoral condyle. (Reprinted with permission from JH Beaty. Fractures and Dislocations of the Knee. Part II: Knee Injuries. In CA Rockwood Jr, KE Wilkins, R King [eds], Fractures in Children [3rd ed]. Philadelphia: Lippincott, 1991;1234.)

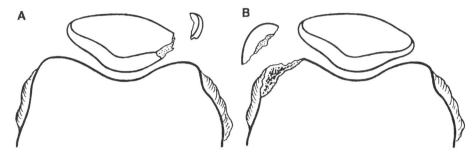

ceps muscle.[23] This fracture should be differentiated from Osgood-Schlatter disease, which is an avulsion of the anterior ossicle of the tuberosity with no involvement of the physis.

Physical examination reveals pain and swelling directly over the tuberosity. If the fracture is a small avulsion, the patient can usually actively extend his or her knee. In more severe cases, however, the extensor mechanism may be disrupted.

X-rays will reveal a fractured tibial tuberosity that may or may not be displaced. The extent of the fracture can best be evaluated on a lateral x-ray.

Treatment should include ice, elevation, immobilization with a knee immobilizer or a long leg splint, no weightbearing on the leg, and urgent referral to an orthopedic surgeon.

Osteochondral Fractures

Osteochondral fractures are usually caused by dislocation of the patella, direct blow to the knee, a sheering force to the medial or lateral femoral condyle, or a flexion-rotation injury of the knee.[22, 23]

Physical examination reveals immediate onset of severe pain and swelling after the injury, with difficulty in weightbearing. The knee is usually held in slight flexion, and any attempt at movement results in severe pain.

X-rays, in general, will not show any abnormalities; however, oblique and skyline views should also be done. Occasionally, a large osteochondral fragment (Figure 15-24) with a small ossified portion may be seen.

Treatment is usually surgical, and referral to an orthopedic surgeon is necessary; however, initial treatment should include immobilization, ice, elevation, and appropriate pain management.

Sinding-Larsen-Johansson Disease

Sinding-Larsen-Johansson disease (Figure 15-25) is a chronic tendinitis accompanied by calcification of the avulsed patellar tendon. It is an overuse injury seen in the 10- to 13-year-old child and presents much like Osgood-

Schlatter disease, except the pain and tenderness are located at the inferior pole of the patella.[24] The pain is worsened by running and stair climbing.

Radiographs of the knee may be normal or may reveal an area of calcification adjacent to the inferior pole of the patella.

Treatment is conservative. In a patient with acute and severe pain, a knee immobilizer or cylinder cast should

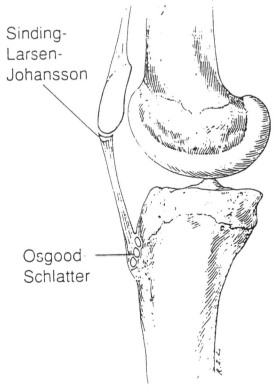

Sinding-Larsen-Johansson

Osgood-Schlatter

FIGURE 15-25
Osgood-Schlatter disease and Sinding-Larsen-Johansson disease are types of traction apophysitis affecting the knees of adolescents. (Reprinted with permission from MD Miller, DE Cooper, JJP Watner. Review of Sports Medicine and Arthroscopy. Philadelphia: Saunders, 1995;61.)

be applied for 3–4 weeks. Patients with milder symptoms can be treated with NSAIDs, along with a prescribed rehabilitation protocol. Rehabilitation should include hamstring and quadriceps stretching exercises. If symptoms persist, referral to an orthopedist may be warranted.

Osgood-Schlatter Disease

Pain is detected over a possibly prominent tibial tubercle in the adolescent with Osgood-Schlatter disease. Lateral x-ray films may reveal enlargement or fragmentation of the tubercle. Treatment is rest, ice, crutches, NSAIDs, and patellofemoral rehabilitation exercises as symptoms subside. The athlete may participate as long as symptoms are minimal. Recurrences may last until skeletal maturity and are very rare thereafter.

GENERAL KNEE REHABILITATION GUIDELINES

Stretching

Stretches are best done after a brief warm-up period. The maximum benefit is gained by stretching after exercise. Directions to the patient for each exercise are as follows:

- *Hamstring stretch*: Lie on your back with your head resting comfortably on the floor with knees bent and feet flat. Raise one leg until your thigh is straight up in the air with your knee bent. Clasp your hands behind that knee to support it, and gently straighten the knee. Point your toes at your nose (dorsiflex your foot). Repeat the exercise with the other leg.
- *Rectus-femoris stretch*: Stand with your back to a table with the toes of your right foot resting on the table top. Hold onto the back of a chair. Slowly flex the knee you are standing on, and lower yourself toward the floor, leaning forward slightly without bending your spine. You should feel the front of your right thigh being stretched. Repeat the exercise for the left thigh.
- *Abductor stretch*: Stand with your right shoulder 12 in. from the wall, with your right hand resting against the wall at shoulder's height. Cross your left leg in front of your right, with your weight mostly on the right. Raise your right hip toward the wall. Repeat the exercise for the left leg.
- *Calf muscle stretch*: Stand facing the wall with your left foot halfway between the wall and your right foot. Place your hands against the wall at shoulder's height. Holding your right knee straight, bend your left knee slightly and lean toward the wall without bending your

spine. Bend your right knee slightly until the right heel just lifts off the ground. Keep your toes and feet pointed directly at the wall throughout the stretch. Repeat the exercise for the left leg.
- *Lateral iliopatellar band stretch*: With your knee fully extended, massage around the patella. Keeping your thigh completely relaxed, gently push the patella toward your other leg. Repeat the exercise for the other leg.

Strengthening

Ankle weights may be added to the following exercises as strength improves.

- *Quadriceps setting exercise*: Lie on your back with your right knee straight and left knee bent. Point your right toes to your nose, and tighten your right thigh muscle for 8 seconds. Do this 10 times, then repeat the exercise with the other leg.
- *Straight leg raises*: Lie on your back with your right leg straight and left knee bent. Lift your right foot 1 ft off the floor for 10 seconds. Repeat this 10 times, then repeat the exercise with the other leg. Exercise each leg for three sets each day.
- *Hip abductors*: Lie on your left side, with your left knee flexed and your right knee extended. Raise your right foot 18 in. off the floor, then gently lower it back to the floor 10 times. Try to keep your pelvis from rocking backward or forward during this exercise. Repeat this with the left leg. Do three sets of 10 lifts with each leg.
- *Hip adductors*: Lie on your right side with your left knee flexed and your left foot flat on the floor and behind your straight right knee. While holding the knee fully extended, lift your right foot 18 in. off the floor, then gently lower it to the floor again. Do this 10 times, then switch legs. Do three sets with each leg.
- *Hip flexors*: Sit on a table with both your knees and hips flexed to 90 degrees. Your right knee is then raised toward the chest 10 times. Repeat with your left knee. Do three sets with each leg.
- *Vastus medialis obliquus strengthening for patellofemoral dysfunction*: Vastus medialis obliquus (VMO) strengthening for patellofemoral dysfunction should start as the quadriceps setting exercise. The VMO should be palpated and the anterior muscles of the thigh tightened until you feel the VMO contract or tighten. This should be held for 8–10 seconds, 10 repetitions.
- *Vastus medialis obliquus advanced training*: Stand with your heels slightly apart and toes pointing outward in a ballet plié position, with your knees slightly bent. Step forward with one foot, keeping the toes pointed outward, and do a deep knee bend until your forward

knee is bent to 90 degrees or less. Return to the beginning position. Repeat the exercise using your other leg. This is an advanced exercise and should not be done while you still have anterior knee pain.

REFERENCES

1. Noyes FR, Bassett RW, Grood ES, Butler DL. Arthroscopy in acute hemarthrosis of the knee: incidence of anterior cruciate tears and other injuries. J Bone Joint Surg Am 1980;62:687–695.

2. Cherney S. Disorders of the Knee. In R Dee, E Mango, L Hurst (eds), Principles of Orthopedic Practice. New York: McGraw-Hill, 1989;1283–1330.

3. Donaldson WF, Warren RF, Wickiewicz T. A comparison of acute anterior cruciate ligament examinations: initial versus examination under anesthesia. Am J Sports Med 1995;13:5–10.

4. Galway RD, Beaupre A, MacIntosh DL. Pivot shift: a clinical sign of symptomatic anterior cruciate insufficiency. J Bone Joint Surg Br 1972;54:763–764.

5. Losee RE, Johnson ETR, Southwick WO. Anterior subluxation of the lateral tibial plateau. J Bone Joint Surg Am 1978;60:1015–1030.

6. Kennedy J, Roth J, Walder D. Posterior cruciate ligament injuries. Orthop Digest 1979;1:19.

7. Butler DL, Noyes FR, Edwards G. Ligamentous restraints to anterior posterior drawer in the human knee. J Bone Joint Surg Am 1980;62:259–270.

8. Clendenin MB, DeLee JC, Heckman JD. Interstitial tears of the posterior cruciate ligament of the knee. Orthopedics 1980;3:764 772.

9. Daniel DM, Stone ML, Barnett P, et al. Use of the quadriceps active test to diagnose posterior-cruciate ligament disruption and measure posterior laxity of the knee. J Bone Joint Surg Am 1988;70:386–391.

10. Boland AL. Soft Tissue Injuries of the Knee. In JA Nicholas, ED Henderson (eds), The Lower Extremity and Spine in Sports Medicine. St. Louis: Mosby, 1986;983–1012

11. Grood ES, Noyes FR, Butler DL, Suntay WJ. Ligamentous and capsular restraints preventing straight medical and lateral laxity in intact human cadaver knees. J Bone Joint Surg Am 1981;63:1257–1269.

12. Noyes FR, Grood ES, Butler DL, Malck M. Clinical laxity tests and functional stability of the knee: biomechanical concepts. Clin Orthop 1980;146:84–89.

13. Swenson TM, Harner CD. Knee ligament and meniscal injuries: current concepts. Orthop Clinic North Am 1995;26: 529–546.

14. Indelicato PA. Non-operative treatment of complete tears of the medial collateral ligament of the knee. J Bone Joint Surg Am 1983;65:323–329.

15. Ogden JA. Subluxation and dislocation of the proximal tibiofibular joint. J Bone Joint Surg Am 1974:56:145–154.

16. Safran M, Fu F. Uncommon causes of knee pain in the athlete. Orthop Clin North Am 1995;26:547–559.

17. Insall J, Falvo KA, Wise DW. Chondromalacia patellae. A prospective study. J Bone Joint Surg Am 1976;58:1–8.

18. Henry JH. Conservative treatment of patellofemoral subluxation. Clin Sports Med 1989;8:261–278.

19. Jacobson KE, Flandry FC. Diagnosis of anterior knee pain. Clin Sports Med 1989;8:179–195.

20. Soren A, Waugh TR. Patella partita. Arch Orthop Trauma Surg 1994;113:196–198.

21. Falk FD. Radiographic observation of incidence of the fabella. Bull Hosp Jt Dis 1963;24:127–129.

22. Beart JH, Kumar A. Current concepts: a review of fractures about the knee. J Bone Joint Surg Am 1994;76:1870–1879.

23. Smit AD, Stantly ST. Knee injuries in young athletes. Clin Sports Med 1995;14:629–650.

24. Gardiner JS, McIrney VK, Avella DG, Valdez NA. Injuries to the inferior pole of the patella in children. Orthop Rev 1990;19:643–649.

16

Lower Leg Pain

William C. Walker

Pain in the lower leg, between the knee and the ankle, is a frequent symptom in the athlete. The differential diagnosis for traumatic injuries (Table 16-1) is different from the one for exercise-induced pain (Figure 16-1). A review of the workup and treatment for each condition (except neoplasm) is presented in this chapter. Emphasis is placed on rehabilitative management.

ACUTE PAIN (TRAUMATIC INJURIES)

Muscle Cramps

Cramps—painful involuntary muscle contractions—occur commonly in the gastrocnemius and may be prevented by proper warm-up and stretching.[1] They often can be interrupted by forceful stretching of the involved muscle or by activation of the antagonistic muscle. The calf muscles are the most commonly involved. Cramps can be relieved by having the patient actively dorsiflex his or her ankle or having an assistant passively dorsiflex the patient's ankle with his or her knee straight. Concomitantly deeply massaging the patient's calf can help.

Muscle Strain

A muscle strain is a partial tear of muscle fibers caused by forceful stretching of an already contracted muscle.[2, 3] Suboptimal flexibility is thought to be a predisposing factor. The gastrocnemius, because it crosses two joints, is especially vulnerable. The high incidence of gastrocnemius strain in tennis players has earned it the nickname "tennis leg."

Tennis leg can present either as acute, severe stabbing calf pain or as mild calf soreness that worsens after rest.[2] Palpation reveals maximal tenderness at the musculotendinous junction of the medial head of the gastrocnemius or sometimes over the muscle belly itself. There may be an associated defect in the muscle. Dorsiflexion of the foot is painful and restricted. If the athlete cannot actively plantarflex to stand on one forefoot, then there is probably a complete tear (rupture).[3] An inhibitory pain response may also prevent active plantarflexion, so a passive test of musculotendinous integrity (Thompson test) should be performed: One forcibly squeezes the calf musculature to cause passive plantarflexion of the foot (negative test) or no response (positive test) (diminished response on symptomatic leg compared with nonsymptomatic leg may indicate partial tear). Ecchymosis and hematoma also usually form with complete tears.[4]

Contusion

Contusions (intramuscular bleeding) commonly occur in the gastrocnemius. They are caused by blunt trauma disrupting muscle fibers and damaging capillaries.[5] An ecchymosis usually becomes evident by 24 hours.[4] After an initial inflammatory response, the contusion heals by scar formation with inelastic, noncontractile connective tissue. Metaplastic ossification (myositis ossificans) occasionally follows and can be a chronic, functionally limiting problem.[6] Early motion and stretching may limit scar formation and prevent myositis ossificans.

Management of Lower Leg Muscle Strains and Contusions

Management uses the standard four-phase treatment of athletic injuries (Table 16-2).

TABLE 16-1
Differential Diagnosis for Acute Injuries to the Lower Leg

Muscle cramp
Heat cramp
Muscle strain
Contusion
Fracture
Acute compartment syndrome
Neoplasm

Phase I

Phase I rest is individualized depending on severity, but it always involves cessation of training. Immobilization is contraindicated in minor injuries; however, crutches or splinting should be used if ambulation is painful. With minor gastrocnemius-soleus strain when the individual has pain with walking, occasionally the addition of heel lifts (to both sides) in shoes will allow pain-free ambulation. The heel lifts allow just enough shortening during ambulation that the injured fibers are not stressed. A significant partial gastrocnemius tear is sometimes treated with long leg cast immobilization with the knee flexed at

60 degrees and the ankle in neutral for 3 weeks. This is followed by another 3 weeks with a boot cast and the ankle plantarflexed 10 degrees.[3] Complete tears may require surgical repair.

In phase I, ice is applied initially for 10–15 minutes with hourly reapplication. The athlete's leg is elevated frequently with compressive wraps. When the athlete's leg is pain free at rest and his or her calf girth has stabilized, the athlete progresses to phase II (motion restoration).

Phase II

The preferred method of motion exercise is a slow and sustained active stretch. The end range is maintained for 20 seconds initially, with a progression to 45 seconds. Some pulling discomfort at the end range is beneficial, but the exercise should not markedly increase pain. Stretching is performed several times per day and is preceded and followed by icing for the first few days. After 72 hours, moist heat or ultrasound may be used before stretching, but ice after stretching should continue. Ultrasound can help resolve a hematoma that limits muscle flexibility. Moist heat and ultrasound increase muscle fiber, flexibility, and blood flow to the area. It is important to cool

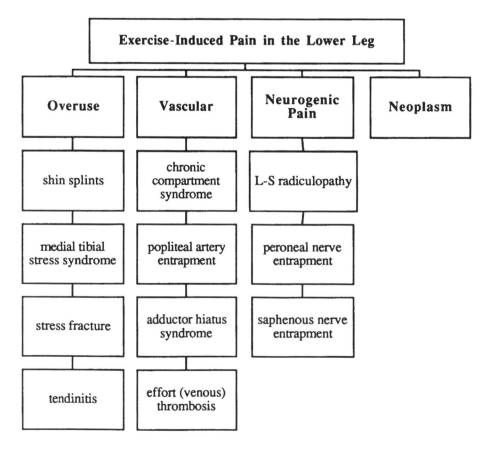

FIGURE 16-1
Algorithm for exercise-induced lower leg pain. (L-S = lumbar-sacral vertebrae.)

TABLE 16-2
Four-Phase Management of Athletic Injuries

I	Initial treatment: rest, ice, compression, elevation (RICE)
II	Motion restoration
III	Functional restoration (strength and endurance)
IV	Return to sport (functional progression using sport-specific tasks)

TABLE 16-3
On-Field Management of Tibial Fracture

Splint
Pressure dressing
Emergency shock management (as needed)
Immediate orthopedic referral

the muscle down (ice) after stretching to cool in the longest position of the muscle fibers reached and to reduce any inflammation or bleeding that may have occurred during the stretching process.

The gastrocnemius-soleus complex should be stretched one side at a time using gravity assistance. The athlete leans forward against a wall, dorsiflexing his or her ankle while keeping his or her knee extended (to stretch the gastrocnemius). The exercises are repeated with the athlete's knee flexed to stretch the soleus. When maximum flexibility is obtained, the athlete progresses to using a slant board. Occasionally, gravity-assisted stretching will be too painful, and the athlete may have to start with manual stretching. If the involved musculature is in the anterior or lateral compartment, then there is no satisfactory alternative to manual stretching. When full, pain-free motion is obtained, the athlete progresses to phase III.

Phase III

Phase III consists of strength and endurance exercises. Isotonic exercises are preferred, but if they are pain provoking, one should begin with isometrics. The athlete can usually tolerate isotonic exercises if elastic tubing is used for resistance. The gastrocnemius-soleus, evertors, and invertors can all be exercised by holding onto the elastic tubing. To exercise the dorsiflexors, the tubing must be secured or held by an assistant. Progression can be made by changing to tubes of decreasing elasticity or by shortening the length of tubing. For maximal resistance to the gastrocnemius-soleus complex, plantarflexion exercises with weight resting on the shoulders should be performed. All exercises should be performed as two sets of 20 repetitions with 30–60 seconds between sets. This method combines strength and endurance training. When gains of strength and endurance reach a plateau, the athlete can progress to phase IV.

Phase IV

In phase IV, the athlete performs progressive sport-specific functional tasks with the goal of full return to the sport (for example, jogging, followed by running, then sprinting, then hopping). In competitive sports, sideline func-

tional progression tasks are used to assess for return-to-play criteria. If the athlete is able to return to play, his or her injury will still need evaluation and proper four-phase management after the event (or contest).

Tibial Fractures

On-field fracture management of tibial fractures is shown in Table 16-3. The diagnosis of tibial fracture is usually obvious when a deformity is present. If there is any doubt regarding the differential of a major contusion from a nondeforming fracture, then immediate radiographic evaluation should take place.

A tibial fracture should be considered an emergency. Bleeding must be controlled with pressure dressings and bandages (no tourniquets). The leg should be splinted, preferably with an air splint. A pillow splint reinforced by boards on three sides is an alternative if an air splint is not available.[7] The athlete should be assessed for shock, and appropriate emergency measures, including surgical consultation, should be instituted.

Acute Compartment Syndrome

Acute compartment syndrome (ACS) begins with bleeding and fluid accumulation within muscle that is compartmentalized by nondeforming fascia.[8] (The four leg compartments are depicted in Figure 16-2.) An increase in tissue pressure causes a reduction in the arteriovenous gradient and consequently a reduction in local blood flow. This relative ischemia initially causes pain and swelling. If allowed to continue, tissue necrosis will develop.

ACS is usually precipitated by osseous fracture or muscle rupture, but it can occur after any injury to the leg.[8, 9] A high index of suspicion is necessary to diagnose ACS in the face of apparent minor injury. The clinical hallmark of ACS is pain out of proportion to the injury. The onset of severe pain is usually immediate but can be delayed 10–12 hours, especially in minor injuries.[10] The pain is usually a deep, throbbing feeling of unrelenting pressure. If ischemia has already progressed to necrosis, however, pain may be absent.

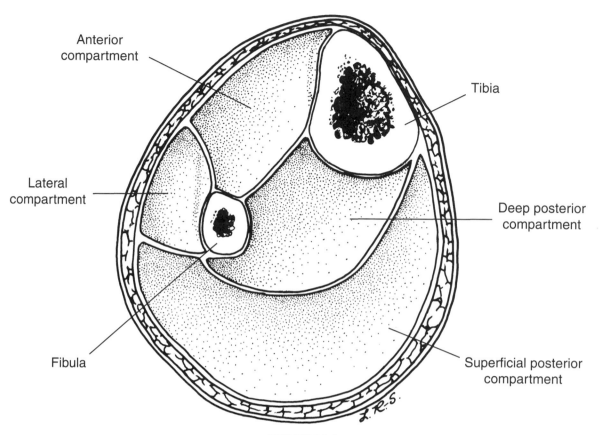

FIGURE 16-2

Cross-section of fascial compartments of the leg. Anterior compartment—nerve: deep peroneal; muscles: tibialis anterior, extensor digitorum longus, extensor hallucis longus, and peroneus tertius. Lateral compartment—nerve: superficial peroneal; muscles: peroneus longus and peroneus brevis. Deep posterior compartment—nerve: tibial; muscles: flexor hallucis longus, flexor digitorum longus, tibialis posterior, and popliteus. Superficial posterior compartment—muscles: gastrocnemius and soleus.

In ACS, the compartment feels tense and swollen and can be accompanied by redness and warmth. Passive stretching of the affected musculature increases pain. There may be paresthesias within the affected nerve distribution (see Figure 16-2). If the condition is allowed to progress, ischemic necrosis causes sensory and motor deficits, and the compartment takes on a woody, hard feeling. Because venous pressure does not rise above arterial pressure, pulses remain intact throughout progression of the syndrome.[8, 9]

Diagnosis of ACS should be made as early as possible to prevent irreversible damage. Clinical findings of ACS are usually so obvious, and time is so precious, that tissue pressure monitoring is of no real importance.[9] In less dramatic cases or in chronic compartment syndrome, measurement of tissue compartment pressures may be useful. The compartment pressure is abnormal if more than 30 mm Hg (normal is 10–20 mm Hg).[4] Once the diagnosis of ACS is

entertained, surgical decompression of the affected compartment(s) should be emergently performed.[8, 9]

EXERCISE-INDUCED PAIN IN THE LOWER LEG

Terminology

The different definitions of shin splint throughout the literature have generated much confusion. The term originated to describe a symptom complex of lower leg pain in marchers and runners. In this chapter, the term *exercise-induced pain in the lower leg* is used to describe this same symptom complex (see Figure 16-1).

The term *shin splint* is used here for an etiologic subset of exercise-induced pain: inflammation that is due to repetitive stress of the broad proximal portion of any of the musculotendinous units originating from the tibia. This narrower definition is consistent with American Medical Association terminology.[11]

Overuse Injuries

Symptoms of overuse injury are precipitated by initiation of training, an increase in training intensity, or a change in surface or equipment. The mechanism for overuse injury is overload of forces on the muscle, tendon, or bone, which leads to an inflammatory reaction.

Shin Splints

Repetitive stress to the lower leg can cause fatigue and failure of the shock-absorbing musculotendinous unit. Musculotendinous injury (shin splint) ensues with partial tearing of muscle, capillary disruption, and inflammation.[4] Initially, the intensity is usually not severe; thus the athlete often attempts to train through the pain, which causes further tissue injury.

Anterior shin splints cause pain and tenderness located lateral to the tibia over the anterior compartment. Posterior shin splints cause symptoms along the posteromedial border of the middle to lower tibia over the posterior compartment.[4] The pain can be reproduced by resisted active movement of the affected muscle. There may be weakness of the affected muscle as well.[4] Diagnostic studies are helpful only in ruling out other conditions, such as stress fracture.

Medial Tibial Stress Syndrome

Medial tibial stress syndrome (MTSS) presents as exercise-induced pain localized to the distal posteromedial border of the tibia. The clinical distinction between posterior shin splints and MTSS is hazy, but the latter is usually more focal and more painful. Stress fractures can also present similarly and often must be ruled out with appropriate plain films and bone scans.[12]

The precise pathophysiology of MTSS is controversial. The most likely explanation is periosteal inflammation (periostitis)[12] near the origin of the posterior tibialis or the medial soleus. Examination reveals a well-localized 3- to 6-cm area of tenderness over the posteromedial edge of the distal one-third of the tibia.[13] The tenderness may increase after exertion. Induration is sometimes present. Active plantarflexion and inversion of the foot against manual resistance may reproduce the pain.[13]

Plain x-ray films in MTSS are always initially negative and usually remain negative. After 3–4 weeks, x-ray films may show hypertrophy of the cortex in a small percentage of patients.[12] Bone scan, while always normal in the angiogram and blood pool phases, can show mild uptake

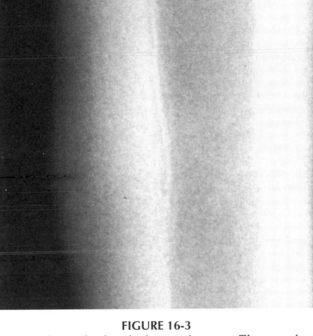

FIGURE 16-3

Plain radiograph of a tibial stress fracture. There are both periosteal and endosteal thickening and a cortical disruption commonly called the "dreaded black line" (due to the prolonged time necessary for healing).

in the delayed phase (Figure 16-3).[14] When the bone scan is positive, the diffuse linear fusiform "stress reaction" pattern is distinguishable from the more focal fusiform stress fracture pattern (Table 16-4).[15]

Stress Fracture

Fractures of the lower extremities account for 95% of all stress fractures in athletes.[16] Approximately one-half occur in the tibia or fibula. Fractures of the fibula, the most common site in runners,[17] usually occur 3–7 cm above the lateral malleolus. The two most common tibial sites are the proximal tibia and the junction of middle and distal thirds of the tibia.[18] Rarely, a combined tibial and fibular stress fracture develops.

Stress fractures result from fatigue failure within bone, although the surrounding muscle may actually fatigue

TABLE 16-4
Bone Scan Findings: Stress Fracture versus Medial Tibial Stress Syndrome (MTSS)

	Stress Fracture	MTSS
Angiogram/blood pool phases (I and II)	Positive (if acute, <1 mo)	Negative
Delayed phase (III)		
Shape	Fusiform, longitudinal	Linear, longitudinal
Location	Posterior tibial cortex, junction mid/distal tibia	Posterior tibial cortex, junction mid/distal tibia
Size	Focal, <⅕ length of tibia	Diffuse, ⅓–¾ length of tibia

first. Increased or different activity results in an altered relationship of bone growth and repair (Wolff law). When remodeling predominates over repair, the cortex transiently weakens and, if stress continues, eventually ruptures. The resulting stress fracture may run the spectrum from a microfracture with simple cortical hypertrophy to rupture of the bony cortices with a fracture line.[19]

Symptoms of stress fracture are usually gradual in onset over a 2- to 3-week period.[19] They are similar to symptoms of the other overuse injuries but are usually more localized and more severe. There is almost always point tenderness.[20] A positive percussion sign (transmission of pain to the fracture site area on percussion of the bone at a distance) is helpful in distinguishing stress fracture from

shin splint or MTSS but is not always present.[19] Sometimes, there is palpable swelling on the bone.

Plain x-ray films taken within 3–4 weeks of onset of symptoms are almost always negative. Multiple views are needed, because seldom is there an obvious fracture line, and often only a single cortex of bone is involved (vague lucent cortical striation).[20] Eventually, x-ray films usually reveal subperiosteal new bone formation (callus) or cortical thickening, demonstrating a healing reaction (Figure 16-4). Because x-ray findings may take as long as 3 months to be evident, and because 67% of initial x-rays are negative,[21] normal x-rays should not preclude the diagnosis of stress fracture as long as symptoms persist.

Bone scan is the gold-standard test to diagnose a stress fracture. The scan may be positive as early as 3 days after injury, and false-positive scans are infrequent.[19] The isotope technetium-99 diphosphonate is incorporated into new bone formation and shows increased activity at the site of stress fracture. A triple-phase study is preferred (see Table 16-4 for specific findings). The angiogram and blood pool phases of the triple-phase bone scan are positive only in acute stress fractures, whereas the delayed scan may remain positive for 6 months to 2 years.[22]

Tendinitis
Another common lower leg overuse injury, tendinitis about the ankle, is discussed in Chapter 18.

Treatment of Overuse Injuries
The principles of initial treatment and rehabilitation of overuse injuries are similar to those for acute injuries (see Table 16-2), but the emphasis on certain components is different. Because the duration of treatment phases is often longer than that for acute injuries, compliance often determines the success of treatment.

Rest of the affected muscle-tendon-bone unit is the mainstay of treatment in phase I, particularly avoidance of impact activities. Any activity that causes pain should be discontinued. If simple weightbearing or walking is painful, then crutches, bracing (such as long pneumatic air stirrup), or even cast immobilization should be used

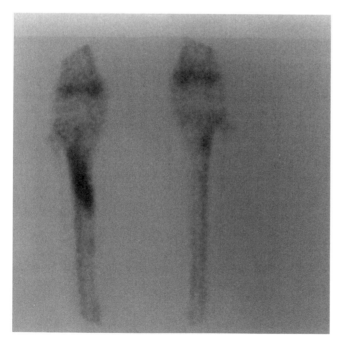

FIGURE 16-4
Bone scan of tibial stress reaction. Radionuclide bone phase image shows asymmetric diffuse increased uptake in the proximal medial tibia.

as needed to achieve pain-free ambulation. The athlete must not try to work through the pain. Both shin splints and MTSS can progress to stress fracture, and stress fractures may progress to complete cortical breaks (see Figure 16-3).[19] Cross-training with nonimpact activities, such as cycling, swimming, and pool running, can begin as soon as walking and daily activities are nonpainful. Cross-training guards against deconditioning and shortens the rehabilitation period, but if symptoms are elicited, it should be modified or discontinued.

The duration of impact avoidance varies from 1 to 2 days for mild shin splints to several months for severe stress fractures. A shin splint may not require a cessation of training but rather a reduction in intensity and duration. Elite athletes may continue to compete if predisposing biomechanical factors can be corrected with in-shoe orthotics and as long as training intensity is lessened and symptoms are monitored closely. MTSS usually requires cessation of training for at least 1 week, followed by a return to training at reduced intensity. Stress fractures, on the other hand, require a much more stringent approach for bone remodeling to take place. A traditional approach involves cessation of running for 3–6 weeks in a fibula fracture and 4–10 weeks in a tibial stress fracture, with 3–4 months before returning to full training in the latter.

Pneumatic leg braces (air splints) are advocated by some authors as a method of shortening the rest period and allowing earlier resumption of training for athletes with shin splints, MTSS, and stress fractures. Subjects in a prospective controlled study who wore leg braces returned to light activity 7 days after the diagnosis of a stress fracture (compared with 21 days for the other traditionally treated group) and returned to full activity at 21 days (versus 77 days).[23] This study and prior uncontrolled air splint studies lack long-term follow-up to assess for possible recurrences. Cast immobilization, although rarely required,[24] has been recommended by some authors for midtibial shaft stress fractures because of their high incidence of delayed union.[25] Duration of casting depends on resolution of pain and radiographic evidence of callus formation.[24] Rarely, midtibial shaft stress fractures require surgery, including intramedullary fixation and lesion excision with bone grafting.[26] Candidates for surgery include elite athletes and patients who have failed 6 months of conservative measures.[27]

Phase I management, analogous to traumatic injuries, also uses ice, compression, and elevation to reduce swelling and inflammation. Icing should continue as long as any symptoms are present. Nonsteroidal anti-inflammatory drugs (NSAIDs) are believed to be beneficial in most types of overuse injury. In stress fractures, however, they may have no advantage over simple analgesics.[17] Hormonal replacement should be considered in thin, amenorrheal female cross-country runners.[19]

Phase II management (motion restoration) begins when there is no pain at rest. Stretching protocols are similar to those discussed under Acute Pain, except that for overuse injuries, emphasis is placed on all muscle groups surrounding the injury, not just the injured one. Gravity-assisted stretching for the gastrocnemius-soleus complex and manual stretching for the dorsiflexors, invertors, and evertors are performed. The hip and thigh muscles should also be included, using standard stretching postures. The athlete should not advance past phase II if there is any local tenderness or pain with daily activities.

Strength imbalance between the powerful plantarflexors and the weaker dorsiflexors may be one of the contributing factors in lower leg overuse injury; thus, phase III strengthening is of paramount importance. Elastic tubing exercises can be used initially (as discussed under Management of Lower Leg Muscle Strains and Contusions). They should be used as resistance against all lower leg muscle groups (plantarflexors, dorsiflexors, evertors, and invertors). When elastic tubing resistance is maximized, the dorsiflexors, invertors, and evertors can be exercised against resistance by strapping weights to the ankle. The powerful plantarflexors may require standing resistive exercises with weights resting on the shoulders. Thigh, hip, and trunk strengthening should proceed using standard isotonic or isokinetic equipment. Phase III exercises should continue at least until strength plateaus, preferably longer.

Phase IV—a sport-specific (functional progression) training program beginning at low intensity—can usually be started before completion of phase III. Any return in local pain is an indication that the program is advancing too rapidly, and the athlete should be reevaluated.

To prevent recurrence of overuse injury, it is imperative to review and correct faulty training methods and to evaluate for biomechanical factors. Of all running injuries, 60% result from training errors such as overzealous training, improper footwear, and running on hard, uneven, or inclined surfaces.[28] Proper footwear cannot be overemphasized, and the reader is referred to Drez's excellent discussion for details.[29]

Direct observation or videotaping of training routines may reveal biomechanical abnormalities that are not noticeable on routine examination. Deviations from the normal leg-heel-forefoot alignment are carefully sought. Malalignment problems include pes planus, tibia vara, tibial torsion, subtalar joint varus, forefoot supination, and heel cord tightness.[4] Overpronation, a very common biomechanical abnormality, may be a primary condition or may be secondary to one of the other alignment problems. Excessive pronation reduces the mechanical efficiency of the lower limb and increases stress on the posterior tibial tendon and muscle.[29]

Overpronation, and perhaps some of the malalignments, may be compensated for with foot orthotics. The goals of in-shoe orthotics include (among others) (1) to maintain the neutral subtalar joint position when the talar head clinically cannot be palpated to bulge asymmetrically on either side of the ankle joint, (2) to decrease overpronation and prolonged pronation using anterior medial or posterior medial wedges, (3) to reduce pressure on the forefoot, and (4) to address leg length discrepancies. Soft orthotics (taping, soft wedges) should be tried before fabrication of custom-molded, rigid orthotics.[12]

Nontraumatic Vascular Conditions

Vascular claudication, another subset of exercise-induced lower leg pain, may occur in athletes in the absence of significant atherosclerotic disease. The reader is referred to Figure 16-1 for the differential diagnosis.

Chronic (Effort-Related) Compartment Syndrome

Chronic compartment syndrome (CCS) is a common cause of lower leg claudication in the athlete. CCS, like ACS, causes an elevation of tissue pressures. Unlike ACS, the elevation occurs only with exercise, the ischemia is reversible, and symptoms resolve after cessation of exercise. CCS occurs most often in the anterior compartment and is frequently bilateral.[8] CCS in the deep posterior compartment is a controversial clinical entity.[30] Distance runners and athletes exposed to significant impact stress to the lower extremities are most likely to develop CCS.[31]

The pathophysiology of CCS is not well understood. In normal individuals, compartment pressures can increase to 3–4 times baseline values after vigorous activity, but rapidly return to normal within a few minutes.[32] In CCS, the elevation is higher and persists longer. Several different factors may contribute to the abnormality, including muscle hypertrophy, fascial compartment that is too small or too inelastic,[8] myofascial scarring, venous hypertension, and posttraumatic soft tissue inflammation.[33]

Symptoms of CCS may be nonspecific, but they are always reproducible for a given amount of exercise and always occur at the same site (usually the anterior compartment muscles) (see Figure 16-2). Typically, there is lower leg pain with muscle tightness or a cramplike feeling and sometimes weakness or numbness. With ACS, the deep peroneal nerve is involved and will cause numbness in the first web space. With lateral compartment

involvement, compression of the superficial peroneal nerve causes paresthesias over the dorsum of the foot. Symptoms usually resolve within minutes if the activity is immediately stopped but can persist for much longer if the activity is continued. Physical examination at rest is almost always unremarkable. A few individuals will have weakness of the involved compartment (see Figure 16-2). Occasionally, a fascial hernia is present.[33] Physical examination after vigorous exercise sometimes reveals tenderness and tenseness of the affected compartment.

Tissue pressure monitoring must be performed to establish the diagnosis of CCS. Pressure measurements are made both before and after a standard exercise test. Postexercise pressure in excess of 15 mm Hg persisting for longer than 15 minutes is abnormal.[4] Electrodiagnostic testing is usually normal, even if performed postexercise, and therefore adds little information.[17]

Unlike the overuse injuries, CCS does not respond to rest, NSAIDs, and therapeutic exercise.[31] Symptoms may improve temporarily with conservative measures but quickly return once vigorous physical activity is resumed. The only effective treatment is surgical compartment release (fasciotomy). Studies in the literature reveal an 85–92% success rate with fasciotomy in relieving CCS symptoms.[34-36] Unsuccessful fasciotomies result when compartments are not adequately decompressed or when the posterior or deep posterior compartments are involved but overlooked.[30, 37, 38] The only alternative to surgery is to quit the sport activity completely or to participate within the limits of pain.[32] If left untreated, there is a risk of developing ACS with irreversible ischemia, especially when attempting to perform through the pain.[32]

Popliteal Artery Entrapment

An unusual cause of lower leg claudication is entrapment of the popliteal artery in the popliteal fossa. This syndrome is usually the result of a congenital abnormality involving the relationship between the popliteal artery and the medial head of the gastrocnemius muscle.[39-41] The anatomic anomaly is bilateral in 25% of cases.[39] Each plantarflexion motion potentially causes reversible occlusion of the popliteal artery. The recurrent pressure can cause splitting of the vessel wall and subsequent premature focal atherosclerosis.[39] Occasionally, there is progression to complete arterial occlusion.[42]

The claudication of popliteal artery syndrome occurs with running or walking and can be exacerbated by going up a ramp.[41] The claudication pain disappears a few minutes after cessation of activity.[40] Other associated symptoms may be coolness, blanching, paresthesias, and numbness of the foot.[39]

Physical examination of the athlete with popliteal artery entrapment may reveal diminution or absence of popliteal, posterior tibial, or dorsalis pedis pulse. Examination of pulses should be performed before and after exercise sufficient to reproduce symptoms. Coolness and pallor are also present if examined during symptoms. When the diagnosis is suspected, noninvasive testing (Doppler ultrasonography or pulse volume recording) should initially be performed. McDonald and colleagues[41] recommended ramped treadmill walking with ankle-brachial arterial pressure measurements taken before and after the exercise. Angiography, the diagnostic gold standard, is indicated when noninvasive testing is positive or when there is a high index of suspicion. The treatment of popliteal artery entrapment is surgical decompression with arterial repair as necessary.[39-41]

Adductor Canal Syndrome

A much rarer cause of lower leg claudication is thrombosis of the superficial femoral artery at the level of the adductor hiatus. The source of constriction is believed to be the vastus medialis or adductor magnus tendon (or hypertrophied band of this tendon).[39] Symptoms are calf claudication, numbness, paresthesias, and coolness of the foot. As with popliteal artery entrapment, distal pulses are absent or diminished, definitive diagnosis is via angiography, and treatment is surgical.

Effort (Venous) Thrombosis

Deep venous thrombosis (effort thrombosis) rarely occurs in the lower extremity of the otherwise healthy athlete. The physical examination, workup, and treatment are identical to those for the nonathlete with deep venous thrombosis.[43]

Neurogenic Pain

Lumbosacral Radiculopathy

Lumbosacral radiculopathies can occasionally cause leg pain without associated back pain. Peripheral nerve entrapments must also be considered in the differential diagnosis. The peroneal nerve is the most likely entrapment to cause primary lower leg pain.

Peroneal (Superficial) Nerve Entrapment

Compression of the peroneal nerve usually occurs at the site where it emerges from the lateral compartment, 8–15 cm proximal to the lateral malleolus.[44] Predisposing factors include fascial herniation, lipoma, prolonged peroneus tunnel, ankle sprain, anomalous course of the nerve, or previous anterior compartment fasciotomy.[44] Overzeal-

ous cryotherapy below the knee can also cause a peroneal neuropathy.

Symptoms of the syndrome are numbness or paresthesias of the dorsum of the foot during exercise and occasionally at rest.[44] Decreased sensation over the dorsum of the foot after exercise is the most consistent finding.[44] Pain on percussion of the compression site (Tinel sign) or pain when the ankle is passively flexed and supinated is sometimes present.

Electrodiagnostic testing (electromyography and nerve conduction velocities) is helpful in diagnosing and assessing the severity of peroneal nerve entrapment. However, one-half of those tested have normal electrodiagnostic studies at rest.[44] Definitive treatment is surgical.[44]

REFERENCES

1. McGee SR. Muscle cramps. Arch Intern Med 1990;150: 511–518.
2. Miller AP. Strains of the posterior calf musculature (tennis leg). Am J Sports Med 1979;7:172–174.
3. Miller WM. Rupture of the musculotendinous junction of the medial head of the gastrocnemius muscle. Am J Sports Med 1977;5:191–193.
4. Nicholas JA, Hershman EB (eds). The Lower Extremity and Spine in Sports Medicine. St. Louis: Mosby, 1986;49–53, 601–655, 1100–1109.
5. Ciullo JV, Zarins B. Biomechanics of the musculotendinous unit. Clin Sports Med 1983;1:71–86.
6. Walton M, Rothwell AG. Reactions of thigh tissues of sheep to blunt trauma. Clin Orthop 1983;176:273–281.
7. Connolly JF (ed). DePalma's The Management of Fractures and Dislocations. Philadelphia: Saunders, 1981;135–141, 1724–1800.
8. Black KP, Shultz TK, Cheung NL. Compartment syndromes in athletes. Clin Sports Med 1990;9:471–487.
9. Mubarak SJ, Hargans AR. Acute compartment syndromes. Surg Clin North Am 1983;63:539–565.
10. Egan TD, Joyce SM. Acute compartment syndrome following a minor athletic injury. J Emerg Med 1989;7:353–357.
11. American Medical Association, Subcommittee on Classification of Sports Injuries. Standard Nomenclature of Athletic Injuries. Chicago: American Medical Association, 1966;122–126.
12. Mubarak SJ, Gould RN, Lee YF, et al. The medial tibial stress syndrome. Am J Sports Med 1982;10:201–205.
13. Jones DC, James SL. Overuse injuries of the lower extremity. Clin Sports Med 1987;6:273–290.
14. Rupani HD, Holder LE, Espinola DA, et al. Three-phase radionuclide bone imaging in sports medicine. Radiology 1985;156:187–196.
15. Datz FL. Handbook of Nuclear Medicine (2nd ed). St. Louis: Mosby, 1993;76–77.

16. Hulkko A, Orava S. Stress fractures in athletes. Int J Sports Med 1987;8:221–226.
17. D'Ambrosia RD, Drez D. Prevention and Treatment of Running Injuries. Thorofare, NJ: Slack, 1982;21–42,89–108.
18. Devas MB (ed). Stress Fractures. London: Churchill Livingstone, 1975.
19. Markey KL. Stress fractures. Clin Sports Med 1987;6:405–425.
20. Detmer DE. Chronic leg pain. Am J Sports Med 1980;8:141–144.
21. Sterling JC, Edelstein DW, Calvo RD, et al. Stress fractures in the athlete—diagnosis and management. J Sports Med 1992;14:336–346.
22. Matire JR. The role of nuclear medicine bone scans in evaluating pain in athletic injuries. Clin Sports Med 1987;6:713–737.
23. Swenson EJ, DeHaven KE, Sebastianelli WJ, et al. The effect of a pneumatic leg brace on return to play for athletes with tibial stress fractures. Am J Sports Med 1997;25:322–328.
24. Monteleone GP. Stress fractures in the athlete. Orthop Clin North Am 1995;26:423–432.
25. Orava S, Karpakka J, Hulkko A, et al. Diagnosis and treatment of stress fractures located at the mid-tibial shaft in athletes. Int J Sports Med 1991;12:419–422.
26. Hershman EB, Mailly T. Stress fractures. Clin Sports Med 1990;9:183–214.
27. Taube RR, Wadsworth LT. Managing tibial stress fractures. Phys Sportsmed 1993;21:123–128.
28. Cook SD, Brinker MR, Poche M. Running shoes: their relationship to running injuries. Sports Med 1990;10:1–8.
29. Drez D. Running footwear: examination of the training shoe, the foot, and functional orthotic devices. Am J Sports Med 1980;8:140–141.
30. Styf J. Diagnosis of exercise-induced pain in the anterior aspect of the lower leg. Am J Sports Med 1988;16:165–169.
31. Turnipseed W, Detmer DE, Girdley F. Chronic compartment syndrome. Ann Surg 1989;210:557–562.
32. Martens MA, Moeyersoons JP. Acute and recurrent effort-related compartment syndrome in sports. Sports Med 1990;9:62–68.
33. Detmer DE, Sharpe K, Sufit RL, Girdley FM. Chronic compartment syndrome: diagnosis, management and outcomes. Am J Sports Med 1989;13:162–170.
34. Wiley JP, Clement DB, Doyle DL, et al. A primary care perspective of chronic compartment syndrome. Phys Sportsmed 1987;15:111–118.
35. Fronek J, Mubarak SJ, Hargens AR, et al. Management of chronic exertional anterior compartment syndrome of the lower extremity. Clin Orthop 1987;220:217–227.
36. Martens MA, Backaert M, Vermaut G, et al. Chronic leg pain in athletes due to a recurrent compartment syndrome. Am J Sports Med 1984;12:148–151.
37. Davey JR, Rorabeck CH, and Fowler PJ. The tibialis posterior muscle compartment: an unrecognized cause of exertional compartment syndrome. Am J Sports Med 1984;12:391–396.
38. Rorabeck CH, Fowler PJ, Nott L. The results of fasciotomy in the management of chronic exertional compartment syndrome. Am J Sports Med 1988;16:224–227.
39. Cohn SL, Taylor WC. Vascular problems of the lower extremity in athletes. Clin Sports Med 1990;9:449–470.
40. Lysens RJ, Renson LM, Ostyn MS, Stalpaert G. Intermittent claudication in young athletes: popliteal artery entrapment syndrome. Am J Sports Med 1983;11:177–182.
41. McDonald PT, Easterbrook JA, Rich NM, et al. Popliteal artery entrapment syndrome: clinical, non-invasive and angiographic diagnosis. Am J Surg 1981;139:318–325.
42. Brener BJ, Alpert J, Brief DK, et al. Limb loss in a young man due to entrapment of the popliteal artery. J Med Soc N J 1975;72:47–51.
43. Harvey JS. Effort thrombosis in the lower extremity of a runner. Am J Sports Med 1978;6:400–402.
44. Styf J. Chronic exercise-induced pain in the anterior aspect of the lower leg. Sports Med 1989;7:331–339.

17

Foot Injuries

Daniel R. Kraeger

Few injuries are more debilitating to the athlete than those of the foot (Figures 17-1 and 17-2). The stress applied to one's foot in running is thee to five times one's body weight.[1] The foot strikes the ground between 1,000 and 2,000 times per mile, depending on the stride length.[2, 3] Injuries involving the foot rank behind only the knee as the most common injuries associated with sports.[3, 4] Statistically, the foot is involved in 30–40% of all running injuries.[5] This chapter is divided into discussions of acute and chronic injuries.

ACUTE FOOT INJURIES

Figure 17-3 shows acute foot injuries.

Metatarsal Fractures

Fifth Metatarsal Fractures

The most commonly fractured metatarsal is the fifth.[6] Acute fractures are caused by a direct blow (for example, having the foot stepped on) or a sudden impact (for example, a faulty dismount in gymnastics). Fractures of the proximal diaphysis of the fifth metatarsal bone are known as *Jones fractures* (Figure 17-4) and should not be confused with metaphyseal or avulsion fractures of the proximal fifth metatarsal (Figure 17-5). Jones fractures are discussed at length under Chronic Foot Injuries. Acute nondisplaced metaphyseal fractures of the fifth metatarsal should be treated nonweightbearing for 1–3 weeks in a short leg cast or, in a reliable patient, a walking boot (e.g., High Tide Walker [Donjoy, Carlsbad, CA]). Weightbearing is allowed when there is no pain with ambulating and immobilization is continuous for a total of 4–6 weeks. Avulsion fractures of the proximal fifth metatarsal usually do well with strapping and a postoperative shoe.

An alternative to strapping is a commercial ankle device; for example, the Air Cast Stirrup (Air Cast, Inc., Summit, NJ) or the ASO ankle stabilizer (Medical Specialties, Inc., Charlotte, NC). When the tenderness resolves, the athlete may begin a gradual return to play.

Lesser Metatarsal Fractures

Nondisplaced fractures of the second through the fourth metatarsals usually do well with a cotton or elastic wrap for 24–48 hours or until the swelling subsides. This is followed by a walking boot or postoperative shoe. Displaced or angulated fractures of the metatarsal neck and shaft should generally be referred for reductions, depending on the degree of angulation and the primary care physician's experience in their management.

Phalangeal Fractures and Dislocations

Fractures and dislocations of the phalanges are caused by kicking an object or by stubbing the toe. Symptoms include localized pain, swelling, and discoloration. Treatment for bone shaft fractures in the toe involves ice, elevation, and buddy taping. The fractured toe is taped to the adjoining toe with a felt or foam pad between the toes. Wearing a postoperative shoe or a shoe with a wide toe box is beneficial. Usually these injuries heal in 3–4 weeks with decreased activity; however, they can remain tender for months. Referral to the orthopedist should be considered if the fracture involves the proximal phalanx of the great toe or the interphalangeal joint.

If recognized early, phalangeal dislocations can usually be reduced with traction on the toe. The toe should be taped, and the athlete should wear a postoperative shoe if bending the toe is painful. Dancers must refrain for several weeks to minimize the likelihood of recurrent subluxations or dislocations. Dislocations of the first

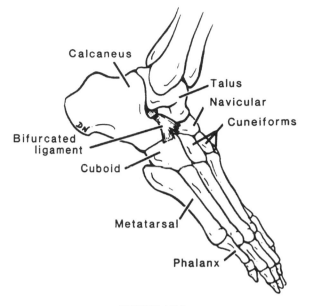

FIGURE 17-1
Normal lateral anatomy of the foot with the bifurcated ligament.

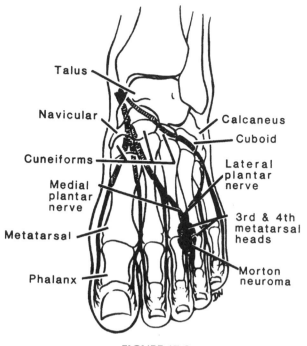

FIGURE 17-2
Normal dorsal anatomy of the foot with Morton neuroma.

metatarsophalangeal joint (MTP) can cause a problem with displacement or secondary fractures of the sesamoids (see Chronic Foot Injuries). Recurrent dislocations should be referred for possible surgery.

Cuboid Subluxation

This may be referred to as the *cuboid syndrome*. The athlete presents with acute, severe pain and sometimes swelling localized to the calcaneocuboid joint. Affected athletes often report lateral midfoot pain that they are unable to

"work through." Palpation of the plantar aspect of the foot over the cuboid produces pain. Roentgenograms are generally unremarkable, and the diagnosis is made clinically.

The treatment is by manipulation of the cuboid and usually brings immediate relief. To manipulate the bone, the athlete is directed to lie prone on a table with his or her affected leg hanging off the table. Standing at the foot end of the table, the examiner grasps the athlete's foot with

FIGURE 17-3
Algorithm of acute foot injuries.

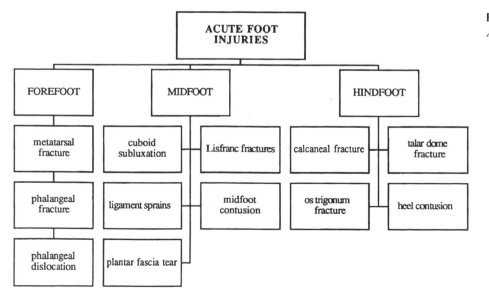

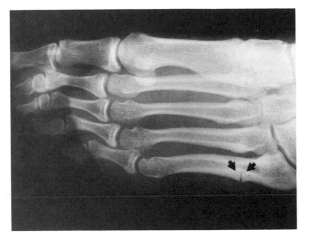

FIGURE 17-4
Jones fracture, proximal diaphysis of the fifth metatarsal (arrows).

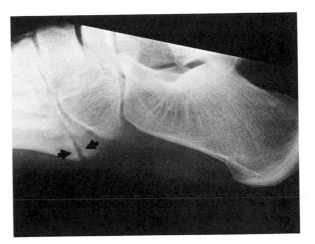

FIGURE 17-5
Avulsion fracture of the fifth metatarsal (arrows).

both thumbs pressing on the plantar surface of the cuboid. With a subtle whip action, the examiner shakes the athlete's leg up and down a few times while pressing hard with the thumbs (Figure 17-6). This action usually allows the cuboid to move dorsally back into place. This should be followed with a LowDye tape procedure to give the arch added support for 1–2 weeks. A gradual return to running may occur when the pain subsides (typically, in 1–2 weeks).

Lisfranc Fractures and Dislocations

A Lisfranc fracture involves the metatarsal head (most notably the second metatarsal) and its associated cuneiform. This fracture is often missed because it is difficult to diagnose on plain radiographs. The athlete presents with the history of having twisted the foot in a fall or having another athlete fall on the foot. This axial loading causes a disruption of the tarsometatarsal joint. Swelling ecchymosis and tenderness are present on the dorsum of the foot.

On the anteroposterior plain film, the most important alignment is the medial margin of the second metatarsal base and the medial border of the middle cuneiform. Roentgenograms should also include an oblique film to examine the medial border of the fourth metatarsal and the medial aspect of the cuboid. A comparison view of the other foot is also recommended. Any malalignment suggests a significant soft tissue injury and should be referred to the orthopedist. A small avulsion fracture, particularly at the base of the second metatarsal, frequently indicates a Lisfranc injury. Magnetic resonance imaging (MRI) or computed tomography (CT) may be needed to make the diagnosis.[7, 8]

Treatment for these fractures frequently involves surgery, so referral is strongly advised. It is now thought that optimum results are achieved with open anatomic reduction.[8]

Ligament Sprains

Ligament sprains can occur to the ligaments of the foot. The calcaneonavicular ligament sprain presents with localized pain on standing or palpation. Treatment is similar to that for an ankle sprain with rest, ice, compression,

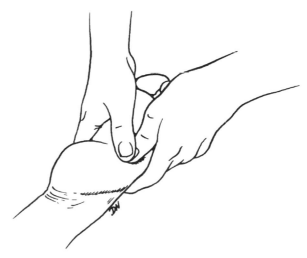

FIGURE 17-6
Proper positioning of the thumbs over the plantar surface of the cuboid. Pressure is exerted dorsally, performing the cuboid squeeze.

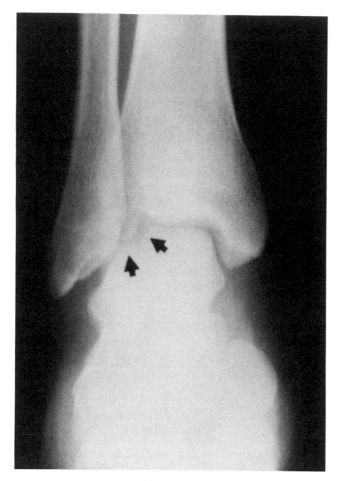

FIGURE 17-7
An obvious fracture of the lateral talar dome (arrows).

and elevation (RICE) and a commercial arch support (1st Step, [Foot Tech, Inc., St. Louis, MO]) or LowDye taping to support the arch. McConnell tape works best when taping the arch if you want it to stay on for several days.

When the bifurcated ligament (see Figure 17-1) is sprained, occasionally a small avulsion fracture is seen from the calcaneal attachment. Midfoot or forefoot sprains occur with excessive dorsiflexion or plantarflexion of the toes or forefoot. The tendons and muscles are usually involved in this soft tissue injury. It is imperative that a significant Lisfranc injury is ruled out before diagnosing this as a sprain.

Significant midfoot sprains should be treated initially with either a cast or arch support and immobilizer for 3–4 weeks. This is followed by progressive rehabilitation and wearing a stiff-soled shoe. For forefoot sprains (MTP sprains), consider using a Turf Toe insole (Foot Management Inc., Pittsville, MD) or postoperative shoe to decrease the bending of the joints. Often, an insert in the shoe of the injured foot is sufficient; however, in athletes

who are runners, use an insert in both shoes to prevent imbalance.[9]

Midfoot Contusion

Often referred to as a *bruised instep*, this injury is commonly the result of a direct blow from a baseball or a hockey puck. Treatment consists of RICE along with decreased weightbearing. Wearing a shoe may be difficult early on, and crutches may be helpful. The athlete may return to play as the symptoms subside. A roentgenogram may be warranted to rule out fracture, depending on the severity of the injury.

Plantar Fascia Tear

Although a gross tear of the plantar fascia is rare, the athlete may present with an acute burning pain in the arch of the foot secondary to microtears of the fascia. The differential diagnosis should include a stress fracture, ligament sprain, and plantar fasciitis. One should always check the dorsiflexion of the ankle to test the length of the Achilles tendon (heel cord). Treatment is similar to that for ligament sprains, with RICE and an arch support. Stretching exercises to improve the flexibility of the plantar fascia and Achilles tendon may be necessary (see also the discussion of treatment under Plantar Fasciitis).

Calcaneal Fracture

Calcaneal fractures are usually due to recurrent stress, unless they are secondary to acute trauma. In an acute fracture, the athlete presents with heel pain, swelling, and ecchymosis. Treatment for a nondisplaced calcaneal fracture consists of RICE, decreased activity, and either a cast or a heel pad for protection. Most athletes are able to return to sports in approximately 8 weeks. Calcaneal stress fractures are discussed under Chronic Foot Injuries.

Talar Dome Fracture

Talar dome fractures occur acutely; however, they are often treated as chronic injuries because they go unnoticed initially (Figure 17-7). The athlete usually presents with anterior ankle and foot pain. The fractures may or may not be associated with ligamentous instability. Roentgenograms often do not demonstrate a fracture because the injury causes a compression fracture of the articular surface of the talus. Six weeks may pass before a plain roentgenogram shows a fracture of the talar dome. The athlete has generally been treated for a sprain and returns to activity 2–3 weeks later.

This entity should be considered if the athlete reports persistent stiffness, instability, or catching and locking of the ankle. Technetium scintigraphy (bone scan) is useful to screen for this injury or other occult fractures. If there is a focal area of increased uptake, the lesion can be defined better with a fine CT scan or MRI. When suspected or diagnosed, referral should be made for consideration of arthroscopy of the ankle to make the definitive diagnosis and treat the injury. An orthopedic referral is warranted if one suspects or diagnoses this injury.[10]

Lateral Talus Fracture ("Snowboarder's Fracture")

Fractures of the lateral process of the talus have been occurring in increasing numbers with the popularity of snowboarding. The mechanism of injury involves severe ankle dorsiflexion and inversion. This force produces a shearing stress transmitted from the calcaneus to the lateral process, resulting in a fracture fragment of variable size. Swelling and ecchymosis occur over the lateral ankle, which can easily be associated with an ankle sprain. As many as 40% of these fractures are missed on initial radiographs because it is difficult to see the fracture on standard views.[11] If clinical suspicion is high, a CT or MRI should be done. A high index of suspicion is needed to find these fractures, and they should be thought of when snowboarders present with an ankle injury.

For a small avulsion fracture that does not involve the articular surface, conservative treatment with nonweightbearing immobilization for 4–6 weeks is appropriate. Fractures involving the articular surface or displaced fractures are best treated by open reduction and internal fixation or excision.[12]

Os Trigonum Fracture

The os trigonum is an accessory bone found posterior to the posterior tubercle of the talus (Figure 17-8). It is present in 5–20% of the population and is unilateral in two-thirds of these individuals.[13, 14] It may be fused to the talus or calcaneus, or both. It is a benign incidental finding until the athlete presents with pain because it is fractured.

Pain is in the posterolateral ankle and is often persistent. Athletes present with tenderness to palpation posterior to the tibia but anterior to the Achilles tendon. Pain is enhanced by forced plantarflexion of the ankle. Swelling is present, and the athlete may report the ankle "giving way." The injured ankle will show a 25% decrease in plantarflexion in comparison with the other side.[14]

Roentgenographic evaluation should include a mortise view in addition to the anteroposterior and lateral views of the ankle. Diagnosis based on the plain film alone may be difficult, and often a bone scan is needed to differentiate between acute and old fractures. Treat-

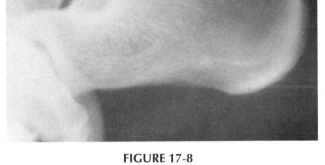

FIGURE 17-8

An example of an os trigonum (arrows). This was an incidental finding on a roentgenogram.

ment consists of a short leg cast for 6 weeks, followed by reexamination. If the ankle remains painful, the cast should be continued for 2–3 more weeks. If symptoms persist for 4–6 months, however, referral for surgical excision is warranted.[10]

Heel Contusion

Heel contusion is, by far, the most disabling contusion that an athlete will ever experience. Hurdlers and long jumpers as well as basketball and volleyball players are prone to this injury. The athlete reports severe heel pain and is unable to bear weight on the affected heel. This condition often develops into a chronic inflammation of the periosteum and can persist for the entire athletic season. A fracture should be ruled out with calcaneal roentgenograms and bone scan if necessary.

Treatment includes RICE and crutches for the first few days to eliminate any weightbearing. If the pain has sub-

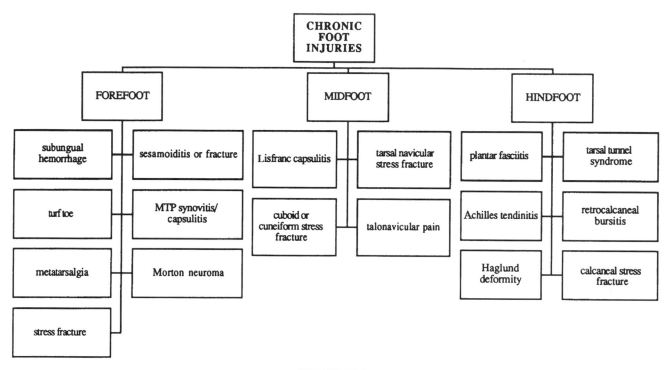

FIGURE 17-9
Algorithm of chronic foot injuries. (MTP = metatarsophalangeal [joint].)

sided after a few days, the athlete may progress to heel cups or pads and eliminate the crutches. The heel cups should be worn in street shoes and athletic shoes. Cold whirlpools along with ultrasound may be beneficial. A slow return to activity, continuing the use of heel cups, begins when the athlete can jog without pain.

CHRONIC FOOT INJURIES

Figure 17-9 lists chronic foot injuries. In the diagnosis and treatment of persistent chronic foot conditions, the biomechanics of the foot in walking and occasionally running should be considered and evaluated for factors that may contribute to the chronic injury. The most common contributing abnormalities are overpronation and prolonged pronation. Intervention ranges from LowDye taping to over-the-counter arch supports to custom-made in-shoe orthotics.

Subungual Hemorrhage and Painful Toenails

Referred to as the "blue toenail syndrome," painful and black toenails are often the result of improper footwear worn by the athlete. Athletes with toes that hyperextend and rub on the underside of the shoe may also present with this injury. Shoes should be analyzed for proper length or

insufficient height within the toe box. A metatarsal pad should be placed beneath the metatarsal heads to straighten the toes. In sports such as tennis and basketball, in which the foot slides forward to jam the toes, a helpful device is the tongue pad. This is an oval felt pad that is placed underneath the tongue of the shoe and acts as a wedge block to keep the foot from sliding forward.[15]

If the hemorrhage is recent, treatment consists of using a disposable, battery-operated cautery device to puncture a hole in the nail. Most emergency rooms throw these away after one use and will be glad to give them away (although it is thought that any virus would be killed on the tip of the cautery with heating, some physicians may prefer not to reuse these). The cautery unit heats in a few seconds and takes less than 1 second to penetrate the nail. They appear less threatening to a patient than a burr or a paper clip heated over an open flame.

Sesamoiditis and Sesamoid Fractures

Athletes present with forefoot pain on the plantar surfaces of the first MTP joint. The differential diagnosis includes stress fractures or osteochondritis of the sesamoids, turf toe, tarsal tunnel syndrome, or entrapment of the medial plantar nerve (seen in the athlete who hyperpronates). With the latter two, even though the athlete feels pain at the sesamoids, there may be no tenderness to palpation directly under the sesamoids. If there is a fracture, the athlete presents with an insidious onset of pain in the first MTP joint that is aggravated by activity and relieved somewhat by rest.[10]

Diagnosis is clinical with the help of the proper roentgenograms. Anteroposterior, lateral, and axial (sesamoid) views should be ordered. The true axial, with the toe maximally dorsiflexed, gives the best view of the sesamoids. Sesamoids often can be bi- or tripartite, and it may be difficult to determine whether there is an acute fracture. If there is doubt about whether a fracture exists, a bone scan will help to confirm the diagnosis.

Treatment of sesamoiditis consists of a metatarsal lift or donut pad placed around the tender area. Turf Toe insoles may be of benefit as well to prevent excess MTP dorsiflexion. Bicycling and swimming are good substitution exercises for the runner. For sesamoid fractures, it is recommended that the foot be placed in a cast for 6 weeks. When the athlete is out of the walking cast, a gradual return to activity should be instituted, using either a metatarsal bar or metatarsal cut-out pad.

Turf Toe

Turf toe is a slang term referring to a hyperdorsiflexion injury to the first MTP joint. It was very common in athletes when artificial turf first came into popular use. The early turfs were unforgiving, and shoes were not developed with rigid soles to support the toes.

The injury occurs when the first MTP joint is forced into extreme dorsiflexion. The athlete presents with pain over the base of his or her great toe. The pain is enhanced with extreme movements in both plantar- and dorsiflexion.

Treatment begins with ice and rest. Taping helps to stabilize the joint and prevent hyperdorsiflexion when the toe is tethered into neutral.

Inserts of either spring steel (Turf Toe Insoles) or plastic laminates can be placed in the shoe to inhibit dorsiflexion of the toe box. Steroid injections are used by some sports medicine physicians when conservative treatment fails in a highly competitive athlete. Caution is advised, however, because the steroid can further weaken the joint capsuloligaments.

Metatarsal Synovitis and Capsulitis

Chronic forefoot pain from an overuse syndrome can present in many different ways. Synovitis differs from bursitis in its lack of visible edema, redness, or outward signs of inflammation. The second metatarsal is most commonly involved in runners with forefoot varus or tennis players with a hallux valgus deformity.[16] *Metatarsalgia* or *neuroma* is often used to describe these con-

ditions, but in this case, the pathology results from a synovitis or capsulitis.

McNerney[16] thought that palpation of the affected joint with the digit fully extended reproduces capsulitic pain. In contrast, a neuroma seldom produces pain at the joint articulation. Also, a neuroma does not benefit from the use of padding under the MTP, whereas a capsulitis may benefit. A stress fracture usually occurs at the neck or shaft of the metatarsal, rather than at the MTP joint like capsulitis. Radiographs are useful to rule out osteochondrosis of the metatarsal head (Freiberg infarction).

Treatment consists of RICE and protective padding. Using ⅛-in. felt, a U-pad is cut to relieve the pressure from the affected MTP joint. Iontophoresis may be helpful as an intracapsular steroid injection in resistant cases. Steroid injection should be used with caution in the young athlete because it may lead to fat pad atrophy and increased capsular laxity.

Metatarsalgia

According to some authors, the term *metatarsalgia* simply refers to pain in the region of the metatarsal heads. The cause may be vascular, avascular, neurogenic, or mechanical.[17] Some of the causes include bunions, arthritis, sesamoid problems, Freiberg infarction (avascular necrosis of the metatarsal head), and perineural fibrosis (Morton neuroma). The more common causes, sesamoid problems and Morton neuroma, are discussed in more detail elsewhere in this chapter.

Generalized metatarsalgia often occurs secondary to a tight Achilles tendon, which restricts dorsiflexion. The loss of full dorsiflexion loads the weight onto the forefoot, thus applying pressure to the MTP joints. If clawing of the toes is present, then subluxation of the MTP joint is probably occurring and may be the cause of the metatarsalgia.

Treatment of the different causes of metatarsalgia is similar, although it must be individualized for the exact problem. Most of the problems with the metatarsals in the athlete can be corrected with a pad placed just proximal to the second or third metatarsal heads. Another option is to place the pad beneath the first metatarsal to allow it to bear more weight. Treatment should include Achilles tendon stretching and a commercial arch support or custom orthosis (particularly for overpronators).

Morton Neuroma

Interdigital Morton neuroma is a thickening of a nerve in the forefoot. It commonly occurs between the third and fourth metatarsal heads (see Figure 17-2), but can involve other metatarsal interspaces. The athlete reports sharp shooting pains extending into his or her toes. Tight-fitting shoes irritate the area, whereas removing the shoes and massaging the toes and foot usually bring some relief. Athletes describe an "after-burning" pain that only gradually resolves with abstinence from weightbearing.

The injury results from an entrapment of the nerve under the intermetatarsal ligament.[18] Diagnosis is made by clinical examination; however, a roentgenogram should be done to rule out a phalangeal stress fracture. Pinching between the metatarsal heads with the index finger and thumb causes intense pain. A mass may be palpable in some patients. A pad placed proximal to and between the involved metatarsals separates the heads and may offer some relief in the early stages. In contrast to a capsulitis, the benefit of this treatment for Morton neuroma is often short-lived. Physical therapy should be tried using iontophoresis along with icing at home. A steroid and anesthetic injection may be helpful, but repeated injections should be avoided. Referral for surgery is often required.

Forefoot Stress Fractures

Metatarsal Shaft Fractures

Stress fractures of the metatarsals are common in runners, as well as in aerobic dancers, tennis players, and gymnasts. Stress fractures occur more commonly in females and are believed to be the result of muscle fatigue.

Muscles are the body's shock absorbers. When they fatigue, the shock is no longer absorbed by the muscle and is passed on to the bone. Over time, the shock will stress the bone, and an increase in bone cell production occurs. This is called a *stress reaction*. When bone cell production cannot keep pace with bone cell destruction, a stress fracture results.

The most common stress fracture of the foot is to the second or third metatarsal shaft.[19] The first metatarsal is the most mobile, and the second is the most stable. These factors contribute to the high frequency of the second metatarsal stress fracture. The examiner requires a high index of suspicion to diagnose these fractures because plain films within the first 2–3 weeks are usually negative. Symptoms include localized pain with weightbearing that has an insidious onset. The pain is often relieved by rest, although some athletes report night pain. The range of motion of the involved metatarsal joint is typically painless, but palpation of the fracture site produces exquisite and pinpoint pain. Usually, the area is not swollen or discolored, and athletes may or may not present with a limp.

Treatment can range from a short leg cast with or without weightbearing to a stiff-soled shoe. Casts are more effective for athletes who are noncompliant with activity restriction. When the athlete is asymptomatic and bone healing is seen on the follow-up roentgenogram at approximately 4 weeks, the athlete can be allowed to gradually resume activity under supervision. Biomechanics, footwear, and training regimens should be reviewed to avoid repeating the same injury. An appropriate shoe with an adequate arch support is important. Commercial arch supports, such as the 1st Steps, should be recommended. Athletes should use pain as a guide as they increase their activity. Cross-training consisting of swimming and bicycling is started before running to maintain fitness during the healing phase. The resulting increase in blood supply to the fracture site will speed the healing as well.

Jones Fractures

Jones fractures involve the proximal diaphysis of the fifth metatarsal (see Figure 17-4). They are more commonly diagnosed as stress fractures. However, the athlete may present with the history of a sudden feeling of a "pop" or increased symptoms. Jones fractures are unpredictable and often progress to delayed union or nonunion. Careers have been shortened by this seemingly simple fracture (such as that of Bill Walton of the Portland Trailblazers). Localized pain with weightbearing and tenderness to palpation are common findings. Diagnosis can often be made with plain films, but occasionally a bone scan is required.

Treatment of a Jones fracture is controversial. There is general agreement that most will heal in a nonweightbearing cast worn for 4–6 weeks followed by 4 weeks in a weightbearing cast or walking boot. Up to 12 weeks of immobilization may be necessary, and full healing occurs at approximately 4 months.[7] Surgical consideration for fractures of the proximal diaphysis is important, because the fracture union is unpredictable. DeLee and colleagues[20] recommended fixing the fracture early with a single long screw. For the very competitive athlete, an early consultation with an orthopedic surgeon is advised. Those who progress well in a cast can usually resume sports activities at approximately 12 weeks.

Lisfranc Capsulitis

Chronic injuries to the midfoot include Lisfranc stress fractures and a capsulitis involving the base of the metatarsals. Stress fractures occur in dancers, and they often present with localized midfoot pain when the dancer is in the pointe position. In this position, the foot is plantarflexed with the full weight on the plantar aspect and tip of the first and second distal phalanges. It is difficult to distinguish a stress fracture from a capsulitis in this area. The injury may even begin as a capsulitis and progress to a stress fracture if the stress continues. Differentiation of the two often requires a bone scan.

Therapy for capsulitis involves RICE and a short course of nonsteroidal anti-inflammatory drugs (NSAIDs). Iontophoresis may offer some relief of the inflammatory responses. Flexibility of the Achilles tendon should be examined and treated if the athlete lacks dorsiflexion. Wearing a postoperative shoe offers some comfort, because it does not allow the midfoot to bend.

When considering Lisfranc or midfoot capsulitis, the examiner must consider the possibility of a posterior tibialis dysfunction. Occasionally, the posterior tibialis, the dynamic stabilizer of the longitudinal arch, avulses from the navicular bone, or the bone itself deteriorates and the athlete presents with pain in the area of the tendon attachment. When suspicion of this exists, the arch should be supported. Once asymptomatic, the athlete should work on toe raises to strengthen the posterior tibialis muscle. A gradual return to play, beginning with bicycling and swimming and progressing to walking and then running, is advised. The importance of good arch supports and heel cord flexibility should be emphasized. If a posterior tibialis tear occurs, the athlete presents with a pronated foot and pain in the arch. With this injury, the static stabilizer of the longitudinal arch, the calcaneonavicular (spring) ligament, is then stressed and may also tear. Acute tears of the posterior tibialis tendon should be referred for possible surgical repair.

Tarsal Navicular Stress Fractures

Tarsal navicular stress fractures are most common in runners and jumpers, although this injury is uncommon in athletes overall. It is difficult to diagnose because the symptoms are mild; the athlete presents with vague pain along the medial dorsum of the foot. The differential diagnosis includes midfoot capsulitis or cuneiform stress fracture. Torg and colleagues[21] described the most common symptom as a cramping sensation in the foot that is aggravated by activity. In a series of 21 of these fractures, they found that the diagnosis was made an average of 7 months after the onset of symptoms.[21]

On physical examination, there is tenderness over the tarsal navicular bone and possibly limited dorsiflexion secondary to pain. There may be no appreciable swelling, and patients may walk without a limp.

Plain films, although part of the workup, may not be diagnostic. In Torg's same series, 12 of the 21 cases (57%) did not demonstrate a fracture on the standard roentgenograms.[21] Bone scans can be helpful. For the navicular, one-third of the bone scans will be negative, and a single photon emission computed tomography scan will be pos-

itive for the fracture. Another option would be to order a triple-phase, pinhole bone scan. The pinhole projection allows for a more specific outline of the individual bones of the foot rather than lighting up the whole foot or ankle. If the bone scan is positive, some physicians think that anteroposterior tomograms or CT should be ordered to demonstrate the fracture.[10, 22] To accomplish this, the foot should be inverted so that the entire mediolateral width of the navicular bone is demonstrated.[22]

Treatment is difficult because of the poor blood supply to the navicular bone and the frequency of delayed unions and nonunions that occur with these fractures. The uncomplicated fracture should be treated with a nonweight-bearing cast for 6–8 weeks. Abstinence from weightbearing is critical, because participation in sports with this fracture often leads to complete fractures with displacement. Lombardo and colleagues[23] recommend a well-molded weightbearing cast for 2 weeks after the initial 6–8 weeks. After the cast is removed, they recommend an oxford-type shoe with an arch support and a gradual return to a walking-only program. Running should not begin for 6–8 weeks after removal of the cast.[23] Any displaced fracture or delayed union should readily be referred because it often requires internal fixation or bone grafting.

Cuboid and Cuneiform Stress Fractures

Although included in the differential diagnosis for tarsal navicular fractures, cuboid and cuneiform stress fractures are comparatively rare. Localization of vague pain on physical examination may be the only clue, initially, that these bones are involved. Diagnosis is made with a bone scan or a CT scan of the foot. Treatment is with cast immobilization or a walking boot initially, followed by a stiff-soled shoe and an arch support. The return to activity is usually sooner than with the tarsal navicular fractures.

Talonavicular Pain

Pain in the region of the talonavicular joint may be due to such entities as accessory tarsal navicular bones or tarsal coalitions (Figure 17-10). The accessory bones are often asymptomatic, but occasionally an athlete presents with pain in this area, and the accessory bone is seen on any one of the standard foot roentgenograms (anteroposterior, lateral, or oblique). If suspicion is high that the accessory bone is causing the symptoms, a triple-phase (three-phase) bone scan is ordered. The triple-phase scan has a vascular and bony phase plus a residual soft tissue labeling. This allows for specificity of abnormal bone activity along with evaluation of soft tissue abnormalities. Surgical excision does not guarantee that the area

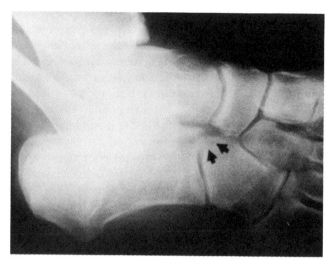

FIGURE 17-10
An oblique view of a calcaneocuboid coalition (arrows).

will improve, so numerous treatment modalities should be tried first (ice, ultrasound, iontophoresis, arch supports, padding, and flexibility training). Patients with significant pain may benefit from short-term casting.

Tarsal coalition is a congenital synostosis between two or more tarsal bones. Most affected athletes present with chronic midfoot or hindfoot pain that is worse after activity. They may have a history of recurrent ankle sprains that are due to the limited subtalar mobility. The symptoms usually first appear in the early teenage years and may result in the inability to participate in sports.[24] There may be peroneal muscle spasm, so one should always check the calf musculature. Subtalar motion may be restricted, and flattening of the longitudinal arch may be noted. The oblique roentgenogram may reveal the coalition, but often CT is needed for the definitive diagnosis (see Figure 17-10). Coronal CT is optimal for talocalcaneal coalition, and a longitudinal study is most effective for the calcaneonavicular coalition. Athletes should be referred if this entity is suspected. Treatment varies with the location and nature of the coalition as well as the athlete's symptoms.[7]

Plantar Fasciitis

Plantar fasciitis is an inflammation of the fascia on the plantar surface of the foot. Chronic stress to the origin of this fascia on the calcaneus causes calcium to deposit, forming a spur. The pain is secondary to the microtears in the fascia and the inflammatory response. Seldom is the pain a result of the spur itself. Patients and medical personnel are often confused about this relationship.

Roentgenograms may show large spurs in athletes without plantar fasciitis or no spurs in an athlete with severe plantar fasciitis. The classic symptom is heel pain with the first few steps in the morning. The pain usually decreases with activity and then recurs with activity after a period of rest.

Physical examination reveals pain at the origin of the fascia on the anteromedial aspect of the calcaneus. Range of motion of the great toe may be limited in dorsiflexion, and ankle dorsiflexion is often less than 10 degrees. To demonstrate gastrocnemius tightness, dorsiflex the ankle with the knee bent (gastrocnemius relaxed) and with the knee straight (gastrocnemius on stretch). Normal dorsiflexion is approximately 25–30 degrees. Demonstrate to the athlete the loss of dorsiflexion with the athlete's knee bent and with his or her knee straight to illustrate the need for stretching. Swelling on the medial heel may occur, and occasionally a small granuloma is palpated on the medial fascia at the origin.

Diagnosis is clinical; however, some medical entities can cause heel pain. The differential diagnosis includes Reiter disease, ankylosing spondylitis, psoriatic arthropathy, and rheumatoid arthritis.[25, 26] Other causes of heel pain include Sever disease (most commonly at ages 9–14 years), a sacral radiculopathy, tarsal tunnel syndrome, and entrapment of the first lateral branch of the posterior tibialis nerve.

Treatment includes stretching of the Achilles tendon and plantar fascia, ice, stress reduction (for example, from running or aerobics by substituting alternative exercises, such as running or swimming in the pool, bicycling), NSAIDs, and friction massage at the origin of the fascia to break down scar tissue. Physical therapy modalities, such as iontophoresis or ultrasound, are useful early. In some patients, night splints may offer relief in the early stages. The arch may be supported with the LowDye taping method, and if this is beneficial, an over-the-counter arch support (1st Step) is recommended. There is also an assortment of heel pads made specifically for heel pain; however, the goal is not to shorten the Achilles long term but to lengthen it.

The actual cause of the injury may not be known, but tight heel cords are a major factor in this injury. Tight Achilles tendons can be remedied with consistent stretching. The athlete should be given a handout demonstrating how to construct an incline board (Figure 17-11) and encouraged to work up to using it for 10 minutes per day. It works best if the back and heels are against the wall; then patients can read or watch television while they stretch. Often, the 6-in. rise (30-degree angle) is too steep, so patients are encouraged to place a book or 2×4 under the back of the box in the beginning to lower the angle.

If they cannot build the box, they can just place a piece of wood on a book or brick and gradually build up the front of the board until it is 6 in. off the ground.

Steroid injections are occasionally needed (e.g., 1 ml of triamcinolone diacetate [Aristocort, 40 mg/ml] is mixed with 2 ml of 0.5% bupivacaine hydrochloride [Marcaine] in a 5-ml syringe). A 27-gauge, ½-in. needle is used to inject the patient's heel from the medial side of the calcaneous to the origin of the plantar fasciae. Be careful not to inject the fat pad of the heel, because it could cause fat atrophy.

Sever Disease

Sever disease (calcaneal apophysitis) is the most common cause of heel pain in children 7–12 years of age. Repetitive loading of the heel combined with tight heel cords overstress the apophysis, leading to a painful heel. Poorly cushioned shoes (e.g., soccer cleats) predispose the athlete to this condition.

The painful heel in a child is often attributed to Achilles tendinitis or plantar fasciitis, but calcaneal apophysis is more commonly the cause of pain in this age group. Pain is reproduced with a medial-lateral squeeze on the calcaneus, and there is often tenderness at the Achilles insertion or plantar fascia origin. Tight heel cords are frequently associated. Radiographs are not necessary but can be useful to illustrate to the parents and child what the problem is.

Treatment depends on the severity. Short-term casting (3–4 weeks) is useful in the child who limps because of the pain. Less severe cases can be treated with a cushioned heel wedge or cup, ice, heel cord stretching, and progressive return to activities as pain abates.

Tarsal Tunnel Syndrome

Tarsal tunnel syndrome is thought to be underdiagnosed by many physicians. It results from an entrapment or stretch of the posterior tibial nerve in the tarsal tunnel. Among runners, it is seen in excessive pronators who stretch the nerve because of their abnormal mechanics. The presentation is similar to that of plantar fasciitis, but there are some key differences. Tarsal tunnel produces more medial heel and arch pain (at the abductor hallucis muscle) rather than at the origin of the plantar fascia. Tarsal tunnel pain increases with running and may produce nocturnal paresthesias and a burning pain. The pain may radiate into the foot and often centers around the first MTP joint. The differential diagnosis includes those listed under Plantar Fasciitis, as well as sciatica, peripheral neuritis, peripheral vascular disease, and an interdigital neuroma.[27]

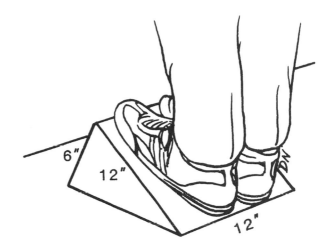

FIGURE 17-11
Example of an incline board or heel cord box.

The physical examination may reveal a positive Tinel sign, weakness of toe flexion, an early loss of 2-point discrimination, and, later, signs of motor loss or paralysis. Besides roentgenograms and blood chemistries, electromyography (EMG) with nerve conduction studies should also be performed if one is suspicious of this entity. EMG must evaluate both the medial and lateral plantar nerves (motor and sensory) as well as the muscles of the foot and leg.[15, 27] Treatment includes rest and ice, NSAIDs, flexibility training, and an examination of the gait on a treadmill. Orthotics are often needed to correct the overpronation. A good running shoe is important, preferably one suited for pronators. Steroid injections are required at times, as is a referral to an orthopedist for surgical intervention when conservative measures fail. Other less common entrapment neuropathies are well described elsewhere and are not covered here.[28]

Achilles Tendinitis

Achilles tendinitis is one of the most common forms of tendinitis seen in athletes. The tendon is formed from the gastrocnemius and soleus muscles. The tendon has a relatively poor blood supply, which can lead to tears in the most severe cases. Athletes with tight Achilles tendons are prone to stress at the insertion of the tendon on the calcaneus. In addition to poor flexibility, many other factors contribute to Achilles tendon breakdown, including training errors and anatomic factors such as overpronation.[28]

Athletes present with pain several centimeters proximal to the insertion of the tendon into the calcaneus, the area of poorest blood supply. Pain is aggravated by activity and relieved by rest. Dorsiflexion causes pain, and crepitus may be felt along the tendon at the most tender area.

Diagnosis is clinical and must differentiate retrocalcaneal bursitis and Haglund disease. The young athlete (9–14 years of age) may present with an apophysitis (Sever disease).

Treatment for Achilles tendinitis begins with RICE. Iontophoresis works well in the acute phase (several days) followed by an effective stretching and eccentric strengthening program. Short-term (2 weeks) use of a ⅜-in. heel lift will often reduce symptoms; however, this must be followed by an aggressive stretching program. Examination of the foot and gait will determine if arch supports or custom orthosis are needed to correct an abnormal pattern. NSAIDs may be used for a short time as well. Severe cases require a walking boot or cast for 2–4 weeks, and occasionally surgery is needed to excise part of a thickened sheath. A rupture of the Achilles tendon requires immediate referral for consideration of surgical repair.

Retrocalcaneal Bursitis

Retrocalcaneal bursitis is seen more frequently in the athlete with a prominent superior tuberosity of the os calcis (calcaneus). The examiner must differentiate this from Achilles tendinitis by the location and the character of the pain. Symptoms include pain that develops early when the athlete begins running. Tenderness is just anterior to the Achilles tendon and posterior to the talus. Hindfoot swelling is often present with bursitis.

Treatment includes ice and a decrease in activity, followed by an effective stretching program and insertion of a heel lift in the shoe. NSAIDs and iontophoresis may provide some benefit. Finally, any postural foot deformities should be corrected.[28] Judicious use of a steroid injection into the bursa can be useful in resistant cases, with care not to inject the tendon. This should be followed by wearing a cast boot for 2 weeks to protect the tendon.

Haglund Deformity

Haglund deformity ("pump bump") is a thickening of the soft tissue at the insertion of the Achilles tendon. There is a bony enlargement of the calcaneus where a low-cut shoe (pump) rubs. It occurs in both sexes and all ages of adults. The clinically detected pump bump is not diagnostic of Haglund deformity. Radiologic criteria are diagnostic and have been well described elsewhere.[29]

Treatment includes ice, padding in the shoes to prevent the heel counter from rubbing the area or shoes with a high-heel counter, arch supports to correct rear foot varus,

and NSAIDs. Athletes return to activity when the proper padding has been made and the acute pain has subsided.

Calcaneal Stress Fractures

Stress fractures of the calcaneus, or os calcis, can often be differentiated from the previous causes of heel pain by the history. Athletes relate a significant change in activity level with severe discomfort. They often present nonambulatory because of the pain shortly after the onset of symptoms. Stress fractures of the calcaneus are diffusely tender with maximum tenderness on the medial and lateral aspects of the heel. This is in contrast to tenderness on the medial and plantar aspect of the heel found with more routine heel pain problems. The heel "squeeze" test is exquisitely tender to these patients in contrast to patients with Achilles tendinitis, retrocalcaneal bursitis, and Haglund deformity. Swelling may be present, much like with retrocalcaneal bursitis.

Diagnosis is difficult to make with plain films, as the callous formation may not be evident for 2–4 weeks. Bone scans are usually diagnostic and should be used when clinical suspicion is high.[8]

Treatment includes rest with some sort of heel padding. A heel cup or cushion is beneficial for the remainder of the season. Athletes usually return to sports in as few as 3 weeks.[22]

REFERENCES

1. Maier T, Pietrocarlo T. The foot and footwear. Nurs Clin North Am 1991;26:223–231.
2. Drez D. Running footwear. Examination of the training shoe, the foot, and functional orthotic devices. Am J Sports Med 1980;8:140–141.
3. Brunet ME, Cook SD, Brinker MR, Dickinson JA. A survey of running injuries in 1,505 competitive and recreational runners. J Sports Med Phys Fitness 1990;30:307–315.
4. Garrick JG, Requa RK. The epidemiology of foot and ankle injuries in sports. Clin Podiatr Med Surg 1989;6:629–637.
5. Sheehan G. Encyclopedia of athletic medicine. Runners World Magazine 1972;1:8.
6. Arnheim DD. Modern Principles of Athletic Training (6th ed). St. Louis: Mosby, 1985;460.
7. Rettig AC, Shelbourne KD, Beltz HF, et al. Radiographic evaluation of foot and ankle injuries in the athlete. Clin Sports Med 1987;6:905–919.
8. Davis AW, Alexander IJ. Problematic fractures and dislocations in the foot and ankle of athletes. Clin Sports Med 1990;9:163–181.
9. Garfinkel D, Rothenberger LA. Foot problems in athletes. J Fam Pract 1984;19:239–250.
10. Keene JS, Lange RH. Diagnostic dilemmas in foot and ankle injuries. JAMA 1986;256:247–251.

11. Mills HJ, Horne G. Fractures of the lateral process of the talus. Aust N Z J Surg 1987;57:643–646.

12. Nicholas R, Hadley J, Paul C, Janes P. "Snowboarder's fracture": fracture of the lateral process of the talus. J Am Board Fam Pract 1994;7:130–133.

13. Ihle CL, Cochran RM. Fracture of the fused os trigonum. Am J Sports Med 1982;10:47–50.

14. Paulos LE, Johnson CL, Noyes FR. Posterior compartment fractures of the ankle. Am J Sports Med 1983;11: 439–443.

15. Rzonca EC, Baylis WJ. Common sports injuries to the foot and leg. Clin Podiatr Med Surg 1988;5:591–612.

16. McNerney JE. Sports-medicine considerations of lesser metatarsalgia. Clin Podiatr Med Surg 1990;7:645–687.

17. Gould JS. Metatarsalgia. Orthop Clin North Am 1989;20: 553–562.

18. Gauthier G. Thomas Morton's disease: a nerve entrapment syndrome. Clin Orthop 1979;142:90.

19. Browne JE. Common running injuries. Hosp Med 1982; 8:13.

20. DeLee JC, Evans JP, Julian J. Stress fracture of the fifth metatarsal. Am J Sports Med 1982;11:349.

21. Torg JS, Pavlov H, Cooley LH. Stress fractures of the tarsal navicular. A retrospective review of twenty-one cases. J Bone Joint Surg Am 1982;63:700–712.

22. Hershman EB, Mailly TD. Stress fractures. Clin Sports Med 1990;9:183–214.

23. Lombardo JA, Bergfeld JA, Micheli LJ. Cross-country runner with pain in the dorsum of the foot. Phys Sports Med 1988;16:85–88.

24. American Academy of Orthopedic Surgeons. Athletic Training and Sports Medicine (2nd ed). Chicago: American Academy of Orthopaedic Surgeons, 1991;429,948.

25. Kwong PK, Kay D, Voner RT, White MW. Plantar fasciitis. Clin Sports Med 1988;7:119–126.

26. Leach RE, Seavey MS, Salter DK. Results of surgery in athletes with plantar fasciitis. Foot Ankle 1986;7:156–161.

27. Jackson DL, Haglund B. Tarsal tunnel syndrome in athletes. Case reports and literature review. Am J Sports Med 1991;19: 61–65.

28. Singer KM, Jones DC. Soft Tissue Conditions of the Ankle and Foot. In JA Nicholas, EB Hershman (eds), The Lower Extremity and Spine in Sports Medicine. St. Louis: Mosby, 1986;514–516.

29. Torg JS, Pavlov H, Torg E. Overuse injuries in sport: the foot. Clin Sports Med 1987;6:291–320.

18

Common Ankle Injuries

ARLON H. JAHNKE, JR., MARK THOMAS MESSENGER,
AND JEFFREY D. PATTERSON

Foot and ankle injuries are endemic to all sports that involve running, jumping, cutting, or kicking. The health care professional involved with the care of the acutely injured athlete must be proficient in diagnosing and treating common injuries to the ankle, as well as in recognizing signs and symptoms of more significant injuries that require referral to specialty care. Ankle injuries are among the most common afflictions seen at all levels of athletic participation and account for approximately 15% of all athletic injuries. In this chapter, a brief review of anatomy is presented, followed by a discussion of various injuries that may involve the ankle joint. A symptoms-oriented approach is presented to familiarize the practitioner with the diagnosis and treatment of each of these injuries.

ANATOMY

An understanding of the anatomy of the tendons, ligaments, and osseous structures about the ankle is necessary to adequately diagnose and subsequently treat injuries that occur. The ankle joint is maintained by the shape of the talus and its tight fit between the mortise formed by the distal aspects of the tibia and fibula. The articular surface of the talus is in the shape of a truncated cone (the width of the talus is narrower posteriorly). This bony anatomy results in stability of the ankle with the foot in a neutral position. In this position, the ankle resembles a mortise and tenon with the talus locking tightly within the distal tibia and fibula. As the foot moves into plantar flexion, the ankle has less bony stability as the narrower posterior portion of the talus rides into the wider area between the medial and lateral malleoli. As the bony stability decreases with plantarflexion, stability of the

ankle relies progressively more on the ligamentous structures about the ankle joint.

The ligaments of the ankle joint can be divided into three anatomic areas: the distal tibiofibular ligaments (syndesmotic ligaments), the lateral ligaments, and the medial ligaments. The lateral ligaments consist of the anterior talofibular ligament (ATFL), the calcaneofibular ligament (CFL), and the posterior talofibular ligament (PTFL) (Figure 18-1).

The ATFL is a broad, flat ligament that courses from the anterior border of the distal fibula to the anterolateral aspect of the talus. With the foot flat on the ground, the ligament courses relatively parallel to the floor. This ligament's primary function is to prevent anterior translation of the talus in the mortise of the distal tibia and fibula. As the foot goes into plantarflexion, the ligament fibers become more perpendicular to the floor and therefore become more of a collateral ligament that prevents inversion of the talus within the ankle mortise.

The CFL is a more tubular structure that courses from the tip of the distal fibula to a small tubercle on the lateral wall of the calcaneus. The CFL lies deep to the peroneal tendons and courses nearly perpendicular to the floor with the foot in a neutral position. The CFL crosses two joints and acts to prevent inversion of both the ankle and subtalar joints.

The PTFL is the strongest of the three lateral ligaments of the ankle and the least frequently injured. It also is a fairly broad, stout ligament that courses relatively horizontal to the floor from the posterior aspect of the lateral malleolus to the talus, posterior and lateral to the articular surface of the talus. This strong ligament prevents forward dislocation of the leg on the foot.

The medial ankle ligament or "deltoid ligament" is a very strong, fan-shaped structure that consists of superficial and

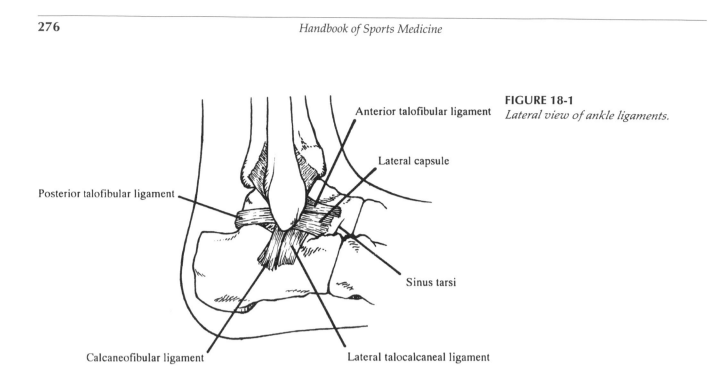

FIGURE 18-1
Lateral view of ankle ligaments.

deep components (Figure 18-2). The medial ligaments of the ankle are much stronger than the lateral and syndesmotic ligaments and are less commonly injured. The superficial portion of the deltoid ligament courses from the medial malleolus to the navicular anteriorly and to the sustentaculum tali posteriorly. This portion of the ligament prevents eversion of the ankle. The deep portion courses relatively horizontal from the deep, posterior surface of the medial malleolus to the medial aspect of the talus. Its relatively horizontal orientation results in its ability to prevent lateral displacement of the talus within the ankle mortise.

The syndesmotic ligaments consist of the anterior inferior tibiofibular ligament, the posterior inferior tibiofibular ligament, and the interosseous membrane. The syndesmotic ligaments are responsible for maintaining the relationship of the distal tibia and fibula. These ligaments hold the distal fibula snug into a small groove on the distal lateral aspect of the tibia. Disruption of this ligamentous complex results in widening of the bony ankle mortise.

ACUTE ANKLE INJURIES

Figure 18-3 is an algorithm for the evaluation of acute ankle injuries.

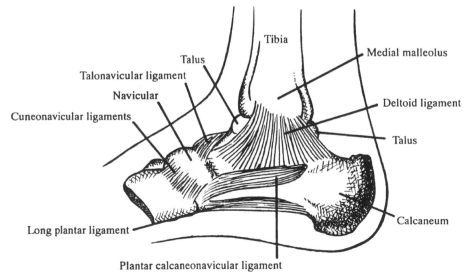

FIGURE 18-2
Medial view of ankle ligaments.

FIGURE 18-3
Algorithm for the evaluation of acute ankle injuries.

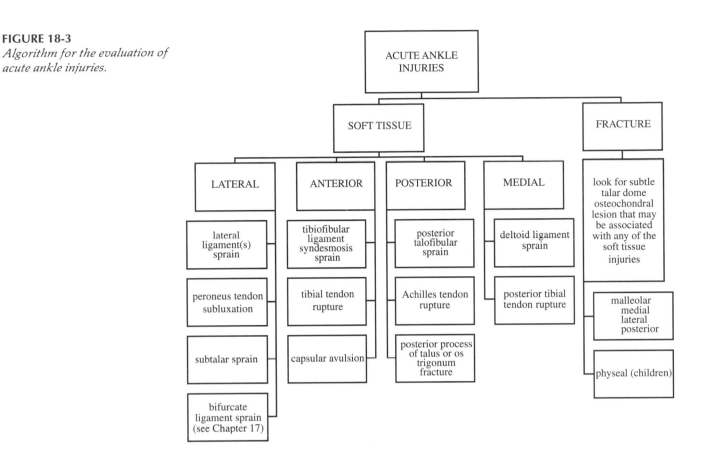

Lateral Pain

Sprains

Injuries to the lateral ligamentous structures of the ankle are the most common injuries seen in sports.[1–3] Sporting activities such as basketball, volleyball, soccer, and football are particularly plagued by these injuries. The majority of these injuries occur in persons younger than 35 years of age, most commonly in the age range from 15 to 19 years.[3] Treatment depends on the severity of the injury. An accurate diagnosis will enable the physician to direct and implement the proper treatment and rehabilitation regimen.

Injuries to the lateral ligamentous structures occur with an inversion mechanism to the tibiotalar joint and hindfoot. In jumping-type sports, the foot is often in a plantarflexed position at the time of injury, resulting in strain to the ATFL. With the foot plantarflexed, the ATFL is the primary stabilizer to inversion stress, because the bony architecture is not as inherently stable. Injuries also occur in cutting-type sports, in which the primary stress is still inversion; however, here the ankle is in neutral position or dorsiflexion. More severe injuries may occur in this position as more stress is placed on all three lateral ligaments.

Traditionally, sprains of the ankle ligaments have been classified in clinical practice as grade I (mild), grade II (moderate), and grade III (severe) injuries.[4] Grade I injuries involve ligament stretching without macroscopic tearing. Clinically, there is little swelling and mild tenderness, minimal functional loss, and no instability symptoms. A grade II injury is a moderate injury involving partial macroscopic tearing of the ligamentous structures. There is moderate swelling and tenderness over the lateral ligamentous structures. There is slight loss of motion and mild to moderate joint instability. A grade III injury is a complete ligament rupture. The patient has severe swelling, ecchymoses, and inability to bear weight on the extremity. There is marked functional limitation and joint instability. The diagnosis of grade I, II, or III lateral ligamentous injuries requires a careful clinical evaluation consisting of an accurate history, thorough physical examination, and radiographic evaluation. Injuries that "mimic" ankle sprains should be recognized and ruled out. These include midfoot sprains, lateral talus (snowboarder's) fracture, Achilles tendon rupture, talar dome fracture, posterior talar process fracture, as well as others.

The athlete can usually describe the mechanism of injury quite well, and from this information the physician may

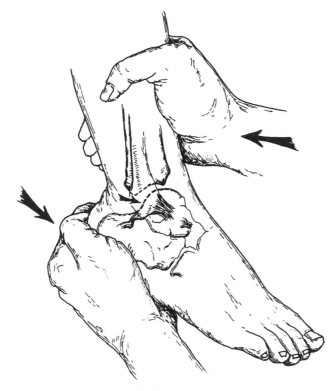

FIGURE 18-4

Anterior drawer test. The examiner places one hand on the anterior aspect of the patient's lower tibia and grasps the calcaneous with his or her other hand. The patient's calcaneus is gently drawn anteriorly while the examiner stabilizes the patient's distal tibia with his or her other hand. Increased translation compared with the contralateral ankle indicates laxity or rupture of the anterior talofibular ligament.

be able to predict which structures have been injured. It is important to determine whether the injury is a first-time injury or a recurrent event. A precise history should include questions regarding previous injuries to the ankle, mechanism of injuries, presence of a "pop" or "snap" at the time of injury, ability to bear weight after the injury, initial treatment given, and the presence and time to development of swelling and ecchymoses. After an injury to the lateral ligaments of the ankle, the patient often experiences a sudden, intense pain localized to the lateral side of the ankle. The pain often improves after a few minutes, only to return as ankle swelling leads to joint distention. Most patients experience pain and discomfort when they try to bear weight on the injured extremity. Swelling occurs in minutes to hours, depending on the severity of the ligamentous tearing. Ecchymoses usually takes 24–48 hours as the hematoma develops both over and dependent to the site of injury. Medial hindfoot swelling suggests an associated sprain to the deltoid ligament or subtalar joint.

The correct diagnosis relies on the ability to perform a thorough and accurate physical examination. The ability to examine the ankle within the first hour or two after injury is advantageous. Initially, the point of maximal tenderness will be localized to the injured structures on the lateral ankle. This is most common over the ATFL or the CFL. If the patient is not seen until several hours after the injury, generalized swelling and pain make the examination more difficult and unreliable. The physical examination begins with inspection of the joint for any deformity, swelling, or discoloration. The entire lower extremity should be undressed to fully evaluate the injury. Examine the skin for abrasions or breaks. The location of abrasions or lacerations will help in understanding the extent of the trauma to the ankle. Palpation should be performed in a systematic manner, beginning with structures believed to be not injured. Laterally, palpate the distal fibula, the ATFL, the CFL, the PTFL, and the base of the fifth metatarsal. Medially, it is important to palpate the medial malleolus, the deltoid ligament, and the navicular bone. For completeness, the proximal fibula and the Achilles tendon to its insertion should be palpated for tenderness or deformity. Range of motion of the ankles should be evaluated, both actively and passively. Normal range of motion for the ankle joint is 20 degrees of dorsiflexion and 50 degrees of plantarflexion.

Several tests have been described to determine the integrity of the ligaments about the ankle. The anterior drawer test (Figure 18-4) is performed with the patient sitting on the edge of the examining table with his or her legs dangling. The injured foot is placed in a few degrees of plantarflexion. The examiner places one hand on the anterior aspect of the lower tibia and grasps the calcaneus with the other hand. The calcaneus is gently drawn anteriorly while stabilizing the distal tibia with the other hand. Normally, the ATFL is tight in all positions of ankle joint motion, and there should be minimal forward movement of the talus. With injury to the ATFL, either acutely or chronically, the test results in abnormal translation of the talus relative to the distal tibia. This is noted as a positive anterior drawer sign.

The second test to determine lateral ligament stability of the ankle is the talar tilt test (Figure 18-5). This test is performed by gently inverting the talus within the ankle mortise while the ankle is in both neutral dorsiflexion and slight plantarflexion positions. If the talus gaps and rocks open while the ankle is in plantarflexion, this indicates laxity of the ATFL. If there is lateral tilt with the ankle in neutral dorsiflexion, then there is laxity of both the CFL and ATFL. If, when performing these stability tests, the patient reports severe pain, the tests can be omitted and performed on subsequent visits because the initial treatment is generally unaffected.

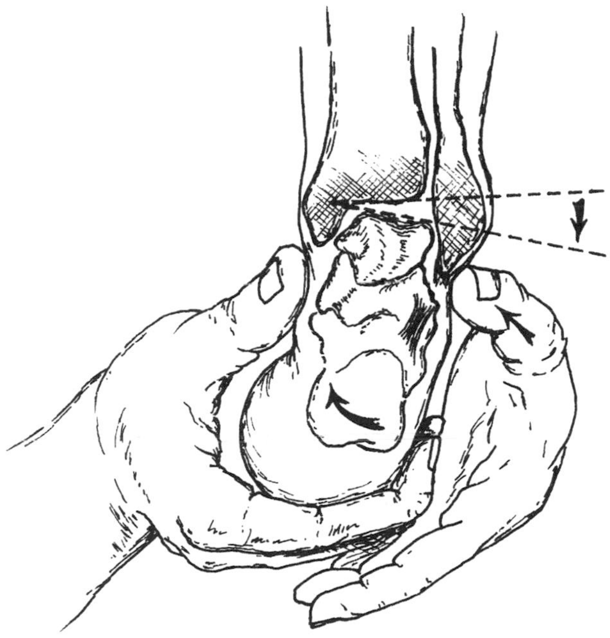

FIGURE 18-5

Talar tilt test. Invert the talus within the ankle mortise. If the talus gaps and rocks open while the ankle is in slight plantarflexion, this indicates laxity of the anterior talofibular ligament.

The physical examination is completed with a neurovascular examination. The dorsalis pedis and posterior tibial pulses should be palpated. Capillary refill to all of the digits should be brisk. A brief sensory examination verifies the integrity of the peripheral nerves. Radiographic evaluation may not be required in relatively minor injuries to the ankle. If there is significant swelling, ecchymosis, or pain present about the ankle, radiographs, including anteroposterior (AP), lateral, and mortise views of the ankle, should be obtained. The mortise view is an AP radiograph taken with the leg internally rotated 15–30 degrees that better profiles the talar dome.

With chronic instability symptoms, specialized AP and lateral stress radiographs may be required. The lateral stress view is a lateral radiograph obtained with an anteriorly applied force to the talus and calcaneus (Figure 18-6). On the lateral stress view, the shortest distance from the posterior lip of the distal tibia to the talar dome is measured. A distance of more than 10 mm, or 3 mm more than the asymptomatic ankle, indicates abnormal laxity of the ATFL.[5] The AP stress radiograph is performed while applying an inversion stress to the talus and calcaneus (see Figure 18-5). An angle is measured between lines drawn parallel to the tibial plafond and the talar dome. An abnormal stress radiograph is obtained if the angle measured is greater than 20 degrees, or 10 degrees more

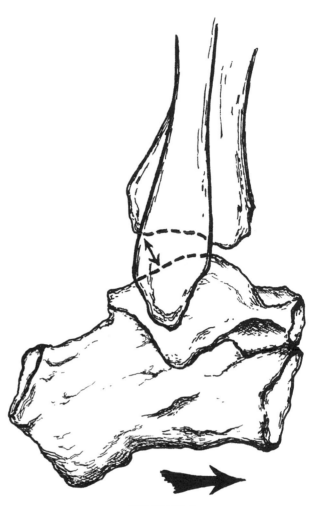

FIGURE 18-6

Lateral stress view. With the talus stressed anteriorly (see arrow), the shortest distance from the posterior lip of the distal fibula to the talar dome is less than 10 mm or 3 mm greater than the asymptomatic ankle, indicating abnormal laxity of the anterior talofibular ligament.

than the asymptomatic ankle.[6, 7] Other specialized studies, including bone scans, arthrography, computed tomography (CT), and magnetic resonance imaging (MRI), are rarely needed to evaluate lateral ligament injuries.

Treatment of acute lateral ligamentous ankle injuries depends on the severity of the injury. Most injuries can be treated initially with rest or immobilization, ice, compression, elevation, and early range of motion. Weightbearing can begin after the initial swelling resolves. Patients should use crutches until they can ambulate with minimal pain. The use of functional braces, such as stirrup braces, elastic sleeves, and laced ankle supports, may be beneficial during the patient's rehabilitation from these injuries. The rehabilitation program should emphasize range of motion early

TABLE 18-1
Ankle Fracture Treatment Guidelines

Location	Fracture Type	Treatment
Lateral malleolus	Nondisplaced	Cast 6–8 wks*
	Displaced	Reduce (probable ORIF)
	Avulsion	Small: rigid sport stirrup and treat as sprain
		Large: ORIF
Medial malleolus	Nondisplaced	Cast 6–8 wks*
	Displaced	Refer for ORIF
Posterior malleolus	Nondisplaced	Cast 6–8 wks*
	Displaced	Refer for possible ORIF
Posterior talar process		Cast 4–6 wks; ankle rehabilitation; excise with late symptoms
Talar dome		See text
Lower leg	Stress	See Chapter 16

*Denotes close monitoring for displacement during treatment.
ORIF = open reduction (with) internal fixation.

followed by proprioceptive training and peroneal muscle strengthening with time (see Appendix A). With more severe injuries, immobilization with casting or a range of motion walker may be required initially. Surgery is reserved for more severe injuries, those associated with fractures, and chronic or recurrent lateral ligament insufficiency. Acute surgical repair of even grade III injuries is rarely needed.

Peroneus Tendon Subluxation

Traumatic dislocation or subluxation of the peroneal tendons, either acute or chronic, is an uncommon injury. This injury most commonly occurs in skiing and less frequently in other athletic activities such as soccer, basketball, and football. The mechanism of injury is a sudden, forceful, passive dorsiflexion of the ankle with the foot in slight eversion. This results in powerful reflex contraction of the peronei, which are the dynamic lateral stabilizers of the ankle. The injury results in tearing of the peroneal retinaculum and subsequent anterior subluxation or dislocation of the peroneal tendons anterior to the lateral malleolus. Tenderness is usually located posterior to the lateral malleolus; however, swelling can be quite severe, and this may obscure the diagnosis. The retinaculum is stressed by eliciting active eversion of the foot with the ankle held in dorsiflexion. In patients with an acute subluxation, this test will produce severe pain and is diagnostic of the problem.

Because of the rapid resolution of symptoms and the difficulty of establishing the diagnosis in the acute state, the patient most commonly seeks medical evaluation when chronic subluxation is established. Patients with recur-

rent subluxation report lateral ankle pain and instability. Treatment of this condition, if diagnosed acutely, consists of a well-molded, nonweightbearing cast with the ankle slightly plantarflexed for 5–6 weeks. Patients with chronic instability usually require surgical reconstruction to prevent recurrent subluxation.

Subtalar Sprain

Injury to the subtalar ligamentous complex results from a mechanism similar to that of lateral ankle ligament injuries. Patients report pain along the lateral aspect of their foot that is localized to the sinus tarsi region. With chronic strains, the symptoms may be identical to that of chronic lateral instability with recurrent inversion instability and lateral pain. Often with isolated subtalar instability, the stress radiographs for ankle instability are normal. Specialized radiographs (Broden views) are necessary to evaluate the subtalar joint.[8] Often, this becomes a diagnosis of exclusion after lateral ankle ligament instability has been eliminated.

Acute injuries are treated similarly to those of lateral ankle ligament sprains with rest, ice, compression, elevation, early range of motion, and peroneal muscle strengthening. Chronic subtalar instability may require surgical reconstruction.

Other Causes

Acute lateral pain can also be caused by fractures of the fibula, lateral talus, and lateral talar dome (Table 18-1).

Anterior Pain

Tibiofibular Ligament and Syndesmosis Sprain

Diastasis of the syndesmosis occurs with partial or complete rupture of the syndesmosis ligament complex. These injuries are often seen with fractures about the ankle. Isolated injuries to the syndesmosis are relatively rare. The injury occurs from sudden external rotation of the ankle, which causes the talus to press against the fibula, thus opening the distal tibiofibular articulation.

An isolated syndesmosis tear can be very difficult to diagnose. Pain and tenderness are located principally on the anterior aspect of the syndesmotic ligaments and the interosseous membrane. Active external rotation of the foot is painful, and the patient usually cannot bear weight on the ankle because of pain. In patients with complete tears, the diagnosis may be recognized with a simple squeeze test. The squeeze test is performed by compressing the fibula to the tibia proximal to the midpoint of the calf. This proximal compression results in pain along the interosseous membrane and its supporting structures. The

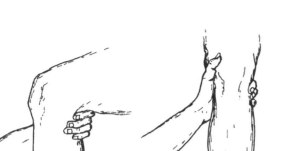

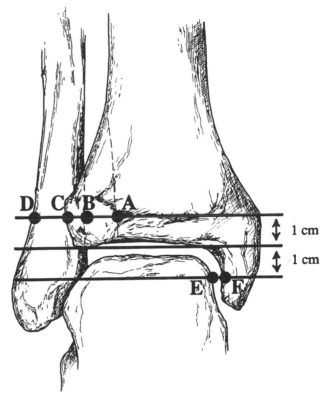

FIGURE 18-7

External rotation stress test. The patient's distal tibia is stabilized with one hand and an external rotation force is applied to the foot with the other hand. If this maneuver reproduces pain in the syndesmosis, it is suggestive of an anterior ankle sprain (also referred to as a syndesmotic ligament sprain or a "high" ankle sprain).

FIGURE 18-8

Anteroposterior radiographic evidence of syndesmosis disruption. Suspicious measures include: (1) medial clear space (E–F) greater than 5 mm, (2) tibiofibular clear space (A–B) greater than 5 mm, and (3) tibiofibular overlap (D–C) 10 mm or less.

external rotation stress test is performed by stabilizing the distal tibia with one hand and applying an external rotational force to the foot with the other hand (Figure 18-7). This maneuver will reproduce pain localized to the area of the syndesmosis.

Routine radiographs to include AP, lateral, and mortise views should be obtained. The diagnosis of syndesmosis disruption is made with widening of the medial space between the medial malleolus and medial talar dome more than 5 mm. With widening of the medial "clear space," it is important to obtain radiographs of the entire fibula to rule out the possibility of a proximal fibular fracture or Maisonneuve fracture. If there is no widening of the clear space on the routine radiographs, stress radiographs should be obtained to ensure integrity of the syndesmotic ligaments. A mortise radiograph is obtained while applying an external rotational force to the foot. An injection of lidocaine hydrochloride (Xylocaine) in to the syndesmosis before this examination may improve the sensitivity of the test. Finally, the diagnosis can be made from evaluating the routine AP radiographs.[9] A measurement is made from the lateral border of the posterior tibial malleolus to the medial border of the fibula (clear space [A–B on Figure 18-8]). This measurement

should be less than 5 mm. Similarly, measurement from the medial border of the fibula to the lateral border of the anterior tibial prominence (tibia-fibula overlap) should be 10 mm or more (C–B on Figure 18-8).

The treatment of syndesmosis sprains depends on the severity of the injury. Less severe strains without complete disruption and no objective widening on radiographic studies should be treated initially with rest, ice, compression, and elevation. Taping or bimalleolar semirigid orthoses can help stabilize the ankle during healing, and crutches are used until the initial pain and inflammation of the injury subside. Progression to normal ambulation is then encouraged. The patient does active resistive and proprioceptive exercises in physical therapy. Gradual return to activity is allowed as symptoms permit, but patients should be informed that these injuries take a considerably longer time to heal than "regular" sprains. For complete tears of the syndesmosis, indicated by widening of the medial clear space on radiographs, referral to

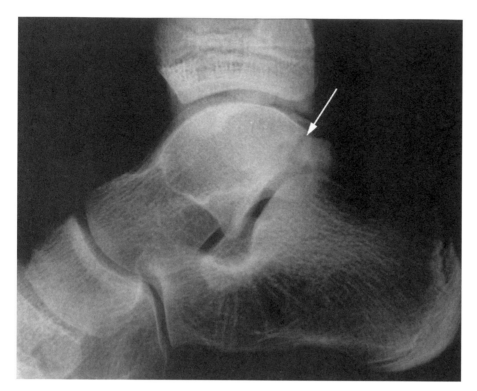

FIGURE 18-9
Fracture of the lateral tubercle of the posterior talar process (Stieda process), indicated by arrow. This can be difficult to differentiate from an os trigonum.

an orthopedic surgeon is necessary. The syndesmosis can be stabilized by either cast immobilization or operatively through the use of sutures or a syndesmosis screw.

Anterior Tibial Tendon Rupture

This is an extremely unusual injury that is caused by forced plantarflexion of the foot and ankle, causing strain or rupture of the anterior tibial tendon. The patient reports loss of strength in dorsiflexion and has difficulty walking because of an unsteady gait (footdrop). Physical examination reveals swelling or a mass (pseudotumor) and a palpable defect of the normal anterior prominence of the tendon with resistive dorsiflexion of the ankle. If the diagnosis is made acutely, then direct repair of the tendon may be possible. However, these injuries often present late and require more complex reconstructive surgical procedures.

Capsular Avulsion

This injury is caused by a plantarflexion force. This force is generally associated with other injury to the ankle, including lateral sprain and malleolar or posterior process of the talus fracture. Physical examination reveals tenderness and a fullness of the anterior aspect of the ankle. Plain radiographs may show a small avulsed fleck of bone off the dorsum of the talus. The instability caused by anterior capsule avulsion may be seen on plantarflexion lateral x-ray films showing anterior talar subluxation on the tibia.

Arthrographic confirmation of the acute injury is possible but unnecessary, because it is treated as an ankle sprain.

Posterior Pain

Posterior Talofibular Ligament Sprain

Injuries to the PTFL occur with external rotational forces to the foot with the ankle in a dorsiflexed position (see Figure 18-2). This ligament rarely tears as an isolated injury. More commonly, it is torn as one component of severe lateral ligamentous ankle sprains with the ATFL and CFL also sustaining injuries. The area of local tenderness will be posterior to the lateral malleolus and is difficult to differentiate from acute peroneal tendon subluxation. Treatment usually is directed as for other ligamentous injuries of the lateral ligamentous complex.

Fracture of the Trigonal Process of the Talus (Os Trigonum)

Fracture of the trigonal process of the talus occurs secondary to forced plantarflexion (Figure 18-9). A fracture line can sometimes show a distinct sharp border versus a nonfused os trigonum. Initially, treatment is conservative, because some cases resolve spontaneously. Initial immobilization for several weeks is helpful for either condition, followed by taping or bracing to prevent plantarflexion and functional rehabilitation. Surgical excision should be considered for persistent symptoms (see Chapter 17).

Achilles Tendon Rupture

Complete ruptures result from a combination of intrasubstance degeneration of the tendon and excessive mechanical forces. Ruptures most commonly occur 3–4 cm proximal to the tendon's insertion on the calcaneus. The precipitating event in nearly all patients who sustain this injury is an active, forceful, sometimes unexpected plantarflexion of the foot. Patients who sustain spontaneous ruptures of the Achilles tendon note a sudden "snap" in the heel region at the time of injury and subsequent pain with active or passive plantarflexion of the foot and ankle. Many patients do not seek immediate treatment because they are still able to plantarflex their ankles through the actions of the posterior tibialis and flexor hallucis tendons. Patients may report a moderate limp and weakness in their ankle.

Physical examination should provide the diagnosis in most patients. With complete ruptures of the tendon, a palpable depression over the area of the rupture will be recognized. The patient will have weakness and pain with active plantarflexion of his or her ankle. The Thompson test is performed with the patient prone or kneeling on the examination table and the patient's feet extending over the end of the table. The calf musculature is gently squeezed in the middle third of the muscle belly, just distal to the widest girth. Normally with this maneuver, there is passive plantar movement of the foot. A positive test is indicated by lack of plantar movement of the foot and indicates a complete rupture of the tendon. Standard radiographs are useful to rule out other osseous conditions.

Treatment of complete ruptures is certainly controversial. Both operative[10, 11] and nonoperative[12, 13] approaches have been advocated with excellent results reported in the literature. Nonoperative approaches involve a period of casting with the foot in a relative equinus position followed by extensive rehabilitation. Surgical treatment consists of repair of the torn tendon followed by rehabilitation. Although the results of these treatment methods are similar, there may be a higher rerupture rate with those patients treated with nonoperative care.[14]

Flexor Hallucis Longus Tears

The repetitive stresses from a forceful toe-off on the great toe (such as occurs in ballet) may lead to injury of the flexor hallucis longus. Affected athletes have sudden onset of pain posteriorly to the medial malleolus and weakness with attempted toe flexion. For high-demand athletes (for example, dancers), a tear of the flexor hallucis longus requires surgical repair to achieve maximum function.

Medial Pain

Deltoid Sprain

Isolated injuries to the deltoid ligament are very rare (see Figure 18-2). Most injuries to this ligament complex occur in conjunction with fractures of the lateral malleolus or proximal fibula (Maisonneuve fracture). These injuries to the deltoid ligament occur as a result of an external rotational force to the planted foot in athletics.

Clinical examination reveals the majority of tenderness to be located on the medial aspect of the ankle. With medial tenderness and suspected injury to the deltoid ligament, it is important to rule out fractures of the lateral malleolus or proximal fibula and injuries to the syndesmosis. Similarly, the proximal aspect of the fibula should be palpated to rule out proximal fracture. On radiographic examination, widening of the medial clear space more than 5 mm on the mortise view (see discussion of syndesmosis injury) is indicative of a deltoid ligament injury.

Most clinicians agree that partial deltoid ligament ruptures should be treated nonoperatively. The treatment is similar to that for lateral ankle ligament injuries. There remains disagreement with respect to the best treatment of complete tears. Most agree that operative repair with stabilization of accompanying fractures is appropriate.[15, 16] Still others believe excellent results can be obtained with cast immobilization and rehabilitation.[17, 18]

Posterior Tibial Tendon Injury

Posterior tibial tendon injuries (Figure 18-10) range from minor strains with subsequent tendinitis symptoms to complete rupture and acquired flatfoot deformities. Strains to the posterior tibial tendon occur in all age groups and are usually associated with athletic activities. In contrast, nearly all complete ruptures of this tendon are associated with degenerative changes within the tendon and consequently occur in older patients.

Acutely, patients report severe pain along the posterior tibial tendon sheath, posterior to the medial malleolus. Symptoms usually resolve shortly after the injury. Patients may then develop symptoms secondary to the flatfoot deformity that ensues over months to years. Chronic symptoms consist of pain along the posterior aspect of the medial malleolus or laterally secondary to impingement of the calcaneus on the lateral talar process or fibula. Patients may or may not notice gradual development of a flatfoot deformity.

Physical examination may reveal tenderness, swelling, inversion weakness, deformity with standing, or pain with

FIGURE 18-10
Medial view of the tarsal tunnel.

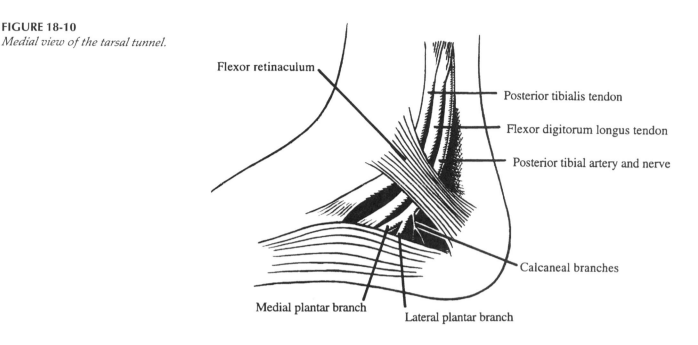

attempted heel rise. A patient with a posterior tibial tendon rupture will usually be unable to perform a single leg toe raise on the affected extremity. This maneuver is performed by asking the patient to lift his or her asymptomatic extremity off the ground, thereby bearing all his or her weight on the symptomatic foot. Then ask the patient to raise up on his or her toes. It is important to stabilize the patient by holding his or her hands during this test, because the patient is often quite unstable. With weightbearing on the symptomatic extremity, the foot obtains a position of hindfoot valgus, talar plantarflexion, and forefoot abduction.

The too-many-toes sign is another examination finding indicative of posterior tibialis tendon rupture. When the standing patient is observed from behind, his or her affected side will reveal more toes visible lateral to his or her heel than the unaffected side (Figure 18-11).

Radiographs in patients with suspected posterior tibial tendon ruptures should be taken while bearing weight on the extremity. These should reveal the flatfoot deformity. There may be degenerative changes recognized in the subtalar, calcaneocuboid, and talonavicular joints in patients with chronic ruptures. MRI is the study of choice for imaging the posterior tibial tendon. Treatment of acute sprains of the posterior tibial tendon consists of a short period of immobilization followed by rehabilitation and strengthening. A temporary orthotic giving medial longitudinal arch support is useful after casting. Complete ruptures with secondary flatfoot deformities may require surgical reconstruction with tendon transfers or arthrodesis of the peritalar joints.

Fractures

Athletes involved in virtually any sport can experience direct or indirect trauma to the ankle, resulting in a fracture (see Table 18-1). A complete description of fractures and dislocations of the ankle is beyond the scope of this chapter. It is important however, to keep in mind that the mechanisms that cause soft tissue injury about the ankle can also frac-

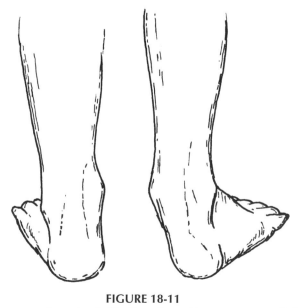

FIGURE 18-11
Too-many-toes sign indicating attenuation or rupture of the posterior tibialis tendon.

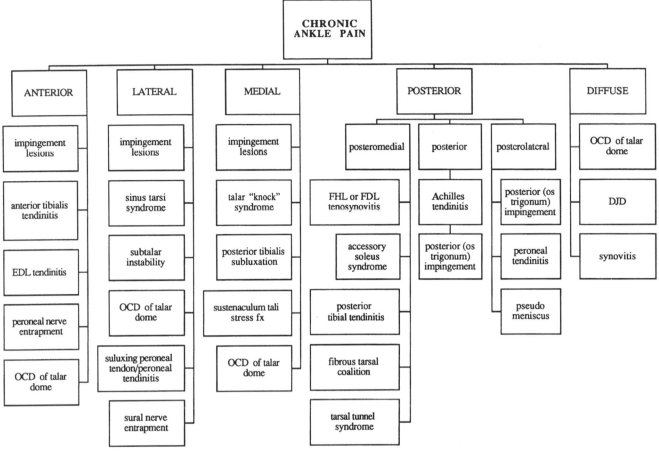

FIGURE 18-12

Algorithm for the evaluation of chronic ankle pain. (EDL = extensor digitorum longus; OCD = osteochondritis dissecans; FHL = flexor hallucis longus; FDL = flexor digitorum longus; DJD = degenerative joint disease; fx = fracture.)

ture components of the bony mortise. The athlete may feel a pop or crack associated with immediate pain. On examination, there is a variable degree of deformity, swelling, and ecchymosis with bony point tenderness over the fracture site. The distal neurovascular status should be assessed and documented. AP, lateral, and mortise radiographs should be obtained for suspected fractures with careful attention paid to the integrity of the mortise.

Fractures are often classified as lateral malleolar, medial malleolar, bimalleolar, and trimalleolar. Isolated fractures occur of either the lateral or medial malleoli. Bimalleolar fractures involve both the lateral and medial malleoli. Trimalleolar fractures include fractures of the lateral, medial, and posterior malleoli. The posterior malleolus is simply the posterior aspect of the tibia where the distal posterior tibiofibular ligament inserts. In general, nondisplaced fractures can be treated with immobilization and casting. This can be accomplished with a padded L or U splint initially, keeping the patient nonweightbearing. When the swelling

subsides, a short leg walking cast is applied, with the total time of immobilization lasting 4–6 weeks. After immobilization, bracing and an aggressive therapy program are instituted, including proprioceptive training, range of motion, and strengthening. If there is any displacement between the fracture fragments, surgical reduction and fixation must be considered.

CHRONIC ANKLE PAIN

Figure 18-12 is an algorithm for the evaluation of chronic ankle pain.

Anterior Pain

Bony Impingement Lesions
Anterior impingement lesions include anterior talar or anterior tibial spurs (Figure 18-13). These spurs are often

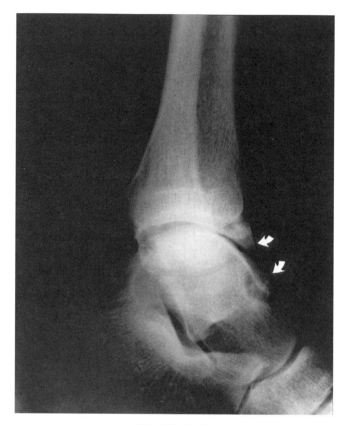

FIGURE 18-13
Anterior ankle bony impingement lesion. Radiograph demonstrates both anterior talar and anterior tibial spurs (arrows).

associated with limited ability to fully dorsiflex the ankle (such as deep squatting or a three-point stance in football, the plié in ballet, or shortening the stride length in running). On examination, spurs over the anterior ankle joint may be palpable and tender, and they cause pain on forced dorsiflexion of the foot. Radiographic findings on oblique and lateral views demonstrate a loss of the normal anterior bevel (angle) of the tibia and the talus (60 degrees) and demonstrate the spurs. If these lesions are symptomatic, a ½-in. heel lift can be used initially, but surgical debridement (often by arthroscope) is often necessary.

Anterior Tibial Tendinitis
Anterior tibial tendinitis often occurs in the dancer after returning from a layoff or in other athletes from shoelace irritation over the anterior ankle. There is local tenderness over the tendon at the level of the inferior retinaculum or at the level of the naviculocuneiform joint. The condition usually responds to a program of padding, rest, ice massage for 10 minutes every 2 hours, gentle strength-

ening and stretching, and nonsteroidal anti-inflammatory drugs (NSAIDs). Iontophoresis or phonophoresis may also be useful (see Chapter 3).

Extensor Digitorum Longus Tendinitis
Extensor digitorum longus tendinitis is similar to anterior tibial tendinitis, except for its location.

Peroneal Neuropathy
Entrapments of the deep peroneal nerve at the ankle can be caused by nerve lesions at the level of the anterior tarsal tunnel (see Figure 18-10), at the superior extensor retinaculum, or at the investing fascia of the ankle. There may be wasting of the extensor digitorum brevis, a positive Tinel sign at the suspected site of entrapment, or a sensory disturbance in the dorsal web space of the great and second toes. Symptoms may increase with plantarflexion, and some of these lesions may be associated with impingement spurs. Electromyography (EMG) or relief with lidocaine hydrochloride injection can support the diagnosis. Surgery may be indicated if avoidance of aggravating positions and steroid injection at the site of neuropathy do not help. Superficial peroneal neuropathy can be caused by compression at the level of the compartmental fascial perforation in the distal third of the lower leg (approximately 11 cm above the lateral malleolus). It is manifested by paresthesias over the dorsum of the foot and occasionally requires fascial release.

Lateral Pain

Impingements
Soft tissue impingement occurs when a soft tissue lesion forms over the anterior aspect of the ankle and impinges between the talus and anterolateral tibia or distal fibula with dorsiflexion of the foot. The soft tissue causing the symptoms is most commonly scar tissue or hypertrophic synovium that becomes pathologic after an injury to the ankle. Another cause of impingement is a "meniscoid lesion" on the inferior border of the distal anterior tibiofibular ligament. Injury to the anterolateral ankle capsule and synovium results in hemorrhage and synovitis, which may cause the formation of a mass of fibrocartilage or scar. Patients most commonly present with chronic anterolateral ankle pain after an inversion injury. They may have symptoms of catching and giving way, although physical examination often does not reveal evidence of instability. There is point tenderness with or without synovial thickening over the anterolateral ankle (between the anterior distal fibula, lateral talar dome, and lateral distal tibia). Pain is often reproduced with forced dorsiflexion of the ankle.

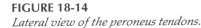

FIGURE 18-14
Lateral view of the peroneus tendons.

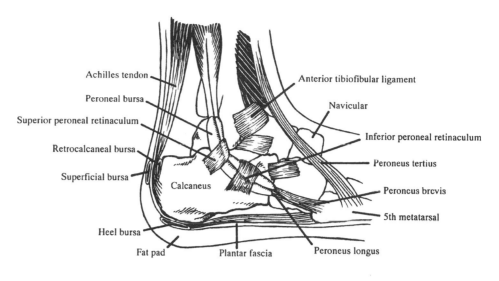

Achilles tendon
Peroneal bursa
Superior peroneal retinaculum
Retrocalcaneal bursa
Superficial bursa
Calcaneus
Heel bursa
Fat pad
Plantar fascia
Peroneus longus
Anterior tibiofibular ligament
Navicular
Inferior peroneal retinaculum
Peroneus tertius
Peroneus brevis
5th metatarsal

Initial treatment includes rest, activity modification, ice, NSAIDs, and physical therapy modalities (iontophoresis, microelectrostimulation), including stretching, strengthening, and proprioceptive exercises. An orthotic with medial longitudinal arch support or medial hindfoot and forefoot posting may be useful to "open up" the lateral ankle, especially in overpronators. If such conservative measures fail to bring relief of symptoms, further evaluation should be instituted. Stress radiographs should be obtained to rule out instability, and a bone scan should rule out occult osseous injury. An injection of corticosteroid combined with a local anesthetic into the thickened synovium or scar and joint should relieve the patient's symptoms if a soft tissue impingement lesion is present. Repeat injections of corticosteroids into the ankle joint should be avoided. Persistent symptoms despite conservative treatment for 4–6 months may warrant surgical consultation.

Sinus Tarsi Syndrome

Sinus tarsi syndrome can occur from injury to the subtalar joint, causing swelling and tenderness in the sinus tarsi. Pes planus and overpronation increase stress in the subtalar area and may aggravate the pain. Symptoms may be improved with lidocaine hydrochloride or steroid injection into the sinus tarsi. Radiographs may show evidence of subtalar arthritis or subtalar instability. Initial treatment includes correction of pronation with orthoses, NSAIDs, and possibly a local steroid injection. Varied results are obtained with synovectomy and debridement of the sinus tarsi. Posttraumatic subtalar instability may require surgical reconstruction. Deep peroneal nerve compression by the tendons of the extensor digitorum longus and the extensor digitorum hallucis brevis under the fas-

cia may also cause pain in this area, and neurolysis may be indicated.

Subtalar Instability

Subtalar instability may present as lateral ankle pain with symptoms similar to those of ankle sprains, such as pain and giving way. Instability may be congenital or may follow trauma. In the unstable congenital variety, many "minor" sprains may occur. The area of swelling and tenderness is distal to that seen with an ankle sprain, and there may be associated pain in the sinus tarsi. With inversion stress testing, there may be a sense of subtle sliding and rotational instability, with the talus subluxating from the calcaneus. A stress Broden view radiograph may show the inferior aspect of the talus going out of parallel with the superior aspect of the calcaneus. An inversion stress view of the ankle may show a similar loss of parallelism. The anterior drawer stress radiograph shows more than 5 mm of slippage of the talus on the calcaneus. Ankle bracing and rehabilitation may help, but persistent symptoms may require surgical stabilization.

Peroneus Subluxation

Subluxations of the peroneal tendons (Figure 18-14) may be due to (1) an incompetent sheath allowing subluxation out of the peroneal groove at the distal fibula (if the groove is too shallow), (2) an incompetent superior peroneal retinaculum, or (3) a bony avulsion of the retinaculum from the fibula. The subluxation of the tendons over the anterior border of the fibula against resisted eversion and dorsiflexion is diagnostic. Elimination of pain with lidocaine hydrochloride injection at the site is helpful in demonstrating peroneal tendon pathology as the source of pain. Conservative management includes ice, NSAIDs, taping the peroneal tendons in a reduced position for sport, orthotics (in a pronated foot to decrease lateral stresses), and ankle bracing. Referral for surgical treatment is indicated if symptomatic subluxation persists.

Peroneus Tendinitis

Tendinitis of the peroneal tendons without subluxation over the fibula can be due to friction between the peroneal tendons within their sheath, partial (longitudinal) tears, accessory slips of tendon in which friction develops, association with avulsion fractures of the CFL, or posttraumatic conditions that narrow the fibulocalcaneal space (enlargement of the peroneal tubercle, old calcaneal fractures, or lateral displacement of the subtalar joint). Initial treatment is ice, NSAIDs, lateral heel wedge for calcaneal varus, iontophoresis or phonophoresis, ankle rehabilitation, and ankle bracing. In resistant cases, CT or MRI may identify the aforementioned conditions, and surgery may be indicated.

Sural Nerve Entrapment

Sural nerve entrapment may be due to local scarring to the nerve along its course as it runs posterior to the peroneal tendons behind the lateral malleolus. There may also be entrapment at the site where the nerve pierces the deep fascia of the leg, usually two-thirds the distance from the knee to the heel. There is local tenderness over the lateral calcaneus with possible referred pain and sensory disturbance. Relief with lidocaine hydrochloride injection and EMG and a nerve conduction study may support the findings. Protective padding around the ankle, steroid injection, or neurolysis may provide relief of symptoms.

Other Causes

Lateral ankle pain can be caused by a lateral talar fracture (nonunited), distal fibular stress fracture, osteochondral fracture of the talus, cuboid subluxation, and tarsal coalitions.

Medial Pain

Impingement Lesions

Impingement lesions may occur after previous avulsion fractures from the tip of the medial malleolus or the medial talus. Examination along the medial edge of the tibiotalar joint reveals local swelling and tenderness and possibly a bony prominence. Ankle radiographs are indicated to assess for fractures, exostoses, or loose bodies, and fine-cut CT may be useful for further definition. If treatment with NSAIDs, padding, orthoses, and local injection fails, then an excision may be necessary.

Medial "Talar Knock"' Syndrome

Pain in medial "talar knock" syndrome is caused by the unstable lateral ankle. Inversion instability allows the talus to make focal contact against the tibia in the medial ankle mortise. Inversion stress testing causes medial pain, and basic treatment is directed to the underlying instability.

Posterior Tibial Tendon Subluxation

This unusual subluxation (see Figure 18-10) can occur secondary to a fracture of the medial edge of the medial malleolus or with attenuation of the retinaculum. Local tendon snapping may be observed over the edge of the medial malleolus with active ankle inversion and dorsiflexion. Lidocaine hydrochloride injection can confirm this as the source of the pain. If bracing, taping, and physical therapy modalities do not relieve pain, referral is indicated.

Other Causes

Sustentacular tali stress fracture, medial malleolar stress fracture, and subtle osteochondral lesions of the talar dome may also cause medial pain and should be considered.

Posteromedial Pain

Flexor Hallucis Longus Tendinitis

This tendinitis is caused by overuse injury or partial tears of the tendon from activities such as ballet or long-distance walking, which require strong plantarflexion of the great toe. Physical examination reveals crepitus or tenderness at the ankle 1–2 cm posterior to the medial malleolus and just posterior to the tibial artery. There may be a more distal tenderness medially over the course of the tendon or pain on standing on tiptoe (en pointe). Passive dorsiflexion or active flexion of the great toe may aggravate the pain. Conservative treatment includes relative rest, physical therapy modalities (iontophoresis, electrical stimulation), NSAIDs, and functional orthotics (to decrease stress on the tendon). Tenolysis is occasionally needed if these measures fail. If an athlete experiences "triggering" of the great toe, partial rupture of the flexor hallucis longus at the ankle should be considered and patients referred.

Flexor Digitorum Longus Tendinitis

Accessory tendons of the flexor digitorum longus can predispose to developing a tendinitis and can be associated with tarsal tunnel syndrome. There may be both a history of mechanical pain (activity-related) and neurogenic pain (at night). Physical examination reveals point tenderness over the tarsal tunnel posterior to the medial malleolus and just behind the posterior tibial tendon, and a

Tinel sign may be present (see Figure 18-10). Active plantarflexion of the lesser toes aggravates the pain. Conservative treatment includes relative rest or even a walking cast for 2 weeks to rest the inflamed tendon (by limiting the flexor digitorum tendon excursion). Orthoses are useful in a pronated foot, and NSAIDs, ice massage, and iontophoresis are helpful. Cautious use of steroid injection into the tendon sheath (not the tendon) may be attempted in resistant cases. This should be followed by short-term immobilization in a range of motion walker to minimize the risk of tendon attenuation or rupture. Referral is indicated if these measures fail.

Accessory Soleus Syndrome

In accessory soleus syndrome, the associated soft tissue enlargement posteromedially is caused by an accessory muscular band, which runs from the soleus to the pre-Achilles bursa. Although the muscle band lies outside of the tarsal tunnel, it may be associated with tarsal tunnel syndrome symptoms and posteromedial pain. CT or MRI confirms a characteristically normal muscle in this location. If measures to decrease local inflammation (NSAIDs, cortisone injection, ice massage, and iontophoresis) fail, surgical referral is indicated.

Posterior Tibial Tendinitis

Posterior tibial tendinitis is more common in the middle-aged athlete with a planovalgus foot and attenuation of local tendon blood flow. There is tenderness over the course of the tendon, swelling, and—if the tendon is ruptured—an inability to perform a single leg standing tip-toe raise. The lack of support from this tendon causes loss of support for the arch and weakness of foot inversion. Viewed from behind, the foot shows "too many" toes laterally, compared with the other foot (see Figure 18-11).

In cases of tendinitis (not rupture), a prominent navicular bone and hypermobile flatfoot are present. If orthotics, NSAIDs, and therapy modalities fail to relieve symptoms, patients should be referred for various surgical options. All acute ruptures should be referred.

Tarsal Tunnel Syndrome

Tarsal tunnel syndrome is caused by entrapment of the posterior tibial nerve within the tarsal tunnel. This tunnel is formed by the flexor retinaculum over the posterior medial malleolus (see Figure 18-10). The tendons of the posterior tibialis, flexor digitorum longus, and flexor hallucis course through the tunnel along with the posterior tibial nerve. Tendinitis from any of these tendons, a tight retinaculum, or overpronation can compress or stretch the nerve and cause symptoms: a burning dysesthesia in the plantar aspect of the foot aggravated by repetitive use.

Physical examination may reveal hypesthesia over the plantar foot, tenderness posterior to the medial malleolus, and a positive Tinel sign over the tarsal tunnel. Associated tendinopathies as discussed in preceding sections should be addressed. EMGs and nerve conduction studies are useful to assess the severity. Treatment is as described for flexor hallucis longus and flexor digitorum longus tendinitis, including orthotics, NSAIDs, therapy modalities, and tarsal tunnel injections. Surgical release and exploration is indicated if these measures fail.

Posterior Pain: Achilles Tendinitis

Overuse injuries to the Achilles tendon include peritendinitis, tendinosis, and partial or complete ruptures. Complete ruptures were discussed under Acute Ankle Injuries. Peritendinitis of the Achilles is one of the more common overuse injuries seen in the athletic population. These injuries result from accumulative impact loading and repetitive microtrauma to the tendon.

The predominant symptom of Achilles tendinitis is pain that is localized to the tendon. Initially, the patient may report pain only with prolonged activity. The pain usually subsides with rest but may be exacerbated by climbing stairs. As the tendinitis progresses, the patient will have pain earlier in the activity being performed. In the later stages of tendinitis or partial rupture of the tendon, the patient will be unable to perform the activity and will report pain at rest. In chronic tendinitis, the patient will report more diffuse pain throughout the tendon substance. Often, there is development of nodularity and fusiform swelling of the tendon.

Physical findings in patients with tendinitis include soft tissue swelling, localized tenderness to palpation, and crepitus with movement of the ankle. Nodularity and diffuse, fusiform swelling should make the examiner suspicious of tendinosis or a partial rupture of the tendon. The lateral radiograph may rarely show calcification of the soft tissues around the tendon or in the tendon itself.

Most cases of tendinitis are successfully managed non-operatively. Treatment principles are aimed at decreasing pain and inflammation and restoring normal function. Symptomatic relief includes decreasing the athlete's activities temporarily. Total rest may not be required, rather, the intensity of training should be decreased or modified. (For example, a runner should avoid hill work or interval training.) Patients with chronic symptoms or more severe acute symptoms may benefit from a short period of immobilization. This usually involves casting for 1–3 weeks. A stretching program is often beneficial. Other useful modalities include the use of a ¼- to ⅜-in. heel lift, oral NSAIDs, physical therapy modalities, ice, and the

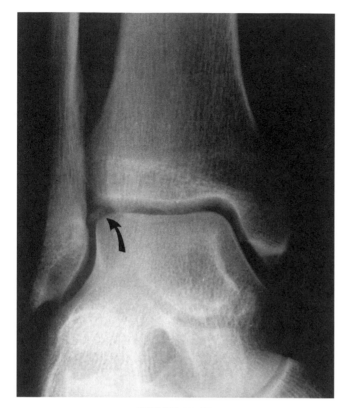

FIGURE 18-15
Osteochondritis dissecans lesion of the anterolateral talus (arrow).

use of orthotics to correct excessive pronation of the foot. The use of corticosteroid injections for the treatment of tendinitis should be discouraged. If an injection is used, it should be placed by an experienced individual and only into the retrocalcaneal bursa. As symptoms improve, an aggressive program of heel cord stretching and balanced muscle strengthening should be instituted. Surgery may be considered for chronic cases of tendinitis that have failed all conservative treatment regimens.

Posterolateral Pain

Posterior Impingement (Os Trigonum Syndrome)
The os trigonum is the nonunited lateral tubercle of the posterior aspect of the talus. Its incidence is estimated to be between 8% and 13% in the general population. In the majority of cases, this bone is considered to be an innocent and asymptomatic finding. In certain athletic endeavors (such as ballet) and kicking sports (such as soccer and football), this bone will impinge on the posterior tibia in plantar flexion of the foot. In these activities, acute or chronic pain can develop along the posterolateral aspect of the ankle.

The clues to the correct diagnosis of posterior impingement on the os trigonum are the location of the pain behind the peroneal tendons and reproduction of the pain with forced plantarflexion of the ankle. Passive dorsiflexion or active flexion of the great toe may cause posterolateral pain that is due to the proximity of the flexor hallucis longus to the os trigonum. Routine radiographs will reveal the os trigonum (see Figure 18-9). An additional lateral radiograph taken with the ankle in maximum plantarflexion may also be beneficial and may show the impingement of the posterior tibia on the posterolateral talus.

As with most conditions affecting the ankle joint, treatment of posterior impingement or os trigonum syndrome should initially be conservative. NSAIDs, rest, ice, and physical therapy modalities should be tried first. It is also important to avoid positions with the ankle in maximum plantarflexion. The use of taping techniques or orthotics may be useful to limit the ankle from extreme plantarflexion. If symptoms persist despite these conservative measures, the patient may be a candidate for surgical excision of the os trigonum.

Peroneus Tendinitis
See the discussion of peroneus tendon injury under Lateral Pain.

Pseudomeniscus Syndrome
Hypertrophic fibrous tissue extending off the posterior tibiofibular ligament of the ankle joint is occasionally seen in dancers. This lesion can cause posterior ankle pain and a sensation of catching or snapping. If physical therapy measures, such as soft tissue mobilization and ultrasound, fail to relieve symptoms, open or arthroscopic debridement may be necessary.

Diffuse Ankle Pain

Osteochondral Lesions
Osteochondral lesions of the talus are disruptions of the normal articular surface of the talar dome. This condition is also known as *osteochondritis dissecans of the talus*. Two types of osteochondral lesions of the talus can be seen. Lesions that occur laterally are usually related to trauma, cause more symptoms, rarely heal spontaneously, and are more likely to require early surgical treatment (Figure 18-15). The lateral lesions are usually thin, wafer-like lesions with a very thin piece of bone involved. The medial lesions are less likely to be associated with trauma and may occur insidiously. These lesions are also less likely to be symptomatic, may heal spontaneously, and usually require surgery only when the lesion becomes dis-

placed from the talus and becomes a loose body in the ankle joint. Morphologically, the medial lesions are more cup shaped and deeper, and they tend to stay in the crater. These two broad categories of osteochondral lesions can be remembered using the acronyms DIAL (*d*orsiflexion, *i*nversion, *a*nterior, *l*ateral) for lateral lesions and PIMP (*p*lantarflexion, *i*nversion, *m*edial, *p*osterior) for medial lesions. The first two words of the acronym refer to the mechanism of injury and the latter two the location of the lesion.

When symptoms associated with a "routine" ankle sprain do not resolve, an osteochondral lesion of the talus should be considered. Symptoms of persistent pain, effusion, locking, or giving way after 5–6 weeks should prompt further investigation. Radiographs should be repeated. Specialized views—including a mortise view with the ankle in maximum plantarflexion—should be performed in attempts to see a fragment from the talus. Bone scintigraphy, using a pinhole collimator, is very sensitive for detecting these lesions of the talus. If a bone scan is negative, it is unlikely that there is significant osteochondral injury. If the bone scan is positive, further investigation with CT or MRI will better delineate the morphology and anatomic location of the lesion. This information is often necessary to direct treatment of this injury.

Treatment of osteochondral lesions depends on the size and severity of the lesions. Small lesions that are not completely detached from the articular surface can be treated conservatively. This usually involves a period of non-weightbearing casting for 4–6 weeks and total immobilization for 8–12 weeks. Larger areas of injury and lesions that are completely detached from the articular surface usually require surgical treatment. Surgical principles include repair of the lesion if the fragment is large enough or excision of the fragment and attempts to induce fibrocartilaginous growth into the remaining defect if the lesion is smaller. Lesions on the anterior one-half to two-thirds of the talus can usually be approached arthroscopically. Lesions on the posterior half of the talus are more difficult to treat arthroscopically and usually require open surgical treatment.

Posttraumatic Arthritis of the Ankle

Posttraumatic arthritis of the ankle can occur after any injury to the ankle. At the time of the acute injury, the cartilage surfaces may be injured microscopically, and gross injury to the articular surface is not recognized. An intraarticular fracture may result in joint incongruities, which over time result in cartilage wear and degeneration. An intraarticular fracture that is reduced anatomically with no subsequent joint incongruity may also develop posttraumatic arthritis because of injury to the articular sur-

face at the cellular level. Posttraumatic arthritis may also develop after repetitive minor injuries to the ankle (repeated ankle sprains). Finally, posttraumatic arthritis can develop as a result of altered biomechanics of the ankle that are due to soft tissue injuries (e.g., posterior tibialis tendon ruptures, contractures about the ankle).

Clinically, patients with posttraumatic arthritis of the ankle present with progressive pain and limited motion of the ankle. A common symptom is pain or inability to fully dorsiflex the ankle. Initially, the pain occurs only with strenuous activities but may progress to pain with activities of daily living and even pain at rest.

Patients with early or mild posttraumatic arthritis can be treated with activity modification and NSAIDs. With more severe symptoms and pathology, the patient may benefit from orthotics to limit motion in the ankle. Intraarticular injections of steroid preparations should be used cautiously. Surgical intervention may be required for severe symptoms and pathology that do not respond to conservative measures. Surgical treatment consists of arthroscopic debridement and excision of osteophytes in mild cases or arthrodesis of the tibiotalar joint in more severe cases.

Synovitis

Chronic ankle pain can be caused by tumor (atypical pain, such as pain at rest or night pain) or systemic rheumatologic conditions (for example, gout and rheumatoid arthritis). After routine examination and plain radiography, evaluation with a bone scan and MRI generally is helpful. The bone scan helps to localize an area of increased osteoclastic activity. MRI can help to diagnose conditions such as pigmented villonodular synovitis, tumor, and osteochondritis dissecans. The MRI findings in many common synovial conditions are often nonspecific, and the cost must be considered. Initial laboratory evaluation for rheumatologic conditions should include an erythrocyte sedimentation rate, antinuclear antibody titer, and rheumatoid factor. Aspirated joint fluid should be sent for crystal analysis, cell count, and mucin clot test to evaluate inflammatory arthropathies. A Gram's stain and culture are performed if infection is suspected. It is most important to consider these additional conditions despite a history of trauma.

PEDIATRIC ANKLE INJURIES

Certain injuries and conditions affecting the ankle are unique to pediatric and adolescent athletes. The physis at the end of the tibia and fibula in children is a weak link and acts as a stress riser when significant force is applied to the pediatric ankle. The physis present at the ends of skeletally imma-

Type I

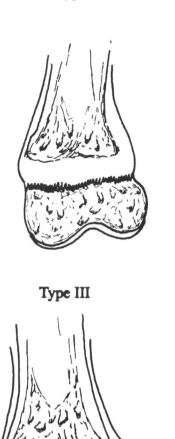

Type II

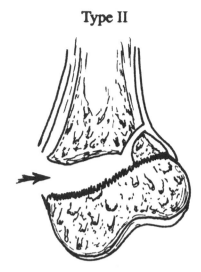

FIGURE 18-16
Salter-Harris classification of pediatric fractures (nondisplaced). Type I is a fracture through the epiphysis, type II involves the epiphysis and metaphysis (arrow), type III involves the physis and epiphysis, type IV involves the physis and metaphysis, and type V (not shown) describes a crush injury to the epiphysis and carries a high risk of early eccentric growth plate closure.

Type III

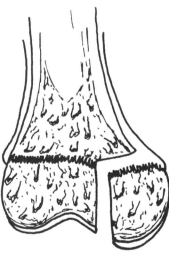

Type IV

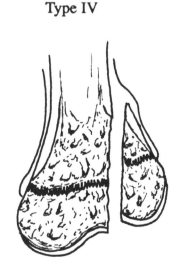

ture long bones is primarily made up of cartilage. Enchondral ossification of this cartilage is responsible for longitudinal growth of the bone. Serious ankle sprains are unusual in the skeletally immature athlete; rather, fractures through the physis occur and must be recognized to minimize the complications of growth arrest to the tibia or fibula.

Pediatric Ankle Fractures

Fractures involving the distal tibia and fibula in the pediatric population often involve the epiphyseal growth plate. Fractures involving the physis have been divided into five types according to the Salter-Harris classification (Figure 18-16). In the pediatric patient, careful examination of the injured ankle is necessary to rule out injury to the physis.

A patient with a nondisplaced fracture through the distal fibular physis may present with similar symptoms to that of a patient with a lateral ankle sprain. The patient with a fracture through the fibular physis plate will be exquisitely tender above the lateral malleolus. The patient with ligamentous injuries that are due to an ankle sprain will have tenderness localized distal to the lateral malleolus.

The distal tibial physis closes at approximately age 15 years in females and age 17 years in males. The closure takes place over approximately 18 months. Closure begins centrally within the physis, extends medially, and finally ends laterally. This asymmetric closure sequence is an important anatomical feature of the growing ankle and is responsible for certain fracture patterns seen in adolescent patients.

The juvenile Tillaux and the triplane fractures are two examples of these fractures unique to the adolescent population. The juvenile Tillaux fracture is a Salter-Harris type III fracture involving the anterolateral distal tibia. The triplane fracture is a complex fracture of the distal tibia that has the appearance of a Salter-Harris type III fracture on the AP radiograph and a Salter-Harris type II fracture on the lateral radiograph. With either of these injuries, it is important to have the patient evaluated by an orthopedic surgeon, because very little displacement of the fracture can be accepted.

Tarsal Coalitions

Tarsal coalition is a bony, fibrous, or cartilaginous connection of two or more tarsal bones. The cause of the anomaly is unknown but occurs in 1–3% of the population. The most common coalitions of the tarsal bones are the talocalcaneal and the calcaneonavicular. A more unusual coalition is the talonavicular coalition. Patients present usually in adolescence when the cartilaginous or fibrous coalition tends to ossify and become less compliant. The patient usually reports vague lateral or diffuse foot pain that may or may not be associated with trauma. Physical findings include localized pain over the subtalar joint, spastic flatfeet, or limited subtalar and transverse tarsal joint motion. The diagnosis can be made with plain radiographs or CT. The oblique radiograph of the foot should reveal the calcaneonavicular coalition. The talocalcaneal coalition is often difficult to see on plain radiographs, and CT is necessary to make the diagnosis.

The initial treatment of these conditions should be conservative measures to relieve the patient's pain. Symptomatic children should be treated with cast immobilization and NSAIDs for 1 month followed by corrective orthotics and functional rehabilitation. Activity modification may be necessary. Patients who continue to report pain despite conservative treatment should be considered for surgical treatment. Surgical treatment consists of resection of the bar and placement of fat or muscle into the defect created to prevent recurrence. For patients with large coalitions and secondary degenerative changes in the subtalar joints, arthrodesis of the joints may be necessary.

SUMMARY

Injuries to the ankle joint continue to be some of the most common injuries seen in athletics. The majority of injuries can be accurately diagnosed with a thorough history and complete physical examination. Judicious use of imaging studies is often necessary to confirm a diagnosis. The treatment of most ankle injuries and conditions is usually nonoperative; however, persistent symptoms after conservative treatment may warrant referral for specialized treatment. Attention to the principles outlined in this chapter will allow individuals with disorders of the ankle to return to activities in the shortest possible time.

REFERENCES

1. Clanton TO, Schon LC. Athletic Injuries to the Soft Tissues of the Foot and Ankle. In RA Mann, MJ Coughlin (eds), Surgery of the Foot and Ankle (6th ed). St. Louis: Mosby, 1993;1095–1224.
2. Garrick JG, Requa RK. The epidemiology of foot and ankle injuries in sports. Clin Sports Med 1988;7:29–36.
3. Smith RW, Reischl SF. Treatment of ankle sprains in young athletes. Am J Sports Med 1986;14:465–471.
4. Lassiter TE, Malone TR, Garrett WE. Injury to the lateral ligaments of the ankle. Orthop Clin North Am 1989;20:629–640.
5. Karlsson J, Bergsten T, Lasinger O, Peterson L. Surgical treatment of chronic lateral instability of the ankle joint. Am J Sports Med 1989;17:266–274.
6. Renstrom PA, Kannus P. Injuries of the Foot and Ankle. In JC DeLee, D Drez (eds), Orthopaedic Sports Medicine. Philadelphia: Saunders, 1994;2:1705–1767.
7. Ryan JB, Hopkinson WJ, Wheeler JH, et al. Office management of the acute ankle sprain. Clin Sports Med 1989;8:477–495.
8. Brantigan JW, Pedegana LR, Lippert FG. Instability of the subtalar joint. Diagnosis by stress tomography in three cases. J Bone Joint Surg Am 1977;59:321–324.
9. Stiehl JB. Complex ankle fracture dislocations with syndesmotic diastasis. Orthop Rev 1990;14:499–507.
10. Beskin JL, Sanders RA, Hunter SC, Hughston JC. Surgical repair of Achilles tendon ruptures. Am J Sports Med 1987;15:1–8.
11. Nistor L. Surgical and non-surgical treatment of Achilles tendon rupture. J Bone Joint Surg Am 1981;63:394–399.
12. Stein SR, Luekens CA. Methods and rationale for closed treatment of Achilles tendon ruptures. Am J Sports Med 1976;4:162–169.
13. Jacobs D, Martens M, Audekercke RV, et al. Comparison of conservative and operative treatment of Achilles tendon rupture. Am J Sports Med 1978;6:107–111.
14. Inglis AE, Scott WN, Sculco TP, Patterson AH. Ruptures of the tendo Achilles. J Bone Joint Surg Am 1976;58:990–993.
15. DeSouza LJ, Gustilo RB, Meyer TJ. Results of operative treatment of displaced external rotation-abduction fractures of the ankle. J Bone Joint Surg Am 1985;67:1066–1074.
16. Yablon IG, Heller FG, Shouse L. The key of the lateral malleolus in displaced fractures of the ankle. J Bone Joint Surg Am 1977;59:169–173.
17. Harper MC. The deltoid ligament: an evaluation of need for surgical repair. Clin Orthop 1988;226:156–168.
18. Chapman MW. Sprains of the ankle. Instr Course Lect 1975;24:294–308.

Appendix A

Ankle Rehabilitation

The following is a sample patient home instruction sheet.

PHASE I: PRICE

In the first 24–72 hours after the injury, the PRICE regimen should be followed:

*P*rotection: Limit motion using an ankle support, such as an air stirrup, canvas, splint, or hinged brace.

*R*est: Use touchdown weightbearing initially; crutches with gradual return to weightbearing. Crutch support can be discontinued when there is no limp with walking.

*I*ce: Fill a plastic zippered bag with water and ice and use in direct contact with injury site. Apply 10–15 minutes every 2 hours until swelling is controlled.

*C*ompression: Ace bandage will often be enough. In more severe injuries, may use taping or a cast. This will limit swelling.

*E*levation: Injured ankle should be elevated above the level of the heart to reduce swelling.

PHASE II: RANGE OF MOTION

Range of Motion Exercises

The following should be performed in sets of 25 repetitions, twice each day.

- Flexion: Pull toes toward ceiling.
- Extension: Push toes downward, pointing toward the floor.
- Inversion: Turn soles of feet inward toward each other.
- Eversion: Turn soles of feet outward, away from each other.
- Foot circles: Trace small circles in the air with toes, clockwise and counterclockwise.
- Alphabet: Sit on a table with your knee straight and ankle extended beyond the table edge. Using your big toe, write all the letters of the alphabet. Do four repetitions of this exercise.

Contrast Baths

Begin these on day 2 or 3, or when swelling resolves. Initially, these exercises should be performed in contrast baths using the following method:

1. Using two containers large enough to comfortably accommodate your foot, fill one with ice and water and the other with warm water approximately 100°–105°F.
2. Place the injured foot in the warm water for 4 minutes, then in the cold water for 1 minute, and alternate 4 minutes warm, then 1 minute cold. Repeat this four times. Always end the session with cold. The range of motion exercises previously described should be done while in the warm water.

PHASE III: STRETCHING AND STRENGTHENING

Wall Lean

Stand approximately 3 ft from the wall with your knees locked, legs straight, and feet flat and slightly turned in. Lean toward the wall until stretching of the calves is felt. Hold this position for 30 seconds; relax and repeat five times. Repeat stretches in the same position, except with knees bent slightly.

Heel Raises

Stand on the edge of a stair with your heels extended over the edge. Raise as high as you can on your toes, and gradually lower your heels as low as possible below the level of the stair. Begin using both feet, 15 repetitions, and progress to using only your injured ankle, gradually increasing the number of repetitions to 50–100.

Stair Step

Using the same starting position as for the heel raise, lower your heels as far as possible and hold for 1 minute. Complete two repetitions of this with your knees straight and two repetitions with your knees slightly bent.

Toe Raises

Stand flat on the floor and raise your toes and forefoot from the floor, standing on your heels for 10 seconds; then lower. Repeat this exercise 10 times.

Exercises with Resistance

Using a 2-ft long strip of elastic tubing or a bike tire inner tube, work your ankle in the following exercises. Begin with sets of 10 repetitions and increase to 25 repetitions.

1. Eversion (out and up). Sit on a chair with the tubing looped over your foot and around the table leg. With your heel on the floor, flex your foot up and out, and hold for 10 seconds.
2. Inversion (in and up). Loop tubing over your foot and table leg, and work your ankle in and up.
3. Dorsiflexion (straight up). Loop tubing over your foot and around the table leg, and pull straight up with your heel on the floor.
4. Plantarflexion (straight down). Hold tubing in your hands, and loop the tubing around the bottom of your foot. With your heel on the floor, work your ankle down.
5. Peroneal muscle strengthening. Lying on your side on a couch with your ankle supported on the couch's arm, loop a belt with 3–6 lb of weight attached over the outside surface of your foot. With your toes and foot pointing down, raise the weight by pulling your ankle outward, leaving your heel on the arm of the couch. Repeat this exercise 25 times, gradually increasing the weight until you can do 15 lb 25 times.

Proprioceptive Training

To improve proprioception (your sense of position and balance), the following exercises are helpful.

1. Stand on your injured leg with eyes closed and arms folded across chest. Hold for 15 seconds, and repeat 15 times.
2. Standing on your injured leg only, perform a half squat. Early in rehabilitation, this should be done with support (use the wall). Progress to doing this exercise with your eyes closed and no support.
3. Balance board. Place an 18-in.×18-in. board over a tennis ball. Step carefully onto board and using both legs, balance the board with edge off the floor 15 times for 10 seconds. Progress to one leg when comfortable.

PHASE IV: SPORT-SPECIFIC EXERCISES

You may begin running while still in a brace. When strength and balance have recovered, and you can walk without pain, a program to return to running should be started. A gradual program should be used to lessen the risk of reinjury. When you can do all of the following exercises without pain, you are ready to return to full sporting activity.

Jog-Walk-Jog

Alternate jog-walk-jog on a smooth, straight surface.

1. Jog 25 yd, walk 25 yd, jog 25 yd; repeat.
2. Jog 50 yd, walk 25 yd, jog 50 yd; repeat.
3. Jog 100 yd, walk 25 yd, jog 100 yd; repeat.

Sprint-Jog-Sprint

Alternate sprint-jog-sprint, as with Jog-Walk-Jog.

Figure Eights

When you can run full speed without a limp or pain, begin gradual direction changes with a figure eight on the full length of a basketball court. When this can be done without pain, condense the figure eight to one-half the court.

Zigzag Cutting

When short-course figure eight running is mastered, begin executing quick, sharp, right-and-left cuts while running.

III

Medical Problems

19

Exercise-Induced Bronchospasm

Wayne A. Schirner

SHORTNESS OF BREATH

A variety of pulmonary problems may present in the athlete as shortness of breath and may result in poor outcomes if not recognized and treated appropriately. Examples include the boxer who has sudden dyspnea during a match and must be evaluated for pneumothorax, or the mountain climber who is brought to the emergency room with severe dyspnea and is considered to have high-altitude pulmonary edema until proved otherwise. The sudden onset of shortness of breath and chest pain must always bring to mind the possibility of a pulmonary embolus. However, most of these cases are easily diagnosed with a quick history and physical examination and are rather sport-specific. This chapter focuses on the much more common problem of exercise-induced bronchospasm (EIB).

EXERCISE-INDUCED BRONCHOSPASM

The prevalence of exercise-induced symptoms in asthmatics has been reported to be 40-90%[1]; therefore, this condition should be anticipated in all asthma patients. Many people will only experience asthma symptoms associated with exercise, however, and these symptoms may not always suggest the diagnosis. Untreated EIB can limit an athlete's performance and significantly disrupt normal life. Although episodes of EIB are short-lived, their severity and impact can be striking. As a result, people with untreated EIB often limit their activities unnecessarily.

Pathophysiology

Although the clinical features of EIB have been clearly described, the pathophysiology is incompletely understood. EIB is characterized by a temporary increase in airway resistance after 5-8 minutes of vigorous exercise. Symptoms may become more severe with the cessation of exercise and usually spontaneously resolve in 30-60 minutes. Uncommonly, a late phase of EIB occurs 4-12 hours after the initial episode. Unlike the late phase of allergen-induced asthma, this reaction in EIB is not considered to be serious and is easily treated with inhaled bronchodilators.

Information about asthma suggests that a significant amount of airway inflammation is occurring in addition to smooth muscle constriction. EIB, however, is thought to be almost exclusively a result of smooth muscle constriction. The development of EIB is influenced by the type and duration of exercise or by air contaminants, especially sulfur dioxide and ozone. Air temperature and humidity have also been recognized as important factors. The severity of EIB is usually increased by poor control of underlying asthma; cold, dry ambient air; viral infections; and allergen exposure.

The character of the exercise performance is an important variable. Strenuous exercise increases the severity of the attack, although both short, intense efforts and long, moderate-intensity workouts may induce an episode. The airway obstruction is typically not as severe with longer sustained exercise (10 minutes or more). This reduced airway obstruction with lower-intensity sustained exercise may be related to a refractory period of 30-90 minutes that develops in some patients after an attack of EIB.[2]

Although some debate remains, it has generally been established that EIB results from loss of heat, water, or both from the small airways during exercise. The chain of events that relates heat and water loss to airway constriction has not yet been clarified. Because the response is far from uniform, it may be that different pathways are involved in different subjects.[3]

Prevalence

There have been no definitive studies on the prevalence of EIB; however, it is thought to affect approximately 12–15% of the general population. Approximately 40% of children with allergic rhinitis who do not have clinical asthma do have EIB.[4]

A screening program developed by the U.S. Olympic Committee that was used before the 1984 Olympic Games in Los Angeles found 67 of 597 Olympic athletes (11%) to have asthma or EIB. With a coordinated medical care approach, these athletes not only competed, but won 41 medals, including 15 gold and 21 silver medals.[5] Of the 667 U.S. athletes in the 1988 Olympic Games in Seoul, South Korea, 52 had confirmed EIB (and another 50 were suspected of having it). In those games, the same percentage of athletes who had and did not have EIB won medals.[6]

One study of a conference championship university football team revealed that 12% of the players admitted to a history of asthma, and 19% indicated that at some time they had chest tightness, cough, wheezing, or prolonged shortness of breath after exercise. A methacholine challenge test was performed on all team members, and positive test results were obtained in 50%. This finding suggests that bronchial hyperresponsiveness is much more common than previously suspected and that the prevalence of EIB may be underappreciated.[7]

Diagnosis

The preseason physical examination required in many states is an excellent opportunity for EIB screening. A previous history of asthma or environmental allergies increases the risk for EIB. A specific yes or no response to a question about coughing or wheezing during or after strenuous sports activity should be required. EIB should be suspected in any athlete with a history of cough, shortness of breath, wheezing, chest pain, chest tightness, or endurance problems during exercise. The diagnosis of EIB can be made based on a therapeutic trial of medication, exercise testing, or bronchoprovocation testing. An algorithm for diagnosing EIB is presented in Figure 19-1.

Therapeutic Trial

Athletes suspected of having EIB may have normal physical findings when they present for evaluation, and baseline pulmonary function testing may likewise be normal. The simplest confirmation of the diagnosis is relief of symptoms after a therapeutic trial of an inhaled beta-adrenergic agonist or cromolyn sodium. Patients must be informed of proper inhalation technique.[2]

Exercise Challenge

When there is still doubt, an exercise challenge test can establish the diagnosis of EIB. In an exercise challenge, the patient exercises at a level of ventilation high enough to produce the intra-airway thermal events that evoke airway constriction. If a patient reports symptoms with exercise, an adequate challenge would consist of having the patient undertake whatever exercise provokes the problem. This can usually be achieved through exercise for 4–8 minutes at an intensity of 50% or more of the patient's maximum predicted oxygen consumption (65% of age-predicted maximum heart rate). A formal exercise challenge test may also be performed with a treadmill exercise capable of raising the patient's heart rate to 80–90% of age-predicted maximum heart rate for a period of 6–8 minutes. Pulmonary function measurements—for example, peak expiratory flow rate (PEFR) or forced expiratory volume at 1 second (FEV_1)—are determined before and after exercise and at 5-minute intervals for 20–30 minutes. Although a drop in PEFR or FEV_1 of more than 10% is compatible with EIB, using a decrease of 15% may be more specific, because it allows for the possibility of confusing variability of spirometry technique with a true drop in pulmonary function. The best of three expiratory maneuvers is taken at each time period.[3]

Having the patient run outdoors for 4–8 minutes at a brisk pace may be more asthmogenic than the treadmill, because air coolness and dryness or environmental triggers will enhance asthmatic response. A 15% drop in PEFR or FEV_1 would, again, be diagnostic of EIB.

For middle-aged and elderly people, it is important to conduct the exercise challenge in a facility with the capability of monitoring heart rate and rhythm as part of the test.

Methacholine Challenge

If an exercise challenge test fails to diagnose EIB when an athlete reports exercise-related symptoms, a bronchoprovocation test with methacholine should be performed before the possibility of EIB is dismissed. A fall in FEV_1 of 20% after inhalation of methacholine is diagnostic of hyperactive airways. Several evaluations demonstrate that a methacholine challenge is more sen-

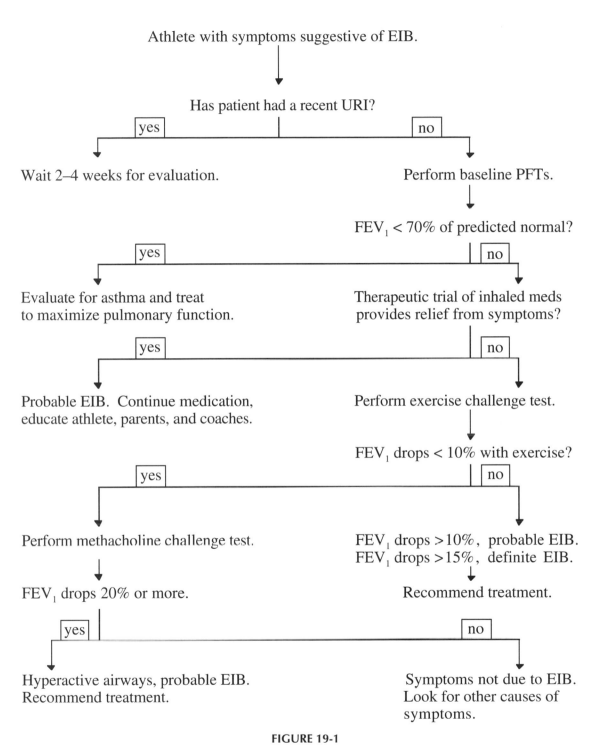

FIGURE 19-1

Algorithm for the diagnosis of exercise-induced bronchospasm (EIB). (PFTs = pulmonary function tests; URI = upper respiratory infection; FEV₁ = forced expiratory volume at 1 second; meds = medications.)

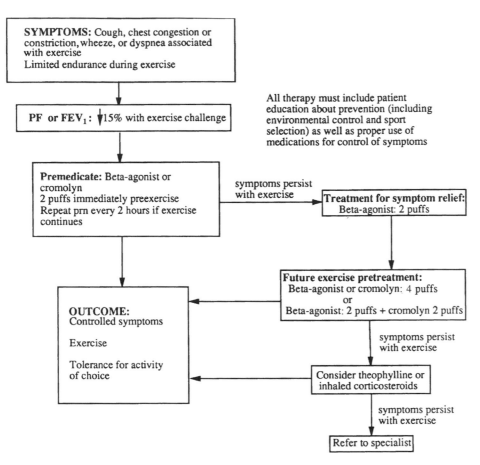

FIGURE 19-2
Algorithm for management of exercise-induced bronchospasm. (PF = pulmonary function; FEV₁ = forced expiratory volume at 1 second; ↓ = decreases by greater than.) (Adapted from National Heart, Lung and Blood Institute. Expert Panel Report: Guidelines for the Diagnosis and Management of Asthma. Publication No. 91–3042. Bethesda, MD: National Institutes of Health, August 1991;121.)

sitive than an exercise challenge for diagnosing hyperactive airways.[8]

Management

Management of athletes with EIB involves sport selection, training regimens, and medications. The goal of treating EIB is to enable patients to participate in any activities they choose without interference from asthma symptoms. Extensive educational programs involving parents, teachers, physical education instructors, coaches, trainers, and athletes should be instituted so that having asthma does not become an exclusion criterion from sports.[9] An algorithm for the management of EIB is presented in Figure 19-2.

Sport Selection

Some sports require skill and coordination more than endurance (for example, baseball, golf, discus, shot put, pole vault, and skiing); some positions are more static (for example, goalies); and some sports are conducted in warm, humid environments that are less likely than others to induce asthma (i.e., swimming). Exercise con-

sisting of approximately 10 seconds of exertion followed by 30 seconds of rest, followed by another 10 seconds of exercise and 30 seconds of rest, may not require any prophylaxis.[10] This type of exercise (for example, badminton, tennis, and football) may be attractive to people with EIB.

Inducing a Refractory Period

Although physical conditioning has not been shown to have a direct effect on EIB, patients in better physical condition can perform a given amount of work at a lower level of ventilation and consequently experience fewer asthma symptoms. A study on the effect of prolonged submaximal warm-up exercise on EIB suggests that refractoriness to EIB can be induced without itself inducing marked bronchoconstriction.[11] Athletes can improve their performance by taking advantage of this refractory period and warming up with 10 minutes or less of vigorous exercise 45–60 minutes before their event. The EIB that will be induced should resolve in 30–40 minutes. Alternatively, they could perform a series of 10–12 short sprints that by themselves do not usually induce asthma but induce a refractory period. Some experimentation on the part of the athlete (with peak flow measurements) will determine the optimal interval between these warm-up exercises and the event.

There are other nonpharmacologic means of managing EIB. Breathing slowly through the nose whenever possible reduces hyperventilation and warms and humidifies the inhaled air. The use of a mask or scarf in cold weather also facilitates rebreathing of warm, humidified air, thus reducing the severity of the EIB.

Pharmacologic Treatment

When choice of sport or nonpharmacologic management is not enough, a variety of medications are available to prevent or treat EIB. These include beta$_2$-agonists, cromolyn sodium, theophylline, glucocorticoids, antihistamines, and anticholinergics. Any physician who treats an Olympic athlete should review the current banned medication list to ensure that the athlete is not taking a medication that might result in disqualification. Because the list of allowed and prohibited drugs may change, the prescribing physician should always check with the U.S. Olympic Committee (USOC) Drug Education Hotline (800-233-0393) for the latest ruling. Asthma medications that are currently approved by the USOC for use in competition include the beta$_2$-agonists albuterol, salmeterol, and terbutaline (all three in inhalant form only); cromolyn sodium; aminophylline; theophylline; ipratropium; nedocromil sodium; and inhaled corticosteroids. Written notification of the use of inhaled beta$_2$-agonists or inhaled corticosteroids must be given in advance by the team physician to the International Olympic Committee Medical Commission or USOC Drug Control Program.

Inhaled beta$_2$-agonists used before exercise will abate EIB in more than 80% of subjects.[12] These may be taken 5–60 minutes before exercise and are generally helpful for several hours. Beta$_2$-agonists are also helpful in relieving EIB after it occurs. The long-acting inhaled beta$_2$-agonist salmeterol has shown efficacy in providing protection against EIB in the majority of subjects for at least 12 hours. Thus, a single inhaled dose of salmeterol in the morning before leaving home may protect susceptible patients against bronchospasm induced by vigorous exercise or other physical activity throughout their work or school hours.[13] Salmeterol is approved by the USOC, but it is not recommended for children younger than age 12 years. Additionally, because of its longer onset of action, salmeterol should not be used in the treatment of acute bronchospasm.

Technique for Use of Inhaled Medications

One of the most important aspects of obtaining relief with inhaled medications is proper technique. The inhalation unit should be held approximately 4 cm from the opening of the mouth and not in the mouth (as most instruc-

tions with inhalers suggest). Inhalation should begin immediately before actuating the inhaler and should continue slowly (approximately 5 seconds) until the chest is maximally expanded. The breath should be held for 10 seconds to allow for particle sedimentation.[14] A second dose should be taken 2–5 minutes later. Patients who experience difficulty with this technique may benefit from use of a spacer device.

Cromolyn sodium inhalation 10–20 minutes before exercise is another acceptable pretreatment and can be used alone or in combination with beta$_2$-agonists. Albuterol and cromolyn appear to act in a synergistic fashion. This combination is ideal for the small number of athletes with mild to moderate EIB who continue to experience bronchospasm despite an adequate trial of either agent alone.[15]

Rapidly absorbed theophylline may be used but requires 1 hour to reach peak levels, may cause gastrointestinal upset or headache when used intermittently, and is less effective than inhaled beta$_2$-agonists. Therefore, theophylline is recommended primarily for EIB patients who require continuous treatment for asthma.

Some studies have demonstrated a beneficial effect of antihistamines in inhibiting or reducing the severity of EIB,[16] but their use is not widely recommended. Glucocorticoids (inhaled or orally) do not prevent EIB, but as with theophyllines, their use may be indicated in the patient who requires continuous asthma therapy.

Anticholinergic agents, such as atropine sulfate and ipratropium bromide, are effective in preventing the symptoms of EIB but not in preventing EIB itself.[17] These agents have generally not been recommended as part of the treatment of EIB but may be useful in selected patients.

Athletes with EIB should be treated aggressively to diminish their symptoms, allowing them to optimize their performance and to be competitive. Teachers and coaches should be notified that an athlete has EIB, then educated about the diagnosis and its treatment. This condition should not limit either participation or success in activities, but it may require the use of inhaled medication before activity and later as needed. Athletes and their coaches may ignore symptoms or abuse medications in their desire to push for optimal performance. Education can help both athletes and coaches to understand the most appropriate management of EIB and the limitations it may impose.

Regardless of the mechanisms that lead to EIB, athletes can be taught to cope with its limitations. Physicians can help by making the proper diagnosis and recommending management strategies that are appropriate for the condition. Exercise is beneficial to individuals of all ages, regardless of whether they have asthma. Most individuals who develop EIB can successfully and safely participate in almost any kind of physical activity. The benefits of regular aerobic exercise are multifaceted and include improved control of EIB symptoms. Asthmatic patients can successfully manage exercise programs through premedication, individualized physical training, and precipitant avoidance. Properly trained and medicated individuals who experience EIB can not only perform exercise at the same levels as nonasthmatics, but can also excel in competitive sports.[18]

REFERENCES

1. McFadden ER. Exercise-induced airway obstruction. Clin Chest Med 1995;16:671–682.
2. American Academy of Pediatrics. AAP issues statement on exercise-induced asthma in children. Am Fam Physician 1989;40:314–316.
3. National Heart, Lung and Blood Institute. Expert Panel Report: Guidelines for the Diagnosis and Management of Asthma. Publication No. 91-3042. Bethesda, MD: National Institutes of Health, August 1991;119–121.
4. Kawabori I, Pierson WE, Conquert LL, Biermann CW. Incidence of EIB in children. J Allergy Clin Immunol 1976;58:447–455.
5. Voy RO. The U.S. Olympic Committee experience with exercise-induced bronchospasm, 1984. Med Sci Sports Exerc 1986;18:328–330.
6. McCarthy P. Wheezing and breezing through exercise-induced asthma. Phys Sportsmed 1989;17:125–130.
7. Weiler JM, Metzger WJ, Donnelly AL, et al. Prevalence of bronchial hyperresponsiveness in highly trained athletes. Chest 1986;90:23–28.
8. Shapiro GG. Methacholine challenge relevance for the allergic athlete. J Allergy Clin Immunol 1984;73:670–675.
9. Nastasi KJ, Heinly TL, Blaiss MS. Exercise-induced asthma and the athlete. J Asthma 1995;32:249–257.
10. Bundgaard A. Exercise and the asthmatic. Sports Med 1985;2:254–266.
11. Rieff DB, Choudry NB, Pride NB, Ind PW. The effect of prolonged submaximal warm-up exercise on exercise-induced asthma. Am Rev Respir Dis 1989;139:479 484.
12. Anderson SD. EIA: new thinking and current management. J Respir Dis 1986;7:48–61.
13. Kemp JP, Dockhorn RJ, Busse WW, et al. Prolonged effect of inhaled salmeterol against exercise-induced bronchospasm. Am J Respir Crit Care Med 1994;150:1612–1615.
14. James TC. Five steps toward better asthma management. Am Fam Physician 1989;40:201–210.
15. Kyle JM. Exercise-induced pulmonary syndromes. Med Clin North Am 1994;78:413–421.
16. Wiebicke W, Poynter A, Montgomery M, et al. Effect of terfenadine on the response to exercise and cold air on asthma. Pediatr Pulmonol 1988;4:225–229.
17. Thompson NC, Patel KR, Kerr JW. Sodium cromoglycate and ipratropium bromide in exercise-induced asthma. Thorax 1978;33:694–699.
18. Gong H Jr. Breathing easy: exercise despite asthma. Phys Sportsmed 1992;20:159–167.

20

Neurologic Injuries

JOSEPH F. YETTER III, JANUS D. BUTCHER,
AND MONTE C. UYEMURA

The common types of neurologic injuries encountered among athletes—brachial plexus injuries, closed head injuries, and headache—are summarized in the algorithm in Figure 20-1.

BRACHIAL PLEXUS INJURIES

The brachial plexus is subject to several types of trauma during sporting activity: penetrating, blunt, traction, compression, and inflammatory trauma. Patterns of injury develop based on the anatomy and mechanism of injury. Certain commonplace patterns are readily recognizable. Most are readily treatable, but some are currently hopeless.

Anatomy

Prebrachial Plexus
Sensory input enters the spinal cord via the dorsal roots (the ganglia of which lie outside the spinal cord) within or near their respective intervertebral foramina (Figure 20-2A). Motor output exits the spinal cord via the ventral roots, which have cell bodies that are the anterior horn cells. Efferent and afferent pathways are joined in the spinal nerves. Each spinal nerve sends off a dorsal ramus; the remaining ventral rami will, at the C5–T1 level, undergo complex rearrangement in the brachial plexus. A lesion of the dorsal root between the dorsal root ganglion and cord is somewhat inaccurately referred to as *preganglionic*; if a preganglionic transection of the axon occurs, sensation is irretrievably lost. If the lesion is postganglionic (distal to the dorsal root ganglion), motor and sensory functions are affected but may recover, depending on the nature and severity of the lesion.

Brachial Plexus
Superior to the clavicle, the five ventral rami of C5 through T1 unite to form three trunks (Figure 20-2B). C5 and C6 form the upper trunk, C7 forms the middle trunk, and C8 and T1 form the lower trunk. Inferior and distal to the clavicle, the trunks divide into anterior and posterior divisions, which reassociate into three cords (medial, lateral, and posterior); these cords further divide and join to form terminal branches that include the radial, median, ulnar, musculocutaneous, and axillary nerves.

Classification of Nerve Injuries

Neurapraxia
Neurapraxia refers to a relatively mild nerve injury involving only demyelinization of the axon sheaths and temporary loss of conduction distal to the injury, followed by remyelinization and recovery of function within several weeks of injury.

Axonotmesis
Axonotmesis is a more severe nerve injury affecting both axon and myelin sheath, but sparing epineurium. Wallerian degeneration of the axon distal to the lesion is followed by regeneration and recovery of function over a time period dependent on the length of axon regeneration (average, 1 mm/day or approximately 2.5 cm/month).

Neurotmesis
Neurotmesis refers to a most severe nerve injury: a laceration, crush, or traction injury causing disruption of axons, sheaths, and endoneurium, with unlikely recovery and consequent permanent denervation.

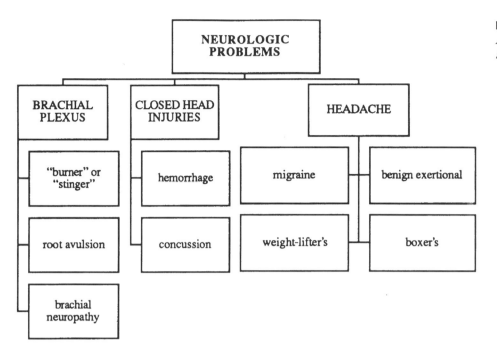

FIGURE 20-1
Algorithm for neurologic problems in the athlete.

Types of Injury

There are distinctive patterns of brachial plexus injury based on mechanism and presentation. The first and most common, the burner or "stinger" syndrome, is presented as a paradigm for the others.

Burner Syndrome ("Stingers")

Traction injuries of the brachial plexus (or, less commonly but more severely, of the cord or roots) are denoted "burners" or "stingers" by athletes describing the sensation. Most common in football players and wrestlers, burners occur when the shoulder is driven forcefully caudad while the neck is often flexed forcefully to the opposite side. Immediate, nondermatomal, circumferential pain radiates down the arm. Stingers from nerve root irritation are caused by either compression (head driven toward the shoulder) or distraction similar to the brachial plexus–type traction injury. These generally involve C5 or C6 dermatomes with variable motor involvement of the deltoid, biceps, supra-, and infraspinatus muscles. The athlete may shake his or her arm and hand to try to get the feeling back or may present supporting the injured arm with the contralateral hand. The pain may resolve in minutes, and neurologic examination may be normal; however, over the succeeding hours to days, weakness may develop.

Clancy[1] has developed a classification of burner injuries. Grade I represents a neurapraxia, with complete recovery of motor and sensory function within 2 weeks. Grade II represents axonotmesis and produces more severe and prolonged sensory and motor deficits. Grade III injuries represent neurotmesis, and the motor and sensory deficits last longer than 1 year.

Diagnosis is based on the characteristic history, mechanism of injury, symptoms, physical findings, and in some cases, electromyography (EMG). Because burner injury syndromes may be produced by injuries of the cord or root rather than the brachial plexus, significant neck pain or muscle spasm of neck muscles indicate cord or root injury (see Root Avulsions). Examination includes both sensory and motor functions, and reexamination occurs over time.

Motor deficits are most common in deltoid, biceps, and shoulder rotators. With any significant neck pain or stiffness, radiographs should be done, including lateral flexion and extension views for instability. Persistent weakness or sensory deficits warrant further evaluation with magnetic resonance imaging (MRI) to evaluate for a compressive neuropathy. EMGs after 3 weeks can help document the location and severity of a nerve injury.

A chronic burner syndrome has been described and appears to be associated with developmentally narrowed cervical canals and disk disease.[2] It appears more commonly in professional and college athletes and results in prolonged and recurrent weakness, although most athletes continue to play.[2]

Management of Burners

Potentially grave injuries must be excluded. Typical burners do not involve neck pain or limitation of neck mobil-

FIGURE 20-2

Nerve anatomy. A. The prebrachial plexus. B. The brachial plexus.

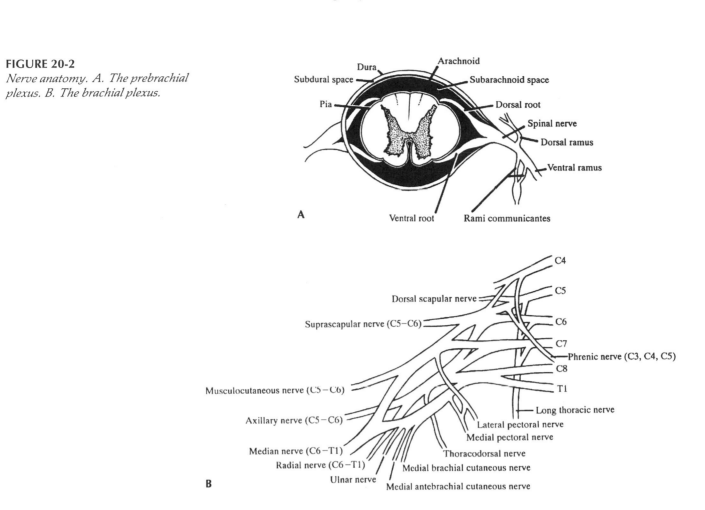

ity, and if these are present or if sensory or motor deficits persist, protection of the cervical spine is essential until definitive diagnosis is achieved. If the burning and temporary loss of strength resolve quickly, the athlete can return to the field. Reexamination is appropriate at the end of the competition and several times during the ensuing week.

Recurrent burners may be prevented by neck and shoulder strengthening and by use of high shoulder pads. In case of recurrence, guidelines to diagnosis and management are similar. Athletes should not be returned to the field until deficits resolve.

Root Avulsions

Root avulsions are more severe traction injuries, usually occurring at higher velocity and impact than burners, but otherwise similar in mechanism. The shoulder is driven forcefully caudad while the head and neck are driven laterally away from the involved shoulder. Diagnosis is aided by EMG showing denervation of posterior cervical muscles (posterior primary ramus) but normal nerve conduction studies and histamine testing (that is, a preganglionic lesion). Imaging studies may also show fractures of transverse processes.[3]

Cervical Cord Neurapraxia (Transient Quadriplegia)

This entity involves an acute transient neurologic episode of cervical cord origin.[4] Symptoms may involve both arms, both legs, all four extremities, or an ipsilateral arm and leg. Sensory symptoms are described as burning pain, numbness, and tingling, and motor symptoms can be paresis or paralysis. Symptoms typically last less than 15 minutes but can take up to 48 hours with return to full neck range of motion and normal motor function.

Affected athletes should undergo a complete workup to rule out bony or ligamentous injury or predisposing spinal abnormalities. Radiographs should include a full cervical spine series with lateral flexion and extension views (to assess for cervical spine instability). An MRI should be done to assess for extrinsic cord or nerve root compression or intrinsic cord damage as well as to determine the presence of congenital or acquired spinal stenosis. Return to play is considered safe if there is full range of motion;

no symptoms; and imaging studies reveal (1) no bony impingement or abnormalities, (2) no ligamentous instability, and (3) no spinal stenosis.[4, 5] The decision regarding safe return to play in an athlete with transient quadriplegia who has a normal workup except for the presence of spinal stenosis is more controversial. Cantu[5] believed that this alone is a contraindication to participation in collision sports. Torg and colleagues[4] stated that athletes with spinal stenosis in the absence of spinal instability or degenerative changes can return to collision sports without an increased risk of permanent neurologic injury. They do, however, have a recurrence rate of transient quadriplegia of 56%, which is strongly related to the degree of stenosis.[4] The decision to allow an athlete with spinal stenosis to participate in collision sports is difficult and should only be made in consultation with a knowledgeable neurosurgeon.

Backpack Paralysis

Backpack paralysis is caused by compression of elements of the brachial plexus by straps of heavy backpacks, coupled with traction on the plexus as the shoulder girdle is pulled posteriorly. The usual injury is a neurapraxia or axonotmesis, with a neurologic distribution corresponding to the involved elements. Relative rest and physical therapy lead to complete resolution.[6]

Healing Clavicle Fractures

Callus formation may impinge on the brachial plexus. Diagnosis is made based on history of fracture and progressive neurologic symptoms as the callus evolves (callus may be particularly exuberant in the case of nonunion). Treatment is resection of the callus, and, if there is nonunion, open reduction and internal fixation.

Acute Brachial Neuropathy

Acute brachial neuropathy is a clinical syndrome of unknown etiology (possibly viral) characterized by the spontaneous onset of shoulder pain, weakness, and atrophy affecting various muscles in the distribution of the brachial plexus and muscles not supplied by the brachial plexus (including serratus anterior, diaphragm, and trapezius). Diagnosis is based on history (usually no specific trauma), examination (weakness of the shoulder muscles—particularly the rotator cuff, deltoid, and triceps—and a variable, usually minor sensory deficit affecting chiefly the axillary nerve distribution), and EMG. Initial therapy consists of relative rest with use of a sling and analgesia. When exercise rehabilitation can be conducted without significant pain, strengthening of all muscle groups of the shoulder area is indicated. Recovery is often slow—

over a period of several years—and may be incomplete. Return to competition and selection of appropriate sports may be limited. Persistent, chronic, and painful symptoms of radicular or peripheral nerve injury (burning, tingling, pins-and-needles sensation) can often be decreased with a low-dose tricyclic antidepressant, such as amitriptyline, or antiseizure medications such as carbamazepine (Tegretol—requires blood count monitoring regularly during course of treatment), phenytoin (Dilantin), or gabapentin. A transcutaneous electric nerve stimulator may also be useful.

ACUTE CLOSED HEAD INJURIES

Head trauma accounts for the most severe and potentially life-threatening injuries experienced on the playing field. Although there have been significant improvements in protective equipment and playing rules designed to maximize safety, these injuries continue to occur with an alarming frequency. Central nervous system trauma has been reported in nearly all athletic activities, but the collision sports (most notably football and boxing) account for the majority of injuries. Data published for American football report that 24% of all injuries to these athletes are concussions, with approximately 250,000 such injuries occurring each year.[7] This translates to an incidence of concussions among high school football players of approximately 20%. Although the majority of these head injuries are minor, several deaths from craniocerebral trauma occur every year in high school football alone.[8]

Hemorrhage

Intracranial hemorrhage can result in devastating brain injury in athletes and is the most common cause of death from head trauma in this group. Four types of hemorrhage are most commonly seen, all of which may be rapidly fatal if not recognized and treated early.

Epidural hemorrhage results from the rupture of the arteries overlying the dura. The resulting hematoma rapidly expands, and if not recognized and treated, can be fatal in 30–60 minutes.[9] A subdural hematoma arises from a tear in a vein, artery, or venous sinus along the inside surface of the dura. The collection of blood beneath the dura can compress the brain parenchyma and cause ischemic injury or herniation.[10] This is the head injury that most often results in death in athletes.[9] Trauma to small vessels in the subarachnoid space results in a subarachnoid hemorrhage. This type of injury is often associated with arteriovenous malformation, aneurysm, or

TABLE 20-1
On-Field Neurologic Assessment of Concussion

Common acute signs and symptoms

Confusion/ disorientation	Athlete appears dazed, walks to wrong bench or huddle, speech halting or incomprehensible, poor performance on subsequent plays (e.g., running wrong pattern, missing cueing events)
Amnesia	Unsure of events before, during, or after injury
Headaches	These may persist as postconcussive syndrome
Dizziness	
Nausea/vomiting	

Mental status examination

Orientation	To person/place/time/events
Memory	Recall of three of three objects at 0 and 5 mins
	Recall of teachers' names, sports figures, specific plays
	Recall of circumstances of injury
Concentration	Serial sevens (100–7, 93–7, etc.)
	Serial digits: give the athlete three to seven digits to repeat
Speech	Character, coherence

Neurologic examination (cranial nerve examination)

Motor function	Exertional testing with wind sprints or other activities such as sit-ups or push-ups
Coordination	Finger-nose-finger, heel-toe walk

TABLE 20-2
Classification of Concussions

Grade	Colorado Medical Society[a]	Cantu[b]
I	Impaired intellectual functioning with confusion but no amnesia and no loss of consciousness	No loss of consciousness and altered memory for <30 mins
II	Confusion with amnesia but no loss of consciousness	Loss of consciousness for <5 mins or amnesia for >30 mins but <24 hrs
III	Loss of consciousness for any duration	Loss of consciousness for >5 mins or amnesia for >24 hrs

[a]Adapted from the Colorado Medical Society: The Sports Medicine Committee. Guidelines for the Management of Concussion in Sports (rev). Denver: Colorado Medical Society, 1991.
[b]Adapted from RC Cantu. When to allow athletes to return to play after injury. J Neurol Orthop Med Surg 1992;13:30–34.

Concussion

Concussion, defined as a traumatically induced alteration in mental status,[11] is the most common brain injury seen in athletes. Clinically, this injury ranges from a short, transient period of confusion to a prolonged loss of consciousness with persistent cognitive deficits. Although a wide range of signs and symptoms may be seen immediately after a concussion (Table 20-1), the initial presentation may be subtle, and the injury may not be apparent until several minutes after impact. This possibility of delayed development of symptoms greatly increases the need for careful evaluation and observation before the athlete is allowed to return to play.[11]

Classification

The classification of concussions has been the topic of considerable debate. As a result, several classification systems have emerged with a range of guidelines for grading severity and recommendations for the return to play (Table 20-2).[12–14] More conservative criteria have been stressed to ensure maximal safety for the athletes. It is important to keep in mind that these are guidelines, and many factors must be weighed in applying them to any given athlete. These decisions are based on the severity of the initial injury, the risk of a second head injury in the chosen sport, and the experience of the treating physician.

Evaluation

On-field evaluation of the athlete must include a careful examination of mental status assessing orientation, con-

other congenital defect. Intracerebral hemorrhage is due to arterial disruption within the parenchyma and is often associated with congenital vascular lesions. Intracerebral hemorrhages can be precipitously fatal.

The crucial first step in the management of these injuries is to establish the diagnosis. An intracranial hemorrhage can follow a seemingly minor head injury. Similarly, the initial presentation may include deceptively minimal symptoms, beginning as a mild headache and nausea with more significant signs, including gait imbalance, severe headache, vomiting, and a focal neurologic examination rapidly developing. All patients with a presentation suggesting an intracranial bleed require emergent imaging with computed tomography (CT) and referral to a neurosurgeon. If intracranial hemorrhage is suspected, even with negative imaging studies, a lumbar puncture to evaluate the cerebrospinal fluid for xanthochromia should be performed.

There are no established guidelines for the return to play following intracranial hemorrhage. This is a decision that has to be individualized for the athlete based on the treatment required, the clinical course, and the risk of subsequent injury. The decision must be made in close consultation with the treating neurosurgeon.

centration, and memory loss (see Table 20-1). Subtle mental status changes can be detected by enlisting the aid of a team member to ask questions regarding plays, call signals, an so forth. Postconcussive symptoms, such as headache, nausea, dizziness, or visual changes, often occur and can indicate more severe injuries with intracranial hemorrhage. Because the injured brain is more susceptible to subsequent injury, the athlete with symptoms suggestive of acute concussion must be closely observed and should not return to play until after an appropriate recovery time after the resolution of symptoms. If these symptoms worsen or persist, further evaluation should be undertaken. Exertional testing with sideline sprints or other activities is useful for uncovering these postconcussive symptoms as well as evaluating coordination and motor function.[11] Athletes should not return to play until they are asymptomatic at rest and after exertion.

In the case of a minor injury without significant cognitive impairment, the athlete may be allowed to ambulate to the sidelines for continued observation. The individual should be reevaluated every 5 minutes for at least 20 minutes for signs of amnesia or other mental status changes. With a grade II injury, the athlete should be removed from play for the remainder of the event. If postconcussive symptoms worsen, or if a focal neurologic examination is observed, transfer to an emergency room for evaluation and observation is advised. In a grade III concussion, the athlete should be transferred immediately to an emergency room for further evaluation.

In the emergency department, all athletes who experienced a loss of consciousness or who have a focal neurologic deficit should be imaged with CT or MRI. Additionally, CT should be performed in those with worsening postconcussive symptoms or a persistent alteration in mental status.

With negative imaging studies and complete resolution of symptoms, the patient can usually be discharged from the emergency room without additional hospitalization.[15] Careful instructions regarding when the athlete can return to play are the responsibility of the treating physician. Some studies, however, have shown that these instructions are most often wrong, inadequate, or not given.[16]

A brief admission for observation should be considered for all athletes who show persistent, severe postconcussive symptoms, including headache, visual changes, confusion, amnesia, or other neurologic deficits.

Postconcussion Syndrome

Postconcussion syndrome describes a constellation of symptoms, including exertional headaches, emotional lability, gait and balance abnormalities, sleep disturbances, and cognitive impairment. These may occasionally persist after head injury and may be related to altered brain neurotransmitter function.[17] Parents and coaches should be instructed about these signs and symptoms to ensure early recognition. Undiagnosed postconcussion syndrome may present initially as depression. Neuropsychologic testing is a sensitive tool for the diagnosis and tracking of this condition and should be performed when available. Referral to a rehabilitation team specializing in brain injury should be considered early in these athletes to facilitate maximal recovery.[18]

Criteria for Return to Play After Concussion

In all major guidelines, the amount of time out of practice or competition is based on the severity of the initial injury. The most commonly used guidelines for return to play after concussion are outlined in Table 20-3. While the three guidelines presented in this table differ in some respects, there is substantial agreement in terms of returning the athlete to play. An athlete sustaining a minor grade I concussion can often return to play following 20 minutes of observation if all symptoms resolve at rest and with exertion. A grade II injury prevents the return until 1 full week after symptoms have resolved. A grade III concussion requires a 1-month symptom-free period out of contact sports before returning to play.

Repeated head injury during recovery from a concussion can result in the second impact syndrome. This poorly understood process leads to malignant cerebral edema and has been associated with a high morbidity and mortality.[19] This emphasizes the need to identify concussion correctly in the athlete and restrict activity based on the degree of injury. Because of the potential cumulative effect of repetitive head injuries, an athlete sustaining multiple concussions in a season requires longer play restrictions. Cumulative effects of repetitive head injuries on cognitive skills are usually grossly underestimated by athletes, coaches, and parents. Education and vigilance are key, especially in young high school athletes. Career options can be greatly limited with cognitive dysfunction.

Severe morbidity has also been described in athletes recovering from viral encephalitis who sustain relatively mild head trauma.[20] Any athlete with a recent history of encephalitis should be restricted from play until fully recovered from the illness.

Concussion Prevention

The major concern in returning the athlete to play is the prevention of repeat head injuries. One study reported that the frequency of concussion in American football is

TABLE 20-3
Return-to-Play Guidelines

	Colorado Medical Society[a]		
Grade	First Injury	Second Injury	Third Injury
I	20 mins of observation with re-evaluation every 5 mins; if no amnesia, athlete may return to play	Out of play for 24 hrs after symptoms resolve	Season terminated; no contact sports for 3 mos
II	Out of play 1 full wk after symptoms resolve	Out of play 1 full mo after symptoms resolve; consider terminating season	Season terminated
III	Out of play for 1 mo with at least 2 wks symptom free	Season terminated	Season terminated

	American Academy of Neurology[b]	
Grade	First Injury	Multiple Injuries
I	May return if symptoms clear completely within 15 mins (while at rest and with exertion)	Out of play for 1 wk after resolution of symptoms
II	Out of play 1 full wk after symptoms resolve	Out of play 2 wks after symptoms resolve
III	Brief LOC (secs): Out of play for 1 wk after resolution of symptoms	
	Prolonged LOC (mins): Out of play 2 wks after resolution of symptoms	Out of play 1 mo or longer based on clinical decision of physician

	Cantu[c]		
Grade	First Injury	Second Injury	Third Injury
I	With a minor injury, may return if normal sideline assessment; often best to hold athlete out until asymptomatic for 1 wk	Out of play for 2 wks after symptoms resolve	Season terminated
II	Out of play 1 full wk after symptoms completely resolve	Out of play 1 full mo after symptoms resolve; consider termination of season	Season terminated
III	Out of play for 1 mo with at least a 1-wk period symptom free	Season terminated	Season terminated

[a]Adapted from the Colorado Medical Society: The Sports Medicine Committee. Guidelines for the Management of Concussion in Sports (rev). Denver: Colorado Medical Society, 1991.
[b]Adapted from Practice parameter: the management of concussion in sports (summary statement). Neurology 1997;48:581–585.
[c]Adapted from RC Cantu. When to allow athletes to return to play after injury. J Neurol Orthop Med Surg 1992;13:30–34.
LOC = loss of consciousness.

six times higher in individuals who had sustained a previous concussion than in those with no previous injury.[21] Rule changes and equipment innovations effected since the 1970s have reduced the incidence of neck injuries, but the incidence of concussion may be increasing.[22] Team physicians and trainers must continue to work with sport governing bodies as well as local sports organizations to further improve the safety of these sports through rule refinement and protective equipment use. In addition, further study in the epidemiology of concussion may uncover differences in the protection of the specific brands of equipment available. The importance of this type of research is emphasized by the results of one study comparing American football helmet brands. In this work, two of the most popular helmet brands showed dramatic differences in concussion rate.[21] Further research in this regard will allow trainers and physicians to select equipment that will maximize safety.

HEADACHE IN THE ATHLETE

Headache is a very common symptom in the general population, and the evaluation of headache in the athlete should follow the same principles as in the nonathlete. A number of headache syndromes related to different athletic activities have been reported.

Migraine

Although exercise often prevents or decreases the severity of migraine headaches, people with known migraine headaches may have exacerbations precipitated by exertion. Exercise may also elicit new migrainous headaches. Migraine headaches are usually described as severe pulsating headaches associated with nausea, photophobia, and phonophobia. They are usually unilateral at onset and may be preceded by a prodromal aura such as transient scotomata, teichopsia, photopsia, paresthesia, or aphasia. They may also be triggered by certain foods or factors such as fatigue, skipped meals, high altitude, and oversleeping.[23] Thompson[24] reported a case of exercise-induced migraine prodrome symptoms without subsequent headache.

Lambert and Burnet[25] described a case in which a controlled warm-up regimen prevented exercise-induced migraine headaches in a competitive swimmer. The pathophysiology of migraine headaches, thought to be related to cerebral artery constriction followed by reflex vasodilation, may also apply to other headache syndromes discussed in the following sections.[26]

Benign Exertional Headache

Benign exertional headaches are throbbing, usually bilateral at onset, and occur suddenly at the peak of physical exertion or immediately after exertion. The headaches last from 5 minutes to 24 hours and have an association with high altitudes, hot weather, and excess exertion.[27] Sands and colleagues[27] reported that these athletes have normal neurologic examinations and do not usually report nausea or vomiting; however, Massey[28] regarded nausea and vomiting a common symptom.

Exertional headaches are most commonly reported in runners. Toshikatsu and Takahashi[29] reported three cases of severe, pulsating headaches precipitated by swimming. Similar to migraine pathophysiology, hyperventilation and hypocapnia associated with exertion or high altitudes may induce cerebral vasoconstriction followed by reflex vasodilation. Breath holding while swimming may cause increased intrathoracic pressures and contribute to headache induction. Exertional headaches may also be related to dehydration, heat load, or hypoglycemia.[26]

Weight-Lifter's Headache

Paulson[30] reported five cases of abrupt onset of occipital, upper cervical, or parietal headaches that occurred as the patient was lifting weights. CT and cerebrospinal fluid studies were normal. The symptoms recurred with lifting for several months and eventually resolved. Weight-lifter's headache may be related to increased intrathoracic pressure with Valsalva or cervical muscle and ligament strain.[26]

Postconcussive Headache

Matthews[31] reported on three football players and one boxer who developed classic migraine headaches believed to be secondary to head trauma. In addition, both chronic subdural bleeds and postconcussive headache may also result from seemingly minor head trauma. Postconcussive headaches may last from hours to years after head trauma and may be associated with vertigo or light-headedness and psychological and cognitive impairment.[32]

Evaluation

In the evaluation of the athlete with headache, the first objective is to rule out ominous etiologies. Subarachnoid hemorrhage, cerebral aneurysm, Arnold-Chiari malformation, and intracranial neoplasm are all associated with exertional headache. In the setting of trauma, of course, neurosurgical problems discussed earlier in this chapter should be considered.

Before the development of the CT scan, Rooke[33] reported on exertional headaches and suggested that certain patients might be managed expectantly without interventional studies, but the current standard of care for sudden exertional headaches includes either CT or MRI. If CT or MRI are normal, Edmeads[34] suggested that a lumbar puncture is not necessary if the headache resolved in less than 1 hour.

Treatment

Once ominous causes of headache have been excluded, symptomatic treatment of the acute headache is appropriate. The treatment of exertional headaches should focus on education and prevention. Strategies include proper warm-up, gradual ascent, acclimatization to altitudes, and proper conditioning. Beta-blockers, tricyclic antidepressants, calcium channel blockers, phenelzine, divalproex sodium, and nonsteroidal anti-inflammatory agents may be used prophylactically for migraines or exertional headaches (Table 20-4). People who develop headaches at higher altitudes may benefit from prophylactic acetazolamide, furosemide, or corticosteroids. Children with migraines have a good response to prophylactic cyproheptadine hydrochloride. Beta-blockers should be used with caution because they may blunt the normal adrenergic response to exertion and decrease exercise tolerance.

TABLE 20-4
Headache Prophylaxis

Class	Medication	Dosage	Frequency
Beta-blockers	Propranolol	20–40 mg	Twice daily
	Atenolol	25–50 mg	Once daily
Tricyclic antidepressants	Amitriptyline	10–25 mg initially; 10–175 mg therapeutic	At bedtime
Calcium channel blockers	Sustained release verapamil	90–360 mg	Once daily
NSAIDs	See Chapter 2; many available	Varies	Varies
Low-dose ergot preparations	phenobarbital with ergotamine tartrate (Bellergal)	One to two tablets	Twice daily
	Ergonovine	0.2 mg oral	Twice daily
Others	Phenelzine	45 mg oral	Once daily
	Methysergide	2 mg oral	1–4 times daily
Altitude prophylaxis	Acetazolamide	125–250 mg oral	Twice daily started 24 hrs before exposure
	Dexamethasone	4 mg oral	2–4 times daily

NSAIDs = nonsteroidal anti-inflammatory drugs.

TABLE 20-5
Medications for Acute Migraine Therapy

Medication	Dosage	Frequency
Ergotamine/caffeine (Cafergot)	Two tablets at onset, then one tablet every 30 mins	Total dose of six tablets in 24 hrs
Dihydroergotamine (D.H.E.-45)	1 mg IV/IM	Repeat every hr as needed
Methysergide (Sansert)	4–8 mg orally	Once daily
Isometheptene (Midrin)	One tablet every hr	Total of five tablets in 12 hrs
Sumatriptan (Imitrex)	6 mg SC	May repeat after 1 hr to a maximum dose of 12 mg/day

IV = intravenous; IM = intramuscular; SC = subcutaneously.

Nonselective beta-blockers should be avoided in people with asthma. Calcium channel blockers may cause fatigue or bradycardia. The anticholinergic side effects of tricyclic antidepressants may cause dry mouth and make athletes more susceptible to heat injury.[23, 27]

Sumatriptan succinate, administered either orally or subcutaneously, is an effective treatment to abort an acute migraine headache (Table 20-5). The ergot preparations are also effective but they should be taken at the onset of a migraine. Nonsteroidal anti-inflammatory agents as well as chlorpromazine and prochlorperazine can also be used for acute migraines. Intranasal butorphanol tartrate should be used with caution because of its addiction potential.[23]

Special considerations must be taken when prescribing medications to athletes. Besides possible adverse effects on performance, many medications are banned or restricted by the National Collegiate Athletic Association (NCAA) and U.S. Olympic Committee (USOC). Diuretics are banned by both the NCAA and the USOC. The USOC requires prior written permission to use corticosteroids other than topical corticosteroids; bans all narcotics except codeine; prohibits the use of phenothiazines in shooting sports; and bans beta-blockers in a number of sports, such as riflery, gymnastics, and diving. Beta-blockers are banned by the NCAA in riflery only.[35]

REFERENCES

1. Clancy WG. Brachial Plexus and Upper Extremity Peripheral Nerve Injuries. In JS Torg (ed), Athletic Injuries to the Head, Neck and Face. Philadelphia: Lea & Febiger, 1982;215–220.
2. Levitz CL, Reilly PJ, Torg JS. The pathomechanics of chronic recurrent cervical nerve root neurapraxia. Am J Sports Med 1997;25:73–76.
3. Leffert RD. Brachial plexus injuries. N Engl J Med 1974;291:1059–1066.
4. Torg JS, Corcoran TA, Thibault LE, et al. Cervical cord neurapraxia: classification, pathomechanics, morbidity, and management guideline. J Neurosurg 1997;87:843–850.
5. Cantu RC. Stingers, transient quadriplegia, and cervical spine stenosis: return to play criteria. Med Sci Sports Exerc 1997;29:S233–S235.
6. Hirasawa Y, Sakakida M. Sports and peripheral nerve injury. Am J Sports Med 1983;11:420–426.

7. Goodwin-Gerberich S, Priest J, Boen JR, et al. Concussion incidences and severity in secondary school varsity football players. Am J Public Health 1983;73:1370–1374.

8. Torg J, Vegso J, Sennet B, Das M. The national football head and neck injury registry. JAMA 1985;254:3439–3443.

9. Cantu R. Head and spine injuries in the young athlete. Clin Sports Med 1988;7:459–472.

10. Lehman L, Ravich S. Closed head injuries in athletes. Clin Sports Med 1990;9:247–261.

11. Kelly J, Nichols J, Filley CM, et al. Concussion in sports: guidelines for the prevention of catastrophic outcome. JAMA 1991;266:2867–2869.

12. Colorado Medical Society: The Sports Medicine Committee. Guidelines for the Management of Concussion in Sports (revised). Denver: Colorado Medical Society, 1991.

13. Cantu RC. When to allow athletes to return to play after injury. J Neurol Orthop Med Surg 1992;13:30–34.

14. Practice parameter: the management of concussion in sports (summary statement). Neurology 1997;48:581–585.

15. Stein S, O'Mally K, Ross S. Is routine computed tomography too expensive for mild head injury? Ann Emerg Med 1991;20:1286–1289.

16. Genuardi FJ, King WD. Inappropriate discharge instructions for youth athletes hospitalized for concussion. Pediatrics 1995;95:216–218.

17. Zasler N. Advances in neuropharmacological rehabilitation for brain dysfunction. Brain Inj 1992;6:1–14.

18. Putukian M, Echemendia RJ. Managing successive minor head injuries: which tests guide return to play? Phys Sportsmed 1996;24:25–38.

19. Saunders R, Harbaugh R. The second impact in catastrophic contact-sports head trauma. JAMA 1984;252:538–539.

20. McQuillen J, McQuillen E, Morrow P. Trauma, sport, and malignant cerebral edema. Am J Forensic Med Pathol 1988;9:12–15.

21. Zemper ED. Analysis of cerebral concussion frequency with the most commonly used models of football helmets. J Athletic Train 1994;29:44–50.

22. Biasca N, Simmen HP, Bartolozzi AR, Trentz O. Review of typical ice hockey injuries: survey of the North American NHL and Hockey Canada versus European leagues. Unfallchirurg 1995;98:283–288.

23. Diamond S. Managing migraines in active people. Physician Sportsmed 1996;24:41–53.

24. Thompson JK. Exercise-induced migraine prodrome symptoms. Headache 1987;27:50–51.

25. Lambert RW, Burnet DL. Prevention of exercise-induced migraine by quantitative warm-up. Headache 1985;25:317–319.

26. Cacayorin ED, Petro GR, Hochhauser L. Headache in the athlete and radiographic evaluation. Clin Sports Med 1987;6:739–749.

27. Sands GH, Newman L, Lipton R. Cough, exertional and other miscellaneous headaches. Med Clin North Am 1991;75:733–746.

28. Massey EW. Effort headache in runners. Headache 1982;22:99–100.

29. Toshikatsu I, Takahashi A. Swimmer's migraine. Headache 1990;30:485–487.

30. Paulson GW. Weightlifter's headache. Headache 1983;23:193–194.

31. Matthews WB. Footballer's migraine. BMJ 1972;2:326–327.

32. Oliaro S. Concussion and post-concussion syndrome. Sports Med Update 1995;10:23–26.

33. Rooke ED. Benign exertional headache. Med Clin North Am 1968;52:801–808.

34. Edmeads J. The worst headache ever: ominous causes. Postgrad Med 1989;86:107–110.

35. Fuentes RJ, Rosenberg JM, Davis A (eds). Athletics Drug Reference '94. Durham, NC: Allen & Hanburys, 1994;25–45, 219–408.

21

Gastrointestinal Problems

JANUS D. BUTCHER

Gastrointestinal (GI) symptoms occur with surprising frequency in athletes at all levels, with a prevalence as high as 81% in certain activities.[1] In spite of this remarkably high prevalence, these problems receive little attention in the lay press and professional literature. GI disturbances are most often reported in runners, with gastroesophageal reflux, abdominal pain, diarrhea, and nausea being the most common symptoms. Other athletes, including swimmers, cross-country skiers, and cyclists, report similar problems, although with a lower incidence.[2–4] In addition to the exertion-related symptoms, the stresses of training and travel for competition may predispose athletes to GI infections.

RUNNER'S DIARRHEA

Exercise has both positive and negative effects on the lower GI tract. Studies have reported a decreased bowel transit time with moderate exercise,[5, 6] and researchers have suggested that this may be responsible for the decreased incidence of colon cancer seen in individuals who exercise regularly.[7] However, this decreased transit time does not occur with low-level exercise.[8]

The more readily apparent negative GI effects of exercise include fecal urgency, loose stools, and frank diarrhea. Numerous studies in long-distance runners indicate that 37–62% of runners experience bowel urgency either during or immediately after a strenuous workout.[1, 6, 9, 10] Frequently, the athlete is forced to interrupt the workout as a result of these symptoms.[9] By these reports, women are more likely to experience lower GI symptoms than men.[9, 10] These symptoms tend to worsen with increasing training mileage or with particularly strenuous workouts and are more likely to occur if the runner has eaten within an hour before running.[11, 12] In addition,

underlying GI conditions, such as irritable bowel syndrome, appear to be a risk factor for this condition. In severe cases, runner's diarrhea may result in significant dehydration and has been implicated in the development of rhabdomyolysis and acute tubular necrosis.[11] Runner's anemia is also a potential complication in cases involving bloody diarrhea.[13]

The precise mechanism for runner's diarrhea is not well understood, although a number of etiologies have been suggested, including GI bleeding, rapid fluid and electrolyte shifts,[9, 14] autonomic nervous system stimulation,[15] stimulation of gastroenteropancreatic hormones,[15, 16] and mechanical trauma. A number of studies have looked at each of these factors without establishing a clear causative relationship.[17, 18] The actual cause of lower GI symptoms in athletes is probably multifactorial, including the preceding issues as well as diet, underlying GI illnesses, and environmental conditions.

Gastrointestinal Bleeding

GI blood loss is a relatively common finding in endurance athletes and may contribute to runner's diarrhea. A study by McCabe and colleagues[19] demonstrated a 20% incidence of occult blood in the stools of runners completing a marathon. Of their respondents, 6% reported frank hematochezia after that race, and 17% reported at least one episode of running-associated bloody diarrhea. Similarly, Yges and colleagues[20] found a 25% incidence of fecal occult blood in runners after a marathon using more specific immunochemical techniques. Even more dramatic is the report of an 87% positive conversion rate on stool occult blood testing in runners after an ultradistance running event.[21] These studies suggest that GI bleeding may be distance or effort related (dose dependent). Several possible mechanisms for this GI bleeding have been suggested.

TABLE 21-1
Evaluation and Treatment of Runner's Diarrhea

Diarrhea Type	Possible Etiologies	Evaluation	Treatment

Bloody	Ischemic enteropathy
	Hemorrhagic gastritis
	Mechanical forces
	NSAID use
		History
		  Training history
		  Pre-existing GI disease
		Laboratory
		  Stool studies (WBC count,
		    cultures)
		  Complete blood cell count
		Other
		  Endoscopy
		  Colonoscopy
		  Barium enema
			Reduce training intensity until
			  symptoms resolve, then gradual
			  return to prior intensity
			H$_2$-blocking agents with gastritis
			Discontinue NSAIDs

Nonbloody	Mechanical trauma
	Fluid shifts
	Gastroenteropancreatic
	  hormones
	Diet/ergogenic aids
	Traveler's diarrhea
		History
		  Training history
		  Pre-existing GI disease
		  Diet and travel history
		Laboratory
		  Stool studies (WBC count,
		    cultures)
		  Complete blood cell count
		  Liver function tests
		  Serum amylase
			Reduce training intensity until
			  symptoms resolve, then gradual
			  return to prior intensity
			Antimotility agents
			Elemental diet before competition

GI = gastrointestinal; WBC = white blood cell; NSAID = nonsteroidal anti-inflammatory drug.
Source: Adapted from JD Butcher. Runner's diarrhea and other intestinal problems of athletes. Am Fam Physician 1993;48:623–627.

Bowel ischemia appears to be the most plausible cause of GI bleeding.[9–11, 22–24] Splanchnic blood flow is reduced by approximately 70–80% of normal with strenuous aerobic exercise.[25] When this low blood flow is maintained for a long period, as in a long-distance run, it leads to local tissue ischemia, necrosis, and superficial mucosal erosions. This then results in intraluminal bleeding.[22] A similar process underlies hemorrhagic gastritis, which is the most common source of GI blood loss in long-distance runners.[21, 24]

Other mechanisms may also contribute to GI blood loss. The mechanical trauma theory suggests that damage occurs to the hollow abdominal viscera because of the repetitive high-impact characteristics of running. This causes jarring of the intestines, resulting in serosal and mucosal injury.[11, 19] A similar pattern has previously been described in the bladder and ureters.[26] Similarly, hemorrhagic gastritis may result from mechanical stress exerted by the diaphragm and gastrophrenic ligaments on the gastric fundus.[21] This mechanical trauma theory is refuted somewhat by the occurrence of GI blood loss in bicyclists.[3]

The relationship between nonsteroidal anti-inflammatory drug (NSAID) use and GI blood loss is not clear. NSAIDs have been associated with the development of gastritis and peptic ulcer disease; however, the studies on GI blood loss in the athlete have not shown any direct correlation.[21]

Perianal disease, including hemorrhoids, fissures, and perianal chafing, is another possible cause of GI blood loss in athletes.

Evaluation

The approach to lower GI symptoms in the athlete should start with a careful history for symptoms of diarrhea, melena, hematochezia, or hematemesis (Table 21-1). Any recent changes in training intensity, duration, or distance should be quantified. NSAID use, any history of recent travel, and pre-existing illness are also important etiologic factors to be considered. Evaluation for inflammatory bowel disease, gastritis, peptic ulcer disease, and other causes of GI bleeding should be undertaken if there is a prior history or if indicated by the patient's presenting circumstances. Laboratory assessment should include stool evaluation for fecal heme content, leukocytes, ovum, and parasites, and stool cultures to determine the presence of inflammatory or infectious etiologies. A complete blood cell count should be done to evaluate for possible anemia. In persons with evidence of bloody diarrhea, further evaluation with a barium enema, flexible sigmoidoscopy, colonoscopy, and esophagogastroduodenoscopy is warranted to determine the source of blood loss.

Treatment: Nonbloody Diarrhea

Treatment of runner's diarrhea begins with a reduction in training intensity or distance for 1–2 weeks with a gradual return to the previous high-intensity workouts. In most cases, this will be effective in stopping the symptoms without recurrence.[11] Exercise substitution and cross-training with low-impact activities also help to reduce the symptoms while allowing the athlete to maintain cardiovascular fitness.

Dietary manipulations may be of some use in the prevention of lower GI symptoms.[27] A complete liquid diet on the day before a long-distance competition or planned strenuous workout may decrease symptoms during the event. This is obviously of limited value in the treatment of long-term running-induced diarrhea; however, a low-residue (low-fiber) diet may be helpful in some athletes.[28]

Treatment: Bloody Diarrhea

The treatment of bloody diarrhea in the athlete includes short-term reduction in training along with exercise substitution.[22] In cases related to hemorrhagic gastritis, the use of H$_2$ antagonist agents (ranitidine 150 mg twice a day or cimetidine 400 mg twice a day) is very effective.[21, 22] It is further assumed that the proton pump inhibitors—omeprazole (Prilosec), 20 mg each day, and lansoprazole (Prevacid), 15 mg each day—are effective, although no controlled studies have been done. Discontinuation of NSAIDs should be advised in most cases of bloody diarrhea. If treatable diseases (inflammatory bowel disease, gastroesophagitis, peptic ulcer disease) are identified during the evaluation, these should be addressed with a combination of appropriate pharmacologic intervention, dietary manipulation, and training restriction or reduction.

TRAVELER'S DIARRHEA

Traveler's diarrhea (TD) is one of the most common health risks among travelers to developing countries. With a large number of international competitions and growing numbers of adventure travelers visiting remote locations, TD can be a major concern for the sports medicine practitioner. Of the 8 million Americans who will travel to a third-world country this year, approximately one-third will develop diarrhea during the trip. The risk varies depending on the destination; however, infection rates range from 20% to 59%.[29–31] The severity of symptoms and the potential for decreased performance make this a particularly important concern for athletes who travel outside the United States for competitions.

The infection is transmitted through the fecal-oral route, generally in food or water. Many pathogens have been described in TD, although in most cases, the specific etiology is not determined. In as many as 50% of those cases studied, the infection was found to be due to enterotoxigenic *Escherichia coli* species.[30] *Shigella*, *Salmonella*, and *Campylobacter* species are other possible bacterial causes. Viral and amebic sources are less commonly implicated in outbreaks. TD usually strikes in the first week of travel with symptoms lasting for 3–7 days. Uncommonly, symptoms may persist for 1 month or more. Diarrhea, vomiting, and abdominal pain are the most common symptoms. Fever, bloody diarrhea, and malaise occur less often but can be quite debilitating. Dehydration is common and is the major concern in the treatment of TD. Although the duration of TD is usually brief, the impact that even a short illness may have in the athlete increases the need for early recognition and treatment.

Prevention

Avoidance of TD is clearly the most effective treatment. Minimizing the risk of exposure to the agents by following a few simple rules has been shown to decrease the incidence of disease. Travelers should be advised to avoid the following sources of infection when traveling: unpeeled fruits, uncooked vegetables, dairy products, ice, and untreated water. Bottled or treated water should be used for drinking and brushing teeth.[31] In addition, bottled soft drinks and beer are generally considered to be safe. These recommendations are often difficult to follow when traveling, and as a result, individuals often ask about prophylactic antimicrobial medications.

The use of bismuth subsalicylate has been shown to reduce the incidence of TD by as much as 65%.[32] Although it is effective, the relatively high dose required for maximal protection—two 262-mg tablets four times a day—has been associated with several side effects, including salicylate-induced tinnitus and a blackened tongue. Prophylactic use of trimethoprim-sulfamethoxazole (one double-strength tablet each day) and doxycycline (100 mg once a day) have previously been shown to reduce the incidence of TD by approximately 50–85%.[33] With growing resistance to these medications and the risk of potentially serious drug reactions, however, their usefulness is limited.

Prophylaxis may be considered in patients with underlying GI illnesses or in other particularly high-risk situations.[34] An argument can easily be made to use prophylactic antibiotics in athletes on short-duration travel for competition to highly endemic regions. This must be weighed against the potential for side effects and adverse reactions for the chosen antibiotic. Currently, the fluoroquinolone antibiotics (ofloxacin 400 mg, ciprofloxacin 500 mg, norfloxacin 400 mg), all in a single dose once a day, have the lowest resistance profiles and are the drug of choice when prophylaxis is indicated.[31]

Treatment

The most important consideration in the treatment of TD is the replacement of fluid losses. Most cases can be satisfactorily managed by the use of noncaffeinated, nonalcoholic oral fluid replacements. More severe illnesses may require intravenous fluids (normal saline or lactated Ringer's solution) in volumes adequate to replace estimated losses.

The course of TD can be significantly shortened by initiating antibiotic therapy early in the infection.[35] Ideally, the antibiotics should be started with the first loose stool but may still shorten the illness if taken as many as 48 hours after symptoms begin. The most commonly used medications are trimethoprim-sulfamethoxazole (Bactrim, Septra), one double-strength tablet twice a day, or doxycycline (Vibramycin), 100 mg twice a day for 3 days.[34] However, growing resistance worldwide has significantly limited the usefulness of both of these medications. Fluoroquinolone antibiotics are currently the antibiotics of choice.[35] Ofloxacin 400 mg, ciprofloxacin (Cipro 500 mg), and norfloxacin 400 mg, each taken twice a day for 3–5 days, are all very effective.

Antidiarrheal agents, such as loperamide (Imodium), two capsules (4 mg) initially and then one capsule (2 mg) after each loose stool, or diphenoxylate (Lomotil), two tablets four times a day, are useful in reducing symptoms in uncomplicated TD. In the presence of fever or bloody diarrhea, however, these agents may actually prolong the course of illness and are contraindicated. These medications are not useful in the prophylaxis against TD. The current recommendation is for combined therapy with both a fluoroquinolone antibiotic and loperamide (Imodium) at the first loose stool, then continuation of the antibiotic for 3–5 days.[35]

GASTROESOPHAGEAL REFLUX

Upper GI symptoms, including belching, nausea, vomiting, and epigastric pain, are often experienced during maximal exertion. These symptoms have been described in running, rowing, cycling, and cross-country skiing and likely occur with most types of strenuous exercise. The symptoms are generally worse with increasing intensity or prolonged duration of exercise and are more severe with immediate postprandial exercise (within 3 hours of eating).[36]

Gastroesophageal reflux (GER) is the most common cause of upper GI symptoms. Several possible causes of GER in athletes have been postulated. Transient relaxation of the lower esophageal sphincter as a result of air swallowing is a likely contributor.[37] Another factor is decreased mucosal secretion resulting from reduced splanchnic blood flow. This reduction in the cytoprotective lining then lowers the resistance to gastric acid secretion.[38] This effect may be accentuated by NSAID use, stress, or any process that increases acid production. Finally, delayed gastric emptying, which is seen with maximal exercise, probably accentuates GER symptoms.[16]

Evaluation

The evaluation of upper GI symptoms in athletes should begin with careful documentation of recent training habits; NSAID use; dietary habits; and prior history of gastritis, peptic ulcer disease, or other GI problems. Care must be taken to rule out more serious causes of epigastric pain, most importantly those of a cardiac etiology. In general, an electrocardiogram should be obtained in all athletes presenting with epigastric pain. Laboratory evaluation includes a complete blood cell count to assess hemoglobin and hematocrit to ensure that there is no significant blood loss. Liver function testing with transaminases, bilirubin, and amylase are relatively inexpensive and will help to exclude other causes of upper GI symptoms, such as hepatitis, pancreatitis, and biliary tract disease. Endoscopy should be performed in patients with recurrent or persistent symptoms in the face of adequate treatment or in those with evidence of upper GI bleeding. Ambulatory pH monitoring has been described in athletes with this condition[39] and may be useful in evaluating patients with refractory symptoms, normal cardiac evaluation, and normal endoscopy.

Treatment

Often, simple changes in dietary and training habits alleviate symptoms. Precompetition fluid loading with low-fat, low-protein liquid calorie and electrolyte solutions is an effective means of supplying immediate pre-exercise calories while minimizing gastroesophageal reflux. Isotonic fluids tend to cause fewer upper GI symptoms.[28] Athletes may also reduce these symptoms by temporarily decreasing training or by alternating running with a lower-impact workout, such as cycling or swimming.[36] Avoidance of immediate postprandial exercise should be advised.

Antacids, such as aluminum hydroxide and magnesium salts, are useful in the treatment of mild symptoms. These should be taken immediately before beginning exercise and can be repeated during the workout as needed. Empiric therapy with H_2 antagonists, such as ranitidine (Zantac), 150 mg twice a day; famotidine (Pepcid), 20 mg twice a day; or cimetidine (Tagamet), 400 mg twice a day, is often effective in decreasing upper GI symptoms in runners.[21, 23, 37] If symptoms persist, further evaluation as outlined in the preceding section is indicated. Alternatively, metoclopramide (Reglan), 10 mg taken 1 hour before running, is effective in reducing gastroesophageal reflux. The proton pump inhibitors—omeprazole (Prilosec), 20 mg, or lansoprazole (Prevacid), 15 mg, each taken once a day—are both effective in the treatment of gastroesophagitis and may be useful in running-related symptoms, although reports of their use in athletes are lacking.

OTHER GASTROINTESTINAL PROBLEMS

Side Stitch

Side stitch is a common symptom associated with running.[40] The character of symptoms varies from a sharp stabbing pain to a dull ache, usually in the right upper abdominal quadrant. Side stitches typically occur as the athlete significantly increases training mileage or on initiating an exercise program. Although the precise etiology is not known, the most likely cause is diaphragmatic muscle spasm related to hypoxia.[41] Other possible explanations include hepatic capsule irritation, pleural irritation, and right colonic gas pains. These symptoms have also been associated with spontaneous intraabdominal adhesions.[42]

The athlete may receive some relief by stretching the right arm over the head or by forced expiration against pursed lips. Stopping exercise nearly always results in immediate cessation of symptoms. Although the frequency and severity of stitches tend to decrease as the overall fitness of the athlete improves, they may be experienced by even the highest level athletes at maximal exertion. Because these pains are often worse with postprandial exercise, delaying exercise until at least 3 hours after a meal may help to avoid them.[40]

Abnormal Liver Function Tests

Athletes may exhibit elevated liver function tests attributable to a wide range of hepatic insults, including trauma, anabolic steroid use, and viral infections. Additionally, liver function may be directly affected by exercise. Liver enzyme elevations have been described in many types of exercise but are most affected by long-distance running. Increased serum glutamic-oxaloacetic transaminase, bilirubin, alkaline phosphatase, creatinine phosphatase, and lactic dehydrogenase are all described in runners.[43] Although these can indicate liver injury, they may also be related to musculoskeletal trauma. More specific indicators of hepatocellular injury—glutamate dehydrogenase and γ-glutamyltransferase—have been found to be elevated in long-distance runners.[44] The gradual serum reductions of albumin seen in ultradistance runners further support the possibility of hepatic injury in these athletes.[44] The injury probably results from decreased oxygen tension in the hepatic blood supply. This ischemic damage to the liver is readily reversible when exercise is stopped, with enzyme levels usually returning to normal within 1 week.

Hepatitis

In the athlete with acute viral hepatitis, no exercise restrictions are indicated. The continuation of exercise in the acute phase may actually allow the athlete to return to pre-illness levels of performance more quickly in the recovery phase of the illness.[45] No specific exercise restrictions are necessary in chronic liver disease; however, the patient's overall condition as a result of the illness must be considered in developing an exercise program.

REFERENCES

1. Worobetz LJ, Gerrard DF. Gastrointestinal symptoms during exercise in enduro athletes. N Z Med J 1985;98:644–646.
2. Strauss R, Lanese R, Leizman D. Illness and absence among wrestlers, swimmers, and gymnasts at a large university. Am J Sports Med 1988;16:653–655.
3. Wilhite J, Mellion M. Occult gastrointestinal bleeding in endurance cyclists. Phys Sportsmed 1990;18:75–78.
4. Butcher JD. Injuries in cross country skiing. Sports Med Primary Care 1996;2:13–16.
5. Oettle GJ. Effect of moderate exercise on bowel habit. Gut 1991;32:941–944.
6. Dapoigny M, Sarna SK. Effects of physical exercise on colonic motor activity [Abstract]. Gastroenterology 1990;98:343.
7. Lee IM, Paffenbarger RS, Hsieh CC. Physical activity and risk of developing colorectal cancer among college alumni. J Natl Cancer Inst 1991;83:1324–1329.
8. Robertson G, Meshkinpour H, Vandenberg K, et al. Effects of exercise on total and segmental colon transit. J Clin Gastroenterol 1993;16:300–303.

9. Keeffe EB, Lowe DK, Goss JR, Wayne R. Gastrointestinal symptoms of marathon runners. West J Med 1984;141:481–484.

10. Riddoch C, Trinick T. Gastrointestinal disturbances in marathon runners. Br J Sports Med 1988;22:71–74.

11. Fogoros R. "Runner's trots." JAMA 1980;243:1743–1744.

12. Sullivan SN, Wong C. Runner's diarrhea: different patterns and associated factors. J Clin Gastroenterol 1992;14:101–104.

13. Stewart J, Ahlquist D, McGill D, et al. Gastrointestinal blood loss and anemia in runners. Ann Intern Med 1984;100:843–845.

14. Rehrer N, Janssen G, Brouns F, Saris WHM. Fluid intake and gastrointestinal problems in runners competing in a 25-km marathon. Int J Sports Med 1989;10(suppl):22–25.

15. Cammack J, Read NW, Cann PA, et al. Effect of prolonged exercise on the passage of a solid meal through the stomach and small intestine. Gut 1982;23:957–961.

16. Read N, Houghton L. Physiology of gastric emptying and pathophysiology of gastroparesis. Gastroenterol Clin North Am 1989;18:359–373.

17. Kayaleh RA, Meshkinpour H, Avinashi A, Tamadon A. Effect of exercise on mouth to cecum transit in trained athletes: a case against the role of runner's abdominal bouncing. J Sports Med Phys Fitness 1996;36:271–274.

18. Swain RA. Exercise induced diarrhea: when to wonder. Med Sci Sports Exerc 1994;26:523–526.

19. McCabe M, Peura D, Kadakia S, et al. Gastrointestinal blood loss associated with running a marathon. Dig Dis Sci 1986;31:1229–1232.

20. Yges C, Chicharro JL, Lucia A, et al. Monoclonal antibodies for exercise induced fecal blood detection—comparison with Hemofec. Can J Appl Physiol 1995;20:78–88.

21. Baska R, Moses F, Deuster P. Cimetidine reduces running-associated gastrointestinal bleeding. Dig Dis Sci 1990;35:956–960.

22. Heer M, Repond F, Hany A, et al. Acute ischemic colitis in a female long distance runner. Gut 1987;28:896–899.

23. Cooper BT, Douglas SA, Firth LA, et al. Erosive gastritis and gastrointestinal bleeding in a female runner. Gastroenterology 1987;92:2019–2023.

24. Moses F. Gastrointestinal bleeding and the athlete. Am J Gastroenterol 1993;88:1157–1159.

25. Clausen JP. Effect of physical training on cardiovascular adjustments to exercise in man. Physiol Rev 1977;57:779–815.

26. Blaklock NJ. Bladder trauma in the long distance runner: 10,000 metres haematuria. Br J Urol 1977;49:129–132.

27. Bounos G, McArdle AH. Marathon runners: the intestinal handicap. Med Hypotheses 1990;33:261–264.

28. Brouns F, Saris W, Reher N. Abdominal complaints and gastrointestinal function during long-lasting exercise. Int J Sports Med 1987;8:175–189.

29. Bruins J, Bwire R, Slootman EJH, van Leusden AJ. Mil Med 1995;160:446–448.

30. Wolfe M. Acute diarrhea associated with travel. Am J Med 1990;88(suppl):34–37.

31. Statement on Traveller's Diarrhea. Can Med Assoc J 1995;152:205–208.

32. Dupont H, Ericsson C, Johnson PT, et al. Prevention of traveler's diarrhea by the tablet form of bismuth subsalicylate. JAMA 1987;257:1347–1350.

33. American Medical Association Consensus Conference. Traveler's diarrhea. JAMA 1985;253:2699–2704.

34. Ferenchick G, Havlichek D. Primary prevention and international travel. J Gen Intern Med 1989;4:247–258.

35. Dupont HL, Erickson CD. Prevention and treatment of traveler's diarrhea. N Engl J Med 1993;328:1821–1827.

36. Clark S, Kraus B, Sinclair J, Castell D. Gastroesophageal reflux induced by exercise in healthy volunteers. JAMA 1989;261:3599–3601.

37. Krause BS, Sinclair JW, Castell DO. Gastroesophageal reflux in runners. Ann Intern Med 1990;112:429–433.

38. Gaudin C, Zerath E, Guezennec C. Gastric lesions secondary to long-distance running. Dig Dis Sci 1990;35:1239–1243.

39. Shawdon A. Gastro-esophageal reflux and exercise: important pathology to consider in the athletic population. Sports Med 1995;20:109–116.

40. Sullivan SN, Wong C, Heidenheim P. Does running cause gastrointestinal symptoms? A survey of 93 randomly selected runners compared with controls. N Z Med J 1994;107:328–330.

41. Pate R. Principles of Training. In D Kulund (ed), The Injured Athlete. Philadelphia: Lippincott, 1988.

42. Lauder TD, Moses FM. Recurrent abdominal pain from abdominal adhesions in an endurance triathlete. Med Sci Sports Exerc 1995;27:623–625.

43. Bunch T. Blood test abnormalities in runners. Mayo Clin Proc 1980;55:113–117.

44. Nagel D, Seiler D, Franz H, Jung K. Ultra-long-distance running and the liver. Int J Sports Med 1990;11:441–445.

45. Ritland S. Exercise and liver disease. Sports Med 1988;6:121–126.

22

Genitourinary Problems

B. Wayne Blount

The genitourinary (GU) system is the source of athletes' symptoms in a variety of circumstances. Cases of GU trauma and of "athletic pseudonephritis"[1] are well known. This chapter highlights the most common GU problems presented to the care provider in sports medicine: proteinuria, hematuria, scrotal enlargement and pain, and sores and discharges.

PROTEINURIA

The most common presentation of proteinuria is an abnormal result on a screening urinalysis. The routine practice of screening urinalyses on healthy athletes as a part of the preparticipation physical examination has been questioned and is generally not recommended.[2] If urinalysis is done, however, proteinuria will be commonly found 5–85% of the time.[2] Proteinuria is defined as more than 150 mg of protein per 24 hours in adults, and more than 140 mg per 24 hours per square meter of body surface area in children.[3] It is more common in males than females, and it is more common in the summer months.[2]

Diagnosis

Proteinuria in childhood and adolescence is benign in 99.2% of cases.[2] The most frequent sources of such benign proteinuria are listed in Table 22-1. These can be either transient (e.g., febrile) or chronic (e.g., orthostatic) in nature.

The history taken from the proteinuric individual should emphasize urinary tract symptoms, drug exposure, recent illnesses, and personal and family history of renal disease. The physical examination should include a search for hypertension and edema as well as any abnormalities found in the history or review of systems.

The frequently benign nature of proteinuria is reflected in the suggested diagnostic workup of this abnormality (Figures 22-1 and 22-2). The algorithms adhere to the principle that the cause of proteinuria is determined by the amount and type of proteinuria and the clinical picture. Transient proteinuria is not often important. Persistent proteinuria requires determination of the cause.

In addition to following the algorithms of Figures 22-1 and 22-2, the athlete should refrain from exercise for 24–72 hours before the repeat testing of urine. Exercise-induced proteinuria is most often secondary to an increased glomerular filtration rate or to transient tubular abnormalities in exhaustive exercise.[4] Such exercise-induced proteinuria is reversible within 24–72 hours.[1, 4] The same caveat for repeat testing holds for febrile illnesses: Wait until the illness is over for 1 week to repeat the urinalysis.

In Figure 22-2, "clinically isolated" proteinuria is defined by the absence of abnormal urinary sediment, diminished renal function, hypertension, urinary tract abnormalities, and systemic disease with renal effects.[3] Nephritic sediment includes red blood cells, white blood cells, or cellular casts.[3]

Summary

Routine preparticipation examination urinalysis may not be warranted. If done and proteinuria is found, the diagnosis is usually benign. Following the algorithms in Figures 22-1 and 22-2 will allow the care provider to assess and care accurately for patients with proteinuria.

HEMATURIA

Hematuria is a frequent occurrence in athletes, with an incidence ranging from 11% to 100% depending on the type and amount of exercise and the state of hydration.[5-7]

TABLE 22-1

Causes of Benign Proteinuria

Orthostatic
Exercise
Febrile
Cold exposure
Emotional stress

The condition can be microscopic or macroscopic, appears in both sexes,[7] and may be benign or a manifestation of serious disease. Because blood in the urine can originate anywhere along the urinary system, the physician presented with an athlete with hematuria must be able to distinguish between those with serious causes (such as neoplasia, hydronephrosis, vasculitides, cystic renal disease, coagulopathies, and nephritides) and those with benign causes (such as exercise-induced hematuria, benign familial hematuria, hypercalciuria, and febrile hematuria).

The past recommendation to perform full urologic workups in all patients with hematuria comes from studies in patients older than 40 years old in whom significant lesions are likely to be found.[8] When there is isolated hematuria in athletes younger than 40 years old, there have been several good studies documenting the overall good prognosis and benignity of the causes.[8–10]

Diagnosis

There have been numerous algorithms proposed for the evaluation of hematuria. The strategy suggested here reflects the demographics of hematuria (Figure 22-3). It attempts to detect serious and treatable problems while limiting unnecessary testing.

Obviously, hematuria must be defined and differentiated from hemoglobinuria, hematospermia, and myoglobinuria. History can then focus on duration and frequency of hematuria; use of medicines; associated symptoms, such as dysuria, fever, or respiratory infection; medications; menses; travel; abdominal pain; trauma; exercise; personal and family history of renal disease and hearing loss; and a review of systems. The physical examination should ascertain the presence of fever, hypertension, costovertebral angle tenderness, rashes, edema, and abdominal masses.

Further workup follows the flow of Figure 22-3. Prompt evaluation is required in anyone with unstable vital signs, hypertension, edema, oliguria, red cell casts, or significant proteinuria. Proteinuria secondary to bleeding alone should not exceed 2+ or 100 mg/dl.[12] At the points in Figure 22-3 that indicate long-term follow-up, a microscopic urinalysis for hematuria and proteinuria and a blood pressure measurement every 12 months are minimal requirements. Two additional tests not contained in Figure 22-3 that could be considered in the workup are spot urine calcium-to-creatinine ratios and phase-contrast microscopy of the red cells. The first test (with a ratio of more than 0.2) suggests obtaining a 24-hour urine calcium excretion to diagnose benign hypercalciuria (urinary calcium more than 4 mg/kg/day).[11] The second test, phase-contrast microscopy, is not yet of proven validity.

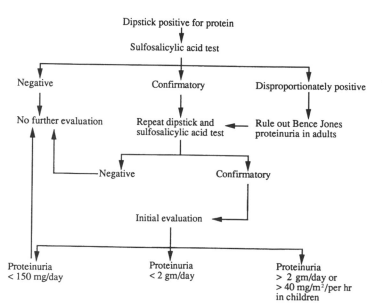

FIGURE 22-1

Initial evaluation of proteinuria. (Reprinted with permission from DW Stewart, JA Gordon, AC Schoolwerth. Evaluation of proteinuria. Am Fam Physician 1984;29: 218–225. Published by the American Academy of Family Physicians. All rights reserved.)

FIGURE 22-2

Characterization of proteinuria. (MCNS = minimal-change nephrotic syndrome; ANA = antinuclear antibody test; C3 = serum level of third component of complement.) (Reprinted with permission from DW Stewart, JA Gordon, AC Schoolwerth. Evaluation of proteinuria. Am Fam Physician 1984;29: 218–225. Published by the American Academy of Family Physicians. All rights reserved.)

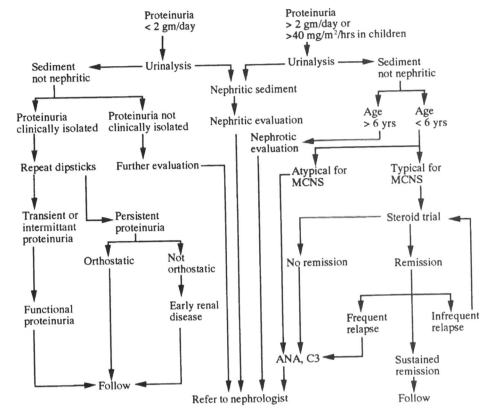

Exercise-Induced Hematuria

Exercise-induced hematuria is a common finding. Its appearance depends on the sport, the vigor with which the sport is pursued, and the state of hydration of the athlete. It has been reported in almost every sport. The etiology can be divided into renal, bladder, and peripheral sources. Peripheral sources are suggested in running and karate, with the proposed cause being mechanical trauma to red cells as they pass through the feet and hands, respectively.[5, 12]

Renal and bladder sources may be involved in any sport of strenuous proportions. Figure 22-4 summarizes the proposed mechanisms involved. Unless the mechanism is a very forceful blow to the kidneys or bladder, the hematuria of exercise is a self-limited and benign condition, micro- or macroscopic, and can recur with further exercise in perhaps 50% of athletes.[7, 13] Causes other than exercise should be sought if any of the following conditions exist: persistence beyond 72 hours without exercise, red cell casts, proteinuria more than 2+, any accompanying symptoms, or a history of renal disease.[5, 7, 13, 14] Further evaluation of the athlete older than 40–60 years old

with recurrent postexercise hematuria may be warranted based on the higher incidence of urologic neoplasms in this age group.[15]

The treatment of exercise-induced hematuria depends on the underlying etiology: better cushioning of shoes or running surfaces, investigation of stride length, fluids before an event, and kidney protection. The athlete with exercise-induced hematuria can safely return to sports. It is prudent to institute some of the preventive measures and to periodically assess kidney function in such athletes.[5]

SCROTAL ENLARGEMENT OR PAIN

Diagnosis of scrotal pain in the athlete can be problematic, and misdiagnosis can be serious. Even though the diagnostic possibilities are numerous (Table 22-2), the major diagnostic possibilities are testicular torsion, testicular rupture, epididymitis, inguinal hernia, urinary calculus, varicocele, and testicular tumor. Orchitis is rare enough today that one should be cautious in making the diagnosis.

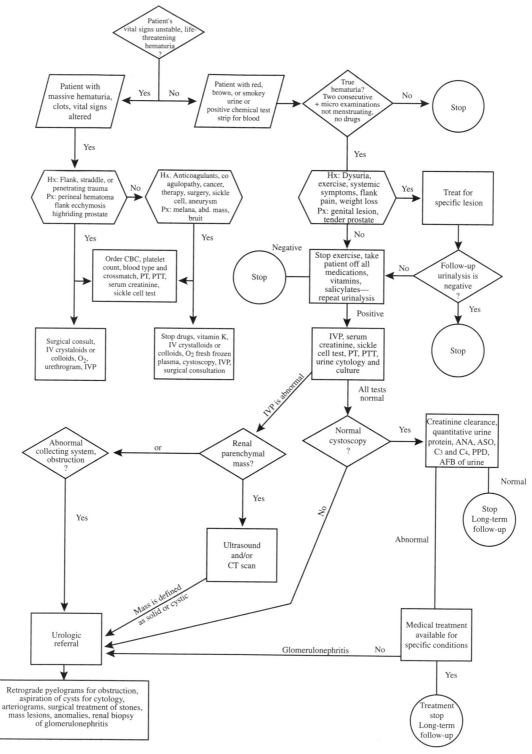

FIGURE 22-3

Primary care of hematuria. (Hx = history; Px = physical examination; CBC = complete blood count; PT = prothrombin time; PTT = partial thromboplastin time; C3 = serum level of third component of complement; C4 = serum level of fourth component of complement; ANA = antinuclear antibody test; ASO = antistreptolysin O test; PPD = purified protein derivative; AFB = acid fast bacilli; CT = computed tomography; IV = intravenous; IVP = intravenous pyelogram; + = positive; abd. = abdominal.)
(Reprinted from CE Driscoll. Hematuria: how to reach an earlier decision. Prim Care Emerg Dec 1985;1:36–37. Copyright 1985, Physicians World Communications Group. All rights reserved.)

FIGURE 22-4

Sports hematuria pathophysiology in kidney and blad-der. (RBCs = red blood cells.) (Adapted from J Abar-banel, A Benet, D Lask, D Kimche. Sports hematuria. J Urol 1990;143:887–890. Copyright 1990 by Williams & Wilkins.)

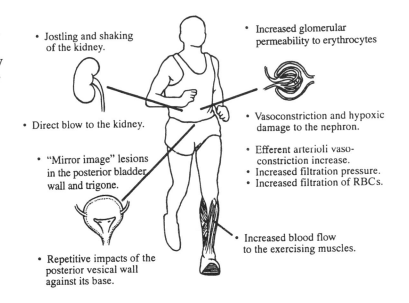

- Jostling and shaking of the kidney.
- Direct blow to the kidney.
- "Mirror image" lesions in the posterior bladder wall and trigone.
- Repetitive impacts of the posterior vesical wall against its base.
- Increased glomerular permeability to erythrocytes
- Vasoconstriction and hypoxic damage to the nephron.
- Efferent arterioli vaso-constriction increase.
- Increased filtration pressure.
- Increased filtration of RBCs.
- Increased blood flow to the exercising muscles.

Musculoskeletal injuries of the groin area are covered in Chapter 14. Most of the preceding major diagnoses can be ruled in or out from the history and physical examination, which consists of inspection, palpation, and transillumination. Palpation should distinguish each component of the scrotum, including testis, epididymis, and cord. If a mass is found, transillumination can help determine if it is cystic or solid.

Varicoceles can be seen and palpated as irregular, worm-like masses on the spermatic cord. Hernia should be apparent on physical examination. If it is not, and other causes of scrotal pain are unlikely, herniography can help in the diagnosis.[16] Surgical consultation is also an alternative. A urinary calculus should present with flank pain and hematuria.

Testicular tumors have one of their bimodal incidence peaks (1 in 10,000) in the common age group for athletes, 15–35 years old.[17] This is particularly true for white males. Other risk factors include a history of an undescended testis or testicular feminization syndrome.[17] In the athlete presenting with subacute scrotal pain, rolling the testicles gently between the fingers and thumb while feeling for hardness, swelling, heaviness, and asymmetry can differentiate this disease. Any area of induration or mass within the testis should be surgically explored.[18]

Ultrasonography plays a role in the diagnosis of testicular rupture. Classically, rupture occurs from a straddle injury or a direct blow to the scrotum during contact sports. A physical examination is generally suboptimal because of tenderness and swelling. Ultrasonography can then be used to assist examination. If the testicle can-not be visualized or if it has poorly defined margins, rupture is likely.[19] If ultrasonography is not readily available or if one is presented with a large, tender, bluish scrotal mass after trauma, urologic referral is warranted. Surgery within 72 hours results in a significant salvage

TABLE 22-2

Causes of Scrotal Pain

Intrascrotal Disease	Extrascrotal Disease
Torsion of	Abdominal aortic aneurysm
Spermatic cord	Ureteral obstruction
Testicular appendage	Ureteral irritation
Epididymitis	Disease of the renal pelvis
Deferentitis	Retroperitoneal disease
Funiculitis	Radicular pain
Epididymo-orchitis	Lower thoracic roots
Orchitis	Upper lumbar roots
Testicular neoplasm	Genitofemoral nerve
Vasculitis	Ilioinguinal nerve
Inguinal hernia	Pudendal nerve
Abdominal abscess	Epilepsy
Varicocele	Prostatitis
Appendicitis in hernia	Prostatodynia
Scrotal fat necrosis	Masturbation interruptus
Scrotal cellulitis	Diabetic neuropathy
Scrotal trauma	Bacterial endocarditis
Sperm granuloma	Hypertriglyceridemia
Ovotesticular ovulation	
Drugs	
Scrotal abscess	
Hydrocele	
Spermatocele	

Source: Adapted from BM Reilly. Practical Strategies in Outpatient Medicine (2nd ed). Philadelphia: Saunders, 1991;1089.

TABLE 22-3
Differentiating between Testicular Torsion and Epididymitis

Features	Torsion	Epididymitis
History		
Onset of pain	Acute	Gradual
Nausea and vomiting	50%	Rare
Voiding symptoms	No	50%
Urethral discharge	No	50%
History of similar pain	35%	Rare
Physical examination		
Epididymal swelling only	10%	Early
Scrotal edema and erythema	Most	Most
Fever	Rare	50%
Laboratory results		
Pyuria	0–30%	20–95%
Urethral culture and Gram's-stained smear	Negative	Often positive
Profusion studies		
Doppler ultrasonography	Decreased flow	Normal or increased flow
Radionuclide scanning	Decreased flow	Normal or increased flow

Source: Reprinted with permission from WO O'Brien. The acute scrotum. Am Fam Physician 1988;37:239–247. Published by the American Academy of Family Physicians. All rights reserved.

rate. Regardless of whether the condition is a rupture or a testicular contusion, the patient will benefit from surgical exploration.[19]

The physician is then left with two major possibilities: torsion and epididymitis. The differentiation between these two is serious and problematic. The signs and symptoms suggestive of epididymitis and testicular torsion are listed in Table 22-3. In torsion, other useful differentiations include an anteriorly situated epididymis, a high-riding testis, and a horizontal contralateral testis. A useful sign is the cremasteric reflex. In one study, if the reflex was present, there was no torsion of the ipsilateral testis.[20] Prehn's sign, pain relief with elevation of the testis, is not reliable.[21] If the diagnosis is epididymitis, besides antibiotics, one can use bed rest, analgesics, ice packs, and scrotal support as supportive measures. Admission to the hospital is warranted for generalized toxicity, severe pain, abscess formation, or an indwelling catheter. Athletes with epididymitis will not want to compete (and should not) because of the pain.

If one diagnoses torsion, immediate surgical referral is mandated. Before surgery, manual detorsion can be attempted; however, even if it is successful, surgery is still a must.

If there is an indeterminate examination, nuclear studies or Doppler ultrasonography can assist in the diagnosis. Doppler ultrasonography is accurate 85% of the time, but it should not be used when there is much scrotal edema.[21] Nuclear scrotal imaging has an accuracy

of 95%.[21] The choice between these two tests is based on availability and the comfort of one's urology consultant. Ready availability is a key factor, because testicular salvage diminishes markedly after 6 hours of torsion. Surgical consultation and exploration should not be delayed beyond that point to wait for a sonographic or nuclear scan confirmation. The principle to follow in distinguishing between torsion and epididymitis is that if the examiner is uncertain, urologic consultation is necessary. It is probably better to operate on patients with epididymitis than not to correct a torsion.[22]

DISCHARGES AND SORES

For discharges and sores, the vast majority of etiologies are the sexually transmitted diseases (STDs). The spectrum of STDs is large, but the two main presentations are urethral discharge or a GU sore. Because the successful management of STDs depends on accurate diagnosis, and clinical diagnosis of STDs without laboratory testing is notoriously inaccurate, the prudent physician uses the laboratory.[23] The approaches presented here account for that. For male athletes presenting with a discharge or dysuria, the algorithm of Figure 22-5 can be used to make a diagnosis.

For athletes presenting with sores in the genital area, the algorithm of Figure 22-6 can be used to diagnose the

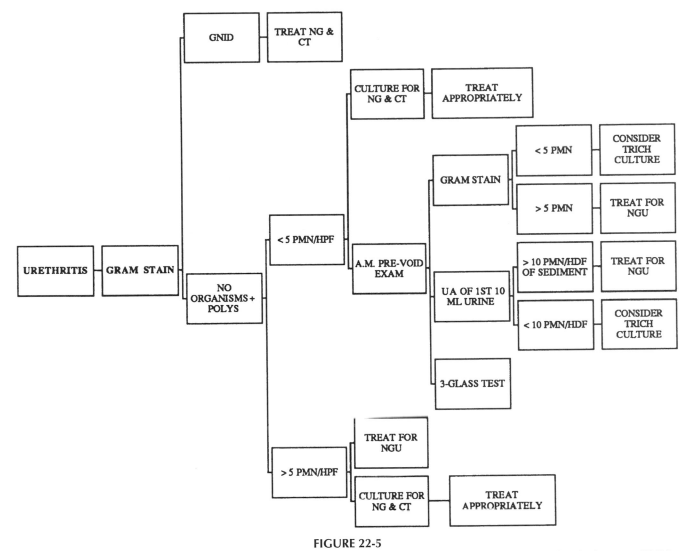

FIGURE 22-5

Evaluation of male urethritis. (GNID = gram-negative intracellular diplococci; polys = polymorphonuclear leukocytes; PMN = polymorphonuclear leukocytes; HPF = high-power field [oil]; NG = Neisseria gonorrhoeae; CT = Chlamydia trachomatis; NGU = nongonococcal urethritis; Trich = Trichomonas; HDF = high dry field; UA = urinalysis.)

cause. The clinical setting must always be considered; for example, in the United States the three most common STD ulcers seen are herpes, syphilis, and chancroid. Syphilis and chancroid are more closely associated with prostitution. With fluctuant inguinal nodes present, one should do a Gram's stain of the ulcer, looking for chancroid. One can also culture to confirm a diagnosis of herpes. Other far less common considerations for genital ulcers are lymphogranuloma venereum, granuloma

inguinale, drug eruption, and trauma. Causes of lumps on the genitalia include condyloma (latum and acuminatum), molluscum, lice, and scabies. Because most STD ulcers are infectious, athletes with exposed STD ulcers should refrain from competition with bodily contact until the ulcers are healed.

Treatment of STDs is summarized in Table 22-4. STDs are reportable. Other STDs frequently accompany one STD, and sex partners must usually also be treated.

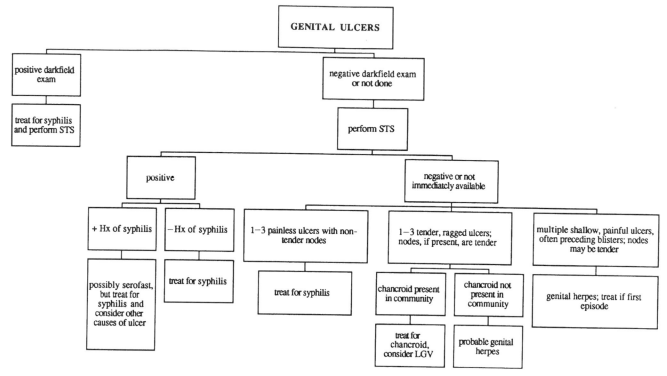

FIGURE 22-6

Evaluation of genital ulcers. (STS = serologic test for syphilis; Hx = history; LGV = lymphogranuloma venereum; + = positive; – = negative.) (Reprinted with permission from GP Schmid. Approach to the patient with genital ulcer disease. Med Clin North Am *1990;74:1569.)*

TABLE 22-4

Treatment of Sexually Transmitted Diseases

Disease	*Recommended Treatment**
Uncomplicated adult gonorrhea	Ceftriaxone, 125 mg IM once, plus doxycycline, 100 mg PO twice daily for 7 days
Uncomplicated childhood gonorrhea (children <45 kg)	Ceftriaxone, 125 mg IM once
Early syphilis	Benzathine penicillin G, 2.4 million units IM once
Late latent syphilis	Benzathine penicillin G, 2.4 million units IM every week for 3 wks
Uncomplicated chlamydial infection	Doxycycline, 100 mg PO twice daily for 7 days
Nongonococcal urethritis	Same as treatment for *Chlamydia*
Epididymitis	Ceftriaxone, 125 mg IM once plus doxycycline, 100 mg PO twice daily for 10 days
Chancroid	Erythromycin base, 500 mg PO four times a day for 7 days, or one dose of IM ceftriaxone, 250 mg
Herpes simplex	
Recurrent infection	Acyclovir 200 mg PO five times a day for 10 days *or* famciclovir 125 mg PO twice a day for 5 days
Suppression	Acyclovir 400 mg PO twice a day
Genital warts	See Chapter 14

*Alternative treatments can be found in Centers for Disease Control and Prevention: 1993 Sexually Transmitted Diseases Treatment Guidelines. IM = intramuscularly; PO = orally.

REFERENCES

1. Fletcher DJ. Athletic pseudonephritis. Lancet 1977;i:910–911.
2. Peggs JF, Reinhardt RW, O'Brien JM. Proteinuria in adolescent sports physical examinations. J Fam Pract 1986;22: 80–81.
3. Stewart DW, Gordon JA, Schoolwerth AC. Evaluation of proteinuria. Am Fam Physician 1984;29:218–225.
4. Campanacci L, Faccini L, Englaro E, et al. Exercise-induced proteinuria. Contrib Nephrol 1981;26:31–41.
5. Abarbanel J, Benet A, Lask D, Kimche D. Sports hematuria. J Urol 1990;143:887–890.
6. Heizer-Julin M, Latin RW, Mellion MB, et al. The effect of exercise intensity and hydration on athletic pseudonephritis. J Sports Med Phys Fitness 1988;28:324–329.
7. Boileau M, Fuchs E, Barry JM, Hodges CV. Stress hematuria: athletic pseudonephritis in marathoners. Urology 1980;15:471–474.
8. Froom P, Ribak J, Benbassat J. Significance of microhematuria in young adults. BMJ 1984;288:20–22.
9. Benbassat J, Gergawi M, Offringa M, Drukker A. Symptomless microhaematuria in school children: causes for variable management strategies. Q J Med 1996;89:845–854.
10. Murakami M, Yamamoto H, Ueda Y, et al. Urinary screening of elementary and junior high-school children over a 13-year period in Tokyo. Pediatr Nephrol 1991;5:50–53.
11. Lieu TA, Grasmeder HM, Kaplan BS. An approach to the evaluation and treatment of microscopic hematuria. Pediatr Clin North Am 1991;38:579–592.
12. Streeton JA. Traumatic haemoglobinuria caused by karate exercises. Lancet 1967;ii:191–192.
13. Fred HL, Natelson EA. Grossly bloody urine of runners. South Med J 1977;70:1394–1396.
14. Siegel AJ, Hennekens CH, Solomon HS, Van Boeckel B. Exercise-related hematuria. JAMA 1979;241:391–392.
15. Gambrell RC, Blount BW. Exercise-induced hematuria. Am Fam Physician 1996;53:905–911.
16. Taylor DC, Meyers WC, Moylan JA, et al. Abdominal musculature abnormalities as a cause of groin pain in athletes. Am J Sports Med 1991;19:239–242.
17. Goldenring JM. Testicular self-examination. Am Fam Physician 1985;32:100–101.
18. Zornow DH, Landes RR. Scrotal palpation. Am Fam Physician 1981;23:150–154.
19. Cass AS. Testicular trauma. J Urol 1983;129:299–300.
20. Rabinowitz R. The importance of the cremasteric reflex in acute scrotal swelling in children. J Urol 1984;132:89–90.
21. O'Brien WO. The acute scrotum. Am Fam Physician 1988; 37:239–247.
22. Brosman SA. Testicular torsion. Med Aspects Human Sexuality 1984;18:21–26.
23. Dangor Y, Ballard RC, Exposto F, et al. Accuracy of clinical diagnosis of genital ulcer disease. Sex Transm Dis 1990;17: 184–189.

23

Hematologic Abnormalities

RICHARD TENGLIN

The many textbooks and journals devoted exclusively to the subject of hematology attest to the extent of this field. This chapter discusses hematologic diseases and conditions associated with participation in athletics. It also briefly addresses other important hematologic conditions.

GENERAL GUIDELINES

Participation in athletics may be undertaken by all but the very young, and this participation in no way limits the hematologic illnesses that an athlete may experience compared with the nonathlete. Although athletes may experience symptoms of disease earlier as a result of athletic stress, participation in athletics does not cause the illness. With few exceptions in the symptomatic patient, the differential diagnosis and diagnostic approach would be the same for the athlete and nonathlete. The challenge for the athlete's care provider is to explain abnormal laboratory values, usually in the pursuit of denied symptoms or physiologic alterations induced by the training environment.

A complete history and physical examination are the foundation on which an additional appropriate workup is built. A careful review of systems must be sought with special emphasis placed on the chronicity of the symptom, drug use or toxin exposure, and family history. In our ever-increasingly drug- and chemical-exposed society, "trivial," "incidental," and illicit drug and toxin exposure must be sought. Many agents are known to damage bone marrow precursors or the bone marrow microenvironment, and many more substances are associated (albeit, some very loosely) with hematologic abnormalities. The ready availability of these agents, their widespread distribution, and their ability to produce severe damage with small amounts or single doses make the history of all chemical, toxin, or drug exposure a vital part of the initial investigation.

Prior laboratory studies—in this case, complete blood counts (CBC)—are critical. Every effort must be made to obtain them, lest an extensive workup be directed at a normal baseline as though it were an acute problem.

As with other athletically induced "injuries," hematologic problems truly associated with athletics improve or resolve with cessation of the athletic program (Table 23-1). Although this solution is distasteful to the dedicated athlete, it is the cheapest and most appropriate diagnostic and therapeutic tool available.

"Normal" laboratory values differ significantly between different laboratories and between patients of different sex, race, or age. It is necessary to ascertain any significant deviation from normal values for that individual before initiation of a workup, based on either the patient's prior laboratory values or established norms for the laboratory currently being used, or the patient's age, sex, and race.

Mild, stable abnormalities in truly asymptomatic individuals more probably represent a normal state for that individual rather than the presence of worrisome disease. Workup can often appropriately consist of building a reassuring series of unchanging CBCs rather than embarking on extensive diagnostic testing. Explanation of the preceding is usually enthusiastically embraced by the patient and assists in obtaining the required periodic visits needed to gather the data.

Most important, laboratory errors do occur. The initiation of an extensive workup based on a single markedly abnormal laboratory value from an asymptomatic patient is seldom appropriate. The cheapest and most effective workup is often a repeat CBC.

TABLE 23-1
Complete Blood Count (CBC) Abnormalities of Athletic Importance

Abnormality	Potential Etiologies	Include in Evaluation
Low WBC	Neutropenia of blacks	Evaluate past CBCs
		Serial CBCs if ANC $>1,000/\mu l$ and other cell lines are normal
	Drug/toxin effect (e.g., NSAIDs)	Detailed questioning, especially ibuprofen, acetaminophen
High WBC	Postexercise granulocytosis	Repeat CBC after 24-hr rest
	Steroid use	Ask patient about steroid use
		Consider urine drug test
Low hemoglobin (reticulocytes $<2\%$)	Anemia of athletes	Evaluate past CBCs
		Serial CBCs if other indices normal—consider discontinuing exercise
	Nutrient deficiency	See text
Low hemoglobin (increased reticulocytes)	March hemoglobinuria	LDH, serum haptoglobin
	Exercise-induced hemolytic anemia	Bilirubin, evaluate peripheral smear, stop exercise
Low hemoglobin (with microcytosis)	Iron deficiency anemia	Stool guaiac, urinalysis
		Iron studies (see text)
High hemoglobin	Blood doping, androgenic steroids, erythropoietin	Ask patient about use
	Carbon monoxide poisoning	Carboxyhemoglobin and history
High platelets	Exercise-induced thrombocytosis	Serial CBCs and stopping exercise
Low platelets	Drug effect (NSAIDs, thiazides)	Ask about use
	DIC/heat stroke	Fibrinogen, fibrin split products, other abnormalities (see text)

WBC = white blood cell; LDH = lactate dehydrogenase; ANC = absolute neutrophil count; NSAIDs = nonsteroidal anti-inflammatory drugs; DIC = disseminated intravascular coagulation.

HEMATOLOGIC LABORATORY ABNORMALITIES

White Cells

Few, if any, persistent white cell abnormalities are attributable to exercise, although transient increases in granulocytes with exercise may be seen.[1] Lymphopenia and granulocytosis may be caused by surreptitious or therapeutic glucocorticoid use. Neutrophil counts as low as $1,000/\mu l$ may represent normal values in blacks and other ethnic populations. Most other causes of leukopenia or leukocytosis are not athletics related or are symptomatic.

A history of drug and toxin exposure should be obtained, and the patient should be evaluated for nonathletics-related viral infections (especially human immunodeficiency virus [HIV]). Common analgesic and anti-inflammatory agents (ibuprofen, acetaminophen) have been associated with neutropenia. Their availability is so ubiquitous that they should be specifically asked about, because their use may not be volunteered when the patient is questioned about "drug use." A lymphatic examination should be performed and bone marrow aspiration and biopsy considered. Further workup, which should continue as clinically indicated, is beyond the scope of this chapter.

Red Cells

Anemia

Anemia results from decreased production of red cells, or increased destruction or loss of red cells, or a combination of these mechanisms. Symptoms, such as decreasing exercise tolerance or shortness of breath, would suggest a new pathologic condition. A "corrected" reticulocyte count of less than 2% would indicate a problem with production, while an increased reticulocyte count would suggest a bone marrow "turned on" in the attempt to compensate for increased destruction or loss. Also called the *reticulocyte index* (RI), the reticulocyte count is calculated as follows: RI = % reticulocytes × (observed hematocrit/normal hematocrit) × "premature release adjustment factor" (0.5 will usually be sufficient).

Anemia Due to Decreased Red Cell Production

The anemia of athletes is a well-known but poorly understood phenomenon.[1] Speculation as to the cause of this condition includes intravascular volume expansion with exercise and improved use of oxygen by tissue, resulting in less demand for oxygen-carrying capacity. The improved rheology of "anemic" blood improves flow (and oxygen delivery) and may decrease the need for higher hemoglobin concentrations. It is vital that this exercise-induced adaptive change be differentiated from athletically induced conditions of red cell destruction or loss.

A microcytic anemia should prompt the search for blood or iron loss. A normocytic anemia may be the initial manifestation of HIV infection.

Anemia Due to Increased Red Cell Loss or Destruction

There is little doubt that exercise-induced trauma can destroy red cells. March hemoglobinuria and other forms of traumatic hemolytic anemia from slapping the feet during running can result in anemia.[2] That swimmers can also traumatize red cells[3] and become anemic suggests the work of other mechanisms more complicated than simply squashing red cells between bone and pavement. An elevated reticulocyte count and bilirubin and a decreased haptoglobin level, along with schistocytes seen on a stain smear of peripheral blood, suggest this diagnosis; resolution when exercise stops virtually confirms it.

Athletes can also lose blood during exercise. Microscopic hematuria in distance runners and heme-positive stools in these and other athletes are common findings. The chronic loss of iron, not the blood loss, is of concern because it may eventually induce an iron-deficient anemia. Menstruating females will develop iron deficient anemia more rapidly from equivalent quantities of blood loss than will males or nonmenstruating females. As with other substances (folate, vitamin B_{12}, protein, and so forth) required for the manufacture of red cells, deficiency of iron may prevent the increase in reticulocytes normally seen with anemia from red cell loss or destruction. With the assurance that the blood loss or iron deficiency is due to exercise and not, for example, malignancy, iron supplementation would be appropriate.

Suggested Workup for Anemia

The workup should begin with a reticulocyte count, which may separate decreased production (low reticulocyte count) from increased loss or destruction (increased reticulocyte count). The red cells are characterized as microcytic (small), which suggests iron deficiency; normocytic (normal); or macrocytic (large), which suggest folate or vitamin B_{12} deficiency. Further testing is done with iron studies (iron, total iron-binding capacity, ferritin), folate levels, and B_{12} levels based on the preceding. Potential sites of blood and iron loss in urine and stool (urinalysis for blood and hemosiderin, and stool guaiac) should be evaluated (see Chapters 21 and 22), and drug or toxin history and stopping exercise with observation for improvement complete the workup. If the workup is unrewarding and stopping exercise for 1 week does not result in reso-

lution of the anemia, referral to a hematologist is appropriate.

Increased Hemoglobin Concentrations (Polycythemia)

The etiologies of increased hemoglobin concentrations in the athlete are numerous. Increases in the reported hemoglobin value can result from increase in the number of red cells, or decreases in plasma volume (hemoconcentration), or both. Blood doping[4] and use of erythropoietin[5] increase stamina and performance and are associated with "polycythemia" that is due to increased red cell numbers. Altitude training and androgens[6] used by weight lifters to increase strength may cause polycythemia through increased red cell production. The use of diuretics[7] (by wrestlers to reduce weight) and smoking decrease plasma volume, resulting in hemoconcentration. Chronic smoking or exposure to other sources of carbon monoxide[8] during training (e.g., hockey and figure skating in ice arenas) can result in similar findings on the hemogram. Meticulous searching of the history is paramount.

Cessation of the possible offending agents followed by observation for normalization of hemoglobin values would be the most appropriate initial step in the asymptomatic patient. Failure to normalize hemoglobin values should prompt continued workup. A normal carboxyhemoglobin concentration, chest radiograph, electrocardiogram, arterial blood gas (to search for cardiopulmonary disease), and normal sonographic or computed tomographic examination of the liver and kidneys (to rule out erythropoietin-producing tumors) minimize the likelihood of other nonathletics-related disease processes. The risks of anticipated workup and of continued abuse of performance enhancers should be emphasized, if it is suspected.

Suggested Workup for Increased Hemoglobin Concentrations

The workup includes drug, training, and smoking history and workup as outlined in Suggested Workup for Anemia.

Platelets

Isolated thrombocytopenia is not commonly recognized as resulting from exercise, although thrombocytosis induced by exercise has been described.[9] Drugs such as sulfonamide antibiotics, thiazide diuretics, nonsteroidal anti-inflammatory drugs, and alcohol all have been associated with thrombocytopenia. Thrombocytopenia as a manifestation of disseminated intravascular coagulation (DIC) has been reported in long-distance runners, and when seen in patients with heatstroke or rhabdomyolysis, it is an ominous sign. Thrombocytopenia in an athlete who has a fracture should raise the suspicion of fat embolus.

Drug and toxin history should be taken as outlined in Suggested Workup for Anemia. A DIC screen should be done when history or suspicion indicates (see sections on coagulopathies and rhabdomyolysis). Severe platelet depression in the acute setting suggests autoimmune mechanisms. As with any cytopenia, thrombocytopenia may be the initial manifestation of HIV infection. In the symptomatic patient with neurologic changes, renal abnormalities, and cell fragments on smear (angiopathic hemolytic anemia), thrombotic thrombocytopenic purpura should be suspected. Multiple-depression of white cells, red cells, and platelets should suggest aplastic anemia. These, and other differential diagnoses, are beyond the scope of this discussion.

In summary, athletically induced hematologic abnormalities involving other than the red cell line are uncommon and would most likely be picked up only on a CBC drawn during the immediate postexercise period.

OTHER HEMATOLOGIC CONDITIONS OF ATHLETIC IMPORTANCE

Coagulopathies

A "bleeding" problem may be discovered at any point in an athlete's career. Although an athletically induced coagulopathy (except DIC) would be improbable, the uncovering of a pre-existing condition during participation in athletics might well be expected.

A bleeding tendency may be uncovered in many ways. A starvation diet for weight loss or a dietary shift to high protein and away from green vegetables could result in vitamin K-dependent factor deficiency. Exposure to trauma could unmask a mild factor VIII or factor IX deficiency. In addition, use of easily available nonsteroidal antiinflammatory agents could increase the bruising or blood loss associated with various sports activities. Prolonged clotting times are seen with DIC. Past history of bleeding or stresses on the coagulation system (such as tooth extractions or surgery) and family history (searching for X-linked factor deficiencies) are critical.

A CBC with platelets and prothrombin time (PT) and partial thromboplastin time (PTT) constitute the basic screening examination. Fibrinogen, fibrin split products, and D-dimer constitute the usual DIC screen and should be ordered when prolonged PT or PTT is discovered in a patient at risk of DIC. The investigation of abnormalities discovered here or the ordering of additional tests in the face of normal CBC, PT, and PTT with strong clinical suspicion should be done only if practitioner and test facility are experienced in the performance and interpretation of these tests.

Sickle Cell Trait

The genetic defect resulting in the substitution of valine for glutamic acid at position six of the beta chain of hemoglobin is called *hemoglobin S*. Sickle cell trait occurs when less than one-half of the hemoglobin is hemoglobin S; the additional hemoglobin A normally prevents sickling under nonexercising, sea-level conditions. Sickling of red cells in hypoxic environments, with the development of pain syndromes and organ damage, does occur in some patients with sickle trait. Sudden death has been reported in individuals with sickle cell trait during severe exercise,[10] and splenic infarction has occurred at high altitudes in these individuals.[11] Abdominal pain and splenic infarction are almost routine syndromes seen in patients with sickle trait by hematologists in areas surrounding the Rocky Mountains in the United States. When an athlete with sickle trait presents in "crisis" in the postexercise period, rhabdomyolysis is frequently part of the presenting syndrome, but whether the sickling caused the rhabdomyolysis or the rhabdomyolysis caused the sickling is uncertain.

Many factors—such as nonblack race,[11] presence of other hemoglobins,[12] glucose-6-phosphate dehydrogenase deficiency (present in 8% of the black population), and red cell cytoskeletal abnormalities (hereditary spherocytosis) (Peter A. Lane, personal communication)—adversely influence the effects of hypoxia on hemoglobin AS red cells. Increasing age and intensity of exercise appear to increase the risk of a sickling event. Maintaining good hydration and good physical condition and acclimatization may decrease the risk.

When an individual with sickle trait is planning vigorous or high-altitude training, the counseling physician should certainly advise the athlete of the preceding. Specific prohibitions in affected individuals are otherwise lacking.

Rhabdomyolysis

Heavy physical exertion always results in some muscle "damage." This stress normally results in compensatory rebuilding and an improved, better-conditioned muscle. Under extreme conditions, the damage to the muscle becomes so severe that released intracellular components overwhelm the body's ability to manage these toxic products. This syndrome is called *rhabdomyolysis*.

Males constitute the vast majority of cases of rhabdomyolysis for unclear reasons. High levels of physical fitness reduce, but do not eliminate, the risk. Initial presentation and workup may be misleading. A minimally symptomatic athlete may be experiencing progressive metabolic and renal deterioration, and even the classic presentation is often not recognized until well after significant damage has occurred. On the other hand, many suggestive laboratory results, such as potassium and creatine phosphokinase levels, may rise as a normal consequence of exercise.

The typical patient has been exercising during hot, humid weather. A history of "pushing" one's self—expending heroic effort, especially at or near the finish—is almost universal. The individual's skin will be pale or gray and moist (although athletes experiencing heatstroke will likely be hot, flushed, and dry), with a weak pulse and altered mental status. Recovery may seem to occur quickly.

Over the next several hours to days, released myoglobin will precipitate in kidneys, causing anuria and renal failure. Hyperkalemia, hypocalcemia, hyperphosphatemia, hyperuricemia, lactic or metabolic acidosis, and DIC may individually, or in combination, produce additional symptoms and organ damage.

The universal risk, potential for missed (especially early) diagnosis, and need for prompt intervention and intensive therapy makes suspicion of rhabdomyolysis mandatory in all athletes exercising under other than their normal conditions or experiencing other than their normal recovery. Its complexity of presentation and course demands management by physicians familiar with this syndrome in facilities equipped to manage its complications. An excellent review has been published.[13]

REFERENCES

1. Dale DC. Neutrophilia. In WJ Williams, E Beutler, AJ Erslev, MA Lichtman (eds), Hematology (4th ed). New York: McGraw-Hill, 1990;816–904.
2. Davidson RJL. Exertional haemoglobinuria: a report on three cases with studies on the haemolytic mechanism. J Clin Pathol 1964;17:536–538.
3. Selby GB, Eichner ER. Endurance swimming, intravascular hemolysis, anemia, and iron depletion: new perspective on athlete's anemia. Am J Med 1986;81:791–794.
4. Cramer RB. Olympic cheating: the inside story of illicit doping and the U.S. cycling team. Rolling Stone 1985;2:25–28.
5. Erslev AJ. Secondary Polycythemia. In WJ Williams, E Beutler, AJ Erslev, MA Lichtman (eds), Hematology (4th ed). New York: McGraw-Hill, 1990;705–715.
6. Gardner FH, Nathan DG, Piomelli S, Cummins JE. The erythrocythaemic effects of androgens. Br J Haematol 1968;14: 611–615.
7. Leth A. Changes in plasma and extracellular fluid volumes in patients with essential hypertension during long-term treatment with hydrochlorothiazide. Circulation 1970;42:479–485.
8. Stonesifer LD. How carbon monoxide reduces plasma volume. N Engl J Med 1978;299:311–312.
9. Dawson AA, Ogston D. Exercise-induced thrombocytosis. Acta Haematol 1969;42:241–246.
10. Jones SR, Binder RA, Donowho EM Jr. Sudden death in sickle-cell trait. N Engl J Med 1970;282:323–325.
11. Lane PA, Githens JH. Splenic syndrome at mountain altitudes in sickle-cell trait. JAMA 1985;253:2251–2254.
12. Witkowska HE, Lubin BH, Beuzard Y, et al. Sickle cell disease in a patient with sickle cell trait and compound heterozygosity for hemoglobin S and hemoglobin Quebec-Chori. N Engl J Med 1991;325:1150–1154.
13. Knochel JP. Catastrophic medical events with exhaustive exercise: "white collar rhabdomyolysis." Kidney Int 1990; 38:709–719.

24

Cardiovascular Problems

John P. Kugler and Francis G. O'Connor

One of the greatest benefits of regular aerobic exercise is its positive impact on the cardiovascular system. It leads to more efficient physiologic functioning and reduces cardiovascular risk because of the potential benefits, including weight and blood pressure control, lipid modification, and smoking cessation.[1] This chapter examines some of the normal physiologic adaptations to vigorous exercise and discusses some clinical issues important for the primary care physician caring for the active athlete.

ATHLETIC HEART

Vigorous athletic training is associated with some specific anatomic and physiologic characteristics. These are not associated with pathology but are distinct from the normal nonathletic heart and represent a normal physiologic adaptation to training.[2]

Cardiac dimensions may increase with sustained training. Left ventricular end-diastolic volume may increase 10%, left ventricular wall thickness may be 15–20% greater, and left ventricular mass may be 45% greater in the athletic heart compared with the normal nonathletic heart.[3]

The heart rate of well-conditioned athletes is usually bradycardic, between 40 to 60 beats per minute. With this bradycardia, normal sinus arrhythmia may be more notable. There is physiologic splitting of S_2, which may be slightly delayed during inspiration. An S_3 may be present and likely results from the increased rate of left ventricular filling associated with the left ventricular dilation often seen with long-distance runners.[4] An S_4 may be normally found in isometric exercisers (e.g., strength training) secondary to concentric left ventricular hypertrophy.[5] Functional systolic murmurs may be found in 30–50% of athletes[5] and should be carefully distinguished from "significant" murmurs on physical examination (see section on heart murmur).

Several electrocardiographic changes are commonly reported in normal athletes.[6–10] These include sinus bradycardia (which may be associated with atrioventricular [AV] junctional escape beats), P-R interval lengthening to 0.18–0.20 seconds, and occasionally Mobitz type I AV block. There also may be altered morphology of the P wave similar to that found in left or right atrial enlargement; increased amplitude of the QRS complex, implying right or left ventricular hypertrophy; widening of the QRS interval, revealing an incomplete pattern of bundle branch block; and changes of early repolarization, including early ST segment takeoff, inversion or elevation of the T wave, and prominent U waves.

Chest x-ray films may show a globular cardiomegaly in endurance athletes with an increase in pulmonary vasculature secondary to enhanced pulmonary blood flow.[5] Echocardiograms in vigorous aerobic exercisers may show left ventricular dilation with little or no wall thickening (eccentric left ventricular hypertrophy). In vigorous isometric exercisers, echocardiograms may show increased left ventricular wall thickening with unchanged chamber size (concentric left ventricular hypertrophy).[3]

These changes reflect normal adaptive changes in a healthy heart. They do not, however, necessarily exclude a pathologic condition in any given patient; therefore, any "abnormal" findings on physical examination, electrocardiogram (ECG), chest x-ray film, or echocardiogram should be interpreted in the context of the individual patient.

SUDDEN DEATH

No activity in life is without some risk. There are very real hazards of physical activity, especially high-intensity competitive activity, the most serious of which is sudden death.

The overall risk of sudden death during athletic training is quite low, however, especially for the young athlete. There have been several incidence studies that have estimated the degree of risk.[11–16] They vary from a low of 1 in 735,000 per year in screened Air Force recruits younger than age 28 years to 1 in 69,000 per year in male college athletes.[11, 12] For older athletes, the incidence estimates are higher, but, again, the actual events are rare. Estimates range from a low of 1 in 18,000 per year in healthy Seattle men between the ages of 25 and 75 years to 1 in 7,620 per year in male Rhode Island joggers between the ages of 30 and 64 years.[13, 14] The physician involved in preparticipation examinations for athletes of all ages must seriously consider the risk for the individual patient, even if the epidemiologic incidence is low. There is no mass-screening mechanism that can effectively select the athletes at highest risk of sudden death.[16, 17] The screening starts with an individually directed history and physical examination.

Since the 1970s, there have been several case studies that have reviewed death certificates or used autopsy procedures to attempt to determine the leading etiologies for sudden death in the athlete.[18–27] It is clear that deaths in younger athletes (younger than ages 30–35 years) are more often associated with congenital cardiovascular structural abnormalities, and deaths in older athletes are more frequently associated with acquired atherosclerotic cardiovascular disease. In the younger age group, estimated death rates in male athletes were fivefold higher than in female athletes.[12] The transition age for the change from congenital to acquired atherosclerotic disease seems to occur between age 30 and 35 years.

Several studies in younger athletes confirm that hypertrophic cardiomyopathy (HCM) is the most common cause of sudden death.[18–20] Coronary artery anomalies, premature atherosclerotic disease, and myocarditis are the next most predominant. Less common etiologies include right ventricular dysplasia, Marfan syndrome, conduction system abnormalities, idiopathic concentric left ventricular hypertrophy, substance abuse (cocaine or steroids), aortic stenosis, mitral valve prolapse, and sickle cell trait.

HCM is an autosomal-dominant congenital disorder manifested by asymmetric septal hypertrophy, marked myocardial cellular disarray, abnormal intramural coronary arteries, and left ventricular outflow obstruction. Using echocardiographic criteria, Maron and colleagues[28] estimated a prevalence of HCM as high as 2 per 1,000 young adults. The condition is usually clinically silent, but it is believed that it predisposes the patient to malignant ventricular arrhythmias resulting in syncope or sudden death. A personal or family history of unexplained syncope (especially effort syncope) or sudden death are key clues to the diagnosis. The chest x-ray may show cardiomegaly but is usually normal. The ECG may show evidence of left ventricular hypertrophy but may also be normal. The diagnosis is best confirmed by two-dimensional echocardiogram. The routine preparticipation history and physical examination process is extremely insensitive in identifying this disorder. In a review of 158 young sudden death victims, medical evaluations, prompted by the usual preparticipation evaluation, failed to identify 47 of 48 cases of HCM.[17]

The coronary arterial disorders include atherosclerotic coronary artery disease and congenital coronary artery anomalies. The latter include anomalous origin of the left coronary artery from the right sinus of Valsalva, the anomalous origin of the right coronary artery from the left sinus of Valsalva, a single coronary artery, the origin of a coronary artery from the pulmonary artery, coronary artery hypoplasia, and a single right coronary artery without a left coronary artery combined with marked cardiac hypertrophy. Less clearly implicated have been tunneled epicardial coronary arteries and coronary artery spasm. These conditions may be difficult to screen for unless suspicion is raised by a history of early exertional fatigue, exertional angina, or exercise-induced syncope. Diagnosis may require cardiac catheterization for confirmation; however, cardiac magnetic resonance imaging is emerging as a useful tool.

The aortic disorder most commonly associated with sudden death has been thoracic aorta dilatation and subsequent rupture secondary to Marfan syndrome.[18]

Valvular disorders implicated include congenital aortic stenosis and Ebstein's anomaly of the tricuspid valve. Mitral valve prolapse has been found at autopsies of sudden deaths and has been implicated in sudden death in at least one long-term study.[22, 23] Its exact etiologic role is unclear; and considering its high prevalence in the young population, the actual risk of sudden death is not established. Its relevance for sudden death may be most important as one of the conditions associated with Marfan syndrome.

Cardiac conduction system disorders may rarely be a cause of sudden death, especially the prolonged QT syndrome.[24] In some rare cases, in which a structural cause was not evident at autopsy in a young person, it has been presumed (but not proved) that a conduction-based arrhythmia was the etiology.

Sickle cell trait may predispose an athlete to sudden death. Kark and colleagues[25] calculated an increased risk of sudden death of 28–40 times for black recruits with sickle cell trait in the U.S. military. The mechanism was unknown, although some believe that hyperkalemia related to renal overload from sudden explosive rhabdomyolysis may play a role. Further studies are needed to clarify the precise nature of the risk.

In the older age group (older than 30 years of age), severe atherosclerotic coronary artery disease is the primary etiology of sudden death events.[26, 27] The combination of a lifetime of atherosclerotic-generating behaviors plus genetic predisposition places a significant number of older individuals at risk of sudden death. Older, novice athletes are at particular risk, and the physician should be thorough and prudent in the evaluation and in exercise prescription. Several studies have confirmed that although chronic exercise lowers the overall risk for cardiac disease and cardiac arrest, individuals with established coronary artery disease are at greater risk of sudden death during exercise.[13, 14, 29] It is essential, therefore, to identify and monitor patients "at risk" of coronary artery disease. Indeed, Thompson and colleagues[29] have shown that prodromal symptoms frequently preceded the sudden death of joggers, suggesting that perhaps careful clinical monitoring may play a role in reducing the risk for older athletes.

What is the physician's role in screening for athletes, young and old, at risk of sudden death? The primary goal of the cardiovascular portion of the preparticipation medical examination is to identify individuals with conditions that put them at higher risk of sudden death. The American Heart Association (AHA) Science and Advisory Committee published consensus recommendations for preparticipation cardiovascular screening for high school and college athletes in 1996.[30] The AHA recommended that a complete and careful personal and family history and physical examination be conducted for athletes regardless of age. This evaluation should be designed to identify those cardiovascular conditions known to cause sudden death or disease progression. The screening should be done every 2 years, with an interim history being obtained in the intervening years. The 26th Bethesda Conference gives guidelines on conditions for which exercise is contraindicated or activity level is limited.[31] These conditions are summarized in Table 24-1. It is the physician's primary responsibility to conduct a thorough history and physical examination to attempt to evaluate for these conditions. If a cardiac condition is identified, the cardiology consultant can then provide expert assistance in definitive diagnosis and severity assessment, as well as assistance in formulating recommendations for specific exercise limitations when indicated.

Patient history should assess risk factors, including a family history of premature coronary heart disease, diabetes mellitus, sudden death, syncope, hypertension, or significant disability from cardiovascular disease in close relatives younger than 50 years of age; a past personal history of the detection of a heart murmur, diabetes mel-

TABLE 24-1

Guidelines on Restriction of Exercise for Cardiovascular Disease

Contraindications to vigorous exercise
  Hypertrophic cardiomyopathy
  Idiopathic concentric left ventricular hypertrophy
  Marfan syndrome
  Coronary heart disease
  Uncontrolled ventricular arrhythmias
  Severe valvular heart disease (especially aortic stenosis and pulmonic stenosis)
  Coarctation of the aorta
  Acute myocarditis
  Dilated cardiomyopathy
  Congestive heart failure
  Congenital anomalies of the coronary arteries
  Cyanotic congenital heart disease
  Pulmonary hypertension
  Right ventricular cardiomyopathy
  Ebstein's anomaly of the tricuspid valve
  Idiopathic long Q-T syndrome
Requires close monitoring and possible restriction
  Uncontrolled hypertension
  Uncontrolled atrial arrhythmias
  Hemodynamic significant valvular heart disease (aortic insufficiency, mitral stenosis, mitral regurgitation)

Source: Adapted from BJ Maron, JH Mitchell (eds). 26th Bethesda Conference. Recommendations for determining eligibility for competition in athletes with cardiovascular abnormalities. J Am Coll Cardiol 1994;24:845–899.

litus, hypertension, hyperlipidemia, or smoking; and a recent personal history of syncope, near syncope, profound exercise intolerance, and exertional chest discomfort, dyspnea, or excessive fatigue. It should also address specific knowledge of a personal or family history of certain cardiovascular conditions, including HCM, dilated cardiomyopathy, Marfan syndrome, prolonged QT syndrome, or significant arrhythmias.[30, 32]

Physical examination should particularly address hypertension, the cardiac rhythm, the presence of a heart murmur, and the findings of unusual facies or body habitus characteristic of a syndrome with an associated cardiovascular defect, especially Marfan syndrome. Specific common features of Marfan syndrome that should alert the clinician include the following[33]: (1) various skeletal features, such as tall stature; relatively long arms, legs, and fingers; highly arched palate; joint hyperextensibility; anterior chest deformity; loss of thoracic kyphosis; scoliosis; and congenital contractures; (2) ocular features, such as flat cornea, myopia, lens subluxation, and retinal detachment; and (3) cardiovascular conditions, such as dilatation of the ascending aorta, mitral valve prolapse, mitral regurgitation, aortic regurgitation, aortic dissec-

TABLE 24-2
Candidates for Stress Test Screening Before Start of an Exercise Program

Males older than age 45 years
Females older than age 55 years
Anyone with total cholesterol >250 or high-density
    lipoprotein <30
Hypertensive patients
Smokers
Diabetic patients
Those with a family history of premature coronary heart
    disease
Anyone with cardiac symptoms (exertional chest discomfort,
    profound exercise intolerance, syncope, and frequent
    premature ventricular contractions)

Source: SP Van Camp. Exercise-related sudden death: cardiovascular evaluation of exercisers (part 2 of 2). Phys Sportsmed 1988;16:47–54. Used with permission of McGraw-Hill, Inc.

tion, and dysrhythmia. Precordial auscultation should be done in the supine and standing positions; femoral pulses should be assessed and blood pressure measured in the seated position.[30]

Laboratory testing should be directed by the patient's history, physical examination, and age. Lipid profiles for a total cholesterol and high-density lipoprotein should be checked in the older athlete and may be useful (although not necessarily economical) at any age. Exercise stress testing is not recommended as a routine screening device for the detection of early coronary artery disease because of its low predictive value and high rate of false-positive and false-negative results. Van Camp,[32] however, recommended that strong consideration be given to certain categories of patients for stress test screening before starting an exercise program (Table 24-2).

A screening echocardiogram is not currently recommended. The echocardiogram is not cost-effective, and the low prevalence of disease has the potential to create high rates of false-positivity. One study did demonstrate that a limited screening echocardiogram can be incorporated into a preparticipation program; however, the validity of the limited echocardiogram as a screening tool remains to be determined.[34] It should be directed at individuals with a family history or symptoms and signs of HCM or aortic stenosis, pulmonic stenosis, Marfan syndrome, or nonfunctional cardiac murmurs that have not been previously assessed. A chest x-ray study is not recommended for screening, and it should be reserved for direct assessment of suspected conditions.

Although there are no firm data supporting the cost-effectiveness of widespread preparticipation cardiovascular evaluations, it is still clinically prudent. When given in the context of an overall health maintenance visit, the preparticipation evaluation can potentially yield benefits far beyond the prevention of the uncommon exercise-related sudden death. Physician endorsement of a sensible lifestyle modification is a highly valuable goal in a preparticipation evaluation, and the astute clinician takes full advantage of this teachable moment in the physician-patient relationship.

HEART MURMUR

The physical finding of a heart murmur necessitates an appropriate, targeted evaluation, whether noted in the clinical record or detected during the careful preparticipation examination. Of young athletes, 30–50% may be found to have a functional murmur, and the critical task for the clinician is to separate clearly functional from organic causes. A family history of syncope or sudden death or an individual's history of syncope or near syncope is important information that supports organicity. On examination, physical maneuvers, such as inspiration, standing, squatting, Valsalva, and isometric hand exercises, may be helpful in the diagnosis.[35] Functional murmurs are usually grade 1 or 2, early- to midsystolic, loudest at the second or third left intercostal space or lower left sternal border, have normal S_2 splitting,[2, 36] and are without accompanying ejection sounds or snaps. They decrease with standing, Valsalva, and handgrip (reflecting decreased preload) and may increase with squatting (reflecting increased preload). They do not vary with inspiration.

Any murmur that is not clearly functional should be further evaluated. Causing special concern are murmurs that increase with Valsalva or standing and murmurs that are diastolic, holosystolic, late systolic, or continuous (except for venous hum) during the cycle. Further evaluation includes ECG, chest x-ray, and, most important, an echocardiogram. If the murmur is clearly not functional despite a normal echocardiogram, or if the chest x-ray film, ECG, or echocardiogram is abnormal, a cardiology consultation for confirmation of diagnosis, possible exercise stress test, assessment of severity, and specific recommendations for exercise limitation is prudent.

As mentioned under Sudden Death, HCM is a particularly dangerous condition that may be associated with sudden death and may be difficult to detect on physical examination. Of patients who die suddenly with HCM, 90% have abnormal but not diagnostic ECGs.[32] Echocardiograms can be diagnostic, demonstrating a thickened ventricular wall, an abnormal ventricular septum to ventricular wall ratio, and diastolic dysfunction.

Table 24-3 is a summary of the characteristics of the most common organic murmurs. As a general rule, however, if the murmur does not clearly sound functional or if the history is suspicious, further evaluation is indicated.

CARDIAC ARRHYTHMIAS

The symptoms of syncope, near syncope, palpitations, rapid heart beat, and exertional chest discomfort or severe dyspnea may be related to a serious cardiac arrhythmia. Athletes with these symptoms should be thoroughly evaluated to rule out structural heart disease (especially coronary heart disease, HCM, aortic stenosis, and congenital heart disease) before being allowed to compete in sports.[31] Evaluation includes history, physical examination, and ECG, followed by chest x-ray examination, echocardiogram, exercise stress test, 24-hour Holter monitoring, and electrolytes or other laboratory tests as indicated. Formal cardiology consultation would be prudent in most cases, as further evaluation that includes electrophysiologic study and tilt table testing may be warranted.

All patients with suspected significant arrhythmias should have a 12-lead ECG, echocardiogram, stress test, and prolonged ambulatory ECG recording. The stress test may need to be customized to match the level of stress under which the particular athlete is training.[31] Arrhythmias may be inconspicuous and require no treatment. They may, in fact, be normal variants of an adaptive athletic heart. If there is no evidence of structural heart disease (that is, normal echocardiogram and exercise stress test), there is less risk of sudden death. Some arrhythmias are compatible with competitive sports once they are controlled, and others are clearly incompatible with vigorous activity. Table 24-4 is a summary of the common dysrhythmias and the recommendations from the 26th Bethesda Conference regarding eligibility for sports.[31]

The primary care physician should ensure that the athlete is fully evaluated and treated. Depending on the experience of the physician and the complexity of the therapy, the primary care physician can manage the patient or refer the patient to someone with more experience with the particular condition. Unexplained syncope, in particular, may require a workup beyond the scope of practice of the typical primary care physician. Early referral for more extensive testing and formal cardiovascular specialty assessment may be the most appropriate course in many of these clinical situations.

HYPERTENSION

Systemic hypertension is one of the most common life-threatening disorders in the United States. People of all ages are at risk, and patients can benefit from early diag-

TABLE 24-3

Characteristics of Common Organic Murmurs

Murmur Type	Characteristics
Aortic stenosis	At least grade III
	Harsh, midsystolic ejection sound
Hypertrophic cardio-myopathy	Harsh, midsystolic
	Increased with Valsalva test and standing
	Decreased with squatting and handgrip
Pulmonic stenosis	Harsh, midsystolic
	Best at second LICS
Mitral regurgitation	Pansystolic if severe
	Mid- to late-systolic with MVP (preceded by midsystolic click)
	At apex radiates to axilla
Ventricular septal defect	Holosystolic
	Best at LLSB
Aortic regurgitation	High-pitched, blowing
	Diastolic heard best at LSB leaning forward after exhalation
Mitral stenosis	Low-pitched rumble
	Diastolic heard best at apex
	Opening snap may precede murmur
Patent ductus arteriosus	Continuous, upper LSB
	Wide pulse pressure
	Bounding pulse

LICS = left intercostal space; MVP = mitral valve prolapse; LLSB = lower left sternal border; LSB = left sternal border.
Source: Adapted from 16th Bethesda Conference. Cardiovascular abnormalities in the athlete: recommendations regarding eligibility for competition. J Am Coll Cardiol 1985;6:1183–1232.

nosis and management. Care should be taken not to over-diagnose this condition in young people.[31] Blood pressures should be compared with normals for age, height, and weight categories. Appropriate-sized blood pressure cuffs should be used, and at least three different blood pressures should be measured on three different days before diagnosis is confirmed.

An appropriate evaluation of the confirmed hypertensive individual is the same for the athlete and nonathlete. It includes a search for secondary causes and an assessment of target organ damage. This evaluation requires a full history, including inquiries about the use of performance-enhancing substances such as anabolic steroids, a physical examination, chest x-ray examination, ECG, urinalysis, complete blood count, serum electrolytes, fasting glucose, lipid profile, blood urea nitrogen and creatinine, and uric acid. It may include an echocardiogram to evaluate for left ventricular hypertrophy and an exercise stress test to assist in a recommendation for sports participation.[31, 36]

Systolic blood pressure increases to higher levels during any type of exercise. Static (isometric) exercise induces

TABLE 24-4
Activity Recommendations for the Common Dysrhythmias

Activity	Recommendations
Disturbances of sinus mode function (includes sinus bradycardia, tachycardia, arrhythmia, arrest, exit block; wandering pacemaker; sick sinus syndrome)	No symptoms, no treatment; if symptoms require pacemaker, then no collision sports
Premature atrial complexes	No restrictions
Atrial flutter and atrial fibrillation	If no structural heart disease and rate is controlled by drugs, then low-intensity sports; if no flutter or fibrillation for 6 mos, then full activity
Supraventricular tachycardia	If episodes are prevented by drugs, then full participation; if structural disease and if syncope or presyncope, no competitive sports; reconsider after 6 mos without recurrence
Ventricular pre-excitation (WPW)	If no structural heart disease and no symptoms, then no limit; if structural heart disease and PVCs worsen with exercise, restrict; PVCs plus prolonged Q-T interval should be restricted (high risk for sudden death)
Heart blocks (first-degree or Mobitz I second-degree)	If no symptoms and no structural disease, then no restrictions
Heart blocks (Mobitz II second-degree or third-degree)	If no symptoms and no structural disease, then no restrictions if rate 40–80; if symptoms, then pacer and avoidance of collision sports
Congenital long Q-T syndrome	At risk for sudden death; restricted from all competitive sports

WPW = Wolff-Parkinson-White (syndrome); PVCs = premature ventricular contractions.
Source: Adapted from BJ Maron, JH Mitchell (eds). 26th Bethesda Conference. Recommendations for determining eligibility for competition in athletes with cardiovascular abnormalities. J Am Coll Cardiol 1994;24:845–899.

a greater elevation of diastolic blood pressure and total peripheral resistance. It is not known whether hypertensive individuals are at any increased overall risk of developing target organ complications when participating in competitive sports.

Treatment

Hypertensive patients are at risk of target organ damage to the brain, eyes, kidneys, and heart. Those who are untreated or poorly controlled are at greatest risk. Both aerobic and resistance exercise have been documented to have a useful role in the therapy of mild to borderline hypertension. Weight reduction and salt limitation may also prove useful in the motivated patient. Drug therapy is not a contraindication to participation, but it does merit close monitoring for potential drug-exercise interactions, especially hypokalemia with diuretics, hyperkalemia with potassium-sparing diuretics and angiotensin-converting enzyme (ACE) inhibitors, bradycardia and bronchospasm with beta-blockers, and fatigue and postexercise blood pressure elevation with adrenergic inhibitors. Generally, ACE inhibitors, calcium channel blockers, and prazosin are best tolerated by athletes. Because of potassium balance issues and the risk of arrhythmias and dehydration, diuretics should be avoided. Likewise, beta-blockers will have an adverse impact on the cardiovascular training effect of exercise. In addition, these medications commonly cause fatigue and impair oxygen consumption and work capacity. Hence, it is preferable to avoid diuretics and beta-blockers as first-line therapy in young athletes. The reader is also encouraged to consult a reference on National Collegiate Athletic Association and U.S. Olympic Committee medication restrictions.[37] Several antihypertensives, including diuretics and beta-blockers, are on the banned drug list for both organizations.

Limitations

Sports participation depends on target organ involvement and overall control of blood pressure. Most patients who have controlled mild to moderate hypertension (less than 140/90 at rest for adults) and no target organ involvement can participate in all competitive sports.[31] Patients with blood pressure not controlled by therapy should be limited to low-intensity sports. Patients with severe hypertension that is controlled and have no target organ damage may participate in low-intensity sports. Some may selectively participate in high to moderate dynamic and low static effort sports (Table 24-5). The exercise stress test may be useful in selecting which patients might safely compete. Patients whose blood pressure is controlled but who have target organ damage should be limited to low-intensity sports.[31]

CHEST PAIN

The workup and evaluation of chest pain in the athlete should be just as diligent and thorough as in the nonathlete. Participation in sports does not immunize against coronary artery disease or genetic misfortune. Indeed, the vigorous nature of some sports places the cardiovascularly vulnerable patient at particular risk.

Exertional chest discomfort relieved by rest is angina, until proven otherwise. The pain may be a vague pressure, a tight squeeze, or a dull ache and may radiate to the neck, shoulders, jaw, or down the arm. There may be no pain at all, just a sense of breathlessness or profound fatigue. The symptoms may be associated with nausea and diaphoresis, or there may be nothing characteristic about them, only an impending sense that "something is not right."

Despite the myriad of symptomatologies, history-taking is still the most critical step in the evaluation. Past medical history is important for cardiovascular risk assessment and a basic understanding of the patient's previous functional baseline. The precise details of the setting and nature of the pain, including the quality, location, duration, factors associated with onset and relief, and accompanying symptoms are crucial to diagnosis. The differential diagnosis of chest pain includes a wide variety of noncardiac etiologies, including gastrointestinal and musculoskeletal disorders. Chest x-ray findings, upper gastrointestinal series, gallbladder ultrasonography, and upper endoscopy may eventually play a role in diagnosis; however, the primary task of the physician is to rule out significant cardiac disease. This can usually be accomplished through a careful history, but it may often require an ECG (which may be normal in the setting of ischemia), an exercise stress test (which may often be abnormal in the setting of nondisease—that is, a false-positive result), an exercise thallium (which may be required to evaluate an equivocal exercise stress test), and finally, a cardiac catheterization to settle questionable cases or to evaluate a strongly positive exercise stress test or thallium.

Echocardiography may be a useful adjunct to evaluate ventricular function and to rule out HCM and valvular disorders that can be associated with chest pain syndromes. The urgency with which the workup is accomplished depends on the clinical circumstances; it may vary from an immediate admission to rule out a myocardial infarction or unstable angina to a purposeful outpatient evaluation for stable symptoms or atypical symptoms in an individual at low risk. The primary care physician should have a low threshold for comanagement with a subspecialty cardiologist.

History or symptoms that should particularly raise concern include the following: a family history of premature heart disease (younger than age 50 years), history of effort syncope or near syncope, a change in exercise tolerance (the so-called prodromal symptoms) that may indicate worsening coronary artery disease, and classic anginal

TABLE 24-5
Intensity Demands of Various Sports

Intensity Demands	Sports
High to moderate dynamic and high static	Boxing, rowing, cross-country skiing, cycling, downhill skiing, fencing, football, ice hockey, rugby, sprint running, speed skating, water polo, wrestling
High to moderate dynamic and low static	Badminton, baseball, basketball, field hockey, lacrosse, orienteering, ping-pong, race walking, racquetball, distance running, soccer, squash, swimming, tennis, volleyball
Low dynamic and high to moderate static	Archery, auto racing, diving, equestrian, field events, gymnastics, karate or judo, motorcycling, rodeoing, sailing, ski jumping, waterskiing, weight lifting
Low dynamic and low static (low intensity)	Bowling, cricket, curling, golf, riflery

Source: Adapted from BJ Maron, JH Mitchell (eds). 26th Bethesda Conference. Recommendations for determining eligibility for competition in athletes with cardiovascular abnormalities. J Am Coll Cardiol 1994;24:845–899.

symptoms in individuals without the risk factor profile of coronary heart disease. Exercise stress test, thallium stress test, echocardiogram, and even cardiac catheterization may be required to settle some questions. The most important diagnostic tool, however, is the alert clinician willing to take the time for a careful history and maintaining a high index of clinical suspicion.

REFERENCES

1. Cantwell JD. Cardiovascular aspects of running. Clin Sports Med 1985;4:627–640.
2. Mukerji B, Alpert MA, Mukerji V. Cardiovascular changes in athletes. Am Fam Physician 1989;40:169–175.
3. Maron BJ. Structural features of the athlete heart as defined by echocardiography. J Am Coll Cardiol 1986;7:190–203.
4. Zeppilli P. The athlete's heart: differentiation of training effects from organic heart disease. Pract Cardiol 1988;14:61–84.
5. Huston TP, Puffer JC, Rodney WM. The athletic heart syndrome. N Engl J Med 1985;313:24–32.
6. Oakley DG, Oakley CM. Significance of abnormal electrocardiograms in highly trained athletes. Am J Cardiol 1982;50:985–989.
7. Sundberg S, Elovainio R. Resting ECG in athletic and nonathletic adolescent boys: correlations with heart vol-

ume and cardiorespiratory fitness. Clin Physiol 1982;2: 419–426.

8. Mumford M, Prakash R. Electrocardiographic and echocardiographic characteristics of long distance runners: comparison of left ventricular function with age- and sex-matched controls. Am J Sports Med 1981;9:23–28.

9. Ferst JA, Chaitman BR. The electrocardiogram and the athlete. Sports Med 1984;1:390–403.

10. Balady GJ, Cadigan JB, Ryan TJ. Electrocardiogram of the athlete: an analysis of 289 professional football players. Am J Cardiol 1984;53:1339–1343.

11. Phillips M, Robiniwitz M, Higgins JR, et al. Sudden cardiac death in Air Force recruits. JAMA 1986;256:2696–2699.

12. Van Camp SP, Bloor CM, Mueller FO, et al. Nontraumatic sports death in high school and college athletes. Med Sci Sports Exerc 1995;27:641–647.

13. Siscovick DS, Weiss NS, Fletcher RH, Lasky T. The incidence of primary cardiac arrest during vigorous exercise. N Engl J Med 1984;311:874–877.

14. Thompson PD, Funk EJ, Carleton RA, Sturner WQ. Incidence of death during jogging in Rhode Island from 1975 through 1980. JAMA 1982;247:2535–2538.

15. Ragosta M, Crabtree J, Sturner WQ, et al. Death during recreational exercise in the state of Rhode Island. Med Sci Sports Exerc 1984;16:339–342.

16. Maron BJ, Poliac LC, Roberts WO. Risk for sudden death associated with marathon running. J Am Coll Cardiol 1996;28:428–431.

17. Maron BJ, Shirani J, Poliac LC, et al. Sudden death in young competitive athletes: clinical, demographic, and pathologic profiles. JAMA 1996;276:199–204.

18. Maron BJ, Roberts WC, McAllister HA, et al. Sudden death in young athletes. Circulation 1980;62:218–229.

19. McCaffrey FM, Braden DS, Strong WB. Sudden cardiac deaths in young athletes. Am J Dis Child 1991;145:177–183.

20. Burke AP, Farb A, Virmani R, et al. Sports-related and non-sports-related sudden cardiac death in young adults. Am Heart J 1991;121:568–575.

21. Corrado D, Thiene G, Nava A, et al. Sudden death in young competitive athletes: clinicopathologic correlations in 22 cases. Am J Med 1990;89:588–596.

22. Waller BF. Exercise-Related Sudden Death in Young (Age < 30 Years) and Old (Age > 30 Years) Conditioned Subjects. In NK Wenger (ed), Exercise and the Heart (2nd ed). Philadelphia: FA Davis, 1988.

23. Duren DR, Becker AE, Dunning AJ. Long-term follow-up of idiopathic mitral valve prolapse in 300 patients: a prospective study. J Am Coll Cardiol 1988;11:42–47.

24. Schwartz PJ, Periti M, Malliani A. The long Q-T syndrome. Am Heart J 1975;89:378–390.

25. Kark JA, Posey DM, Schumacher HR, Ruehle CJ. Sickle-cell trait as a risk factor for sudden death in physical training. N Engl J Med 1987;317:781–787.

26. Virmani R. Jogging, marathon running, and death [Abstract]. Hosp Phys 1982;18:28–39.

27. Waller BF, Roberts WC. Sudden death while running in conditioned runners aged 40 years or over. Am J Cardiol 1980;45: 1292–1300.

28. Maron BJ, Gardin JM, Flack JM, et al. Prevalence of hypertrophic cardiomyopathy in a general population of young adults: echocardiographic analysis of 4111 subjects in the CARDIA study. Circulation 1995;92:785–789.

29. Thompson PD, Stern MP, Williams P, et al. Death during jogging or running. A study of 18 cases. JAMA 1979;242: 1265–1267.

30. Maron BJ, Thompson PD, Puffer JC, et al. Cardiovascular preparticipation screening of competitive athletes: a statement for health professionals from the Sudden Death Committee (Clinical Cardiology) and Congenital Cardiac Defects Committee (Cardiovascular Disease in the Young), American Heart Association. Circulation 1996;94:850–856.

31. Maron BJ, Mitchell JH (eds). 26th Bethesda Conference. Recommendations for determining eligibility for competition in athletes with cardiovascular abnormalities. Am J Cardiol 1994;24:845–899.

32. Van Camp SP. Exercise-related sudden death: cardiovascular evaluation of exercisers (part 2 of 2). Phys Sportsmed 1988;16:47–54.

33. Pyeritz RE. The Marfan syndrome. Am Fam Physician 1986;34:83–94.

34. Lembo NJ, Dell-Italia LJ, Crawford MH, O'Rourke RA. Bedside diagnosis of systolic murmurs. N Engl J Med 1988;318: 1572–1578.

35. Weidenbener EJ, Kraus MD, Waller BF, et al. Incorporation of screening echocardiography in the preparticipation examination. Clin J Sport Med 1995;5:86–89.

36. Strong WB, Steed D. Cardiovascular evaluation of the young athlete. Pediatr Clin North Am 1982;29:1325–1339.

37. Fuentes RJ, Rosenberg JM, Davis A (eds). Athletic Drug Reference '96. Durham, NC: Clean Data, Inc., 1996.

25

The Diabetic Athlete

ROBERT E. JONES

Diabetes mellitus is the most common metabolic disorder encountered by health care professionals. Diabetes is characterized by hyperglycemia and is associated with several serious, potentially fatal complications, including retinopathy, nephropathy, neuropathy, and macrovascular disease. Nevertheless, many amateur and professional athletes with diabetes engage in competitive sports. The goals of health professionals should be to advise the diabetic athlete how to participate safely in sports and how to minimize any potential complications that could arise from his or her involvement in these activities.

The diagnostic criteria and classification of diabetes mellitus have been revised.[1] Diabetes mellitus is still classified into several types, and the most frequently encountered categories are type 1 (previously called *insulin-dependent diabetes*) and type 2 (formerly designated as *non–insulin-dependent diabetes*). Type 2 diabetes is the most prevalent form and affects approximately 10% of the adult population, whereas type 1 diabetes is diagnosed in as many as 1 in 500 children. Diabetic children are as likely as nondiabetic children to participate in sports, as demonstrated by a European survey.[2]

Management decisions must be based on the understanding of the physiology of diabetes and are therefore dependent on the correct classification of the patient. Each of these different forms of diabetes has its own unique problems and potentially different approaches to therapy.

TYPE 1 DIABETES MELLITUS

Type 1 diabetes is generally thought to occur as a result of destruction of the pancreatic islet cells resulting in an absolute deficiency of insulin. The loss of islet cell function may be due to a primary autoimmune process or may

be idiopathic. Nonetheless, because of the beta-cell injury and loss of insulin secretion, these patients typically present with weight loss and ketosis in addition to the symptoms of hyperglycemia (polyuria, polydipsia, and fatigue). The onset of the illness is usually abrupt, although a hyperglycemic prodromal phase may be seen.[3, 4] Type 1 diabetes more frequently occurs in younger individuals, but new-onset type 1 diabetes can be recognized at any age. These patients are absolutely dependent on insulin to maintain anabolic processes; within hours of insulin withdrawal, they can rapidly develop ketosis and eventually proceed into diabetic ketoacidosis. Therefore, these patients need a continuous source of exogenous insulin to stave off ketosis.

TYPE 2 DIABETES MELLITUS

Type 2 diabetes is characterized by the coexistence of peripheral insulin resistance coupled with a defect in the secretion of insulin. In contrast to patients with type 1 diabetes, these patients have a relative—rather than an absolute—insulin deficiency and maintain enough endogenous basal insulin secretion to prevent ketosis. As a result, the onset may be insidious, and the condition may go unrecognized for many years. Type 2 diabetes is usually an illness of middle age; however, a phenotypically similar but genetically distinct variant[5] previously called *maturity-onset diabetes of the young*[6] may be seen in young adults and adolescents. Type 2 diabetes is frequently associated with obesity, but it can also occur in slender individuals. Occasionally, the prodrome of type 1 diabetes can be confused with that of type 2 diabetes, and, if sufficiently stressed either by concurrent illness or trauma, patients with type 2 diabetes may develop diabetic ketoacidosis, which may complicate the distinction between these diabetic forms. Type 2 diabetes is initially managed using a combination of diet and exercise to control the hyperglycemia. If these measures fail, a variety of oral agents— sulfonylureas, metformin, acarbose, or troglitazone—may be used either as monotherapy or in selected combinations to control hyperglycemia. Occasionally, insulin may be added to the regimen. A frequent error is the assumption that a patient who requires insulin has type 1 diabetes; however, the addition of insulin should be viewed as a therapeutic adjunct instead of a factor complicating the diagnosis. The diagnosis of patients with type 2 diabetes who require insulin for control should not be changed to type 1 diabetes.

Although this classification scheme is relatively straightforward, some patients encountered in clinical practice are difficult to categorize. Typically, these patients have the physiology of type 2 diabetes but the phenotype of type 1 diabetes. In other words, they are young and slender but do not become ketotic or present with significant weight loss. These patients may represent a prolonged prodrome of type 1 diabetes and are frequently managed as having type 1 diabetes. Occasionally, screening for the presence of autoantibodies to islet cell antigens may prove helpful in management.[7]

METABOLIC RESPONSES TO EXERCISE

An in-depth review of the physiology of exercise and the biochemistry of substrate fluxes during exercise is beyond the scope of this chapter (see Vranic and colleagues[8] for a complete discussion). Because the most common complications of exercise in diabetic patients are related to blood glucose levels, however, a brief overview is offered to emphasize the differences in the effects of exercise on glucose homeostasis between diabetic and nondiabetic people.

Hormonal and biochemical responses to exercise are dependent on the intensity and duration of the activity. Energy demands are met through the use of depot fuels: carbohydrates are stored in muscle and liver as glycogen, and fatty acids are stored as triglycerides. The synthesis and maintenance of these depots are critically dependent on the presence of insulin. During exercise in nondiabetic subjects, insulin secretion is suppressed, which in conjunction with the glucose counterregulatory hormones (growth hormone, cortisol, glucagon, and catecholamines) facilitates substrate mobilization (lipolysis, gluconeogenesis, and glycogenolysis). This process allows blood glucose levels to remain relatively constant and provides additional metabolic substrates in the form of free fatty acids.

The fall in insulin levels coupled with the rise in counterregulatory hormones also spares glucose for use by non–insulin-dependent tissues such as the central nervous system. The overall result is careful integration between substrate synthesis and oxidation.

In contradistinction to normal individuals, insulin levels in type 1 diabetic patients are essentially unregulated, because these patients rely on injected insulin for survival. If the patient is underreplaced with insulin, substrate production is unchecked because of the lack of opposition of the counterregulatory hormones. This results in an exaggeration of the pre-existing hyperglycemia and may predispose to the development of ketoacidosis. On the other hand, patients who are well insulinized may experience hypoglycemia because of inappropriately high insulin levels. An elevated insulin level during exercise causes suppression of hepatic gluconeogenesis and an enhancement of muscle glucose uptake. The net effect is a reduction in serum glucose levels. Additionally, the suppression of lipolysis results in an impaired substrate delivery to actively metabolizing myocytes.

Mild reactions may be manifested simply as fatigue. More significant reactions activate the sympathetic nervous system, and severe reactions may result in neuroglycopenia culminating in seizures. The symptoms and suggested treatments of hypoglycemia are summarized in Table 25-1. The metabolic and hypoglycemic effects of exercise may last for many hours after completion of the activity secondary to increased insulin sensitivity and to replenishment of hepatic or muscle glycogen. Indeed, postexercise hypoglycemia may occur up to 24 hours after strenuous exercise; therefore, it is prudent to advise athletes to anticipate the possibility of a late hypoglycemic reaction.

The metabolic effects of exercise in patients with type 2 diabetes are similar, but the risk of provoking ketoacidosis is lower because of their ability to secrete basal levels of insulin. If the patient is poorly controlled before exercise, an exacerbation of the pre-existing hyperglycemia may be observed. Hypoglycemia may occur in patients who require either insulin or sulfonylureas to assist in diabetic control. On the other hand, hypoglycemia is extremely rare in patients using metformin and has not been observed in patients treated with either troglitazone or acarbose.

GUIDELINES FOR PREPARTICIPATION EVALUATION

The recommendations for evaluating diabetic athletes before participation in sports activities are summarized in Table 25-2. Specific suggestions are predicated on the

TABLE 25-1
Symptoms and Treatment of Hypoglycemia

Degree of Hypoglycemia	Symptoms	Treatment	Activity Resumption
Mild	Fatigue, weakness, nausea, hunger, anxiety, tremor, palpitations	10–15 g of oral carbohydrate	15 mins after symptoms improve
Moderate	Tachycardia, diaphoresis, headache, mood and personality changes, lethargy, inattentiveness, somnolence	10–20 g of oral carbohydrate May need to repeat treatment and monitor the patient closely for recurrence Patient may require help in managing this level of hypoglycemia	15 mins after symptoms completely resolve
Severe	Unresponsiveness, unconsciousness, seizures	Use buccal glucose gel, glucagon (1 mg IM/SC), IV dextrose Patient will require help for this degree of hypoglycemia	Medical evaluation before returning

IM = intramuscular; SC = subcutaneous; IV = intravenous.
Note: The appropriate amount (10–20 g) of carbohydrate can be obtained by ingesting 4–8 oz of sweetened soda pop, sport drink, or juice; 5–8 small pieces of candy (e.g., Lifesavers); 4 teaspoons of table sugar; or 6 sugar cubes. Because of the risk of aspiration, oral glucose repletion should never be given to a diabetic patient who is unresponsive or has an impaired gag reflex.

type of diabetes, the duration of the illness, and the age of the patient. Duration of illness is a more critical parameter in dealing with type 2 diabetic patients because of the likelihood that relatively asymptomatic hyperglycemia may precede the diagnosis of diabetes by several years.

General Assessment

The annual preparticipation evaluation should include a general assessment of health and a search for other coexisting conditions that could influence athletic performance or affect medical clearance for sports activities. Specific information critical in evaluating a diabetic athlete before his or her participation in sports activities should include an evaluation of the frequency and duration of hypoglycemic events, an appraisal of the patient's diabetic control, and an effort to detect any diabetic complications or a potential predisposition for aggravating pre-existing complications.

Hypoglycemia unawareness is usually manifested as repeated, severe episodes of neuroglycopenia (lethargy, confusion, inappropriate behavior, unconsciousness, or seizures) without the patient sensing an adrenergic prodrome (rapid heartbeat, sweating, anxiety, tremor). Frequently, these patients also have difficulty in counterregulation of blood glucose and may have prolonged episodes of hypoglycemia. Clearly, these diabetic patients should be excluded from individual sports activities, such as swimming, and should be directed toward events that would allow close supervi-

sion by a coach or "buddy." One should also obtain historic hints to suggest unusual insulin absorption kinetics or delayed gastric emptying, because alterations in insulin dose and supplemental feedings are used as prophylaxis against exercise-induced hypoglycemia.

Glycemic Control

Glycemic control is assessed by a careful review of the results of self-monitoring of blood glucose and by obtaining a hemoglobin A_{1c} (glycosylated hemoglobin and hemoglobin A_1 are slightly different tests and yield different results[9]). The hemoglobin A_{1c} gives an average index of the blood glucose level over the preceding 2 months. Because of its long half-life, the hemoglobin A_{1c} should not be checked more frequently than every 3–4 months. If the mean blood glucose on home glucose monitoring is 155 mg/dl (8.6 mmol/L) or less and the hemoglobin A_{1c} is 7.2% or less, the patient is under good control.[10] A careful history of the frequency, duration, and prodromal symptoms of hypoglycemic events is also essential. Changes in weight or symptoms of hyperglycemia should be sought. If the diabetes is clearly poorly controlled (hemoglobin A_{1c} greater than 10%), participation in sports activities should be postponed until an adequate degree of metabolic regulation is achieved. The care of a diabetic patient is unique because of the central role of patient self-management in controlling blood glucose levels, and, on occasion, delaying participation in sports to tighten metabolic control serves as the sole factor to stimulate an otherwise unmotivated patient.

Exercise-Induced Hypertension

Vital signs taken before and after moderate exercise may identify previously normotensive diabetic patients who develop exercise-induced systolic hypertension.[11] Exercise-induced hypertension is defined as a peak systolic blood pressure of more than 210 mm Hg in men and 190 mm Hg in women.[12] If the exercise response is normal, yearly re-evaluation is warranted. There is no consensus concerning the medical approach to these individuals, but it has been recommended that they avoid sports activities that could further elevate their blood pressure.

Retinopathy

Because of the risk of vitreous hemorrhage, retinal detachment, and subsequent blindness, diabetic patients with proliferative retinopathy should be excluded from contact sports with high static demands or events such as weight lifting that predictably raise blood pressure. A routine funduscopy may be inadequate to detect peripheral lesions, and, therefore, a consultation and routine follow-up with an ophthalmologist is usually necessary. It is unnecessary to restrict activity in diabetic athletes without retinopathy.

Nephropathy

Diabetic nephropathy, another condition aggravated by hypertension, can usually be detected by finding albuminuria or proteinuria on screening. Initial screening should be accomplished using a simple urinalysis, and, if gross proteinuria is not present, proceeding with an assay for microalbumin excretion. Grossly elevated urine protein levels may overwhelm the assay used for microalbumin detection, which may lead to a report of falsely low microalbumin excretion rates (the "Hook effect"). Therefore, prescreening the urine for the presence of gross proteinuria prevents the clinician from making a false assumption based on errant laboratory results. If gross proteinuria is present, a 24-hour urine collection for total protein quantification is the test of choice. It is clear, however, that the screen for microalbuminuria is the most sensitive test to detect the presence of diabetic nephropathy. Nonetheless, there is no evidence that exercise permanently aggravates diabetic nephropathy, although it does temporarily increase protein (especially microalbumin) excretion. Prudence should be used in advising diabetic patients with proteinuria about participation in sports, and frequent monitoring of creatinine and urinary protein or albumin excretion is indicated in individuals who are exercising.

Neuropathies

The neurologic evaluation should be directed toward the detection of both peripheral sensory and autonomic neuropathies. Normal vibratory and position senses in the lower extremities essentially exclude the presence of a clinically significant sensory neuropathy. Similarly, a normal blood pressure and pulse-rate response to Valsalva and orthostatic maneuvers virtually eliminate the possibility of significant autonomic dysfunction. Sensory neuropathy may predispose one to joint injury because of an elevated pain threshold resulting in repeated overuse of the extremity or because of joint laxity from impaired proprioception. Autonomic insufficiency is associated with gastroparesis and with dramatic, inappropriate fluctuations in blood pressure.

Atherosclerosis

Stress testing is warranted in all type 2 diabetic patients older than age 40 years or those with a longer than 10-year history of the illness. It should be considered in type 1 diabetic patients older than 30 years of age or those with more than a 15-year duration of the disease (see Table 25-2). In addition to evaluating the diabetic patient for the possibility of coronary artery disease, care should be taken to assess the possibility of peripheral vascular insufficiency by paying attention to peripheral pulses, capillary refill times, and the presence of bruits over major arteries.

Conditions mandating precautions or limitations in participation are summarized in Table 25-3.

PREVENTION OF HYPOGLYCEMIA

One of two simple approaches can be used to prevent hypoglycemia during exercise: addition of dietary supplements or a reduction in insulin dose (Table 25-4).[13] These approaches can be used singly or in combination, but there is no substitute for glucose monitoring before, during, and after exercise to assist in modifying the regimen. Each regimen must be individualized. It is common for diabetic athletes to evaluate a regimen in practice before using it in actual competition. If possible, periods of exercise should be scheduled when the blood glucose levels are highest (for

TABLE 25-2
Guidelines for Preparticipation Evaluation of Athletes with Diabetes

Type of Diabetes	Age (Yrs)	Duration (Yrs)	Special Evaluations
Type I	<30	<10	Assess glycemic control
	<30	10–15	Assess glycemic control
			Careful funduscopy
			Vital signs with exercise
	30+	<15	Assess glycemic control
			Careful funduscopy
			Vital signs with exercise
			Urinalysis
			Neurologic evaluation
			Consider stress test
Type II	<40	<10	Assess glycemic control
			Careful funduscopy
			Vital signs with exercise
	40+	<10	Assess glycemic control
			Careful funduscopy
			Vital signs with exercise
			Urinalysis
			Neurologic evaluation
			Stress test

example, between 1 and 3 hours after eating). Before exercise, blood glucose levels should range between 100 and 200 mg/dl (5.5–11.1 mmol/L). If the blood glucose is less than 80 mg/dl (4.4 mmol/L), the diabetic athlete should consume 15–20 g of readily absorbed carbohydrate. On the other hand, it may be appropriate to delay activity if the blood glucose exceeds 300 mg/dl (16.7 mmol/L) or if urine ketones are positive before exercise.

Caloric supplements are taken just before and every 30–60 minutes during the event. Simple carbohydrates, up to 40 g for adults and up to 25 g for children, may be used (see note to Table 25-1); however, this approach may be associated with an excessive glycemic excursion and may tend to exaggerate the normal fluid losses that occur

during exercise. A better alternative would be to use a supplement containing a mixture of nutrients. A snack derived from complex carbohydrates and protein should be sufficient. Dietary supplementation is usually all that is required to prevent hypoglycemia during less strenuous exercise of modest duration (less than 45 minutes).

More strenuous or prolonged exercise may require an adjustment in insulin dose. Any reduction in insulin dose is dependent on the insulin regimen and the time of day the event or exercise is planned. A 15–25% reduction in the dose of the insulin anticipated to peak during the event usually prevents hypoglycemic reactions; however, elite athletes participating in exhaustive competitions may reduce their insulin dose up to 40%.[12] For example, ath-

TABLE 25-3
Diabetes-Associated Conditions Requiring Precautions for Participation in Sports Activities

Hypoglycemia unawareness
Active proliferative retinopathy
Poor metabolic control
Hypertension
Sensory/autonomic neuropathy
Coronary artery disease
Peripheral vascular disease
Nephropathy (uncertain)
Noncompliance

TABLE 25-4
Recommendations for Prevention of Hypoglycemia during Exercise

Schedule exercise 1–3 hrs after a meal
BG should be between 100 and 200 mg/dl
If BG <80 mg/dl, consume 15–20 g carbohydrate
If BG >300 mg/dl or urine ketones are positive, delay activity
Eat carbohydrate supplement immediately before exercise and every 30–60 mins during exercise
Reduce the insulin dose that is anticipated to peak during the exercise by 15–25%

BG = blood glucose.

letic events that are scheduled before noon would require a reduction in the amount of rapid-acting insulin administered that morning. Similarly, a midafternoon game or practice could be managed by reducing the dose of the morning intermediate-acting insulin. To avoid recurrent episodes of hypoglycemia in patients who are controlled on a single daily amount of insulin, their insulin dose may need to be split into morning and evening injections. Patients controlled on a regimen of extended insulin zinc suspension (Ultralente) and multiple injections of a rapid-acting insulin (regular insulin or insulin lispro) generally do not require a reduction in their Ultralente dose but should not inject rapid-acting insulin before the event. Similarly, patients using an insulin pump for the continuous delivery of subcutaneous insulin should continue their basal insulin rate and avoid bolusing insulin before exercise. The pump should be disconnected and the tubing capped before participation in water or contact sports. Extreme care should be taken, however, to limit the amount of time off the pump because of the risk of developing ketosis secondary to the decline in circulating insulin levels and the concomitant rise in counterregulatory hormones induced by exercise. Because insulin lispro has a particularly short half-life, patients using insulin lispro should be advised to limit their time off the pump to less than 3 hours.[14] If the patient is using regular insulin in his or her pump, time off the pump can be extended for as long as 4 hours.

Other caveats exist concerning the use of insulin. Because local factors, such as blood flow, can influence the absorption of insulin, insulin should not be administered in an extremity that will be exercised.[15] Also, physical conditioning results in increased insulin sensitivity, which translates into lower insulin requirements. A 20–50% reduction in total insulin requirements is common.

There are few data concerning the use of oral antidiabetic agents in athletes. Because sulfonylureas can cause prolonged or recurrent episodes of hypoglycemia, it may be wise to try diet therapy alone. If this fails, it would be prudent to switch these patients to insulin or to other oral agents not associated with hypoglycemia. The use of metformin in this circumstance, however, may be unwise because of the possibility that lactic acidosis may develop if the patient becomes either hypoxic or acidemic during the event.[16]

The phenomenon of postexercise hypoglycemia[17] can be avoided by increasing caloric intake and close monitoring of capillary blood glucose. If the patient is unaccustomed to the degree of physical activity or is just beginning a conditioning program, a prophylactic reduction in the evening insulin dose may also be required.

LONG-TERM EFFECTS OF EXERCISE ON DIABETIC CONTROL AND COMPLICATIONS

Despite the beneficial effects of exercise on glucose homeostasis and insulin sensitivity, several studies[2, 18, 19] have documented that regular exercise or participation in sports does not improve long-term glycemic control, although short-term improvement has been noted.[20] Whether this is due to pre-event carbohydrate loading and subsequent hyperglycemia before and during the initial portion of the event,[21] or to overcorrection of hypoglycemia[2] either during an event or for prevention of postexercise hypoglycemia, or to physiologic barriers[22] is unclear. It is clear, however, that regular physical activity in type 1 diabetic patients may decrease the risk of macrovascular complications[23] without increasing their risk for microvascular complications such as retinopathy.[24]

MANAGEMENT TEAM

Care for the diabetic athlete requires a team approach. The central member is the diabetic athlete, who must be educated concerning symptoms, hazards, precipitating events, and self-help measures to abort hypoglycemia. The diabetic athlete should also carry an appropriate medical identification tag and a source of carbohydrate. In addition to the diabetic athlete and the physician, the team should incorporate coaches and trainers who must be able to recognize and treat hypoglycemia, including the emergency use of glucagon. The trainer's box should include glucagon, buccal glucose gel, and chewable glucose tablets, candy, or sweetened soda.

Any treatment plan must be individualized and reviewed periodically. Frequent alterations, based on the results of self-glucose monitoring or performance, may be necessary and should be anticipated.

REFERENCES

1. Expert Committee on the Diagnosis and Classification of Diabetes Mellitus. Report of the expert committee on the diagnosis and classification of diabetes mellitus. Diabetes Care 1997;20:1183–1197.
2. Weiliczko MC, Gobert M, Mallet E. The participation in sports of diabetic children: a survey in the Rouen region. Ann Pediatr Paris 1991;38:84–88.
3. Groop LC, Bottazzo GF, Doniach D. Islet cell antibodies identify latent type I diabetes in patients ages 35–75 years at diagnosis. Diabetes 1986;35:237–241.

4. Zimmer PZ, Tuomi T, Mackay R, et al. Latent autoimmune diabetes mellitus in adults (LADA): the role of antibodies to glutamic acid decarboxylase in diagnosis and prediction of insulin dependency. Diabet Med 1994;11:299–303.

5. Byrne MM, Sturis J, Menzel S, et al. Altered insulin secretory response to glucose in diabetic and nondiabetic subjects with mutations in the diabetes susceptibility gene MODY3 on chromosome 12. Diabetes 1996;45:1503–1510.

6. Fajans SS, Cloutier MC, Crowther RI. Clinical and etiologic heterogeneity of idiopathic diabetes mellitus. Diabetes 1978;27:1112–1125.

7. Schott M, Schatz D, Atkinson M, et al. GAD65 autoantibodies increase the predictability but not the sensitivity of islet cell and insulin autoantibodies for developing insulin dependent diabetes mellitus. J Autoimmun 1994;7:865–872.

8. Vranic M, Wasserman D, Bukowiecki L. Metabolic Implications of Exercise and Physical Fitness in Physiology and Diabetes. In H Rifkin, D Porte (eds), Diabetes Mellitus: Theory and Practice (4th ed). New York: Elsevier, 1990;198–219.

9. Santiago JV. Lessons from the diabetes control and complications trial. Diabetes 1993;42:1549–1554.

10. American Diabetes Association. Implications of the diabetes control and complications trial. Diabetes Care 1993;16:1517–1520.

11. Blake GA, Levin SR, Koyal SN. Exercise-induced hypertension in normotensive patients with NIDDM. Diabetes Care 1990;7:799–801.

12. Lauer MS, Levy D, Anderson KM, Plehn JF. Is there a relationship between exercise systolic blood pressure response and left ventricular mass? Ann Intern Med 1992;116:203–210.

13. Horton ES. Role and management of exercise in diabetes mellitus. Diabetes Care 1988;11:201–211.

14. Holleman F, Hoekstra JBL. Insulin lispro. N Engl J Med 1997;337:176–183.

15. Kiovisto V, Felig P. Effects of acute exercise on insulin absorption in diabetic patients. N Engl J Med 1978;298:79–83.

16. Bailey CJ, Turner RC. Metformin. N Engl J Med 1996;334:574–579.

17. MacDonald MJ. Postexercise late-onset hypoglycemia in insulin-dependent diabetic patients. Diabetes Care 1987;10:584–588.

18. Selam JL, Casassus P, Bruzzo F, et al. Exercise is not associated with better diabetes control in type 1 and type 2 diabetic subjects. Acta Diabetol 1992;29:11–13.

19. Sackey AH, Jefferson IG. Physical activity and glycemic control in children with diabetes mellitus. Diabet Med 1996;13:789–793.

20. Stratton R, Wilson DP, Endres RK, Goldstein DE. Improved glycemic control after a supervised eight week exercise program in insulin-dependent diabetic adolescents. Diabetes Care 1987;10:589–593.

21. Koivisto VA, Sane T, Fhyrquist F, Pelkonen R. Fuel and fluid homeostasis during long-term exercise in healthy subjects and type I diabetic patients. Diabetes Care 1992;15:1736–1741.

22. Regensteiner JG, Sippel J, McFarling ET, et al. Effects of non–insulin-dependent diabetes on oxygen consumption during treadmill exercise. Med Sci Sports Exerc 1995;27:875–881.

23. LaPorte RE, Dorman JS, Tajima N, et al. Pittsburgh insulin-dependent diabetes mellitus morbidity and mortality study: physical activity and diabetic complications. Pediatrics 1986;78:1027–1033.

24. Cruickshanks KJ, Moss SE, Klein R, Klein BE. Physical activity and proliferative retinopathy in people diagnosed with diabetes before age 30 years. Diabetes Care 1992;15:1267–1272.

26

Acute Minor Illnesses in the Athlete

William F. Miser

THE ATHLETE AND INFECTION

Exercise affects the immune system. The immune system is enhanced with moderate exercise, whereas intensive exercise, especially overtraining, depresses it.[1-4] The athlete involved in a demanding training program is more susceptible to infections and viral illnesses than the nonathlete.[5-10] Exercising strenuously during the incubation phase of an infection (characterized by fever, malaise, myalgias, and so forth) may actually worsen the severity of the illness.[8] Sometimes the desires of the athlete to train through an illness or to minimize the layoff time conflicts with the need to avoid strenuous exercise during an acute illness. Those who provide health care to the athlete must recognize and correctly manage these illnesses to avoid unnecessary complications and to speed the athlete's recovery. This chapter highlights common acute minor illnesses that may occur in the athlete. Space prohibits an exhaustive dissertation on each illness, and the reader is encouraged to refer to the reference list, which has several excellent reviews.

RUNNY OR CONGESTED NOSE (RHINITIS, RHINORRHEA)

The evaluation of the athlete who reports a runny or stuffy nose requires a systematic approach, including a careful history, physical examination, and appropriate laboratory and x-ray studies.[11-13] In addition to the common causes of a runny or congested nose (Table 26-1), the athlete may also have nonspecific causes that are due to recurrent exposure to polluted air or to formaldehyde, glues, paints, cleaners, and vinyls commonly found in indoor gymnasiums.[14]

The overall goals in treating the athlete with a runny nose are to (1) gain as much relief as possible from discomfort without affecting performance and (2) design a treatment plan that meets the criteria of the National Olympic governing bodies.[14] For example, antihistamines that are approved for international competition may be appropriate, but side effects, such as drowsiness, may impair performance, anticholinergic effects, such as impaired sweating, may predispose the athlete to a heat injury, and the combination with other medicines may cause a life-threatening cardiac arrhythmia.[15] Combining the antihistamine astemizole (Hismanal) with erythromycin can prolong the QT interval leading to a potentially malignant dysrhythmia. Neither topical nor systemic decongestants are approved for use by Olympic athletes, although they may be approved for use in other athletic competitions. Thus, it is important to weigh the discomfort and effects of the runny nose on the athlete against the potential side effects and disqualifying nature of the medical therapy. If the athlete has relatively mild to moderate symptoms that do not impair performance, it may be better to avoid any pharmacotherapy. However, if the symptoms do impair performance, then drug therapy should be individualized.

Common Cold (Coryza, Viral Upper Respiratory Infection)

The common cold, a benign, self-limited viral infection of the upper respiratory tract, causes more disability among athletes than all other diseases combined.[6, 7, 16, 17] During the 1992 Winter Olympics, upper respiratory infections (URIs) prevented a number of athletes from competing and caused others to have subpar performances.[18] More than 200 different viruses can cause a cold, the chief

TABLE 26-1

Most Common Causes of a Runny or Congested Nose (Rhinorrhea and Rhinitis)

Inflammatory
   Infectious
      Common cold (coryza)
      Sinusitis
   Noninfectious
      Seasonal allergic rhinitis
      Perennial allergic rhinitis
      Nonallergic (vasomotor) rhinitis
      Nonallergic rhinitis with eosinophilia
Noninflammatory
   Drug-induced rhinitis
      Rhinitis medicamentosa
      Aspirin and nonsteroidal anti-inflammatory drugs
      Oral contraceptives
      Beta-blockers
   Anatomic abnormalities
      Deviated nasal septum
      Nasal polyps
      Atrophic rhinitis

TABLE 26-2

Examples of Medicines Permitted and Prohibited by the U.S. Olympic Committee[a]

Medicines permitted
   Analgesics such as aspirin, acetaminophen, and non-steroidal anti-inflammatory drugs
   Antihistamines such as chlorpheniramine
   Anticholinergics such as ipratropium bromide
   Cough suppressants such as dextromethorphan
   Corticosteroids used as nasal or inhalation therapy
   Expectorants such as guaifenesin
   Throat lozenges such as domiphen bromide
Medicines prohibited
   Caffeine[b]
   Codeine[b]
   Ephedrine[b]
   Oral corticosteroids
   Phenylpropanolamine[b]
   Propylhexedrine[b]
   Pseudoephedrine[b]

[a]For an up-to-date listing of permitted and prohibited drugs, visit the Internet Web site of the International Olympic Committee (http://www.olympic.org/), or write to the U.S. Olympic Committee, 1750 E. Boulder St., Colorado Springs, CO 80909-5760; or the National Collegiate Athletic Association, Box 1906, Mission, KS 66201.
[b]Common ingredients found in decongestant cold and sinus medications; as a general rule, avoid combination products that may contain caffeine (analgesics); codeine (analgesics and cough remedies); mild stimulants, such as ephedrine (decongestants and cold remedies); and alcohol (many liquid cough and cold preparations).

of which is rhinovirus. The athlete with a common cold typically has sneezing, a watery nasal discharge, nasal congestion, a sore or scratchy throat, and a nonproductive cough. Constitutional symptoms, if present, include headache, myalgias, and low-grade fever. The acute symptoms last 2–7 days, with complete resolution expected by 7–14 days. Potential complications of the common cold are acute otitis media, pharyngitis, sinusitis, bronchitis, pneumonia, and precipitation of asthma attacks.

Because it is a self-limited viral illness, treatment of the common cold is symptomatic and includes rest, humidification, and warm fluids. Antibiotics are not indicated. Although currently not available, effective antivirals for treating the common cold may soon be developed.[19] Both aspirin and acetaminophen may actually worsen or prolong symptoms and should be avoided.[16, 17] Nonsteroidal anti-inflammatory drugs, such as naproxen or ibuprofen, do not have this effect and are preferred for treating myalgias and headaches.

There are more than 800 cold medicines on the market, and most include mixtures of antihistamines and decongestants. The majority of these medicines may be ineffective,[16, 20, 21] and many are prohibited by the International Olympic Committee (Table 26-2). If needed, decongestants (pseudoephedrine, phenylpropanolamine, and oxymetazoline), chlorpheniramine, and guaifenesin may provide some relief. Ipratropium bromide nasal spray provides specific relief of rhinorrhea and sneezing associated with the common cold.[22] The use of vitamin C

(1 g per day or more) to both alleviate and prevent common cold symptoms is controversial—some studies have shown it to be effective, and others have suggested it has no proved benefit.[16, 17, 23] Zinc gluconate throat lozenges, and Echinacea, an herbal remedy, started within the first few days of symptoms, may shorten the duration of the common cold.[24, 25] Chicken soup improves mucociliary clearance and may provide some relief.[16]

Allergic Rhinitis (Hay Fever)

Allergic rhinitis (AR) is a common recurrent condition affecting 20–30% of the U.S. population. It is manifested by sneezing, clear runny nose, nasal congestion, and itchy watery eyes and nose.[11, 26–28] The athlete with AR may also have either a personal or a family history of other allergic problems such as urticaria, eczema, or asthma. Typically, the runny nose is either a seasonal or a perennial problem and is a result of inhalants such as cigarette smoke, perfumes, pollen from trees, grasses and weeds, dust, molds, and animal dander. Physical examination of the external nose typically shows the "allergic salute," a transverse nasal crease that is due to the patient pushing up the tip of the nose to relieve nasal itching. The nasal turbinates are typically pale, blue, and edematous with a clear, watery discharge. Nasal polyps, which are smooth, pale, gelatinous-appearing growths, may sometimes be found along the middle meatus or the middle and superior turbinates. The eyelids are typically puffy, and the eyes are injected. "Allergic shiners," a bluish discoloration in the infraorbital areas, may also be present.

Typically in AR, the percentage of eosinophils seen on the nasal smear will be between 10% and 100%. However, a negative nasal smear does not rule out AR. Testing for peripheral eosinophilia and serum immunoglobulin E levels is usually not helpful. Allergy skin testing may be helpful, but a positive test does not confirm that the given allergen is the cause of the symptoms. In some individuals, a sinus x-ray (Waters view) or a limited coronal computed tomography (CT) scan may be helpful to rule out the possibility of chronic sinusitis. When anatomic problems, such as a deviated nasal septum, adenoid hypertrophy, or nasal polyps, are suspected, rhinoscopy may be useful.

The International Rhinitis Management Working Group has developed guidelines for the rational treatment of AR.[29] After a thorough history and physical examination are performed, the primary treatment is avoiding the precipitating factors (environmental control). Often, these factors cannot be found, however, or they may be unavoidable. In these cases, the next step in the management of AR is pharmacotherapy, which includes antihistamines, decongestants, anticholinergics, cromolyn sodium, and topical or systemic corticosteroids.[27, 30]

Antihistamines rapidly relieve sneezing, itching, and runny nose, but not congestion. As a group, they are the first drugs of choice for treating AR; however, their use may result in sedation and may predispose the athlete to a heat injury during extreme exercise. Today, there are more than 100 antihistamine agents available on the market (Table 26-3).[27, 31-34] The first-generation antihistamines are effective and inexpensive, but often cause sedation, diminished alertness, slowed reaction time, and impaired cognitive function and have anticholinergic side effects such as dry mouth or blurred vision. The newer second-generation antihistamines are more expensive, but are just as effective without the sedation and anticholinergic side effects. Despite the additional costs, nonsedating antihistamines provide a safer alternative and improved patient satisfaction compared with the first-generation sedating agents.[35] One of the nonsedating second-generation antihistamines (astemizole) can on rare occasion cause fatal arrhythmias if used in combination with certain other drugs such as erythromycin. Of the four nonsedating second-generation antihistamines currently available, ceti-

TABLE 26-3

Selected Treatment Options for Allergic Rhinitis*

Treatment	Adult Daily Dosage
Oral antihistamines	
First generation	
Chlorpheniramine maleate (Chlor-Trimeton)	8–12 mg bid
Hydroxyzine hydrochloride (Atarax)	25–50 mg tid
Diphenhydramine hydrochloride (Benadryl)	25–50 mg qid
Second generation	
Astemizole (Hismanal)	10 mg qd
Cetirizine (Zyrtec)	5–10 mg qd
Fexofenadine (Allegra)	60 mg bid
Loratadine (Claritin)	10 mg qd
Nasal sprays	(each nostril)
Corticosteroid nasal sprays	
Beclomethasone	
Beconase	1 spray bid
Vancenase Pockethaler	1 spray bid
Beconase AQ	1–2 sprays bid
Vancenase AQ	1–2 sprays bid
Budesonide (Rhinocort)	4 sprays qd
Flunisolide (Nasalide, Nasarel)	2 sprays bid
Fluticasone propionate (Flonase)	1–2 sprays qd
Triamcinolone acetonide (Nasacort)	2 sprays qd
Antihistamine nasal spray	
Azelastine hydrochloride (Astelin)	2 sprays bid
Anticholinergic nasal spray	
Ipratropium bromide (Atrovent)	2 sprays bid
Cromolyn sodium (Nasalcrom)	1 spray qid

*These are representative agents of more than 100 antihistamines and topical corticosteroids available on the market in 1997.

rizine is reported to have the quickest onset of action and highest efficacy.[36]

Decongestants can be given orally (phenylephrine, pseudoephedrine, and phenylpropanolamine) or topically (phenylephrine, oxymetazoline, and xylometazoline). As a group, they are useful in treating the nasal congestion of AR, but their use in Olympic competition is prohibited. The most common side effects include insomnia and irritability, and the topical forms may cause rebound congestion and rhinitis medicamentosa if used for more than 3 days.

Cromolyn sodium, given intranasally as a 4% spray metered dose inhaler, is similar to antihistamines in relieving sneezing, nasal itching, and runny nose. Because of its mode of action, it may take 2–4 weeks before symptoms are relieved, and it is best used prophylactically before the onset of seasonal symptoms.[27] Its major drawback is patient compliance because of its frequent dosing (one spray in each nostril every 3–4 hours).

Corticosteroid aerosols (see Table 26-3) are generally safe and are the most potent medicines available for treating AR.[37] The usual starting dose is one to two sprays in each nostril three times a day. After 3 days, the symptoms are usually relieved. After the symptoms of AR have been controlled, it is recommended to decrease the sprays to the lowest effective dose by gradually decreasing the dose by one puff each week until either the patient is off this medicine or the symptoms recur. New preparations of steroid nasal sprays are less irritating and better tolerated.

Oral corticosteroids can be used for treatment of acute and severe symptoms of AR, but are most effectively given as a short course (for example, prednisone 50 mg given orally for 5 days). Their long-term use is not recommended because of the harmful side effects and because they are prohibited by the U.S. Olympic Committee.

Immunotherapy is the last step in the treatment of AR and is reserved for those who fail to find relief from the environmental controls and pharmacotherapy. At this point, it is recommended to refer the athlete to an allergist for further evaluation and treatment.

Nonallergic (Vasomotor) Rhinitis

The athlete with nonallergic (vasomotor) rhinitis has nasal congestion and an excessive watery runny nose that may be precipitated by smoke, odors, noxious fumes, exercise, emotion, or environmental changes. It is often difficult to differentiate this condition from AR. Unlike AR, it is not allergic or seasonal in nature, and itching is usually not present. The nasal turbinates are typically swollen and vary in color from dark red to blue with a watery nasal discharge. Nasal smear for eosinophils and allergy skin testing are usually negative. The treatment is similar to that for AR. Obvious precipitating factors should be avoided. If symptoms are particularly bothersome, decongestants, antihistamines, and intranasal corticosteroids are the primary medical treatments (see section on allergic rhinitis). In addition, the newly released anticholinergic agent ipratropium bromide (Atrovent nasal spray) effectively clears nasal discharge.[38]

Rhinitis Medicamentosa

Nasal congestion may be caused by certain drugs such as oral contraceptives, beta-blockers, prazosin, hydralazine, reserpine, methyldopa, and guanethidine. However, the most common cause of drug-induced rhinitis is the abuse of topical nose drops and sprays.[39] Topical decongestants, although useful for up to 3 days, may on a long-term basis cause rebound congestion. The nasal mucosa is markedly red, swollen, and friable. Treatment is often difficult and requires total cessation of the topical decongestant. Intranasal corticosteroids (see Table 26-3) or systemic steroids may help during the withdrawal period.

Sinusitis

All of the above-listed conditions may predispose athletes to sinus infection, especially those involved in water sports such as swimming, diving, surfing, and water polo. Sinusitis should be suspected if the symptoms of a common cold fail to resolve, if the nasal discharge is thick and yellow or green in color, if fever or chills occur, or if pain is present over the cheek or teeth, especially if worsened by bending forward.[13] It is often difficult to differentiate sinusitis from perennial rhinitis.[40–42] A combination of maxillary toothache, poor response to nasal decongestants, colored nasal discharge by history or examination, and transillumination are the most useful clinical findings of sinusitis.[13] Sinus x-rays (occipitomental Waters and occipitofrontal Caldwell) may show mucoperiosteal thickening, opacification, or air-fluid levels of the affected sinus and are helpful in those with confusing or recurrent symptoms. If plain films do not help, CT is the most sensitive but expensive test for detecting sinusitis.

In treating sinusitis, analgesics are often needed for control of pain. Decongestants, saline nasal spray, and hot tea with lemon are useful to promote drainage of the sinuses. Guaifenesin 1,200 mg orally twice a day is effective in thinning nasal secretions.[43] Because they may thicken the nasal mucosa, antihistamines should be avoided. Nasal corticosteroids (see Table 26-3) used for a minimum of 3–5 days are effective and safe. Although this has been questioned,[44, 45] antibiotics are still considered the mainstay of therapy, with an efficacy of as much as 90%.[41] For the majority of cases, 7–10 days of a first-line antibiotic (Table 26-4) is effective most of the time;[46] one study reported success with a 3-day treatment course.[47] If there is incomplete resolution or early relapse of symptoms, perform an x-ray (if not already done) to confirm the diagnosis, and treat the athlete with another 10- to 14-day course of a second-line antibiotic. If no significant improvement occurs after the second course of antibiotics, consult an otolaryngologist. For those with an isolated frontal sinusitis or those with severe symptoms and fever, hospitalization may be required. The athlete should avoid diving below the water surface until the sinusitis is completely cured.

PAINFUL EAR (OTALGIA)

Pain felt in the ear either may arise from disease within the ear or may be referred from disease occurring in other

TABLE 26-4
Oral Antibiotics Used for Treating Sinusitis in Adults

Antibiotic	Dosage
First-line therapy	
Amoxicillin*	500 mg tid
Ampicillin*	500 mg tid
Doxycycline	100 mg bid
Trimethoprim-sulfamethoxazole	160/300 mg bid
Second-line therapy	
Amoxicillin-clavulanate (Augmentin)	875/125 mg bid
Cefaclor (Ceclor)	500 mg bid
Cefixime (Suprax)	400 mg qd
Cefpodoxime proxetil (Vantin)	200 mg bid
Cefprozil (Cefzil)	250–500 mg bid
Ceftibuten (Cedax)	400 mg qd
Cefuroxime axetil (Ceftin)	250 mg bid
Clarithromycin (Biaxin)	500 mg bid
Levofloxacin (Levaquin)	500 mg qd
Loracarbef (Lorabid)	400 mg bid

*In some parts of the United States, bacterial resistance to these drugs is high.

TABLE 26-5
Common Causes of Ear Pain (Otalgia)

Diseases of the ear
    Infection of auditory canal (external otitis—swimmer's ear)
    Acute auricular hematoma (cauliflower ear)
    Foreign body in auditory canal
    Cerumen impaction of auditory canal
    Eustachian tube dysfunction
    Infection of middle ear (otitis media)
Causes of referred ear pain
    Dental and periodontal disease
    Infectious causes (sinusitis, pharyngitis, salinitis)
    Temporomandibular joint dysfunction
    Vascular causes (carotodynia, temporal arteritis)
    Skeletal causes (cervical arthritis)
    Neurologic causes (trigeminal and glossopharyngeal
      neuritis)

areas of the head and neck (Table 26-5).[48] If after a thorough ear examination the cause for the ear pain is not found, a more thorough head and neck examination must be performed. Referral to an otolaryngologist may be necessary if the cause of referred ear pain is not easily found.

Cerumen Impaction

Impaction of cerumen (earwax) is especially common in athletes involved in water sports. When attempting to remove the earwax with a cotton-tipped applicator, the athlete may cause the cerumen to become impacted deep in the ear canal, making the problem worse.[49] Therefore, athletes should be counseled against such a practice.

Cerumen may be removed in the office by several methods.[50] If a perforated tympanic membrane or acute otitis media is not present, a wax softener—such as olive or mineral oil, triethanolamine polypeptide oleate-condensate, or carbamide peroxide—makes cerumen removal easier. Earwax can then be removed by either gentle irrigation, suction, or cerumen curette under direct visualization. Once the earwax is removed, it is important to evaluate the function of the tympanic membrane and hearing to ensure both are normal.

Acute Otitis Externa

Commonly known as "swimmer's ear," acute otitis externa is the most common infection related to water activi-

ties.[48, 51] Symptoms include itching, acute ear pain, muffled hearing, and a scant watery discharge from the ear. The pathognomonic sign of acute externa is pain with manipulation of the auricle. The ear canal is often edematous and red, and is often occluded with debris and purulent material.

To treat acute otitis externa, the ear canal is cleansed to improve treatment and to ensure the patient does not also have an otitis media. If the tympanic membrane cannot be seen, treatment must be directed at both external and middle ear infections (see section on acute otitis media). The most effective topical antibiotic medicines are mixtures: neomycin, and bacitracin or polymyxin with hydrocortisone. Both are mixed with a vehicle that is either glycerin-based (solution) or water-based (suspension). If no eardrum perforation is present, the solution is ideal. However, glycerin is irritating to the middle ear mucosa and should not be used if a perforation is present. If the eardrum cannot be seen, the suspension should be used. The topical antibiotics are given in dosages of four to five drops four times per day for at least 7 days. In particularly occluded ears, a wick of cotton soaked with antibiotic suspension may be inserted into the external canal. During treatment, the ear canal must be kept dry.

The athlete should abstain from water sports for 2–3 days after beginning treatment and preferably for 7–10 days until the infection is cleared. Future infections may be prevented by proper removal of cerumen (avoid touching or scratching the ear) and by thoroughly drying the ear canal after a water event using a handheld hair dryer, set on a low setting, followed by the use of 70% ethyl alcohol drops as a drying agent.[51] In addition, the ear canal can be temporarily occluded by inserting a cotton ball coated with petrolatum (Vaseline) or by using the newer silicone earplugs (wax-type earplugs should be avoided).

Middle Ear Disease

Middle ear pathology represents the true continuum of disease, which often has indistinct and overlapping features.[52, 53] Otitis media denotes inflammation of the middle ear, which includes the middle ear cavity, the eustachian tube, and mastoid.

Eustachian Tube Dysfunction

Eustachian tube dysfunction refers to any condition that interferes with the ability of the eustachian tube to permit equilibration of air and middle ear pressure. Common causes include URIs, allergies, anatomic deformities, and barotrauma (for example, scuba diving). This dysfunction causes a middle ear effusion that results in popping sounds or intermittent pressure sensation in the ear. The tympanic membrane is typically thickened with a gray or amber fluid seen in the middle ear. Occasionally, bubbles may be seen. The membrane is immobile by pneumatic otoscopy and tympanometry.

Usually, acute middle ear effusions are self-limited and resolve within 2 weeks. In the absence of other illness (sinusitis or purulent rhinitis), decongestants and antibiotics are not effective.[54, 55] Autoinflation maneuvers, such as forcefully blowing the nose while the mouth and nares are kept closed, may help hasten the recovery. If the effusion persists beyond 2 weeks, a chronic, low-grade bacterial infection may be present, and a trial of antibiotics and corticosteroids may be warranted.[56] Prednisone, 50 mg given once daily for 7 days, in combination with an antibiotic (trimethoprim-sulfamethoxazole [Bactrim DS] given orally twice a day, or amoxicillin, 250 mg, given orally three times a day) for 21 days typically will cure the chronic effusion that is caused by an infection. If the effusion persists beyond 12 weeks, an otolaryngologist should be consulted. To prevent worsening of the effusion and possible rupture of the tympanic membrane, diving below water should be avoided until the effusion is resolved. Surface swimming does not increase the risk of infection, even in those who have tympanostomy ventilating tubes.[57] However, earplugs should be used when ocean swimming to avoid getting sand grains in the middle ear.

Acute Otitis Media

Although considered a disease of childhood, acute otitis media (AOM) does occur in teenagers and adults.[58] There is a paucity of research in treating AOM in this older age group. Unlike children, athletes usually present within 1 day of symptom onset. They typically report a severe, deep throbbing pain in the ear, temporomandibular joint, or throat, usually after a viral URI. Decreased hearing and a low-grade fever may be present. The most valuable diagnostic test is inspection of the middle ear with a pneumatic otoscope.[59, 60] The tympanic membrane typically is red, dull or opaque, and immobile. Vesicles present on the tympanic membrane (bullous myringitis) suggests a *Mycoplasma* infection. Tympanometry is also a useful diagnostic aid. A flat (type B) tracing on the tympanogram provides objective evidence of otitis.

Although there is a growing consensus that antibiotics may not be beneficial, the mainstay of treatment for AOM remains amoxicillin, 250 mg three times a day, or trimethoprim-sulfamethoxazole double-strength tablets twice a day, given for 10 days.[56, 61] In the case of bullous myringitis, erythromycin, 250 mg given three times a day for 10 days, is the drug of choice. Treatment with cefuroxime axetil, 250 mg twice a day for 5 days, is just as effective, as is a 10-day course of the other antibiotics.[62] Ear drops with benzocaine (local anesthetic) and antipyrine (analgesic), such as Auralgan Otic Solution, are helpful in relieving pain. With these medications, the fever and pain is typically improved within 2 days. If fever persists or the pain has not improved, the antibiotics should be changed to either amoxicillin-clavulanate, 250 mg given three times a day; cefaclor, 250 mg given twice a day; or cefixime, 400 mg given once a day. There is no proved efficacious role for antihistamines or decongestants in the treatment of otitis media. If the athlete becomes asymptomatic, there is no need for reevaluation. However, as many as 25% of adults with AOM develop a middle ear effusion that may persist for as long as 3 months.[58] The treatment for this effusion should be that described in the section on eustachian tube dysfunction. During the illness, the athlete should not dive below the surface of the water. If the infection fails to clear or if the effusion persists beyond 12 weeks, the athlete should be referred to an otolaryngologist.

SORE THROAT

Sore throat is one of the most common symptoms seen by primary care physicians, with nearly 40 million visits made each year in the United States.[63] There are numerous causes for an athlete to have a sore throat, the majority of which are infectious (Table 26-6). Typically, the athlete will report pain that is aggravated by swallowing, which may also radiate to the ears. Associated features may include cough, runny nose, tonsillar enlargement, pharyngeal or tonsillar exudate, tender anterior or pos-

TABLE 26-6
Common Causes of Sore Throat

Viral causes (30–60% in adults)
  Adenovirus (most common)
  Rhinovirus
  Influenza viruses
  Epstein-Barr virus
  Parainfluenza virus
  Respiratory syncytial virus
  Coxsackievirus
  Herpes simplex virus
  Coronavirus (uncommon)
Bacterial causes (5–15% in adolescents and adults)
  Group A beta-hemolytic streptococcus
  Group B, C, and G streptococci
  Neisseria gonorrhoeae (uncommon)
  Corynebacterium diphtheriae (rare)
  Arcanobacterium haemolyticus
  Chlamydia pneumoniae
  Chlamydia trachomatis
  Mycoplasma pneumoniae
Noninfectious causes
  Postnasal drip or sinusitis
  Allergies
  Irritant exposure—cigarette smoke, smog
  Mouth breathing
  Lack of ambient humidity at home or work
  Trauma—accidents, burns, other thermal injuries

terior cervical adenopathy, and fever. Nearly every step in the management of pharyngitis is controversial. Because more than 60% of cases of sore throat are caused by a virus, the challenge is to determine, in a cost-effective manner, which athletes require antibiotic therapy.[63, 64]

Viral Pharyngitis

Viruses, especially adenovirus and rhinovirus, are the most common causes of sore throat. Typically, the athlete experiences irritation or scratchiness of the throat with mild edema and erythema of the pharynx. Fever, tender cervical adenopathy, and tonsillar exudates are not commonly found. The athlete also may have other symptoms of the common cold, such as runny nose and dry cough. These viruses are typically self-limited and benign. Treatment is symptomatic and includes lozenges, sprays, warm saltwater gargle, and anti-inflammatories (ibuprofen and naproxen).

Acute Epiglottitis

In contrast to the common cold, the athlete who has acute epiglottitis is severely ill, with abrupt onset of high fever, dysphagia, drooling, dysphonia, and dyspnea.[65] Although the cardinal sign is a cherry-red, edematous epiglottis, direct visualization may precipitate complete airway obstruction. When one examines an individual who may have epiglottitis, someone experienced in intubation must be present. The diagnosis is sometimes made by a lateral neck x-ray film, which demonstrates a swollen epiglottis ("thumb sign"). Caused by *Haemophilus influenzae,* acute epiglottitis is a medical emergency that requires hospitalization and antibiotic treatment with cefuroxime or third-generation cephalosporin.

Gingivostomatitis and Herpangina

Primary infection with herpes simplex virus types 1 or 2 often causes a sore throat. Examination of the pharynx demonstrates the characteristic painful, superficial vesicles and ulcers on an erythematous base. Fever and tender cervical adenopathy are commonly present. In contrast, 1- to 2-mm vesicles located on the soft palate may represent herpangina, which is usually caused by coxsackievirus A or B. Gingivitis and cervical adenopathy do not occur, but fever and sore throat are usually present. This condition is important to recognize because the coxsackievirus has been identified as a cause for myocarditis in the athlete.[66] In both conditions, treatment is symptomatic, and complete recovery is expected within 2 weeks.

Group A Beta-Hemolytic Streptococcus

The classic features of group A beta-hemolytic streptococcus (GABHS) pharyngitis include the sudden onset of sore throat and moderate fever (39.0°–40.5°C); headache; anorexia; nausea; vomiting; abdominal pain; malaise; tonsillopharyngeal erythema; patchy, discrete tonsillar or pharyngeal exudate; soft palate petechiae; tender cervical adenopathy; or scarlet fever.[67, 68] However, these "classic" features occur in only 33–50% of patients. The majority of patients have mild or asymptomatic disease, and there is much overlap with these features and those of viral pharyngitis.

The presence of GABHS must be recognized, because antibiotics accomplish four goals: (1) patients clinically improve more quickly; (2) they become noninfectious within 24 hours, thus preventing transmission of infection; (3) suppurative complications, such as peritonsillar abscess, are avoided; and (4) acute rheumatic fever and heart disease is prevented.[63] GABHS can often be confused with viral pharyngitis, however, and even the most experienced physician may miss the diagnosis based on clinical findings alone.

The gold standard for diagnosing acute GABHS pharyngitis is a properly processed and interpreted throat cul-

TABLE 26-7

Treatment Options for Group A Beta-Hemolytic
Streptococcal Pharyngitis

Antibiotic	Adult Dosage*
First-line treatment	
Benzathine penicillin G	1,200,000 units IM once
Benzathine/procaine PCN	900,000/300,000 IM once
Penicillin VK	500 mg bid
Penicillin allergic	
Erythromycin estolate	250 mg bid
Erythromycin ethylsuccinate	400 mg tid
Second-line treatment	
Amoxicillin	250 mg qd–tid
Cephalexin	250 mg tid
Cefadroxil	1,000 mg qd
Cefaclor	250 mg tid
Cefuroxime axetil	125 mg bid
Cefixime	200 mg qd
Amoxicillin/clavulanate	250 mg tid
Clarithromycin	250 mg bid
Azithromycin	500 mg on day 1, then 250 mg days 2–5

*Unless otherwise indicated, antibiotic is given orally for 10 days.
IM = intramuscularly.

ture, but obtaining the results may take 48 hours, and as many as 10% may be falsely negative.[69] There are more than 25 different streptococcal rapid antigen tests available commercially. Most are highly specific (90–96%), but not as sensitive (41–93%) as throat cultures.[70] If a rapid antigen test is positive, one can almost be certain that GABHS is present in the pharynx. If the test is negative, most authors recommend obtaining a throat culture in those whom one suspects has GABHS infection.[71]

There is no consensus on the best cost-effective approach to treating patients with a sore throat.[63, 70, 72] The conservative approach is to treat only individuals with positive throat cultures. Others suggest treating the patient only on the basis of clinical findings because of the high rate of false-positive results, false-negative results, and cost of testing. At this time, it is not unreasonable to treat the athlete for presumed GABHS who presents with a sore throat and fever, pharyngeal or tonsillar exudates, and enlarged or tender cervical adenopathy. For those who might have GABHS but do not appear ill, a throat culture may be obtained to confirm the diagnosis before beginning antibiotics.

The choice of antibiotic for GABHS pharyngitis (Table 26-7) should consider cost, side-effect profile, and patient compliance. Penicillin remains the drug of choice, with erythromycin for those who are penicillin allergic. In addition to antibiotics, pain can be relieved with ibuprofen or naproxen, warm liquids, and in those with severe inflam-

matory symptoms, a short course of oral prednisone or a single 10-mg injection of dexamethasone.[73]

Peritonsillar abscess, a local complication of GABHS, is manifested by a severe unilateral sore throat associated with fever, dysphagia, referred otalgia, pain with lateral movement of the neck, rancid breath, trismus, drooling from a partially opened mouth, and a "hot potato" voice. There is generalized erythema of the pharynx and tonsils, with a deeper dusky redness overlying the involved area, swelling of the anterior pillar and soft palate above the tonsil, and uvular deviation to the opposite side. Referral to an otolaryngologist is recommended. In addition to intravenous penicillin, treatment options include repeated needle aspiration, incision and drainage, abscess tonsillectomy, and delayed (2–4 weeks) tonsillectomy.[74]

Infectious Mononucleosis

Infectious mononucleosis (IM) is an acute, nearly always self-limited, lymphoproliferative disease with autoimmune features caused by the Epstein-Barr virus (EBV).[75–78] IM may occur at any age, but the highest incidence occurs in the 15- to 19-year-old age group. On college campuses, 1–3% of all students each school year develop symptomatic IM. Typically, the athlete with IM experiences a 3- to 5-day prodromal period of malaise, fatigue, myalgias, low-grade headache, anorexia, and nausea. This is soon followed by moderate fever; chills; severe—sometimes incapacitating—exudative pharyngitis; and tender, enlarged, posterior cervical lymphadenopathy. As many as 10% may also develop clinical jaundice or a transient, morbilliform rash similar to rubella.

During the acute phase, laboratory evaluation will reveal a modest leukocytosis of 10,000–20,000/μl with a striking absolute lymphocytosis (more than 50% of the total white blood cell count) and more than 10–20% atypical lymphocytes. A transient neutropenia and thrombocytopenia may occur during the second week of illness, but it is rarely severe. Anemia is not a common feature and if present may suggest splenic rupture. As many as 90% of those with IM will by the third week of illness have mild elevations of their liver function tests consistent with mild hepatitis, which usually resolves by the fifth week.

The diagnosis of IM is suggested by the preceding typical clinical and laboratory findings and is confirmed by serologic tests. As many as 90% of individuals with IM have a positive heterophile test (Monospot) by the end of the third week of illness. However, 10% repeatedly have a negative Monospot; in these individuals, EBV-specific antibody studies would be needed to confirm the diagnosis of IM.[78]

The acute phase of IM (fever, pharyngitis, malaise, and fatigue) typically lasts for 15 days, with complete recovery expected within 8 weeks. However, the highly trained athlete may not attain the pre-illness level of fitness for as long as 3 months.[75] Most athletes with IM recover without problems, but complications can occur. As many as 30% of those with IM also have a throat culture positive for GABHS. These individuals require treatment with penicillin or erythromycin; ampicillin should be avoided because it causes a florid, diffuse, maculopapular eruption in those with IM. Potential life-threatening complications, although uncommon, include upper airway obstruction, granulocytopenia, and autoimmune hemolytic anemia.

Almost all patients with IM have splenomegaly to some degree, although it is often missed on physical examination.[79, 80] The most accurate method of detecting splenomegaly is radiography, which includes a plain abdominal x-ray film, ultrasonography, CT, and radionuclide scan. Spontaneous rupture of the enlarged spleen, a rare but potentially fatal complication of IM, typically occurs spontaneously between the days 4 and 21 of symptomatic illness.[81, 82] All spleens that rupture are enlarged, but the spleen is clinically palpable in less than one-half. The characteristic pattern of splenic rupture includes left upper quadrant abdominal pain, which may radiate to the top of the left shoulder (Kehr's sign), and leukocytosis with absolute neutropenia. The diagnosis of splenic rupture is confirmed by ultrasonography or CT in those who are hemodynamically stable, or by diagnostic peritoneal lavage in those more emergent. Current treatment options for this complication include splenectomy (presently the preferred treatment), partial splenectomy, splenorrhaphy, and observation in selected individuals.[82, 83]

Therapy for the athlete with IM consists of (1) providing supportive care, (2) identifying and treating potential complications, and (3) giving safe yet rational guidelines for resumption of training and competition, especially in contact sports. Because the duration of the most symptomatic part of the illness lasts for only 5–7 days in the majority of those with IM, treatment is primarily supportive. Analgesia with acetaminophen, 650 mg given orally every 4 hours as needed, is preferable to aspirin, which may inhibit platelet function. For those with refractory pain, codeine, 30–60 mg every 4–6 hours, may be required. All patients with IM should have a throat culture done, and those with GABHS should be treated accordingly. Those who develop a very severe pharyngitis with impending airway obstruction and those in extremis may require hospitalization, treatment with intravenous corticosteroids, and evaluation by an otolaryngologist. Routine use of corticosteroids in uncomplicated IM is not recommended.

The athlete with IM during the acute phase should limit activity to what can be tolerated. Strict bed rest or isolation is not required. Light duties and work typically can resume within 5–7 days. If the athlete has obvious splenic discomfort and an enlarged spleen, then walking should be limited and stool softeners given until the symptoms resolve and the spleen returns to normal size.

The most difficult decision facing the team physician is when to allow the athlete to resume training. Recommendations have ranged from 3 weeks to 6 months.[84] The most feared complication is that of splenic rupture, especially in individuals involved in strenuous contact sports such as football, ice hockey, lacrosse, rugby, wrestling, basketball, judo, karate, diving, and gymnastics. The current recommended return-to-play criteria for the athlete with IM are as follows:

- Easy jogging or swimming—but not weight lifting, diving, or other strenuous activity—may be resumed any time after day 21 of illness if the athlete subjectively feels ready to resume easy training and if marked or symptomatic splenomegaly is not present.
- For those with clinically enlarged or tender spleens, most activity and all athletic training should be restricted until the splenic discomfort and splenomegaly have totally resolved.
- For those not in strenuous contact sports, full participation can be resumed 1 month after onset of symptoms.
- For those in strenuous contact sports, especially football, early easy training is allowable as energy permits; contact is delayed for at least 1 full month after onset of symptoms if no splenomegaly is present; if splenomegaly is present, ultrasonography should be done at 1- to 2-week intervals until the spleen returns to normal size.

COUGH

Cough is one of the most common reasons for seeking medical care.[85–88] The cause of a cough of short duration is usually easy to find and is typically the result of either a viral URI or a bacterial lower respiratory infection (acute bronchitis or pneumonia). The latter, if accompanied by fever and sputum production, should be treated with antibiotics. Erythromycin, 333 mg given orally three times a day for 10 days, along with the use of an albuterol inhaler, effectively treats uncomplicated community-acquired bronchitis or pneumonia.[89] The diagnostic challenge occurs when the cough becomes persistent, recurrent, or chronic, which is defined as lasting longer

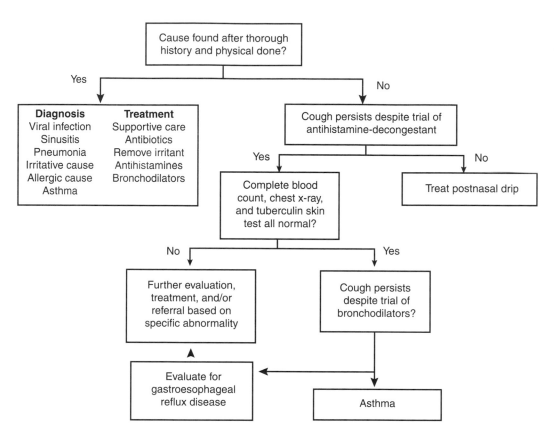

FIGURE 26-1
Evaluation of the chronic cough.

than 3 weeks. The differential diagnosis for a chronic cough is quite long and requires a systematic approach, as outlined in Figure 26-1.[90]

A carefully performed history usually provides most of the critical information for evaluating a chronic cough. Certain medicines, such as angiotensin-converting enzyme (ACE) inhibitors, propranolol, aspirin, and nonsteroidal anti-inflammatory agents, can cause a cough.[91] Fever, weight loss, or decreased energy may indicate a more serious systemic illness. A cough that worsens with exercise suggests reactive airway disease. The physical examination should include a thorough evaluation of the head, neck, and cardiopulmonary system. In nonsmokers who are not taking ACE inhibitors and have normal or nearly normal and stable chest radiographs, 99.4% have postnasal drip syndrome, asthma, or gastroesophageal reflux disease.[92]

Every effort should be made to determine the cause of the cough. The optimal approach to therapy of the cough is first to determine its cause and direct treatment specifically at eliminating it.[87, 93] For example, smokers should be encouraged to stop smoking. An important cause of chronic cough that should not be overlooked is cough-variant asthma.[94, 95] The diagnosis for this common condition should be considered in any athlete who has a cough

lasting more than 2 weeks without an obvious cause, especially if the cough is dry, nocturnal, induced by exercise or cold air, or if there is a family or personal history of atopic disease. In this form of asthma, wheezing is usually not present. Athletes with this history should be given a trial of albuterol, which should ease the cough. The diagnosis can then be confirmed with either an exercise pulmonary function test, which may fail to reproduce the symptoms, or a methacholine challenge pulmonary function test.[90, 96, 97]

Influenza is an acute febrile infection of the respiratory tract that typically occurs during the winter months and is characterized by an abrupt fever, prominent myalgias, headache, and cough. Complications can include pneumonia and myocarditis. The athlete who competes in winter sports and lives in close quarters with other athletes may benefit from receiving the influenza virus vaccine. This vaccine is given annually and is 70–90% effective in preventing the occurrence of disease.[98] The virus in the vaccine is killed and does not cause influenza or produce viremia. Those who have an anaphylactic reaction to eggs should not receive the vaccine. If the athlete develops symptoms suggestive of influenza and there is a known influenza type A outbreak in the area, the duration of the fever and symptoms may be shortened by 1–2 days by starting amantadine or rimantadine within the first 48 hours of symptoms. The usual dosage of both drugs is 100 mg given twice daily for 3–5 days. Common side effects may include loss of appetite, nausea, difficulty in concentrating, nervousness, insomnia, and light-headedness.

If no specific cause for the chronic cough can be found, then nonspecific therapy is directed at the symptom itself (the cough), with the aim being to control but not totally eliminate it. The three most common cough suppressants with proved efficacy are codeine, dextromethorphan, and guaifenesin.[99] The use of codeine is prohibited in international competition. Dextromethorphan is equivalent to codeine and is generally safe at lower dosages, such as 15–30 mg given orally four times a day. However, excessive use at higher doses may cause death.[100]

RETURN-TO-PLAY CRITERIA

Except for those described under the section on infectious mononucleosis, there are no absolute rules on when an athlete should return to play after an acute minor illness. No well-controlled studies have been performed to help elicit return-to-play criteria. However, several considerations should be addressed. First, although it is difficult to prove that an intercurrent viral illness increases the risk of death during exercise, there are numerous anecdotal reports of young athletes dying while vigorously exercising during an acute viral illness.[5, 18] Besides sudden death, it is now well known that during prolonged exercise certain common viruses—such as coxsackievirus, adenovirus, and influenza virus—may cause a myocarditis with subsequent cardiomyopathy.[18, 66] Exercising during subclinical myocarditis has caused some arrhythmia-associated deaths.[101] In addition, acute illnesses, especially when accompanied by fever, and the medicines used to treat them, such as antihistamines, predispose the athlete to a heat injury.[102, 103] Therefore, severe exertion during an acute viral febrile illness or in early convalescence is potentially dangerous and should be avoided.

In addition to the potential serious complications in the athlete, viruses also affect performance with decreased endurance and isometric strength.[18] Also, exercise during an acute illness actually prolongs the condition and may increase its severity. On the other hand, periods of as much as 10 days of inactivity have been shown not to alter the fitness levels of endurance athletes.[104]

Based on these facts, the following general guidelines for return to training are offered, with the realization that they are quite conservative and are not based on well-controlled studies:

- For the athlete who has signs or symptoms of an impending viral infection, the intensity of training should be reduced for 1–2 days.
- For the athlete who has symptoms of a common cold with no other constitutional symptoms, such as fever or myalgias, training can safely be resumed a few days after the symptoms have resolved.
- For the competitive athlete who does not want to miss training days even when ill, a "neck check"[105] can be done. If symptoms are confined to the head (stuffy or runny nose, sneezing, or scratchy throat) with no constitutional symptoms, the athlete can proceed through the scheduled workout at half-speed. After a few minutes, the athlete can gradually increase the intensity and finish the workout if the symptoms improve; however, if the symptoms worsen, the athlete should rest.
- For the athlete who has suspected coxsackievirus or influenza virus infection, or who has a viral infection with myalgias and fever, full training can safely be resumed 2–4 weeks after the symptoms have resolved. It is hoped that this extra time will avoid the complication of myocarditis, cardiomyopathy, and arrhythmia.
- For the athlete who has a documented bacterial infection, full training may resume once the fever has resolved and the athlete feels well.

Of course, the best way for an athlete to ensure no training is missed is to prevent illness. This is best accomplished by eating a well-balanced diet, minimizing life stresses, avoiding overtraining and chronic fatigue, obtaining adequate sleep, avoiding individuals who are ill, and spacing vigorous workouts as far apart as possible.

REFERENCES

1. Lewicki R, Tchorzewski H, Denys A, et al. Effect of physical exercise on some parameters of immunity in conditioned sportsmen. Int J Sports Med 1987;8:309–314.
2. Gabriel H, Kindermann W. The acute immune response to exercise: what does it mean? Int J Sports Med 1997;18 (suppl):28–45.
3. Garagiola U, Buzzetti M, Cardella E, et al. Immunological patterns during regular intensive training in athletes: quantification and evaluation of a preventive pharmacologic approach. J Int Med Res 1995;23:85–95.
4. Stiene H, Black W. Pericarditis in a collegiate basketball player. Clin J Sport Med 1996;6:251–254.
5. Roberts J. Viral illnesses and sports performance. Sports Med 1986;3:296–303.
6. Strauss R, Lanese R, Leizman DJ. Illness and absence among wrestlers, swimmers, and gymnasts at a large university. Am J Sports Med 1988;16:653–655.

7. Weidner T. Reporting behaviors and activity levels of intercollegiate athletes with a URI. Med Sci Sports Exerc 1994;26:22–26.

8. Fitzgerald L. Overtraining increases the susceptibility to infection. Int J Sports Med 1991;12(suppl):5–8.

9. MacKinnon L, Chick T, van As A, Tomasi TB. The effect of exercise on secretory and natural immunity. Adv Exp Med Biol 1987;216:869–876.

10. Nieman D. Exercise, upper respiratory tract infection, and the immune system. Med Sci Sports Exerc 1994;26:128–139.

11. Guarderas J. Rhinitis and sinusitis: office management. Mayo Clin Proc 1996;71:882–888.

12. Knight A. The differential diagnosis of rhinorrhea. J Allergy Clin Immunol 1995;95:1080–1083.

13. Williams J, Simel D. Does this patient have sinusitis? Diagnosing acute sinusitis by history and physical examination. JAMA 1993;270:1242–1246.

14. Katz R. Rhinitis in the athlete. J Allergy Clin Immunol 1984;73:708–711.

15. Milgrom H, Bender B. Adverse effects of medications for rhinitis. Ann Allergy Asthma Immunol 1997;78:439–446.

16. Spector S. The common cold: current therapy and natural history. J Allergy Clin Immunol 1995;95:1133–1138.

17. Lorber B. The common cold. J Gen Intern Med 1996;11:229–236.

18. Sevier T. Infectious disease in athletes. Med Clin North Am 1994;78:389–412.

19. Mainous A, Hueston W, Clark J. Antibiotics and upper respiratory infection: do some folks think there is a cure for the common cold? J Fam Pract 1996;42:357–361.

20. Smith M, Feldman W. Over-the-counter cold medications: a critical review of clinical trials between 1950 and 1991. JAMA 1993;269:2258–2263.

21. Luks D, Anderson M. Antihistamines and the common cold: a review and critique of the literature. J Gen Intern Med 1996;11:240–244.

22. Hayden F, Diamond L, Wood P, et al. Effectiveness and safety of intranasal ipratropium bromide in common colds: a randomized, double-blind, placebo-controlled trial. Ann Intern Med 1996;125:89–97.

23. Hemila H. Vitamin C supplementation and common cold symptoms: problems with inaccurate reviews. Nutrition 1996;12:804–809.

24. Zinc for the common cold. The Medical Letter 1997;39:9–10.

25. Blackwelder RB. Alternative Medicine. Monograph, Edition No. 219, Home Study Self-Assessment Program. Kansas City, MO: American Academy of Family Physicians, August 1997.

26. Naclerio R. Allergic rhinitis. N Engl J Med 1991;325:860–869.

27. Pedinoff A. Approaches to the treatment of seasonal allergic rhinitis. South Med J 1996;89:1130–1139.

28. Noble S, Forbes R, Woodbridge H. Allergic rhinitis. Am Fam Physician 1995;51:837–846.

29. International Rhinitis Management Working Group. International consensus report on the diagnosis and management of rhinitis. Allergy 1994;49(suppl 19):5–34.

30. Milavetz G, Smith JJ. Pharmacotherapy of asthma and allergic rhinitis. Prim Care 1990;17:685–701.

31. Simons F, Simons K. The pharmacology and use of H_1-receptor-antagonist drugs. New Engl J Med 1995;330:1663–1670.

32. Peggs J, Shimp L, Opdycke R. Antihistamines: the old and the new. Am Fam Physician 1995;52:593–600.

33. Montgomery L, Deuster P. Effects of antihistamine medications on exercise performance: implications for sportspeople. Sports Med 1993;15:179–195.

34. Fireman P. Treatment strategies designed to minimize medical complications of allergic rhinitis. Am J Rhinol 1997;11:95–102.

35. Nolen T. Sedative effects of antihistamines: safety, performance, learning, and quality of life. Clin Ther 1997;19:39–55.

36. Day J, Briscoe M, Clark R, et al. Onset of action and efficacy of terfenadine, astemizole, cetirizine, and loratadine for the relief of symptoms of allergic rhinitis. Ann Allergy Asthma Immunol 1997;79:163–172.

37. Kobayashi R, Kiechel F III, Kobayashi A, Mellion M. Topical nasal sprays: treatment of allergic rhinitis. Am Fam Physician 1994;50:151–157.

38. Georgitis J, Banov C, Boggs P. Ipratropium bromide nasal spray in non-allergic rhinitis: efficacy, nasal cytological response and patient evaluation on quality of life. Clin Exp Allergy 1994;24:1049–1055.

39. Voght H. Rhinitis. Prim Care 1990;17:309–322.

40. Druce H. Emerging techniques in the diagnosis of sinusitis. Ann Allergy 1991;66:132–136.

41. Willett L, Carson J, Williams J. Current diagnosis and management of sinusitis. J Gen Intern Med 1995;9:38–45.

42. Diaz I, Bamberger D. Acute sinusitis. Semin Respir Infect 1995;10:14–20.

43. Ferguson B. Acute and chronic sinusitis: how to ease symptoms and locate the cause. Postgrad Med 1995;97:45–57.

44. van Buchem F, Knottnerus J, Schrijnemaekers V, Peeters M. Primary-care-based randomised placebo-controlled trial of antibiotic treatment in acute maxillary sinusitis. Lancet 1997;349:683–687.

45. Stalman W, van Essen G, van der Graaf Y, de Melker R. Maxillary sinusitis in adults: an evaluation of placebo-controlled double-blind trials. Fam Pract 1997;14:124–129.

46. Poole M. Antimicrobial therapy for sinusitis. Otolaryngol Clin North Am 1997;30:331–339.

47. Williams J, Holleman D, Samsa G, Simel D. Randomized controlled trial of 3 vs 10 days of trimethoprim/sulfamethoxazole for acute maxillary sinusitis. JAMA 1995;273:1015–1021.

48. Amundson L. Disorders of the external ear. Prim Care 1990;17:213–231.

49. Macknin M, Talo H, Medendrop S. Effect of cotton-tipped swab use on ear-wax occlusion. Clin Pediatr (Phila) 1994;33:14–18.

50. Freeman R. Impacted cerumen: how to safely remove ear-wax in an office visit. Geriatrics 1995;50:52–53.

51. Bojrab D, Bruderly T, Abdulrazzak Y. Otitis externa. Otolaryngol Clin North Am 1996;29:761–782.

52. Kemp E. Otitis media. Prim Care 1990;17:267–287.
53. Goycoolea M, Hueb M, Ruah C. Definitions and terminology. Otolaryngol Clin North Am 1991;24:757–761.
54. Cantekin E, Mandel E, Bluestone C, et al. Lack of efficacy of a decongestant-antihistamine combination for otitis media with effusion ("secretory" otitis media) in children: results of a double-blind, randomized trial. N Engl J Med 1983;308:297–301.
55. Cantekin E, McGuire T, Griffith T. Antimicrobial therapy for otitis media with effusion ("secretory" otitis media). JAMA 1991;226:3309–3317.
56. Berman S. Otitis media in children. New Engl J Med 1995;332:1560–1565.
57. Cohen H, Kauschansky A, Ashkenasi A, et al. Swimming and grommets. J Fam Pract 1994;38:30–32.
58. Bartelds A, Bowers P, Bridges-Webb C, et al. Acute otitis media in adults: a report from the International Primary Care Network. J Am Board Fam Pract 1993;6: 333–339.
59. Jordan M. Clinical approach to treatment of otitis media. Otolaryngol Clin North Am 1991;24:901–904.
60. Weiss J, Yates G, Quinn L. Acute otitis media: making an accurate diagnosis. Am Fam Physician 1996;53: 1200–1206.
61. Kligman E. Treatment of otitis media. Am Fam Physician 1992;45:242–250.
62. Gooch W, Blair E, Puopolo A. Effectiveness of five days of therapy with cefuroxime axetil suspension for treatment of acute otitis media. Pediatr Infect Dis J 1996;15:157–164.
63. Evans P, Miser WF. Sinusitis and Pharyngitis. In R Taylor (ed), Family Medicine: Principles and Practice (5th ed). New York: Springer-Verlag, 1997;337–344.
64. Denny F. Tonsillopharyngitis 1994. Pediatr Rev 1994;15: 185–191.
65. Loos G. Pharyngitis, croup, and epiglottitis. Prim Care 1990;17:335–345.
66. Burch G. Viral diseases of the heart. Acta Cardiol 1979;1:5–9.
67. Vukmir R. Adult and pediatric pharyngitis: a review. J Emerg Med 1992;10:607–616.
68. Kiselica D. Group A beta-hemolytic streptococcal pharyngitis: current clinical concepts. Am Fam Physician 1994; 49:1147–1154.
69. Rabinowitz H. Upper respiratory tract infections. Prim Care 1990;17:793–809.
70. Pichichero M. Group A streptococcal pharyngitis: cost-effective diagnosis and treatment. Ann Emerg Med 1995;25:390–403.
71. Dajani A, Taubert K, Ferrieri P, et al. Treatment of acute streptococcal pharyngitis and prevention of rheumatic fever: a statement for health professionals. Pediatrics 1995;96:758–764.
72. Perkins A. An approach to diagnosing the acute sore throat. Am Fam Physician 1997;55:131–138.
73. O'Brien J, Meade J, Falk J. Dexamethasone as adjuvant therapy for severe acute pharyngitis. Ann Emerg Med 1993;22:212–215.
74. Epperly T, Wood T. New trends in the management of peritonsillar abscess. Am Fam Physician 1990;42:102–112.
75. Maki D, Reich R. Infectious mononucleosis in the athlete: diagnosis, complications, and management. Am J Sports Med 1982;10:162–173.
76. Chetham M, Roberts K. Infectious mononucleosis in adolescents. Pediatr Ann 1991;20:206–213.
77. Haines J. When to resume sports after infectious mononucleosis: how soon is safe? Postgrad Med 1987;81:331–333.
78. Bailey R. Diagnosis and treatment of infectious mononucleosis. Am Fam Physician 1994;49:879–885.
79. Dommerby H, Stangerup S, Stangerup M, Hancke S. Hepatosplenomegaly in infectious mononucleosis, assessed by ultrasonic scanning. J Laryngol Otol 1986;100: 573–579.
80. Grover S, Barkun A, Sackett D. Does this patient have splenomegaly? JAMA 1993;270:2218–2221.
81. Safran D, Bloom G. Spontaneous splenic rupture following infectious mononucleosis. Am Surg 1990;56:601–605.
82. Farley D, Zietlow S, Bannon M, Farnell M. Spontaneous rupture of the spleen due to infectious mononucleosis. Mayo Clin Proc 1992;67:846–853.
83. Schuler J, Filtzer H. Spontaneous splenic rupture: the role of nonoperative management. Arch Surg 1995;130:662–665.
84. Rutkow I. Rupture of the spleen in infectious mononucleosis: a critical review. Arch Surg 1978;113:718–720.
85. Kamei R. Chronic cough in children. Pediatr Clin North Am 1991;38:593–605.
86. Fuller R, Jackson D. Physiology and treatment of cough. Thorax 1990;45:425–430.
87. Irwin R, Curley F. The treatment of cough: a comprehensive review. Chest 1991;99:1477–1484.
88. Johnson D, Osborn L. Cough variant asthma: a review of the clinical literature. J Asthma 1991;28:85–90.
89. Hueston W. Albuterol delivered by metered-dose inhaler to treat acute bronchitis. J Fam Pract 1994;39:437–440.
90. Pratter M. An algorithmic approach to chronic cough. Ann Intern Med 1993;119:977–983.
91. Meeker D, Wiedemann H. Drug-induced bronchospasm. Clin Chest Med 1990;11:163–175.
92. Mello C, Irwin R, Curley F. Diagnosis of chronic cough. Arch Intern Med 1996;156:997–1003.
93. Lalloo U, Barnes P, Chung K. Pathophysiology and clinical presentations of cough. J Allergy Clin Immunol 1996;98 (suppl):91–96.
94. Miser WF. Variant forms of asthma. Am Fam Physician 1987;35:89–96.
95. Katz R. Exercise-induced asthma/other allergic reactions in the athlete. Allergy Proc 1989;10:203–208.
96. Eggleston P. Methods of exercise challenge. J Allergy Clin Immunol 1984;73:666–669.
97. Shapiro G. Methacholine challenge: relevance for the allergic athlete. J Allergy Clin Immunol 1984;73:670–675.
98. Zimmerman R, Ruben F, Ahwesh E. Influenza, influenza vaccine, and amantadine/rimantadine. J Fam Pract 1997; 45:107–124.
99. Croughan-Minihane M, Petitti D, Rodnick J, Eliaser G.

Clinical trial examining effectiveness of three cough syrups. J Am Board Fam Pract 1993;6:109–115.

100. Pender E, Parks B. Toxicity with dextromethorphan-containing preparations: a literature review and report of two additional cases. Pediatr Emerg Care 1991;7:163–165.

101. Burke A, Farb V, Virmani R, et al. Sports-related and non–sports-related sudden cardiac death in young adults. Am Heart J 1991;121:568–575.

102. Feinstein R. Heat-related illnesses in the athlete. Compr Ther 1985;11:31–37.

103. Squire D. Heat illness. Pediatr Clin North Am 1990;37: 1085–1109.

104. Cullinane E, Sady S, Vadeboncoeur L, et al. Cardiac size and VO$_2$max do not decrease after short-term exercise cessation. Med Sci Sports Exerc 1986;18:420–424.

105. Eichner E. Neck check. Runner's World 1992;27:16.

27

Dermatologic Problems in Athletes

MARK A. CROWE AND GREGORY W. SORENSEN

Dermatologic problems are frequently found among athletes. To diagnose and manage the common dermatologic disorders, one must have a basic understanding of the skin and the terms used to describe it. The skin is the largest organ in the body and has many valuable functions. It serves as a protective layer and fluid barrier, protecting the body against the outside elements while keeping fluids within the body. It has an important role in heat regulation, in body metabolism, and as a sensory organ. The skin is composed of three layers: the epidermis, the dermis, and the subcutis. The epidermis, the thinnest and outermost layer, consists mainly of keratinocytes and is responsible for the barrier function of the skin. The dermis is the middle layer and consists mainly of connective tissue and of vessels and nerves. The subcutis is the bottom layer and is composed primarily of fat cells. Each layer of the skin varies in thickness, depending on which area of the body it covers.

To provide appropriate care to athletes with skin disorders, practitioners must be familiar with the terms used to describe the primary and secondary lesions that occur on the skin. The following are terms for primary lesions:

- *Macule*—a nonpalpable circumscribed change in skin color of any size or shape
- *Patch*—most commonly defined as a very large macule
- *Papule*—a raised, circumscribed lesion 1 cm or less in diameter
- *Nodule*—a raised lesion more than 1 cm in diameter
- *Plaque*—a generally flat elevation more than 1 cm in diameter
- *Vesicle*—a fluid-filled elevation 1 cm or less in diameter
- *Bulla*—a fluid-filled elevation more than 1 cm in diameter
- *Pustule*—an elevated pus-filled lesion
- *Wheal (hive)*—a transient elevated lesion caused by an increase in localized interstitial fluid

The common secondary lesions are defined as follows:

- *Crust*—the dried residue of blood, pus, or other fluid.
- *Comedo*—a sebaceous follicle with a keratin plug.
- *Scale*—an excess of keratin material on the skin.
- *Excoriation*—an erosion secondary to scratching.
- *Erosion*—a partial thickness loss of epidermis that does not extend into the dermis.
- *Ulcer*—a deeper lesion that extends into the dermis, usually appearing sunken.
- *Fissure*—a cracklike break in the skin that extends into the dermis.
- *Scar*—a fibrous lesion caused by healing of a wound.
- *Eczema*—a superficial inflammatory process involving primarily the epidermis, characterized early by redness, itching, minute papules and vesicles, weeping, oozing, and crusting, and later by scaling, lichenification, and often hyperpigmentation. It is not a disease entity or an acceptable diagnosis.

Dermatologic problems in athletes have many causes, ranging from infections of the skin by bacteria, viruses, and fungi, to dermatoses secondary to physical factors (such as sunshine and friction) and endogenous dermatoses (such as dyshidrotic eczema). Most of these conditions can be treated by the primary care provider. This chapter covers the common skin disorders seen in the sports medicine clinic. Many disorders discussed in this chapter are not peculiar to athletes; however, they may either be exacerbated by athletic activities or are particularly common in athletes. Most of the disorders are presented according to their location on the body. Basic treatment plans are discussed.

Many dermatologic disorders classically present in specific regions of the body. The disorders listed in Table 27-1 are grouped according to the most common distri-

TABLE 27-1
Simplified Regional Differential Diagnosis

Region	Diagnosis	Region	Diagnosis
Generalized dermatoses	Acne vulgaris	Trunk	Folliculitis (classical and hot tub)
	Contact dermatitis		Herpes zoster
	Folliculitis		Jogger's nipple
	Miliaria		Paget's disease
	Urticaria		Pityriasis rosea
	Xerosis		Psoriasis
Scalp	Alopecia areata		Tinea versicolor
	Folliculitis	Buttocks	Folliculitis (hot tub)
	Green hair		Furunculosis
	Pilar cyst		Herpes simplex
	Psoriasis		Scabies
	Seborrheic dermatitis		Tinea
	Tinea	Groin	Condyloma (warts)
Face	Erysipelas		Contact dermatitis
	Herpes simplex/zoster		Herpes simplex
	Impetigo		Hidradenitis suppurativa
	Lupus erythematosus		Molluscum contagiosum
	Molluscum contagiosum		Pearly penile papules
	Rosacea		Pediculosis (lice)
	Seborrheic dermatitis		Scabies
	Tinea		Tinea
	Warts (flat)	Leg	Abrasions
Lips	Allergic contact dermatitis		Bites
	Angioedema		Cellulitis
	Aphthous ulcer		Erythema nodosum
	Herpes simplex		Granuloma annulare
	Mucous cyst		Xerosis
Ear	Seborrheic dermatitis	Foot	Calcaneal petechiae (black heel)
	Swimmer's ear		Contact dermatitis
	Nickel contact dermatitis		Corn (clavus)
Axillae	Acanthosis nigricans		Dyshidrotic eczema
	Erythrasma		Granuloma annulare
	Hidradenitis suppurativa		Immersion foot
	Striae distensae		Onychomycosis
	Tinea		Pernio
Arms and forearms	Atopic dermatitis		Piezogenic papules
	Insect bite		Pitted keratolysis
	Keratosis pilaris		Psoriasis (pustular)
Hand	Calluses		Scabies
	Contact dermatitis		Subungual hematoma
	Dyshidrotic eczema		Subungual melanoma
	Herpes simplex (whitlow)		Syphilis (secondary)
	Onychomycosis		Tinea—dry, toe web, bullous
	Paronychia		Turf toe
	Scabies		Wart
	Syphilis (secondary)		
	Tinea (two foot—one hand)		
	Wart		

butions. Not all of these disorders are discussed in this chapter. However, this table may serve to widen your differential diagnosis when evaluating difficult cases.

Table 27-2 contains a list of differential diagnoses based on the primary lesion type or symptom. It is an abbrevi-

ated list but may also serve to direct you to the more common disorders that present with these classic lesions. There are several general rules to keep in mind when evaluating the athlete with a rash. Because occult or partially treated fungal infections are exceedingly common and frequently misdiagnosed, always consider this diagnosis when evaluating any localized area of eczema. Allergic or irritant contact dermatitis should also be included in the differential diagnosis of localized eczema, particularly if pruritus is a chief symptom. Scabies should always be considered in the patient with severe pruritus and nonspecific papular dermatitis.

GENERALIZED DERMATOSES

Dry Skin

Dry skin, or xerosis, is a disorder often seen in swimmers and in athletes who shower frequently. It is also more common in dry environments and cold winter months. Very low humidity and repeated cycles of wetting and drying contribute greatly to this condition. The most commonly affected areas include the hands, face, and lower legs. Xerosis is characterized by superficial fissures and fine, dry scales. Patients should avoid prolonged hot showers or baths. Short showers or baths in lukewarm water with limited use of soap are the preferred bathing method. When leaving the shower or pool, patients should liberally apply emollients while the skin is still moist. Mild to moderate potency topical steroids may be used to reduce associated erythema and pruritus.

Papules and Pustules

Acne vulgaris and folliculitis are two pustular diseases prevalent in the athletic population.

Acne Vulgaris

Acne vulgaris is characterized by multiple comedones and erythematous papules and pustules. These lesions are usually distributed on the face, neck, back, and chest. Acne is most common in the teenage years, but can persist throughout adult life. It is a complex disorder of the pilosebaceous unit, controlled largely by genetics, hormones, and bacteria. Physical factors in athletes, such as pressure, occlusion, friction, and heat acting on the skin, either separately or in unison, may also exacerbate acne. Despite the complexity of the disease, treatment is straightforward and usually effective. Patients should be counseled that foods and cleanliness are not etiologic factors in acne. Mild cases should be treated with topical therapy. A combination of topical antibiotics solutions (such as clindamycin 1% or erythromycin 2%) along with either 5% benzoyl peroxide gel or tretinoin (Retin-A) 0.05% cream is usually very effective. Tretinoin should be applied in the evening and benzoyl peroxide in the morning or twice a day. Therapy for 6–8 weeks is needed before improve-

TABLE 27-2
Differential Diagnosis by Lesion or Symptom Type

Lesion or Symptom Type	Diagnosis
Macules	Black heel
	Tinea versicolor
	Vitiligo
Papules	Acne
	Cherry angiomas
	Dermatofibroma
	Keratosis pilaris
	Molluscum contagiosum
	Nevi
	Scabies
	Tinea
	Warts
Nodules	Athlete's nodules
Plaques	Lichen simplex chronicus
	Pityriasis rosea
	Psoriasis
	Tinea
Vesicles	Bug bites
	Chickenpox
	Dyshidrotic eczema
	Herpes simplex
	Herpes zoster
Bulla	Contact dermatitis
	Epidermolysis bullosa
	Tinea pedis
	Traumatic blisters
Pustules	Acne
	Bug bites
	Folliculitis
	Impetigo
	Tinea
Eczema	Atopic dermatitis
	Contact dermatitis
	Seborrheic dermatitis
	Tinea
Pruritus	Allergic contact dermatitis
	Bug bites
	Scabies
	Urticaria

ment in the symptoms occurs. In moderate and severe cases, an oral antibiotic is added to the regimen. Tetracycline, 500 mg twice a day, is considered first-line oral therapy. Severe cases of cystic acne vulgaris should be referred to a dermatologist for evaluation and treatment.

The provider should also be aware of steroid-induced acne. High dosages of testosterone and anabolic-androgenic steroids, often self-administered by athletes, increase the cutaneous population of *Propionibacterium acnes* and the cholesterol and free fatty acids of the skin surface lipids. Acne, oily hair and skin, sebaceous cysts, a receding hair line, hirsutism, androgenic alopecia, striae atrophicae, seborrheic dermatitis, and secondary infections, including furunculosis, may occur in persons using these drugs. Linear keloid formation has been reported in adolescent male weight lifters 8–14 months after the use of anabolic steroids. This skin damage is caused by the rapid development of underlying muscle groups, especially the deltoids.

Acne Mechanica

Acne mechanica is a papulopustular eruption caused by the physical factors of pressure, occlusion, friction, and heat. This disorder is the result of the friction and heat caused by the contact between athletic apparel (from leotards to football helmets) and the underlying skin. The eruption is particularly common in football players where bulky padding comes in direct contact with the skin. This includes areas of the forehead, shoulders, and back. The disorder has also been reported in weight lifters whose backs are in contact with plastic-covered weight benches. The simplest form of prevention is the use of a clean cotton T-shirt under uniforms and equipment.[1, 2]

Folliculitis

Folliculitis presents as small pustules centered around hair follicles. This condition usually arises on the extremities or scalp. *Staphylococcus aureus* is the etiologic organism. If only a few lesions are present, treatment consists of washing with soap and water twice a day and applying a topical antibiotic (bacitracin or mupirocin). In widespread cases, an oral antibiotic is added to the therapy. A penicillinase-resistant penicillin, erythromycin, or cephalosporin (such as cephalexin, 250–500 mg given orally four times a day) is appropriate. "Hot tub" folliculitis is a common form of the disease found in young athletes. Several days after using a hot tub, pustules develop on the trunk and buttocks. *Pseudomonas aeruginosa*, the etiologic agent, thrives in improperly treated water. Hot tub folliculitis will resolve spontaneously by avoiding the contaminated hot tub.

Vesicles and Bullae

The most common lesions of vesicles and bullae in athletes are contact dermatitis and miliaria. Pruritic patches of vesicles on a weeping erythematous base are characteristic of contact dermatitis, whereas groups of discrete 1- to 3-mm pruritic vesicles on the trunk, antecubital and popliteal fossa, and groin are found in miliaria.

Contact Dermatitis

Dermatitis produced by an environmental exposure to either an irritant or allergen is exceedingly common. Contact dermatitis is generally subdivided into irritant contact dermatitis and allergic contact dermatitis. Irritant dermatitis is due to a nonallergic reaction resulting from exposure of the skin to an irritating substance. With a high enough concentration, an irritant will cause dermatitis in any patient and may occur during the first exposure. Patients with an irritant contact dermatitis may develop symptoms within minutes of the exposure. The dermatitis is often localized to the site of exposure and a burning sensation is more common than the intense pruritus associated with allergic contact dermatitis. The severity of dermatitis is dependent on the concentration and dwell time of the irritant and the site and condition of the skin. Areas of the body with thick, dry skin are the most resistant to the effects of irritants.

Examples of an irritant dermatitis include the reaction that results from contact with acids, alkalis, and metal salts. Bromine and chlorine (commonly used in hot tubs and swimming pools), as well as many hydrocarbons produce an irritant dermatitis. The dermatitis produced by excessive use of harsh soaps or detergents is most frequently an irritant reaction, but can represent an allergic reaction to perfumes, dyes, lanolin, deodorants, or antiperspirants in soap.

Allergic contact dermatitis is an acquired hypersensitivity response generated after exposure to an allergen. Not all patients will react to the allergen, and the allergic response does not occur during the primary exposure unless the patient has been exposed to a closely related compound in the past. Symptoms of allergic contact dermatitis usually develop hours to days after exposure. The dermatitis associated with allergic reactions is frequently very pruritic and may extend beyond the borders of the region exposed to the allergen. Allergic contact dermatitis is generally much more edematous than that seen in an irritant contact dermatitis and vesiculation is much more common. Compared with irritant contactants, very small quantities of allergens are required to stimulate the dermatitis.

Patch testing can often confirm the etiology of allergic contact dermatitis. By placing standard concentrations of common allergens or specific ingredients of an implicated product on the skin and leaving them covered for 2 days, one may identify the cause of the dermatitis.

When contact dermatitis is suspected and the contactant is not obvious, the provider must specifically question the patient regarding environmental exposures. An environmental exposure history should include a detailed description of daily activities with emphasis on exposures to materials, such as paints, dyes, cleaning solutions, and soaps, and protective gear such as eyewear and gloves. Protective gear with black rubber seals are particularly common causes of allergic contact dermatitis. Often, a site visit is very productive. The patient should be asked whether symptoms improve or worsen over weekends or vacations. It is important to ask about exposures in the home and in recreational activities. The patient should be asked about exposures related to hobbies and if any topical or oral therapy is being used. The information contained in Table 27-3 may also suggest a line of questioning that might prove helpful.

In acute contact dermatitis, the involved areas should be thoroughly cleansed with plain water to prevent further dermatitis. Calamine lotion or wet dressings with Burow solution may be applied to an allergic contact dermatitis to ease the symptoms. An oral antihistamine, such as hydroxyzine or diphenhydramine, will also help control symptoms. Vesicles may be drained, but the roof should be left intact. As the vesicles subside, a topical corticosteroid should be applied (triamcinolone spray is quite effective). In moderate to severe cases, a 10- to 14-day course of prednisone, 40–60 mg per day, is recommended.

Miliaria

Miliaria, or "heat rash," occurs when sweat cannot reach the surface of the skin because the sweat duct is occluded. It is common in hot, humid environments or any time a person perspires heavily. Treatment involves placing the patient in a cool, dry area and avoiding further sweating. Hydrophilic ointments, such as Eucerin (Beiersdorf, Inc., Norwalk, CT), can be applied to help open the occluded ducts. Athletes should be aware that hypohidrosis may follow a case of miliaria. This can last for several weeks and places the athlete at risk of heat injuries; it can also impair performance.

Wheals

Urticaria is a disease process characterized by episodes of pruritic wheal formation. These transient lesions may occur anywhere on the body. They may appear acutely or recur chronically. An anaphylactic reaction is acute urticaria associated with respiratory or cardiovascular symptoms and should be treated appropriately. Most cases of urticaria, however, are not associated with anaphylaxis. The etiology of urticaria includes foods, drugs, autoimmune disease, and physical factors such as cold, sun, and pressure. Although multiple etiologies have been identified, often a causative agent is not discovered. The most effective treatment is to avoid the causative agent, if known. Antihistamines, such as hydroxyzine, 25–50 mg given orally every 4–6 hours, are frequently effective at suppressing the urticaria, but daily therapy for several weeks or months may be required.

TABLE 27-3
Allergic Contact Dermatitis: Clues by Distribution

Location	Material
Scalp and ears	Shampoo, hair dyes, metal earrings, eyeglasses, ear plugs, bathing caps
Eyelids	Nail polish (transferred by rubbing), cosmetics, contact lens solution, swim goggles
Face	Airborne allergens (poison ivy from burning leaves, ragweed), cosmetics, sunscreens, nose clips
Lips	Lip balms, lipstick, toothpaste, mouthwash, bubble gum
Neck	Necklaces, perfumes, aftershave lotion, rubber or leather supporting straps
Trunk	Topical medication, sunscreens, poison ivy, clothing, undergarments (e.g., spandex bras, elastic waistbands), metal belt buckles, dive suits
Axillae	Deodorant (axillary vault), clothing (axillary folds)
Hands	Soaps and detergents, foods, poison ivy, solvents and oils, cement, metal, topical medications, rubber or leather gloves, athletic tape
Arms	Same as hands; watch and watchband
Genitals	Poison ivy (transferred by hand), rubber condoms
Anal region	Hemorrhoid preparations (benzocaine, dibucaine)
Lower legs	Topical medication (benzocaine, lanolin, neomycin, parabens), dye in socks
Feet	Shoes (rubber or leather), topical medications, fins, fin straps, athletic tape

Many forms of urticaria may be induced or exacerbated by athletic activity. These include cold urticaria, cholinergic urticaria, dermatographism, pressure urticaria, aquagenic pruritus, aquagenic urticaria, solar urticaria, heat urticaria, papular urticaria, and exercise-induced urticaria.

Cold Urticaria

Cold urticaria can occur in winter athletes and swimmers. Urticarial plaques do not develop in the cold environment, but shortly after rewarming. Wheals can be generalized or confined to the area exposed to the cold. Application of ice to the skin for 5 minutes and the development of wheals immediately on warming confirms the diagnosis. Treatment includes avoiding cold, wearing protective clothing, and using antihistamines.

Solar Urticaria

Solar urticaria is a form of photosensitivity. Itching and burning are followed by erythema, and then wheals.

Symptoms develop within minutes after exposure to sunlight and usually clear within 1 hour after exposure. The reaction is most severe in normally unexposed areas (such as the trunk) and occurs less commonly on the face and hands. All wavelengths of ultraviolet light can cause solar urticaria. Complete sunblock or protective clothing is required to prevent the disorder.

Cholinergic Urticaria

Cholinergic urticaria is also known as heat-induced or stress-induced urticaria. It consists of pinpoint erythematous wheals surrounded by an erythematous flare and extreme pruritus after exposure to heat or during exercise. Cholinergic urticaria may be very resistant to therapy. Treatment consists of antihistamines, usually hydroxyzine. In some individuals, avoiding heat and exercise may be the only means of obtaining relief.

Aquagenic Pruritus and Urticaria

Rarely, individuals may develop pruritus or wheals on exposure to water at any temperature. Antihistamines may provide relief.

Pressure Urticaria

In patients with pressure urticaria, severe swelling and deep pain occur 3–12 hours after local pressure has been applied. Unlike other urticarial reactions, there may be a latent period of as much as 12 hours before the symptoms develop, with the symptoms lasting for 8–24 hours. It can be very resistant to therapy. Antihistamines are ineffective, and chronic oral corticosteroids may be required in severe cases.

Papular Urticaria

Papular urticaria consists of pruritic lesions found most commonly on the extremities. Lesions are usually more pruritic at night and are most commonly the result of hypersensitivity to insect bites. Treatment includes antihistamines and exposure prevention with protective clothing or insect repellents.

Exercise-Induced Anaphylaxis

The most severe form of exercise-induced urticaria is exercise-induced anaphylaxis. Symptoms develop shortly after the start of exercise with cutaneous warmth progressing to pruritus, erythema, urticaria, angioedema, respiratory distress, and possible vascular collapse. Acute episodes are treated as any anaphylactic episode (i.e., epinephrine and antihistamines). Patients with this disorder should never exercise alone, and an epinephrine injection should be on hand at all times during exercise. Episodes may be prevented by taking a long-acting nonsedating antihistamine 1 hour before exercise or 40 mg of prednisone 12 hours before exercise if the antihistamine is ineffective.

ENVIRONMENTAL DERMATOSES

Skin disorders, such as sunburn and frostbite, which are caused by environmental factors, occur frequently among athletes. Prevention is the most effective treatment for these dermatoses.[3]

Sunburn

Sunburn is an avoidable injury. Ultraviolet radiation from the sun causes both acute and long-term skin damage. Acute reactions range from mild erythema to intense erythema with blistering and edema. Sunburn should be treated with cool compresses, a low- to midpotency topical corticosteroid, and avoidance of further exposure. Patients with severe burns may also receive a 3- to 7-day course of prednisone, 40–60 mg given orally, once a day. Sun exposure significantly increases the risk for skin cancer and produces changes such as wrinkling, thinning of the skin, and solar lentigos frequently misinterpreted as "old skin." It is recommended that all persons apply a sunscreen with a sun protection factor of at least 15 before any sun exposure.

Photosensitivity Reactions

Photosensitivity reactions may also occur in athletes. Certain drugs can cause patients to have abnormal reactions to the sun. These reactions range from sunburns to eczematous dermatitis and usually occur on sun-exposed areas of the body. Commonly used drugs, such as tetracyclines, sulfonamides, and thiazides, can cause these reactions. Treatment involves local measures, withdrawal of the drug, and use of sunscreens. Urticarial reactions to sun exposure were discussed earlier in this chapter.

Seabather's Eruption

Seabather's eruption occurs in athletes who participate in saltwater sports along the Gulf Coast of Florida, off the coast of Long Island, and in many parts of the Caribbean. The condition begins as a pruritic, urticarial, erythematous, maculopapular eruption in a bathing suit distribution and progresses to itchy papules, wheals, and pustules that resemble insect bites. These lesions develop into eschars. Chills, fever, swelling, headache, nausea, and vomiting may develop. The eruption may take 1–2 days to develop and, if untreated, will last 2–14 days. The causative agents vary, but all appear to be stinging larvae of species such as jellyfish, man-of-war, sea anemone, or fire coral. Prevention includes closure of the offending beach area by public health officials until the threat clears, thorough cleaning of swimwear, and showering after swimming in potentially infected waters. Treatment includes cool compresses, antihistamines, and topical steroids. Not all patients respond to these measures, and severe cases may require oral corticosteroids or thiabendazole.[3, 5]

Swimmer's Itch

Swimmer's itch is similar to seabather's eruption, developing after swimming in fresh water of the northern United States and Canada. An urticarial reaction is caused by the cercarial form of nonhuman schistosomes or flukes. The acute reaction clears and is replaced by a papular eruption. Swimmer's itch occurs on exposed areas, whereas seabather's eruption is usually on skin covered by a bathing suit. Treatment is symptomatic, and the lesions regress spontaneously, clearing completely in 1–2 weeks.

Grain Itch

Athletes, such as equestrians, who work in or around stables that contain dry hay or barley, are at risk for grain itch. Grain itch is caused by a small mite, *Pyemotes tritici*. This small mite produces a pruritic papular urticarial eruption in exposed individuals. Lesions are most common on the trunk, often with a central vesicle or hemorrhagic punctum. Because the mites do not live on human skin, therapy is symptomatic. Prevention includes limiting exposure and prompt showering after exposures. Work areas may be treated with 2% deodorized malathion emulsion to eliminate the offending mites.

Cold Injuries

Local cold injuries are divided into chilblain, frostbite, and immersion foot (see discussion under Foot Problems). The ears, nose, fingers, and toes are the areas most commonly affected by cold injury.

Chilblain

Chilblain, the mildest form of cold injury, is a recurrent localized erythema and swelling caused by exposure to cold. Blistering and ulcerations may develop in severe cases. Patients are usually unaware of the injury at first, but later burning, itching, and redness may develop. The areas are bluish red and are cool to the touch. Involved areas should be warmed, massaged gently, and protected against further injury and exposure to cold or dampness. If the feet are affected, woolen socks should be worn at night during the cold months.

Frostbite

Frostbite occurs when tissue becomes frozen. Superficial frostbite involves the skin and subcutaneous tissues, whereas deep frostbite may include muscles, tendons, and nerves. Frostbitten tissue appears cold, white, and firm but there is little or no pain until thawing occurs. Frozen areas should be rewarmed as rapidly as possible in warm water (100°–110°F). However, rewarming should be accomplished only when the patient is not at risk of refreezing the affected part. Analgesics are generally needed during the thawing. After the injured tissue is rewarmed, edema and blistering may occur. The affected area may be kept dry and open to the air. In all but the most superficial cases, it is recommended that patients be evaluated by a surgeon experienced in the treatment of frostbite.

TRAUMATIC DERMATOSES

Acute trauma to the skin may produce contusions, black heel or petechiae of the heel, black toe (bleeding under the nail), "jogger's nipple" caused by chafing, and foot blisters. Chronic trauma may result in sport-specific calluses and corns.

Hard fibrous nodules developing as a result of recurrent trauma and friction in certain sports have been called *athlete's nodules*.[2-4] Surfers, boxers, marble players, and football players are some athletes in whom these lesions have been observed. The nodules can be found on the dorsal aspects of the feet, knees, or knuckles and can usually be readily differentiated from other conditions by clinical history. These lesions result from recurrent trauma and friction to the involved areas. Treatment options include avoidance of the repetitive skin trauma, padding, or surgical excision.

The peculiar sport-specific lesions discussed in the following pages are just a few of the repetitive motion injuries reported. Many of these lesions may be corrected by using proper equipment or technique. Although some of these disorders are of little or no clinical significance, they serve to demonstrate the types of unusual injuries produced by athletic activities.

FOOT PROBLEMS

Papules and Nodules

Three problems commonly present with rough papules and nodules on the foot: corns, calluses, and plantar warts. Corns and calluses are responses to chronic friction and pressure to the skin; plantar warts are caused by the human papillomavirus.

Corns and Calluses

Corns and calluses are commonly found over the bony prominences of the foot and between the toes. Corns are small, hard conical lesions. Calluses are larger, circumscribed, hyperkeratotic lesions. Corns and calluses can be differentiated from plantar warts by paring the lesion in question with a sharp blade. Warts reveal small black dots (thrombosed capillaries), corns reveal a translucent core, and calluses show a thickened epidermis with normal skin lines apparent. The most critical aspect of treatment is removing the source of pressure—by modifying footwear or by using moleskin or foam rubber pads on the foot to redistribute pressure. The lesions may be removed by paring with a sharp blade, abrading with a pumice stone or emery board, or applying a keratolytic such as salicylic acid (plaster or solution). Patients should be taught to rub these lesions with a pumice stone regularly. Surgical excision of the lesion or correction of an underlying bony abnormality is rarely necessary.

Plantar Warts

Plantar warts are found on the plantar surface of the foot and are often resistant to therapy. They are most effectively treated with a combination of keratolytic therapy and paring. Keratolytic solutions, such as 17% salicylic acid in collodion (Duofilm, Occlusal, Compound W) or 40% salicylic acid plaster (Mediplast) should be applied and occluded overnight. The wart should then be pared the next day. This should be repeated on a daily basis until a satisfactory result is achieved; this often takes several weeks. Cryotherapy with liquid nitrogen can be repeated every 2–3 weeks. This is frequently effective but painful and may take many applications. Electrosurgery and surgical excision can all be used in resistant cases; however, scarring is a possible side effect of these treatments, and recurrence in the region of the scar is common.

Surfer's Nodules

In athletes, clinically similar nodules each produced by different pathophysiologic processes may arise and are somewhat sports specific. Five different types of surfer's nodules, ulcers, or knots have been described based on clinical appearance and underlying pathology. They appear on the anterior tibia, knee, or dorsum of the foot. Another example is a nodular lesion appearing on the dorsum of the foot observed in a woman who wore tight-fitting athletic shoes. This was termed "Nike nodules." Similar lesions, referred to as "skate bites," have been described in hockey players.[3]

Piezogenic Papules

Piezogenic papules are multiple 2- to 5-mm skin-colored herniations of subdermal fat on the lateral or medial surfaces of the heel. They are usually noticeable only on standing. They are most common in long-distance runners and may be so painful that running must be discontinued. A heel cup in the athlete's shoe may help to reduce pain.[3]

Papulosquamous Disease

Tinea Pedis (Athlete's Foot)

Tinea pedis, athlete's foot, a superficial dermatophytic fungal infection, is by far the most common papulosquamous disease involving the foot. It usually presents with pruritus and scaling on the sole and lateral aspects of the foot, often with maceration and fissures between the toes. Vesicles and bullae may also be found. The diagnosis is confirmed by potassium hydroxide (KOH) preparation or fungal culture. Most cases respond promptly to topical antifungal agents, such as miconazole or clotrimazole. Severe or recalcitrant cases can be treated with oral griseofulvin. Severe, foul-smelling, watery dermatitis involving the toes may indicate secondary gram-negative infection.

Immersion Foot

Trench foot and tropical immersion foot are two forms of injury usually restricted to the military. However, with the increasing popularity of activities, such as environmental endurance races, these types of injuries are becoming more common in athletes. Trench foot results from prolonged exposure to cold water without actual tissue freezing. The term is derived from trench warfare during World War I, when soldiers stood, sometimes for hours, in trenches with a few inches of cold water in them. Cold-induced circulation changes produce edema and pain. In severe cases, gangrene may occur. Treatment is similar to that for chilblain and frostbite.

Tropical immersion foot results from immersion of the feet in warm water for 48 hours or more. It was common among military personnel in Vietnam who were exposed to prolonged or repeated wading in paddy fields or streams. Immersion foot presents as maceration, blanching, and wrinkling of the soles and sides of the feet. Itching and burning with erythema and swelling may persist a few days after moving to a drier environment. Immersion foot can be prevented by allowing the feet to dry for a few hours each day. Recovery is usually rapid if the feet are allowed to dry.

Macules: Black Heel

Black heel is a condition often seen in running athletes. Small black macules form on the heel secondary to the mechanical shearing stress of sports. This stress damages vessels, causing minute bleeding. The macules are asymptomatic and resolve without treatment.[3]

Vesicles and Bullae

Friction blisters and dyshidrotic eczema are two disorders commonly found on the foot. Minimally inflamed blisters on the plantar surface of the feet with no specific history of frictional trauma are commonly seen in vesicular tinea pedis (discussed under Papulosquamous Disease). Localized epidermolysis bullosa simplex is an autosomal dominant disorder producing recurrent bullous eruption of the hands and feet. The lesions are exacerbated by hot weather and prolonged walking or running. This uncommon disorder may present in infancy or early adulthood.

Friction Blisters

Friction blisters are usually caused by the pressure and friction of poorly fitting shoes. Hot spots and small blisters can be treated with moleskin donuts and taping. If the blisters are very large or uncomfortable, they should be drained, leaving the roof of the blister in place to serve as a dressing. If the blister is unroofed, the application of a hydrocolloidal dressing (DuoDerm) will reduce symptoms and speed recovery. Friction blisters may be prevented by wearing correctly fitted, well-broken-in footwear.

Dyshidrotic Eczema

Dyshidrotic eczema is an endogenous eczematous eruption of unknown etiology. It usually presents as small pruritic vesicles on the sole in a bilaterally symmetric distribution. Dyshidrotic eczema must be differentiated from bullous tinea pedis (by KOH preparation) and from allergic contact dermatitis. Dyshidrotic eczema is chronic and often difficult to treat. Repeated wetting and drying cycles exacerbate the condition; therefore, one must keep the feet dry and wear clean, dry socks. These actions combined with twice daily applications of medium- to high-potency topical corticosteroid creams usually keep the condition under control.

Toe and Toenail Disorders

Ingrown Toenail

An ingrown toenail usually occurs on the large toe and is caused by nail growth into the lateral nail fold. Often, wearing shoes with a larger toe box or placing a small piece of cotton under the corner of the nail to allow drainage will rectify the problem. If these measures are ineffective, the affected one-third to one-half of the nail may be surgically excised.

Black Toenails

Black toenails occur most commonly in tennis, jogging, skiing, hiking, and climbing. Trauma or pressure from repetitive slippage of the foot anteriorly against the shoe or frequent dorsiflexion of the toes in a shoe with a limited toe box causes a subungual hematoma. The hematomas are often accompanied by nail dystrophy, especially onycholysis and periungual hyperkeratosis. Often, no treatment is necessary and the hematoma resolves spontaneously. However, if the condition is acutely painful, the hematoma may be drained by drilling the nail plate with an 18-gauge needle. To avoid this problem, footwear should have an adequate toe box. Trimming the toenails to their shortest point in a straight tangential line that does not cause discomfort may also be preventive. A linear black streak running from the proximal nail fold to the distal edge of the nail may represent a subungual melanoma and should be evaluated by a dermatologist. Multiple such streaks in an individual may represent a benign process known as *melanonychia striata* and is particularly common in blacks.

Onychomycosis

Onychomycosis is a fungal infection of the nail that persists as a discoloration and thickening of the nail, sometimes causing it to separate from the toe. This infection is difficult to treat. Local twice-daily application of topical antifungals or 3% thymol in alcohol may help control some cases and even produce significant cosmetic improvement but is seldom curative. Oral griseofulvin has been replaced by several more effective oral therapies. The two most commonly used oral antifungal regimens are itraconazole (Sporanox) 400 mg daily for 1 week, repeated 1 week each month for 3 months, or terbinafine (Lamisil) 250 mg daily for 12 weeks. The cure rate with these regimens is 70–80%, but relapses are common. Itraconazole may produce significant adverse effects when given concurrently with many other medications (see package insert) and may very rarely produce hepatotoxicity. Terbinafine has been reported to produce temporary loss of taste in approximately 1% of patients and rare cases of severe pancytopenia. A course of therapy with either of these medications is expensive. Because of these limitations, many clinicians do not recommend therapy of mild, "cosmetic" onychomycosis.

LEG CONDITIONS

Abrasions

Also known as "turf burn," "rug burn," and "strawberry," the abrasion is a highly common injury among athletes.

Treatment is simple and consists of washing the area with soap and water and applying a topical antibacterial ointment, such as bacitracin. Deeply imbedded rock and debris should be removed to prevent epidermal overgrowth with resultant "tattooing" of the skin. A simple nonadherent dressing should then be placed over the abraded area. Contrary to popular belief, these wounds will heal faster and with less discomfort if they are kept moist with a thin covering of bacitracin or white petrolatum. The use of a hydrocolloidal dressing (DuoDerm) will also speed recovery but is more costly.

Cellulitis

Cellulitis is a bacterial infection of the subcutaneous tissue that presents as an erythematous, tender, warm plaque. It appears suddenly and slowly enlarges. It often occurs in the lower extremities and is usually caused by streptococcal or staphylococcal bacteria. Often, a break in the skin or fungal infection precedes the onset of cellulitis and serves as a portal of entry for the bacteria. In debilitated patients and children, lymphangitis and sepsis can occur, but this is unusual in healthy adults and adolescents. Treatment consists of rest, heat, elevation, and a 10- to 14-day course of antibiotics that covers staphylococcal and streptococcal organisms (for example, dicloxacillin, erythromycin, cephradine). Compromised or very ill patients should be hospitalized for intravenous antibiotics. Athletes with cellulitis should not participate in their sports until the condition is completely healed.

GROIN

Papules and Nodules

Papular conditions in the groin among athletes include umbilicated papules found in molluscum contagiosum, papules and burrows in scabies, and verrucous papules in venereal warts.

Molluscum Contagiosum

Molluscum contagiosum, which is caused by a poxvirus, is characterized by small, firm, skin-colored or white umbilicated papules. In children, the papules occur more commonly on the face and extremities, rather than in the groin. The virus is spread from person to person through direct contact and on the patient through autoinoculation. Treatment involves removal of the lesions. This may be accomplished by curettage, trichloroacetic acid, topical tretinoin, cryotherapy with liquid nitrogen, or electrodesiccation. Athletes with this condition may resume close-contact sports 48–72 hours after curettage of all the lesions.

Scabies

Scabies presents as multiple, very pruritic papules and burrows that are usually found on the genitals, waistline, finger webs, wrists, axillae, and buttocks. Often, the lesions are excoriated at presentation. The mite *Sarcoptes scabiei* is the cause of scabies, and it spreads through close personal contact. Diagnosis is confirmed by identifying the mite with microscopic examination of skin scrapings from burrows. The treatment of choice is 5% permethrin cream. It is applied over the entire skin surface from neck to toes at bedtime and rinsed off 8 hours later. Bed linen and clothing should be washed in hot water. All individuals in the home should be treated even if they are symptom free. Treatment with permethrin cream is considered curative, and athletes may resume close-contact sports the day after this treatment.

Venereal Warts

Venereal warts, or condyloma acuminatum, can appear as asymptomatic, small, smooth papules or verrucous pedunculated papules. They can cluster or form cauliflowerlike projections and are found on the genital organs and perianal region. Genital warts are caused by the human papillomavirus and spread through close personal contact. They should be treated with cryotherapy using liquid nitrogen. They may also be treated by applying 25% podophyllin solution or podophyllotoxin to the warts, rinsing the solution off the skin several hours after application. This regimen should be repeated weekly until the lesion disappears. Patients with this disorder must always receive appropriate counseling on sexually transmitted disease.

Vesicles: Herpes

Small, grouped, painful vesicles on the genitals usually indicate genital herpes, a sexually transmitted disease. Herpes simplex virus (HSV) is the etiologic agent. The first presentation of this disease is usually the most painful and prolonged. The diagnosis should be confirmed by Tzanck preparation, which shows multinucleated giant cells, or by viral culture. In most individuals, genital herpes recurs. Currently, it cannot be eradicated, but control is possible with the antiviral drug acyclovir. Therapy for the primary outbreak consists of analgesics for pain control (opiates are occasionally necessary) and acyclovir 200 mg given orally five times a day for 5 days. Famciclovir is also effective with less frequent dosing: 250–750 mg three times a day for 5 days. Athletes with frequent, recurrent outbreaks (more than six per year) may take 200 mg acyclovir two or three times a day to reduce the frequency of outbreaks. Otherwise, patients with infrequent outbreaks may take acyclovir, 200 mg orally five times a day for 5 days, at the outset of symptoms to reduce the duration of the outbreak. All patients should receive appropriate counseling on sexually transmitted disease. It is recommended that patients do not participate in close-contact sports during an outbreak. The National Collegiate Athletic Association (NCAA) Wrestling Committee recommends no tournament participation unless (1) the athlete is free of new lesions for 3 days, (2) there are no active lesions, (3) all lesions are crusted, (4) the athlete is on an antiviral medication, and (5) all lesions are covered.

Papulosquamous Disease: Tinea Cruris

An erythematous, marginated, pruritic groin rash with a scaling border usually means tinea cruris, or "jock itch." It is a superficial dermatophytic infection treated effectively with twice-daily applications of a topical antifungal agent (miconazole or clotrimazole) for 2 weeks. The diagnosis should be confirmed with a KOH preparation. Moist, eczematous dermatitis in the inguinal area may also represent a combination of maceration from chronic moisture and friction and irritation from harsh soaps. This will respond to drying agents such as Domeboro soaks, air drying, and mild topical steroids. As the area heals, recurrence may be prevented with the use of drying powders.

BUTTOCKS

Papules and Pustules

Multiple, small, pruritic papules and burrows on the buttocks are highly suspicious for scabies (see section on the groin). On the other hand, an individual acutely tender erythematous nodule is characteristic of a furuncle.

Furuncles

Furuncles are staphylococcal abscesses that are commonly found on the buttocks but do occur elsewhere. Treatment involves warm compresses and antibiotics. A 10-day course of either a cephalosporin (cephalexin, 500 mg four times a day), erythromycin (250 mg four times a day), or penicillinase-resistant penicillin (dicloxacillin, 500 mg four times a day) should be administered. When the furun-

cle becomes fluctuant and points, it should be incised and drained. A carbuncle is similar to a furuncle but has multiple points. Patients should not participate in close contact sports, such as wrestling, until the furuncle is sufficiently healed.

Folliculitis

See Generalized Dermatoses.

Macules: Runner's Rump

Runner's rump consists of small ecchymoses on the superior portion of the gluteal cleft in long-distance runners and is thought to result from constant friction at this site. It is of no consequence.[3]

Plaques: Rower's Rump

Rower's rump results from rowing while sitting on an unpadded seat for long periods. It appears as a thickened, lichenified plaque and is a form of lichen simplex chronicus. Treatment consists of substituting a padded seat and the use of a potent steroid cream.[3]

TRUNK

Papules and Pustules: Acne

See Generalized Dermatoses.

Hypo- or Hyperpigmented Macules: Tinea Versicolor

Tinea versicolor is exceedingly common in warm, humid months. Lesions are usually macular with areas of hypo- or hyperpigmentation with little or no obvious scale. Lesions occur most commonly on the chest and back but may occasionally involve the lateral neck and upper extremities. Patients are usually asymptomatic. Tinea versicolor may be treated with selenium sulfide shampoo. The shampoo is applied to the skin from the neck down to the waist and out to the wrists. It is allowed to dry and left on overnight. The shampoo is showered off in the morning. Because *Pityrosporum orbiculare* is part of the normal flora, it often recurs, necessitating regular treatment. During summer months, when tinea versicolor flourishes, applications of selenium sulfide during routine showering may adequately suppress recurrent infections. In extensive or recurrent disease, ketoconazole (400–800 mg) as a single dose is a very effective alternative therapy. One hour after taking the ketoconazole, the patient should exercise to the point of sweating. The sweat is allowed to dry on the skin and washed off after several hours. Patients should be notified that residual discoloration may take several weeks to resolve even after successful therapy.[6]

Eczema

Jogger's Nipples

Jogger's nipples are painful, fissured, eroded nipples that occasionally bleed. This condition occurs in long-distance runners from constant irritation and friction of hard fabrics against the unprotected nipple and areola. Preventive measures include wearing soft fiber shirts, application of adhesive bandages, or the application of petroleum jelly to the nipples immediately before running.[3]

Swimmer's Shoulder

Swimmer's shoulder is an erythematous plaque on the shoulder resulting from irritation from an unshaven face during freestyle swimming. Shaving before swimming prevents the problem.[3]

HANDS

Macules

Mogul Skier's Palm

Mogul skier's palm consists of hypothenar ecchymoses resulting from the repetitive planting of ski poles. The ecchymoses, which may have a golden hue because of the presence of hemosiderin from past hemorrhages, usually clear after the end of the skiing season.[7]

Ping-Pong Patches

Ping-pong patches are erythematous macules 2–3 cm in diameter caused by the high-velocity impact of the ball on the forearms and dorsal aspect of the hands.[3]

Papules and Nodules

Warts

Warts, or verrucae vulgaris, are prevalent throughout all populations. They are caused by the human papillomavirus. Untreated warts usually resolve spontaneously, especially in children. Because they can be painful to the athlete and are contagious and unsightly, warts can be treated. Common warts can be treated effectively in several ways. Cryotherapy with liquid nitrogen, and keratolytic therapy with salicylic acid preparations are frequently effective. Persistence with these therapies is usually more rewarding than progression to more aggressive therapies. Discomfort can be reduced by having the patient flatten thickened lesions with sandpaper or a nail file.

Calluses

Calluses, as described under Foot Problems, are areas of thickened skin secondary to repeated applications of friction and pressure. Most calluses on the hand are treated effectively by light rubbing with a pumice stone.

Pulling-Boat Hands

Pulling-boat hands occur in crew team members and consist of subcutaneous vascular injuries combined with epidermal blister formation. They are thought to be the result of mechanical injury in combination with cold exposure. Calluses soon form in place of the acute lesions and may serve as a competitive advantage.[3]

Hooking Thumb

Hooking thumb occurs exclusively in competitive weight lifters and consists of abrasions, hematomas, bullae, denudation, calluses, and subungual hematomas on the distal third of the thumb. Hooking is a method of gripping the weight bar with the thumb under the index and middle finger to provide a better grip. Hooking thumb may hamper performance because of pain but resolves after discontinuation of the hooking maneuver.[3]

Vesicles and Bullae

Dyshidrotic Eczema

Dyshidrotic eczema, which is described in the preceding section on foot problems, is even more common on the hands. Typically, small vesicles are found on the tips and sides of the fingers. Effective therapy involves keeping the hands dry, using moisturizing lotion liberally, and applying medium- to high-potency corticosteroid creams twice daily. If the patient has an active tinea pedis infection, a dermatophytid reaction should be considered.

Herpetic Whitlow

Herpetic whitlow presents as a tender, erythematous papule, vesicle, or bulla near the distal finger. This eruption is caused by HSV and is treated with acyclovir (see the section on vesicles under Groin). Patients should be counseled on the transmissibility of this disease.

Dermatophytid

Dermatophytid, or "id" reaction, is a skin reaction to a fungal infection at a distant site, most commonly a vesicular outbreak on the hands that is due to a tinea pedis infection. It responds to treatment of the remote fungal infection. Severe "id" reactions may require a 10- to 14-day course of oral prednisone (40–60 mg daily) to achieve control of symptoms.

Contact Dermatitis

Hands are exposed to many products that can produce pruritic eczema, vesicles, or bullae. Potential offending agents to consider include hand creams, leather or rubber gloves, plant materials (poison ivy, poison oak), adhesives, and rosins. These are discussed in more depth under Generalized Dermatoses.

Nail Disorders

Onychomycosis

Onychomycosis is a fungal infection that can involve both the fingernails and the toenails (see section on nail disorders under Foot Problems). Fingernail onychomycosis responds more readily to oral antifungals than the toenail variety. Therapy is expensive, however, and relapses are common. Other conditions, such as nail psoriasis and horizontal ridging of the nails resulting from trauma, may closely mimic onychomycosis. Fungal cultures or KOH preparations are used to confirm the diagnosis of onychomycosis before treatment.

Paronychia

Paronychia is an inflammation of the nail fold surrounding the nail and is caused by bacterial or yeast infections. An acutely inflamed paronychia may present with superficial abscess formation that should be incised and drained. Chronic paronychia is usually caused by a yeast infection and is frequently related to activities that keep the athlete's hands wet. Treatment of chronic paronychia consists of diligent efforts to keep the hands dry and twice-daily application of nystatin or ketoconazole topically. Occasionally, oral ketoconazole is necessary. Several months of therapy may be needed to achieve a complete cure.

Golfer's Nails

Golfer's nails are splinter hemorrhages or linear dark streaks of the fingernails that occur in golfers who grip the shaft of the club too tightly. Prevention involves learning proper techniques to grip the club.[3]

HEAD AND NECK

Papules and Pustules: Acne

See Generalized Dermatoses.

Vesicles

Herpes Labialis

Herpes labialis and herpes gladiatorum are vesicular disorders found on the face. Both are caused by HSV. Herpes labialis, also known as a *cold sore*, is one of the most common HSV infections and can be treated with acyclovir as described previously (see section on vesicles under Groin). Athletes with this condition should always wear sunscreen on their lips, because ultraviolet radiation is a common trigger for recurrence.

Herpes Gladiatorum

Herpes gladiatorum is the term given to an HSV-1 outbreak occurring on the face or elsewhere on the body of wrestlers, rugby players, and other athletes.[8-11] Herpes gladiatorum is a common problem, and morbidity associated with this skin disease can be significant. Lesions appear 1–2 weeks after exposure in an athletic event. Classic lesions consist of a crop of pruritic vesicles, most commonly on the right side of the face or neck. Symptoms may include regional lymphadenopathy, fever, chills, sore throat, and headache. A national survey of athletic trainers showed that 7.6% of college wrestlers and 2.6% of high school wrestlers had HSV skin infection during the 1984–1985 season. The virus is passed between athletes during the close skin contact of athletic competition. Therefore, contact sports are contraindicated until the lesions resolve. Clinical appearance of this disorder may be unreliable, however, and all suspicious skin and eye lesions should be cultured for HSV-1. Treatment is the same as for other HSV infections (see section on vesicles under Groin for treatment and return-to-play guidelines). Topical acyclovir is probably no more effective than routine wound care. Prevention of infection consists of inspection of all participants before competition and showering before and after events.

Yellow Crusted Lesions

Yellow crusted lesions on a red weeping base are signs of the bacterial infection impetigo. Impetigo may be transmitted in a manner similar to herpes gladiatorum.[11, 12] It is classically described as a streptococcal infection, but many infections with both *Streptococcus* and *Staphylococcus* are common. Treatment consists of removal of the crusts and either twice-daily application of mupirocin ointment for 10 days or a 10-day course of an oral cephalosporin, penicillinase-resistant penicillin, or erythromycin. The oral antibiotic may be combined with topical bacitracin. As with herpes gladiatorum, close contact sports should be avoided until the lesions clear. NCAA guidelines suggest that before competition, wrestlers must have completed 3 days of antibiotic treatment or have no new lesions 48 hours before competition. All lesions must be covered.

Eczema of the External Ear Canal

Swimmer's ear is an otitis externa caused by gram-negative organisms such as *Pseudomonas*. Excessive water exposure produces maceration of the external ear canal, decrease of normal cerumen, and decrease in pH, all of which promote inflammation and secondary infection. Treatment consists of avoiding water exposure until the problem resolves, gentle cleansing, placement of a wick into the external ear canal, and application of an antibiotic or anti-inflammatory solution such as polymyxin neomycin hydrocortisone drops (two drops four times a day). In very severe cases, oral antibiotics and oral steroids may be indicated. Recurrences may be prevented with the use of 2% acetic acid in propylene glycol applied before and after swimming.

Hair Discoloration

Green hair is another disorder seen in swimmers.[13] The copper contained in swimming pool water can produce a green tinge in the hair of fair-haired swimmers. The green tinge may be removed either by shampooing with a copper-chelating shampoo, such as Ultraswim (Chattem, Inc., Chattanooga, TN), for 30 minutes, or 3% hydrogen peroxide soaks for 3 hours.

RETURN TO PLAY

An issue that must be addressed for athletes with dermatologic problems is the time within which participation in the sport is restricted. Many conditions discussed in this chapter do warrant excluding the athlete from sports for periods—some because of pain or other symptoms, and others because of the potential spread of infectious organisms. In the former case, the decision to return to play depends on the symptom. For example, an athlete who is unable to train because of painful corns may return as symptoms permit. Similarly, an athlete with a severe drug photosensitivity reaction may return to action when symptoms resolve and precautions against recurrence are

taken. Athletes with infectious conditions should be given approval to return to play only when healing has reached the point at which competing would not worsen the condition and fellow competitors are not at risk of infection. The decision is condition and sport dependent. For example, an athlete with a herpes outbreak on the shoulder may not compete in the close-contact sport of wrestling until the lesion is healed, yet would be cleared to throw the shot put at a track meet.

REFERENCES

1. Basler RS. Acne mechanica in athletes. Cutis 1992;50:125–128.
2. Basler RSW. Skin injuries in sports medicine. J Am Acad Dermatol 1989;21:1257–1262.
3. Pharis DB, Teller C, Wolf JE Jr. Cutaneous manifestations of sports participation. J Am Acad Dermatol 1997;36:448–459.
4. Cohen PR, Eliezri YD, Silvers DN. Athlete's nodules: sports-related connective tissue nevi of the collagen type (collagenomas). Cutis 1992;50:131–135.
5. Burnett JW. Seabather's eruption. Cutis 1992;50:98.
6. Berger TG, Elias PM, Wintroub BU. Manual of Therapy for Skin Diseases. New York: Churchill Livingstone, 1990.
7. Swinehart JM. Mogul skier's palm: traumatic hypothenar ecchymosis. Cutis 1992;50:117–118.
8. Becker TM. Herpes gladiatorum: a growing problem in sports medicine. Cutis 1992;50:150–152.
9. Belongia EA, Goodman JL, Holland EJ, et al. An outbreak of herpes gladiatorum at a high school wrestling camp. N Engl J Med 1991;325:906–910.
10. Goodman RA, Thacker SB, Solomon SL, et al. Infectious disease in competitive sports. JAMA 1994;271:862–866.
11. National Collegiate Athletics Association. NCAA Sports Medicine Handbook. Skin Infections in Athletes. Benser, MT: NCAA Publications, 1996.
12. Levine N. Dermatologic aspects of sports medicine. J Am Acad Dermatol 1980;3:415–424.
13. Person JR. Green hair: treatment with a penicillamine shampoo. Arch Dermatol 1985;121:717–718.

28

Thermal Illness and Exercise

ROBERT C. GAMBRELL

Athletes exercising in hot environments are faced with physiologic challenges that frequently impair their performance and may place them at risk for serious thermal injury. In spite of excellent health and conditioning, athletes frequently succumb to the effects of high temperature and heat stress. It may be surprising to learn that heat stroke continues to be the third most common cause of death in athletes each year.[1] There were 84 deaths from heat stroke in American football reported between 1955 and 1990,[2] and each year as many as 30 cases of heat stroke are expected at the Marine Corps Recruit Depot, Paris Island, South Carolina.[3] The majority of serious thermal illnesses and their complications can be prevented. Athletes, as well as those training and caring for them, should be knowledgeable in the prevention and treatment of thermal illnesses.

Heat exhaustion and heat stroke are hyperthermic syndromes that are life-threatening and require immediate treatment. Heat stroke is further classified as either classic or exertional. Classic heat stroke generally occurs in epidemics after heat waves and affects debilitated individuals who become overwhelmed by high environmental temperature. It is typically associated with the triad of hyperthermia (generally 40°C [104°F] or higher), anhydrosis, and central nervous system (CNS) dysfunction. Exertional heat stroke (EHS) occurs sporadically in young, healthy individuals exercising and working in hot environments. EHS is associated with hyperthermia and CNS dysfunction but is frequently accompanied by profuse sweating.

In the larger picture, heat stroke is responsible for 400 deaths per year in the United States alone.[4] The vast majority of these deaths occur in elderly or debilitated individuals. In addition to heat exhaustion and heat stroke, a variety of other thermal illnesses also occur. Heat cramps, heat edema, and heat syncope are mild thermal illnesses that occur without compromise of thermoregulation (hyperthermia) and generally respond to rest and hydration. The thermal illnesses most commonly seen among athletes and individuals exercising in hot environments are heat cramps, heat exhaustion, and EHS.[5]

THERMOREGULATION

A knowledge of human thermoregulatory mechanisms is necessary to understanding thermal illnesses. Heat exhaustion and EHS are caused by overloading or overwhelming the body's usual thermoregulatory mechanisms. Hyperthermia results when heat production exceeds the body's ability to dissipate heat. Heat is produced in the body from both endogenous and exogenous sources. Endogenous heat comes from body metabolism and muscle activity. During exercise, muscles can expend more than 20 times as much energy as at rest. Exogenous heat transfers thermal energy to the body from the environment.

Nearly all of human heat dissipation comes from radiation, convection, or evaporation, with less than 2% of heat loss being the result of conduction.[5, 6] When environmental temperature is below body temperature, heat loss occurs principally through convection and radiation. When environmental temperature exceeds body temperature, sweating provides compensatory heat loss through evaporation. During exercise in a hot, dry environment, the athlete relies almost exclusively on evaporative heat loss through sweating to regulate body temperature.[6] The ability to lose heat through evaporation of sweat is diminished in hot, humid environments, especially when the relative humidity exceeds 70%. This creates an increased demand for heat loss through radiation and convection and requires a greater portion of cardiac output to be directed to cutaneous vessels, thereby decreasing venous return to the heart and increasing cardiovascular strain.

TABLE 28-1
Risk Factors for Thermal Illness in Athletes

Environmental	Individual
Temperature	Dehydration
Humidity	Drug/alcohol use
Air velocity	Sunburn
Radiant heat load	Increased percent body fat
Air pollution	Diarrhea, vomiting
Terrain	Fever
Clothing, equipment	Sleep deprivation, fatigue
Mode of exercise	Low cardiopulmonary fitness
Group vs. solitary exercise	Lack of heat acclimatization
	Extreme or imprudent effort
	Residual heatstroke injury
	Age extremes
	Skin disease, anhydrosis
	Cardiovascular disease
	Endocrine disorders

Source: Adapted from FL Allman Jr. The effects of heat on the athlete. J Med Assoc Ga 1992;81:307–310; LE Armstrong, CM Maresh. The exertional heat illnesses: a risk of athletic participation. Med Exerc Nutr Health 1993;2:125–134; MD Bracker. Environmental and thermal injury. Clin Sports Med 1992;11:419–436; and PA Tom, GM Garmel, PS Auerbach. Environment-dependent sports emergencies. Med Clin North Am 1994;78:305–325.

Humans have the capacity to adapt to hot environments by improving the heat-dissipating mechanisms of thermoregulation. Heat acclimatization is defined as the improved ability to exercise or work in a naturally hot environment. Repeated exposure to a hot environment for 60–90 minutes per day for 1–2 weeks results in physiologic adaptations that improve heat transfer from the body's core to the skin.[7–9] Once acclimatized, an individual experiences a smaller rise in rectal temperature at any given workload in the heat.[1, 10] Physiologic changes that lead to acclimatization include increased cardiac output, extracellular fluid volume expansion, diminished sweat sodium concentration, and increased sweat volume.[6, 8] Acclimatization not only enhances performance in the heat but also places the athlete at decreased risk for experiencing a thermal illness.[1, 5, 6, 8, 9, 11]

Improved cardiovascular conditioning also decreases the risk for thermal illness in athletes. Improvements in VO_2max have been shown to be associated with enhanced heat tolerance and appear to be independent of the physiologic changes that occur with heat acclimatization.[5, 9] Accordingly, factors leading to impairment of the cardiovascular system will increase the risk for thermal illness. Dehydration leading to volume contraction and decreased circulatory volume will impair the ability to transfer heat peripherally and diminish heat dissipation. Progressive dehydration is believed to cause hyperthermia in proportion to the fluid deficit. As little as 2%

decrease in effective circulating volume impairs performance, and further deficits place the athlete at risk for heat exhaustion and EHS.[10]

RISK FACTORS

A number of environmental and individual factors interact to place athletes at increased risk for EHS by either increasing heat production or decreasing heat dissipation (Table 28-1). Environmental heat stress is influenced by temperature, humidity, wind, and degree of cloud cover and is measured by the wet-bulb globe temperature (WBGT) index. The WBGT is calculated by the following equation:

$$WBGT = 0.7\,NWB + 0.2\,GT + 0.1\,DB$$

where NWB = natural wet-bulb temperature, DB = dry-bulb (air) temperature, and GT = globe thermometer temperature.

Increased relative humidity greatly inhibits the ability to sweat and lose heat through evaporation and is reflected in its large contribution (70%) to the WBGT index.

For utmost accuracy, the WBGT index should be measured at the site where athletes are competing or practicing, because conditions vary markedly within geographic regions. Determination of WBGT requires the use of a black globe thermometer, a natural wet-bulb thermometer, and a dry-bulb thermometer. The wet-bulb thermometer measures the evaporative heat loss capacity of the environment and reflects an athlete's ability to lose heat by sweating. The wick of the natural wet-bulb thermometer should be kept wet with distilled water. The dry-bulb thermometer measures ambient temperature, and the globe thermometer measures radiant heat energy. The dry-bulb thermometer must be shielded from the sun without restricting air flow around the bulb. A globe thermometer consists of a 6-in. diameter hollow copper sphere painted black with the bulb of the thermometer fixed in the center of the sphere. A stand should be used to suspend the three thermometers so that they do not restrict air flow around the bulbs and so that the wet-bulb and globe thermometers are not shaded. If making your own WBGT device is impractical, commercial devices are available and convenient to use.[12]

Heat tolerance may be influenced by more than 30 different factors and predispose the athlete to heat illness (see Table 28-1). Insufficient heat acclimatization, low cardiopulmonary fitness, dehydration, pyrexial illness, lack of sleep, and extreme effort are frequently associated with EHS.[5] Restrictive clothing, equipment, obesity, age extremes, cardiovascular diseases, residual heatstroke injury, endocrine disorders, skin diseases, and various medications may predispose to heat illness by interfering with heat dissipation.[1, 5, 11]

HEAT EXHAUSTION

Heat exhaustion is defined as the inability to continue exercise in the heat and is the most common thermal illness among athletes and soldiers.[5] Heat exhaustion occurs from excessive sweating in a hot environment leading to volume contraction (depletion) and decreased cardiac output. The competing demands of perfusion to the skin for heat loss and to the muscle for continued exercise cannot be maintained. Core body temperature rises but usually remains below 40°C (104°F), and the athlete cannot continue activity in the heat.

Heat exhaustion has been described as a diagnosis of exclusion because the signs and symptoms are often vague and similar to those seen with EHS. Common symptoms include malaise, weakness, headache, hyperirritability, anxiety, tachycardia, dizziness, nausea, vomiting, diarrhea, and hypotension.[1, 2, 5, 11] Major neurologic impairment is absent. Treatment of heat exhaustion requires rest, cooling, and rehydration. Adequate rehydration requires replacement of both fluids and electrolytes. Oral electrolyte solutions usually suffice, but some athletes may require 3–4 L of intravenous fluid.[5] Most athletes recover quickly.

EXERTIONAL HEAT STROKE

EHS is an emergency that requires immediate treatment. Core body temperatures in excess of 40°C (104°F) may rapidly cause irreversible CNS damage. The severity of EHS is primarily related to the degree of temperature elevation and the length of time before cooling measures are initiated. Extreme or prolonged periods of elevated core body temperature exceeding 40°C (104°F) may cause widespread cellular injury and multisystem organ failure.

Symptoms of EHS include hypotension, vomiting, diarrhea, and mental status changes such as headache, confusion, agitation, seizures, stupor, or coma.[1, 2, 5, 11] Evidence of CNS dysfunction distinguishes EHS from heat exhaustion. Early mortality results from CNS injury, but complications from heat stroke also include liver injury, rhabdomyolysis, acute renal failure, pulmonary edema, and disseminated intravascular coagulation.[1, 2, 11] Whenever the diagnosis is unclear, individuals should be treated for EHS. Poor prognostic indicators are core body temperatures more than 42.2°C (107.6°F), aspartate amino-transferase greater than 1,000 during the first 24 hours, and coma more than 2 hours in duration.[2, 5, 11]

DIAGNOSIS

The diagnosis of heat stroke is suspected in any individual exhibiting symptoms. Heat exhaustion and EHS are commonly thought of as a continuum of the same process of progressive volume depletion. Athletes may demonstrate prodromal symptoms, but commonly do not, and frequently maintain a high level of performance up until they collapse. The differentiation between heat exhaustion and EHS is very difficult, with the primary clinical parameter being CNS dysfunction. A core body temperature of 40°C is frequently used to diagnose heat stroke, but temperatures exceeding this have been recorded in athletes demonstrating no symptoms of thermal illness.[13] Nonetheless, an accurate core body temperature is crucial in the diagnosis and treatment of EHS. Core body temperature must be measured rectally to insure accuracy. Oral, axillary, and aural temperatures do not reliably reflect core body temperature and should not be used.[1, 11, 14] Measurement of serum enzymes, aspartate aminotransferase, alanine aminotransferase, lactic dehydrogenase, and creatine phosphokinase may assist in making the diagnosis of EHS.[5] Evidence of cellular injury may exist even without documented core body temperature exceeding 40°C.

The differential diagnosis of hyperthermia with CNS changes includes meningitis, encephalitis, malaria, typhoid, delirium tremens, thyrotoxicosis, malignant hyperthermia, acute hepatic necrosis, and drug intoxication.[1, 2, 5, 11] Cooling should not be delayed whenever heat stroke is suspected and will not harm patients with hyperthermia from other causes. Hyponatremia should also be considered in athletes who present with mental status changes but are not hyperthermic. Symptomatic hyponatremia initially develops in less competitive athletes who have maintained high rates of fluid intake during endurance events lasting at least 5 hours.[15]

TREATMENT

The key element and initial step in the treatment of EHS is rapid cooling of the core body temperature to below 39°C (102°F). A variety of cooling measures are available based on either cold-water immersion or evaporative heat loss, which may be used in combination. Cold-water immersion has been the standard technique for rapid cooling and is based on the ability of water to conduct heat better than air. Heat loss occurs by radiation and conduction across the thermal gradient that is established between the cold-water bath and the body core. Variations on this technique include ice packs, ice water blankets, partial body cold-water immersion, and total body cold-water immersion.

Evaporative heat loss measures were probably first developed by South African mining personnel and came into standard use in Saudi Arabia for treatment of heat stroke victims during the annual hajj pilgrimage.[16] This process is based on the evaporative properties of water and takes advantage of the large amount of heat released when water transitions from a liquid to a gaseous state. Treatment consists of suspending the patient in a cot and spraying them with water mist. Large fans then blow air across the skin and facilitate evaporation of the water, thus simulating sweating. This process is very effective and has led to the development of the body cooling units used by the Saudi authorities.

Internal cooling measures are infrequently used because of their invasiveness and inherent risks of complications. Methods include peritoneal, gastric, bladder, and rectal ice saline lavage, as well as cardiopulmonary bypass.[1, 2, 5, 11] There is no evidence that internal cooling measures are superior to external measures, and they should be reserved for cases in which external measures fail.[17, 18]

Controversy exists over which cooling method is superior. Advocates of cold-water immersion note that it is a time-tested method that has proved to be safe and may be the only practical method in the absence of electricity to drive fans. The medical team at the Falmouth Road Race (Falmouth, MA) has successfully used plastic wading pools that immerse the trunk but not the arms and legs.[19] Critics site theoretical concerns that peripheral vasoconstriction and reflexive shivering from cold-water immersion may actually increase the core body temperature, a phenomenon not seen in actual practice.[5] Additional objections to the use of immersion include extreme discomfort for the patient as well as decreased access for evaluation, monitoring, or performance of cardiopulmonary resuscitation. The difficulty in maintaining large quantities of ice and water may limit the effectiveness of immersion in military or field settings.

Evaporative heat loss may have the advantage of increased access to and comfort for the patient. Research conducted with healthy volunteers shows evaporative heat loss to be superior to cold-water immersion, but advocates of immersion question the value of comparison between healthy volunteers and actual patients with EHS.[17] No treatment modality has been shown to be more effective than cold-water immersion in preventing death from EHS.[3, 5] In practice, combinations of the two methods are frequently used. A review of cooling measures used worldwide indicates that evaporative heat loss techniques are preferred in the Middle East and Africa, whereas physicians in the United States are equally split in their preference.[18] The topic deserves further research with controlled studies on comparable patients using each technique.

Overzealous cooling may actually lead to hypothermia. The monitoring of vital signs and placement of a rectal thermistor to continuously measure core body temperature are both essential to avoid this serious complication. Replacement of intravascular fluids is indicated if the patient remains hypotensive or volume contracted. Intravenous fluids should be replaced carefully, but large volumes are frequently necessary.

RETURN TO ACTIVITY

Most athletes exhibit normal heat acclimatization responses 2 months after recovering from EHS.[5, 7] A gradual return to competitive activities may then be attempted while ensuring adequate hydration and avoiding extreme environmental conditions. Some individuals remain heat intolerant for more than 1 year.[7] Based on these findings, it has been recommended that all clinically normal EHS patients should undergo heat tolerance evaluation in a controlled laboratory setting before return to physical training.[5] This may be unrealistic in most cases but could be useful in elite athletes or individuals attempting to return to training less than 2 months after EHS. Additionally, individuals successfully treated for heat exhaustion should not immediately resume training activities. After 24–48 hours of rest, rehydration, and replenishment of electrolytes, they may gradually return to activities if they are asymptomatic.

MINOR THERMAL ILLNESSES

Minor thermal illnesses include heat cramps, heat edema, and heat syncope. They occur in individuals with intact thermoregulatory mechanisms and are not associated with hyperthermia. Minor heat-related illnesses result from physiologic changes associated with acclimatization to heat stress and respond well to rest and hydration.

Heat cramps are painful spasms that occur as the result of excessive salt and electrolyte loss from sweating. They occur most commonly in poorly acclimated individuals but may also occur in highly acclimatized athletes who drink large volumes of water to replenish fluids lost by sweating. Heat cramps usually affect the large muscles of

TABLE 28-2

Guidelines for Team Activities Based on Wet-Bulb Globe Temperature (WBGT)

WBGT	Activity
< 65°F (18°C)	Follow regular schedules; allow full access to fluids
65°–72°F (18°–22°C)	Add quarterly fluid breaks; allow free access to fluids
73°–82°F (23°–28°C)	Shorten games or allow unlimited substitutions; add quarterly fluid breaks; allow full access to water
82°–85°F (28°–30°C)	Establish an alternate schedule in advance to move midday games to earlier and later hours; allow unrestricted substitution at all age levels; shorten game times; add quarterly fluid breaks; allow fluid breaks during play
> 85°F (31°C)	Cancel all exertion and avoid sun exposure at rest

Source: Reprinted with permission from MD Bracker. Environmental and thermal injury. Clin Sports Med 1992;11:431.

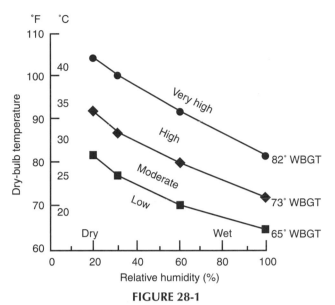

FIGURE 28-1

Risk of thermal illness while exercising in hot environments. (WBGT = wet-bulb globe temperature.) (Adapted from American College of Sports Medicine. Position stand: heat and cold illnesses during distance running. Med Sci Sports Exerc 1996;28:i–x.)

the legs but may involve any of the skeletal muscles. Treatment consists of rest, massage, and removal from heat, in addition to fluid and salt replacement. Heat cramps respond quickly to intravenous normal saline solution or a 1% oral salt solution.[1, 2, 5]

Heat edema is swelling of the extremities that frequently occurs in unacclimatized individuals when they are initially exposed to a hot environment. The swelling results from peripheral vasodilation, decreased intravascular volume, and increased hydrostatic pressure in response to aldosterone-mediated sodium retention.[1] Heat edema is a self-limited process and should not be treated with diuretics. Treatment includes elevation of the extremities, temporary removal from the heat, and continued acclimatization.

Heat syncope occurs from the same mechanisms as heat edema. Syncope results when the peripheral vasodilation and decreased intravascular volume lead to orthostatic hypotension and loss of consciousness. Heat syncope may be avoided by sitting or lying down whenever symptoms occur and avoiding prolonged standing in a hot environment. The most effective treatment for heat syncope is rest and rehydration.

PREVENTION

Once armed with the knowledge of factors predisposing to thermal illnesses, a number of steps can be taken toward prevention. Athletes should be advised of the early symptoms of thermal illness. Before vigorous exercise in the heat, individuals should allow for adequate heat acclimatization and be in good physical condition. Exercise in hot environmental conditions should be avoided when illnesses associated with fever, respiratory symptoms, or diarrhea are present.

The risk for thermal illness increases proportionally with increasing heat stress. The WBGT should be frequently monitored and activities modified accordingly (Table 28-2). Precautions should be taken to avoid periods of extreme heat stress by scheduling events and practices for cooler times in the day. The American College of Sports Medicine recommends rescheduling or delaying events when the WBGT is above 29°C.[12] If a WBGT device is not available, heat stress may be approximated based on a knowledge of the relative humidity and ambient temperature (Figure 28-1). Additional preventive measures may include modifications in rules to allow for unlimited substitutions during tournaments, shedding of restrictive clothing and equipment, and avoiding extreme efforts or attempts at a personal best during extremely hot conditions.

Heat exhaustion and EHS are primarily due to dehydration, and a well-hydrated individual is less susceptible to thermal illness. Ensuring free access to adequate amounts of water is essential in preventing serious thermal illnesses. Athletes participating in team sports should be monitored closely for dehydration by measuring their weight before and after practices. Individuals losing more than 5% of their base line body weight should be held out of practice to rest and rehydrate.[2] An adequate supply of fluids for distance races must be available at the start of the race, along the race course, and at the end of

TABLE 28-3
Recommendations for Fluid Replacement with Exercise

1. It is recommended that individuals consume a nutritionally balanced diet and drink adequate fluids during the 24-hour period before an event, especially during the period that includes meals before exercise, to promote proper hydration before exercise or competition.
2. It is recommended that individuals drink approximately 500 ml (approximately 17 oz) of fluid 2 hours before exercise to promote adequate hydration and allow time for excretion of excess ingested water.
3. During exercise, athletes should start drinking water early and at regular intervals in an attempt to consume fluids at a rate sufficient to replace all the water lost through sweating (i.e., body weight loss) or consume the maximal amount that can be tolerated.
4. It is recommended that ingested fluids be cooler than ambient temperature (between 15° and 22°C [59°–72°F]) and flavored to enhance palatability and promote fluid replacement. Fluids should be readily available and served in containers that allow adequate volumes to be ingested with ease and with minimal interruption.
5. Addition of proper amounts of carbohydrates and electrolytes to a fluid replacement solution is recommended for exercise events of duration >1 hour because it does not significantly impair water delivery to the body and may enhance performance. During exercise lasting <1 hour, there is little evidence of physiologic or physical performance differences between consuming a carbohydrate-electrolyte drink and plain water.
6. During intense exercise lasting longer than 1 hour, it is recommended that carbohydrates be ingested at a rate of 30–60 g/hour to maintain oxidation of carbohydrates and delay fatigue. This rate of carbohydrate intake can be achieved without compromising fluid delivery by drinking 600–1,200 ml/hour of solutions containing 4–8% carbohydrates (4–8 g per 100 ml water). The carbohydrates can be sugars (glucose or sucrose) or starch (e.g., maltodextrins).
7. Inclusion of sodium (0.5–0.7 g per liter of water) in the rehydration solution ingested during exercise lasting longer than 1 hour is recommended because it may be advantageous in enhancing palatability, promoting fluid retention, and possibly preventing hyponatremia in certain individuals who drink excessive quantities of fluid. There is little physiologic basis for the presence of sodium in an oral rehydration solution for enhancing intestinal water absorption as long as sodium is sufficiently available from the previous meal.

Source: Reprinted with permission from American College of Sports Medicine. Position stand: exercise and fluid replacement. Med Sci Sports Exerc 1996;28:i.

the race. Surprisingly, athletes and soldiers exercising and working in the heat and given free access to water, may not consume enough fluids to maintain adequate hydration. Fluids should be cooled and may be flavored to improve their palatability and promote their consumption. Electrolyte- or carbohydrate-containing solutions have not been proved to be superior to water for fluid replacement in athletes exercising for less than 1 hour.[10] For vigorous exercise lasting more than 1 hour, the addition of carbohydrates and sodium are recommended in the rehydration solution. Salt tablets are unnecessary and discouraged. Although sodium lost during bouts of exercise must be replaced to ensure complete rehydration, adequate amounts are contained in a regular diet. Specific recommendations concerning oral rehydration for athletes are contained in the American College of Sports Medicine's Position Stand on Exercise and Fluid Replacement (Table 28-3).

SUMMARY

Thermal illnesses commonly seen in athletes include heat cramps, heat exhaustion, and EHS. Heat exhaustion and EHS may be difficult to distinguish clinically and require rapid cooling to prevent serious sequelae. Multiple factors have been found to decrease heat tolerance or increase heat stress and predispose to thermal illnesses. Identifying athletes at risk, monitoring the WBGT index, ensuring adequate hydration, and rapidly treating athletes exhibiting symptoms of thermal illness can help prevent EHS.

REFERENCES

1. Bracker MD. Environmental and thermal injury. Clin Sports Med 1992;11:419–436.
2. Allman FL Jr. The effects of heat on the athlete. J Med Assoc Ga 1992;81:307–310.
3. Costrini A. Emergency treatment of exertional heatstroke and comparison of whole body cooling techniques. Med Sci Sports Exerc 1990;22:15–18.
4. US Department of Health and Human Services. Heat-related illnesses and deaths—United States, 1994–1995. MMWR Morb Mortal Wkly Rep 1995;44:465–468.
5. Armstrong LE, Maresh CM. The exertional heat illnesses: a risk of athletic participation. Med Exerc Nutr Health 1993;2:125–134.
6. Nadel ER. Temperature regulation and hyperthermia during exercise. Clin Chest Med 1984;5:13–20.
7. Armstrong LE, DeLuca JP, Hubbard RW. Time course of recovery and heat acclimation ability of prior exertional heatstroke patients. Med Sci Sports Exerc 1990;22:36–48.

8. Armstrong LE, Maresh CM. The Induction and Decay of Heat Acclimatisation in Trained Athletes. Sports Med 1991;12:303–312.

9. Nielsen B. Heat stress and acclimation. Ergonomics 1994;37:49–58.

10. American College of Sports Medicine. Position stand: exercise and fluid replacement. Med Sci Sports Exerc 1996;28:i–vii.

11. Tom PA, Garmel GM, Auerbach PS. Environment-dependent sports emergencies. Med Clin North Am 1994;78:305–325.

12. American College of Sports Medicine. Position stand: heat and cold illnesses during distance running. Med Sci Sports Exerc 1996; 28:i–x.

13. Hubbard RW. Exertional heatstroke: an international perspective. Med Sci Sports Exerc 1990;22:2–5.

14. Hansen RD, Olds TS, Richards DA, et al. Infrared thermometry in the diagnosis and treatment of heat exhaustion. Int J Sports Med 1996;17:66–70.

15. Noakes TD. The hyponatremia of exercise. Int J Sport Nutr 1992;2:205–228.

16. Weiner JS, Khogali M. A physiological body-cooling unit for treatment of heat stroke. Lancet 1980;1:507–510.

17. White JD, Kamath R, Nucci R, et al. Evaporation versus iced peritoneal lavage treatment of heatstroke: comparative efficacy in a canine model. Am J Emerg Med 1993;11:1–3.

18. Harker J, Gibson P. Heat-stroke: a review of rapid cooling techniques. Intensive and Critical Care Nursing 1995;11:198–202.

19. Armstrong LE, Crago AE, Adams R, et al. Whole-body cooling of hyperthermic runners: comparison of two field therapies. Am J Emerg Med 1996;14:355–358.

29

Drugs and Sports

TED EPPERLY

The consumption of ergogenic aids to enhance athletic performance is as old as the history of man. The earliest reported usage dates back to the third century B.C., when Greek athletes reportedly used stimulants to improve their athletic performance.[1] Similarly, through time, Incas chewed coca leaves, berserkers ate mushrooms, and ancient Olympians ate opium-soaked bread to help them achieve their maximum athletic performance.[2] With the discovery of androgenic steroids, such as testosterone in 1935, came the gradual appearance of steroid use among athletes. The first known use was by a Soviet weight-lifting team in the 1950s.[3] Since the 1960s, the use of anabolic steroids has crept into endurance sports, such as running, swimming, and cross-country skiing, and into the recreational athlete who just wants an improved appearance.[3]

The term "doping" came from the Dutch *doop*, which means viscous opium juice, and today signifies any stupefying drug—or in the athletic parlance, any ergogenic drug.[2]

As the illicit drug explosion of the late 1960s rocketed into the 1970s, 1980s, and 1990s, it is little wonder that the sports community has also developed a major drug use-abuse problem. With the mentality of "win at all cost" has come an era of unnatural and dangerous substance abuse.

This chapter provides a review of the currently used ergogenic aids (Table 29-1) and discusses their efficacy, risks, and benefits. Additionally, practical means of detection and intervention as they apply to the physician, therapist, or trainer are discussed.

ANABOLIC AGENTS

In 1992, the category of anabolic-androgenic steroids (AASs) was renamed "anabolic agents." This was done primarily to include the anabolic effects of the beta$_2$-agonists[4]:

salbutamol (albuterol), terbutaline sulfate, and clenbuterol. These drugs, as well as AASs, are explicitly prohibited. At the time of the ban, clenbuterol had been gaining much acclaim as a potent anabolic drug in the cattle industry.[4]

The normal adult male testes produce approximately 4–10 mg of testosterone per day.[5] AASs are synthetic derivatives of testosterone and possess both anabolic (growth) and androgenic (masculinizing) properties. The anabolic and androgenic effects of testosterone and these synthetic derivatives are not the result of different actions but of the same action in different tissues.[6] Two forms of AASs are on the market. The oral form is alkylated at the 17-alpha position, which results in rapid absorption, slow hepatic inactivation, and increased hepatotoxicity.[6] The parenteral forms consist of 19-nortestosterone derivatives and testosterone esters; they are taken intramuscularly and absorbed slowly with long serum half-lives.[6] Table 29-2 lists some of the common oral and parenteral agents.

That these agents are abused is an understatement when reported doses are anywhere from 10 to 1,000 times larger than those prescribed for medical purposes.[7] Not only are the doses large, but many athletes take multiple anabolic steroids concurrently ("stacking") and cycle the drugs by tapering the dose upward or downward for 4- to 18-week periods.[6, 7] This is usually followed by a drug-free interval of 2–3 months, although some steroid abusers take these drugs year-round.

The cost of oral steroids is variable, depending on source, quantity, and location, and ranges from $30 per 100 tablets of stanozolol to $75 for 60 tablets of testosterone undecenoate.[6] The parenteral steroids range from $15 per vial of nandrolone phenpropionate (Durabolin) to $140 per vial of trenbolone acetate (Finajet).[6] The U.S. Food and Drug Administration estimates black market sales at $300 million to $500 million a year.[7] Approxi-

TABLE 29-1
Currently Used Ergogenic Drugs and Aids

Anabolic-Androgenic Steroids	Newer Drugs
Human growth hormone	Creatine
Caffeine	Carnitine
Beta-blockers	Sodium bicarbonate
Stimulants	Phosphates
Alcohol	Branched-chain amino
Marijuana	acids
Diuretics	Cyproheptadine
Nonsteroidal anti-inflammatory	Ginseng
drugs	Methylating drugs
Antiasthmatic drugs	Local anesthetics
Erythropoietin	Octacosanol
Blood doping	Guarana
Beta-agonists (e.g., clenbuterol)	Gamma oryzanol
	Proteolytic enzymes
	Dimethyl sulfoxide
	Bee pollen
	Protein supplements
	Vitamins

mately 80% are believed to be purchased through the black market, involving mail order and gymnasiums, and roughly 20% through health professionals (physicians, pharmacists, or veterinarians).[7, 8]

Epidemiology

AAS abuse is widespread in society and affects both men and women at the high school, college, professional,

Olympic, and amateur levels. Studies indicate that usage is as high as 80% among weight lifters and bodybuilders[7] and is approximately 100% at the level of national and international bodybuilding, weight lifting, power lifting, and power events.[5] Another study focusing on men and women bodybuilders in Kansas and Missouri found steroid use on a regular basis in 54% of the male and 10% of the female competitors.[9] At the high school level, studies indicate AAS use ranging from 0.8% to 1.4% for females and from 4.5% to 6.6% for males.[2, 10, 11]

Benefits

AASs do have clear-cut medical indications in which they have been found to be clinically useful. These conditions are anemia of renal disease, breast cancer, bone marrow failure, bone resorption during space flight, hereditary angioneurotic edema, hypogonadism, Turner's syndrome, hyperlipidemias, and osteoporosis.[2, 12]

Presently, there are believed to be three mechanisms of action for the increase in muscle strength caused by AASs: (1) increased muscle protein synthesis, (2) blocking of the catabolic effects of glucocorticoids, and (3) steroid-induced aggressiveness, which promotes more frequent and demanding muscular workouts.[13]

Many studies have been performed to establish whether AAS use is beneficial. The most thorough and comprehensive review concluded that consistent improvements in strength, body size, and body weight would result from AAS administration if the following criteria were met: (1) intensive weight training was used immediately before

TABLE 29-2
Commonly Used Anabolic-Androgenic Steroids

Oral Anabolic-Androgenic Steroids		Parenteral Anabolic-Androgenic Steroids	
Trade Name	Generic Name	Trade Name	Generic Name
Anadrol	Oxymetholone	Anatrofin	Stenbolone
Anavar	Oxandrolone	Bolfortan	Testosterone nicotinate
Dianabol	Methandrostenolone	Deca-Durabolin	Nandrolone decanoate
Halotestin	Fluoxymesterone	Durabolin	Nandrolone phenpropionate
Maxibolin	Ethylestrenol	Delatestryl	Testosterone enanthate
Nilevar	Norethandrolone	Depo-Testosterone	Testosterone cypionate
Primobolan	Methenolone acetate	Dianabol	Methandrostenolone
Proviron	Mesterolone	Enoltestovis	Hexoxymestrolun
Winstrol	Stanozolol	Equipoise	Boldenone
	Testosterone undecenoate	Finajet	Trenbolone acetate
		Oreton	Testosterone propionate
		Parabolan	Trenbolone
		Primobolan	Methenolone enanthate
		Winstrol V	Stanozolol

Source: Adapted from RH Strauss, CE Yesalis. Anabolic steroids in the athlete. Annu Rev Med 1991;42:449–457; and MD Johnson. Anabolic steroid use in adolescent athletes. Pediatr Clin North Am 1990;37:1111–1123.

and during the steroid regimen, (2) the athletes used a high-protein and high-calorie diet, and (3) strength measurements were determined by simple free-weight measurements rather than isometrically with dynamometers.[12]

The majority of studies not using these criteria have failed to show gains in strength from AASs.[5] One review of 25 trials on male subjects produced conflicting results and concluded "evidence for enhancement to be inconclusive or at best indicative of small increases."[2] There have been no data to demonstrate that AAS use improved aerobic capability.[12] As Catlin and Hatton pointed out, "it is unlikely that the efficacy question will be definitively answered with conventional study designs."[2] One report on the effect of anabolic steroids on lean body mass demonstrated that there is a typical dose-response curve.[14] This report showed that a low dose of AAS produces a very modest effect, whereas large doses result in a greater augmentation of lean body mass. Studies that do show some differences between the steroid and placebo group after 3–12 weeks of training demonstrate an improvement of approximately 8 kg in maximal lifts in the bench press and 11 kg in maximal lifts in the squat.[5]

A fair conclusion to draw from the confusing literature is that AASs by themselves probably do not improve muscular strength. When coupled with high-intensity weight training and an adequate diet in a previously trained athlete, however, AASs will produce an increase in muscle strength.[15] As Lombardo has said, "rarely, if ever, is there a solitary factor that contributes to success; success is a result of optimal development of many factors."[16] The factors Lombardo cited include level of conditioning, skill, diet, psyche, opponent, arena, sleep, drugs, and genes.[16]

Risks

Most athletes, trainers, coaches, and physicians are aware of some of the side effects of AAS use. The truth of the matter is that almost all organ systems are in some way affected. Table 29-3 summarizes these deleterious effects.

As a result of a careful review of the literature, the American College of Sports Medicine took an official stand on the use of AASs in sports and concluded that "the use of AASs by athletes is contrary to the rules and ethical principles of athletic competition" and this organization "deplores the use of AASs by athletes."[13]

HUMAN GROWTH HORMONE

Human growth hormone (hGH) is a polypeptide neurohormone that is secreted by the anterior lobe of the pituitary. Until 1985, the only source of hGH was cadaveric collection. Currently, hGH is synthetically manufactured using recombinant DNA techniques. This recombinant hGH has similar efficacy to cadaveric sources, but the molecule contains a methionyl group on the amino-terminal end that causes antibody formation in approximately 30–40% of users.[1]

As a growth promoter, hGH induces tissue growth, stimulates protein synthesis, accelerates linear growth, and increases body weight and mass.[2] In addition, performance may be enhanced through hGH-mediated lipid mobilization. Serum growth hormone levels are artificially increased by two means: (1) direct injection of hGH or (2) the use of oral drugs that stimulate the release of endogenous growth hormone from the pituitary.[17] Drugs that may cause endogenous hGH release include propranolol, vasopressin, clonidine, levodopa, and amino acids, most notably arginine, lysine, ornithine, and tryptophan.[17]

The serum half-life of hGH is very short, ranging from 15 minutes to 1 hour, and is not currently detectable through available testing. Recombinant hGH is reported to be available without a prescription in many countries and is widely available on the black market.[18, 19] One major factor that limits hGH from becoming pandemically abused is its astronomic wholesale cost of approximately $210 per 5-mg dose (or approximately $1,000 per month).[20] In 1996, the International Olympic Committee (IOC) in conjunction with other groups launched a $2 million project to develop and implement a validated test for hGH before the Sydney Olympics in 2000.[4]

Epidemiology

Few studies have been done to determine the prevalence of hGH abuse. In one study of high school students, the majority of these students were familiar with the hormone and its effects, 31% claimed they knew someone using growth hormone, and 5% reported using this drug themselves.[18] Because of the difficulties in detecting the use of hGH, this has the potential to become the drug of choice in many power athletes.[17]

Benefits

Human growth hormone is medically indicated to treat growth hormone–deficient conditions in children (dwarfism). Additionally, it is being investigated for use in speeding fracture healing, treating osteoporosis, and reversing the catabolic changes seen in debilitating disease and aging.[17] There are numerous anecdotal claims from bodybuilders and weight lifters that hGH has caused 30- to 40-lb increases in lean body weight.[17] Other users,

TABLE 29-3
Deleterious Effects of Anabolic-Androgenic Steroids

System	Effects	System	Effects
Central nervous system	Aggressive behavior ("roid rage")	Endocrine	Testicular atrophy
	Homicide[a]	Male	Decreased reproductive hormones
	Depression		(LH, FSH, testosterone)
	Suicide[b]		Oligospermia/azoospermia
	Acute psychosis		Prostatic hypertrophy
	Irritability		Prostatic carcinoma
	Manic episodes		Gynecomastia
	Increased or decreased libido	Female[c, 41]	Masculinization
	Cerebrovascular accidents		Breast tissue reduction
	Headache		Voice deepening
	Euphoria		Hirsutism
	Dependence/addiction		Clitoral hypertrophy
Hepatic	Increased liver function tests		Increased or decreased libido
	Hepatic carcinoma		Male pattern hair loss
	Peliosis hepatis		Menstrual irregularities
	Cholestatic jaundice	Skin	Striae
Cardiac	Hypertension		Acne
	Decreased HDL cholesterol		Temporal hair loss
	Increased LDL cholesterol		Alopecia
	Increased triglycerides		Oily skin
	Clotting abnormalities		Folliculitis
	Myocardial infarction	Miscellaneous	Dizziness
Renal	Edema		Nausea
	Increase in BUN and creatinine		Scrotal pain
	Wilms' tumor		Small bowel obstruction[2] secondary to iliopsoas hypertrophy
	Urinary frequency		
	Urethritis		AIDS (sharing needles)

LH = luteinizing hormone; FSH = follicle-stimulating hormone; HDL = high-density lipoprotein; LDL = low-density lipoprotein; BUN = blood urea nitrogen; AIDS = acquired immunodeficiency syndrome.
[a]Pope HG, Katz DL. Homicide and near homicide by anabolic steroid users. J Clin Psychiatry 1990;51:28–31.
[b]Brower KJ, Blow FC, Eliopulos GA, et al. Anabolic androgenic steroids and suicide. Am J Psychiatry 1989;146:1075–1078.
[c]Strauss RH, Liggett MT, Lanese RR. Anabolic steroid use and perceived effects in ten weight-trained women athletes. JAMA 1985;253:2871–2873.
Source: Adapted from DH Catlin, CK Hatton. Use and abuse of anabolic and other drugs for athletic enhancement. Adv Intern Med 1991;36:399–424; DO Hough. Anabolic steroids and ergogenic aids. Am Fam Physician 1990;41:1157–1164; and MD Johnson. Anabolic steroid use in adolescent athletes. Pediatr Clin North Am 1990;37:1111–1123.

however, are not as impressed and think that these effects are overrated. The current evidence does not show a clear benefit from hGH and supports that its major effect may be to increase muscle bulk and mass (primarily by increases in connective tissue and not contractile elements) without an increase in strength.[17]

Risks

The adverse effects of hGH are similar to those of gigantism in children and acromegaly in adults. These effects consist of hyperglycemia, hyperlipidemia, heart disease, impotence, arthrosis, hypothyroidism, muscle weakness, and bony enlargement of the forehead, jaw, hands, and feet, producing a Frankenstein-like appearance.[2, 21, 22] Additionally, people with acromegaly have a shortened life span. Risks that have been reported in

the pediatric population include slipped femoral capital epiphysis, hGH antibody formation, insulin resistance, sodium and fluid retention, acromegaly, and leukemia.[23] Because black market preparations are often from cadaveric collection from former eastern bloc countries, there is a real risk of Creutzfeldt-Jakob disease.[19] Additional risks are those of shared needles, such as hepatitis and acquired immunodeficiency syndrome (AIDS).[17]

CAFFEINE

Caffeine and other xanthine-containing foods and beverages are mild stimulants. Caffeine is commonly ingested in coffee (100 mg per cup), soft drinks (30–45 mg per can), and analgesic and cold medications (32–64 mg per tablet).

Abusers use tablet, suppository, and intravenous caffeine in doses approaching 1 g.

Caffeine was added to the list of substances banned by the IOC in 1982 at the limit of 15 mg/L, which was subsequently reduced to 12 mg/L, where it now stands.[2] Some have called for this level to be lowered to 8 mg/L.[24] An athlete would have to consume approximately 1,000 mg of caffeine within 3 hours to exceed this level of 12 mg/L.[25] This would equate to approximately 7–8 mg/kg.[24]

Epidemiology

Caffeine is used and consumed by many citizens as well as athletes. Good data on abuse are lacking, although one study purports that misuse of caffeine is more pronounced in both professional and amateur classes than in younger categories.[26] The Center for Drug Free Sport found that 26% of 16,000 Canadian youth (ages 11–18) had reported using caffeine to enhance their athletic performance.[24]

Benefits

Being a stimulant, caffeine can cause a heightened sense of arousal and alertness. Its postulated effect as an ergogenic aid is the result of increased mobilization and oxidation of free fatty acids and relative sparing of muscle glycogen.[27] A facilitation of neuromuscular function is also postulated.[27]

Whether caffeine is effective as an ergogenic aid is controversial. Some studies have shown improved performance in endurance sports—such as cycling, Nordic skiing, and running—whereas others have shown no beneficial ergogenic aid.[2, 27-29] Several studies have found that high caffeine dosage (9 mg/kg) increased the endurance times of both well-trained competitive runners and recreational athletes by 50% and 27% respectively.[24] Similarly, doses of 5–13 mg/kg improved endurance cycling and swimming times.[24]

Risks

Modest use of caffeine carries no serious side effects. In addition to increased heart and respiratory rate and diuresis, caffeine results in bronchodilation, increased gastric acid secretion, and less fatigue. Decreased coordination and increased blood pressure are also seen, and their extent is dependent on dose. Higher doses can lead to nervousness, irritability, tremulousness, insomnia, irregular heartbeat, delirium, and seizures. Physical dependence can occur, and withdrawal headaches are common.[2]

BETA-BLOCKERS

The beta-blockers—such as propranolol (Inderal) and metoprolol (Lopressor)—have been used by marksmen, archers, golfers, ski jumpers, ballet dancers, musicians, and other athletes since the early 1970s.[2, 30] Their use appears to be in sports in which fine motor control is desired. They work by blocking the stimulant action of the catecholamines and thus decrease heart rate and tremor. In a study of 33 marksmen, metoprolol was compared with placebo, and it was clearly evident that shooting scores improved by 13.4%.[30] This improvement was most pronounced in the most skilled marksmen and thought to be the result of decreased hand tremor. The beta-blockers are now banned by the IOC in such sports as the modern pentathalon, diving, archery, shooting, bobsled, freestyle skiing, sailing, synchronized swimming, and ski jumping.[2, 4] Beta-blockers have been shown to reduce performance in endurance events by as much as 50%.[2]

STIMULANTS

The class of compounds known as *stimulants* acts on the central nervous system and the neuromuscular system by stimulating the effects of the body's catecholamines. Agents in this class include amphetamines, cocaine, and the more commonly used phenylpropanolamine and ephedrine. The prevalence of their use is estimated to be approximately 1% in athletes.[2] The stimulants cause euphoria, increased alertness, aggressiveness, anorexia, increased confidence, and fatigue reduction. Usage is seen primarily in running, swimming, cycling, and speed skating and among athletes competing in weight categories, who use them as anorectics.[2] Of 11 studies, eight demonstrated that amphetamines improved performance in running, swimming, and cycling time, most likely by decreasing fatigue.[2] The adverse effects of these agents in high enough doses include psychosis, seizures, hypertension, arrhythmias, heat stroke, tolerance, dependence, and even one report of a cyclist's death.[2] Ephedrine has one-fifth the potency of amphetamine, and one double-blind study showed no significant improvement in athletic performance while using that agent.[31] However, the use of over-the-counter drugs containing ephedrine and pseudoephedrine in high doses is similar to that of amphetamines.[4]

ALCOHOL

Alcohol is probably the most frequently used drug in this review. There appears to be no evidence that alcohol usage before or during athletic performance enhances abilities. Conversely, the decremental loss of fine motor skills and coordination speaks against its use.[31] Two studies evaluating alcohol as an ergogenic aid in well-trained runners revealed that it does not enhance endurance or improve performance.[32, 33] The only sport that bans ethyl alcohol is the modern pentathalon because of its potential aid in the shooting event secondary to its potential antitremor effect in low dose.[4]

MARIJUANA

The active ingredient in marijuana, delta-9-tetrahydrocannabinol (THC), impairs coordination and can lead to apathy, decreased concentration, loss of ambition, declined work performance, and reduction in plasma testosterone, oligospermia, and gynecomastia.[31] This review found no substantiation of any evidence supporting THC as an ergogenic aid.

DIURETICS

Diuretics, such as furosemide (Lasix), are most often abused by athletes in judo, karate, boxing, and wrestling who are trying to "make" weight by diuresing water from their bodies. Additionally, bodybuilders try to "cut" their physique before competition by use of these agents. Not only can the diuretics lead to dehydration, dizziness, hypokalemia, and heat injury, but they can also decrease muscular work and performance. Diuretics are also used to conceal banned substances by diluting them in urine. However, this practice can be overcome by keeping athletes until their urine-specific gravity reaches 1.005 or 1.010 or by freeze-drying their urine to concentrate it. Additionally, the diuretics themselves are banned and easily detected in the urine.[2]

NONSTEROIDAL ANTI-INFLAMMATORY DRUGS

Nonsteroidal anti-inflammatory drugs (NSAIDs) are commonly used by physicians and trainers to treat a wide variety of injuries. No evidence could be found that they enhance performance other than by relieving pain. NSAIDs, however, are associated with adverse effects that can decrease athletic performance: dyspepsia, gastrointestinal bleeding, sedation, reduced renal perfusion, hyperkalemia, and salt and water retention. They can also interfere with thermoregulatory function, such as increas-

ing sweating and predisposing to dehydration and heat injury. These agents are not banned by the IOC.[31]

ANTIASTHMATIC DRUGS

All sympathomimetic amines with alpha or beta stimulation are banned. There is minimal evidence to suggest that other medications to control asthma or exercise-induced bronchospasm—such as $beta_2$-agonists, cromolyn sodium, and glucocorticoids administered by inhalation—are ergogenic. Conversely, theophylline's ability to enhance both cardiac and respiratory muscle function could be ergogenic, and further studies to determine this effect are warranted.[31]

Although the $beta_2$-agonists have an anabolic effect, three agents (terbutaline, salbutamol, and salmeterol) are allowed by the National Collegiate Athletic Association and IOC if declared in advance and used only by inhalation.[4] Similarly, inhaled corticosteroids may be used if declared in advance. Theophylline, cromolyn sodium, and anticholinergics can be used as well. If a team's or individual's usage of antiasthma medicines is questioned, then spirometry or other diagnostic tests may be performed.[4]

INDUCED ERYTHROCYTHEMIA (BLOOD DOPING)

Anecdotal reports of blood doping have existed since the 1950s. This technique has traditionally involved the precompetition transfusion of 1–2 units of type- and cross-matched blood from a donor (homologous) or the athlete's own blood (autologous) harvested 8–12 weeks earlier and given 1–2 days before the event.

Blood doping is thought to improve performance through two effects: (1) an increase in the red cell mass that accentuates oxygen delivery to muscle, and (2) an increase in blood volume leading to increased cardiac output and improved thermoregulation and lactate buffering.[34] More than 20 clinical trials have been reported on the performance aspects of blood doping.[2] Although early research did not show clear-cut improvements, several more recent studies have demonstrated significant increases in hemoglobin concentration, VO_2max, and endurance.[1, 2] One study that used a double-blind, sham infusion–controlled, crossover design showed significant increases in run times to exhaustion (35%), VO_2max (5%), and hemoglobin (7%).[2] Five-mile-run time was improved by 49 seconds after infusion of 920 ml of blood in another controlled and placebo-designed study.[1] Another study showed that when the hematocrit was elevated by 10% with transfusion, VO_2max increased 11%, and 3-mile–run time improved by 23.7 seconds.[1] The consensus of the literature confirms that autologous red blood cell transfusion significantly improves endurance.[2]

Erythropoietin

The practice of blood doping was revolutionized with the synthesis of recombinant erythropoietin (EPO). Endogenous EPO is a glycoprotein hormone produced by the kidney to stimulate hemoglobin and red blood cell production. Its production is increased in response to hypoxic stress, such as with anemia or altitude. Recombinant human EPO (r-Hu-EPO) has been available since 1988 and is currently indicated for use in patients with anemia secondary to chronic renal failure, zidovudine-induced anemia, and anemia associated with cancer chemotherapy. r-Hu-EPO has been shown to significantly increase hematocrit in these patients. Some studies have shown a similar effect in healthy athletes treated with r-Hu-EPO.[35] These hematologic changes are accompanied by improvements in performance.[36] Not surprisingly, r-Hu-EPO has found its way into the endurance sport communities of bicycling, swimming, and cross-country skiing, although epidemiologic studies of its use are lacking.

Risks of Blood Doping

The most important risks of induced erythrocythemia are those associated with hyperviscosity that is due to the expanded total red blood cell mass and hemoconcentration associated with dehydration. Several deaths in cyclists have been anecdotally linked to the practice of doping (both transfusion and r-Hu-EPO administration), although this relationship has not been proved (Undetectable dialysis drug is tied to athlete's death. *Los Angeles Times*, May 22, 1990). Other medical risks of doping include those of homologous blood transfusion, such as minor transfusion reactions (in 3–4%, fever, chills, malaise) and the risk of infection transmission (less than 1%), primarily that of malaria, hepatitis, AIDS, and cytomegalovirus. The reported risks of r-Hu-EPO administration include hypertension, thrombotic events, and seizures, all postulated to be secondary to an expanded blood volume and increased viscosity.[2]

Testing and Detection

Neither r-Hu-EPO abuse nor autologous blood transfusion is directly detectable by present methods. Although serum EPO levels can be measured using sensitive immunoassays, the levels indicating illicit r-Hu-EPO are not defined.[37] This is further complicated by the fact that the EPO levels return to baseline in 4–7 days after administration, but the effects of the drug last for the life of the newly synthesized red blood cells, which is approximately 120 days.[38]

Efforts to test for blood doping in athletes has led several sports governing bodies to investigate the use of hematologic indices (hemoglobin, hematocrit, and serum iron) as a screening test.[35, 38] The use of hematocrit level is currently being adopted by the international governing bodies of both cycling and Nordic skiing and will likely be used for most national and international competitions in the near future.

The American College of Sports Medicine revised its position on blood doping as an ergogenic aid and concluded that "the use of blood doping as an ergogenic aid is unethical and unjustifiable, but that autologous red blood cell infusion is an acceptable procedure to induce erythrocythemia in clinically controlled conditions for the purpose of legitimate scientific inquiry."[39]

NEW DRUGS

Many other drugs have been tried and are presently being used and introduced at all levels of athletic competition. These drugs are mentioned here for completeness, but the scope of this text prevents a more detailed description. Some of the newer agents that have gained attention are creatine, carnitine, sodium bicarbonate, phosphate, and branched chain amino acids. The literature on these agents is somewhat conflictual. Future studies should be well-defined, double-blind, placebo-controlled trials to determine these new agents' true efficacy. Some other agents are cyproheptadine (Periactin); ginseng (an oriental herb); methylating drugs, such as trimethylglycine and dimethylglycine (pangamic acid or vitamin B_{15}); local anesthetics (Novocain, Xylocaine); and agents that decrease recovery time between heavy exercise, such as octacosanol (alcohol from wheat germ oil), guarana (Brazilian herb), gamma oryzanol (alcohol from rice bran oil), and proteolytic enzymes (trypsin, chymotrypsin, papain). Additionally, other drugs to consider are dimethyl sulfoxide, bee pollen, and a whole list of nutritional supplements (proteins and vitamins B, C, and E). All of these agents have no proved efficacy as ergogenic acids.

DETECTION

The astute physician, therapist, or trainer may be able to detect potential ergogenic drug use from a variety of sources, including the patient, friends, and "locker room talk." Odd or atypical behavior on the part of an athlete should raise suspicion. Another excellent source of information comes from the preparticipation sports examination, as well stated by Johnson.[6]

History

A useful approach to addressing drug use is to ask whether the athlete has any friends who use steroids or other performance-enhancing drugs. This can then be followed by asking whether the athlete has used or is using any of these drugs. Be open, honest, and nonjudgmental, and remind the individual of your confidentiality as the situation dictates. If the patient admits to ergogenic drug use, ask about what types, doses, frequency, duration of use, when last used, and side effects. Answers to questions about rapid weight gain, rapid maturation, and rapid muscular growth are important to obtain from the athlete or the athlete's parents. Mood swings, increased aggressiveness, sudden emotional or violent outbursts, and personality changes are potential tip-offs.

Physical Examination

Observation for hypertension, edema, facial puffiness, acne, scleral icterus, and hepatic enlargement and tenderness are important. Additionally, height and weight, body habitus, muscle mass, and Tanner staging should be done. For males, signs of testicular atrophy, prostatic hypertrophy, gynecomastia, temporal hair loss, and deepened voice are findings consistent with potential anabolic steroid use. In females, checking for signs of masculinization may detect covert steroid abuse.

Laboratory

If ergogenic drug use is suspected, the following tests should be performed: hemoglobin and hematocrit (for blood doping, EPO), glucose (hGH), creatinine and blood urea nitrogen (steroids, diuretics), high-density lipoprotein and low-density lipoprotein cholesterol (steroids, hGH), and urinalysis (steroids). Additionally, liver function tests to include alkaline phosphatase, lactate dehydrogenase, and bilirubin should be obtained (steroids, alcohol). Tests of alanine aminotransferase (serum glutamate pyruvate transaminase), aspartate aminotransferase (serum glutamic-oxaloacetic transaminase), and creatine phosphokinase are also helpful but may be elevated secondary to skeletal muscle breakdown. Early epiphyseal closure (hGH, steroids) may be determined by bone-age x-ray studies. Sodium and potassium (diuret-

ics, NSAIDs) and uric acid (protein supplements, steroids) may also be useful.

Special Drug Testing

Urine can be initially screened for many of these substances (steroids, caffeine, stimulants), and serum can be checked for others (alcohol). In the case of anabolic steroids, urine screen by radioimmunoassay followed by gas chromatography (GC) with mass spectrometry (MS) for specific identification is often the diagnostic protocol.[6] These steroid assays using GC/MS, however, are expensive: the cost of a single test is more than $100.[40] The IOC has adopted the use of testosterone to epitestosterone (T/E) ratio to detect the use of endogenous testosterone supplements. Current guidelines consider a T/E ratio less than 6 to be negative, a T/E ratio between 6 and 10 to warrant further testing, and a T/E ratio more than 10 to be positive indication of AAS abuse.

Follow-Up

Reviewing with the athlete the results of the history, physical, and laboratory tests is very important. If patients are using ergogenic aids, the demonstration of how these drugs are affecting them can be made in an extremely valuable and timely "teaching moment" to persuade them to stop. If a patient denies ergogenic drug use (but you still strongly suspect it), then revealing the abnormalities on examination or laboratory results may be enough to persuade the individual to stop using the drug. If the patient decides to continue the drug use, then follow-up examination and laboratory work are recommended every 6 months; however, the physician should make every reasonable attempt to halt the drug use and remind the athlete that it is detrimental to his or her health and is unpredictable.[6]

PREVENTION

Education is the most effective tool for deterring ergogenic drug abuse. The physician, therapist, and trainer can become involved with this education at multiple levels. The "teaching moment" (when one is with the athlete alone) is very important. One should try to take advantage of these opportunities to educate the athlete about risks in an effort to provide the information necessary for an informed and wise choice. Similarly, discussions and lectures to parents, coaches, teachers, teams, and students are beneficial in providing information.

There are many myths and half-truths concerning these agents, and education is key to shattering them. Especially important is education focused on parents, coaches, and teachers, because they have such a large impact on young, impressionable students. One such example of an organized effort to decrease adolescent athletes' use of AASs is the Adolescents Training and Learning to Avoid Steroids (ATLAS) program.[41] This program was developed in Oregon and used seven weekly, 50-minute class sessions delivered by coaches and student team leaders that addressed AAS effects, sports nutrition, strength training alternatives to AAS use, drug-refusal role play, and anti-AAS media messages. A study of this intervention by Goldberg and colleagues[41] compared 702 players in the experimental group and 804 players at control schools on 31 high school football teams. Questionnaires before and after the intervention and at 9- and 12-month follow-up showed the ATLAS program enhanced healthy behavior, reduced factors that encourage AAS use, and lowered intent to use AASs.[41] Most important, these behavioral changes were sustained over a period of 1 year.

Along with adequate and timely education, there must be appropriate drug testing that is consistently and fairly applied, as well as clearly stated penalties and sanctions to athletes found to be using these agents. This combined approach of education, appropriate drug testing, and fair penalties and sanctions will, one hopes, eventually lead to a major change in a detrimental behavior and dangerous medical problem. This change is also necessary to preserving the integrity of sports and sport competition.

REFERENCES

1. Wooley BH. The latest fads to increase muscle mass and energy. Postgrad Med 1991;89:195–205.
2. Catlin DH, Hatton CK. Use and abuse of anabolic and other drugs for athletic enhancement. Adv Intern Med 1991;36:399–424.
3. Strauss RH, Yesalis CE. Anabolic steroids in the athlete. Annu Rev Med 1991;42:449–457.
4. Catlin D, Murray T. Performance-enhancing drugs, fair competition, and Olympic sport. JAMA 1996;276;3:231–237.
5. Hough DO. Anabolic steroids and ergogenic aids. Am Fam Physician 1990;41:1157–1164.
6. Johnson MD. Anabolic steroid use in adolescent athletes. Pediatr Clin North Am 1990;37:1111–1123.
7. Council on Scientific Affairs. Medical and nonmedical uses of anabolic-androgenic steroids. JAMA 1990;264:2923–2927.
8. Breo DL. Of MDs and muscles—lessons from two "retired steroid doctors." JAMA 1990;263:1697–1705.
9. Tricker R, O'Neill MR, Cook D. The incidence of anabolic steroid use among competitive bodybuilders. J Drug Educ 1989;19:313–325.
10. Windsor R, Dumitra D. Prevalence of anabolic steroid use by male and female adolescents. Med Sci Sports Exerc 1989;21:494–497.
11. Scott D, Wagner J, Barlow T. Anabolic steroid use among adolescents in Nebraska schools. Am J Health Syst Pharm 1996;53:2068–2072.
12. Haupt HA, Rovere GD. Anabolic steroids: a review of the literature. Am J Sports Med 1984;12:469–484.
13. American College of Sports Medicine. Position stand on the use of anabolic-androgenic steroids in sports. Med Sci Sports Exerc 1987;19:540–543.
14. Forbes GB. The effect of anabolic steroids on lean body mass: the dose response curve. Metabolism 1985;34:571–573.
15. Nelson MA. Androgenic-anabolic steroid use in adolescents. J Pediatr Health Care 1989;3:175–180.
16. Lombardo JA. Anabolic-androgenic steroids. NIDA Res Monogr 1990;102:60–73.
17. McIntyre JG. Growth hormone and athletes. Sports Med 1987;4:129–142.
18. Deyssig R, Frisch H. Self-administration of cadaveric growth hormone in power athletes. Lancet 1993;341:768–769.
19. Riskert VI, Pawlak-Morello C, Sheppard V, Jay MS. Human growth hormone: a new substance of abuse among adolescents? Clin Pediatr (Phila) 1992;25:723–726.
20. Drug Topic, Red Book. Montvale, NJ: Medical Economics Co., Inc., 1997.
21. White GL, Murdock RT, Richardson GE, et al. Preventing growth hormone abuse: an emerging health concern. Health Educ Q 1989;4–10.
22. Council on Scientific Affairs. Drug abuse in athletes: anabolic steroids and human growth hormone. JAMA 1988;259:1703–1705.
23. Neely EK, Rosenfeld RG. Use and abuse of human growth hormone. Annu Rev Med 1994;45:407–420.
24. Clarkson P. Nutrition for improved sports performance. Sports Med 1996;6:393–401.
25. Van Der Merwe PJ, Muller FR, Muller F. Caffeine in sport: urinary excretion of caffeine in healthy volunteers after intake of common caffeine-containing beverages. South African Med J 1988;74:163–164.
26. Delbeke FT, Debackere M. Caffeine: use and abuse in sports. Int J Sports Med 1984;5:179–182.
27. Tarnopolsky MA, Atkinson SA, MacDougal JD, et al. Physiological response to caffeine during endurance running in habitual caffeine users. Med Sci Sports Exerc 1989;21:418–424.
28. Flinn S, Gregory J, McNaughton LR, et al. Caffeine ingestion prior to incremental cycling to exhaustion in recreational cyclists. Int J Sports Med 1990;11:188–193.
29. Sasaki H, Maeda J, Usui S, et al. Effect of sucrose and caffeine ingestion on performance of prolonged strenuous running. Int J Sports Med 1987;8:261–265.
30. Kruse P, Jorgen L, Nielsen U, et al. Beta blockade used in precision sports: effect on pistol shooting performance. J Appl Physiol 1986;61:417–420.
31. Puffer JC. The use of drugs in swimming. Clin Sports Med 1986;5:77–89.

32. Houard JA, Langenfeld ME, Wiley RL, et al. Effects of the acute ingestion of small amounts of alcohol among 5-mile run times. J Sports Med 1987;27:253–257.

33. McNaughton L, Preece D. Alcohol and its effects on sprint and middle distance running. Br J Sports Med 1986;29:56–59.

34. Jones M, Tunsfall DS. Blood doping—a literature review. Br J Sports Med 1989;23:84–88.

35. Casoni I, Ricci G, Borsetto C, et al. Hematologic indices of erythropoietin administration in athletes. In J Sports Med 1993;14:307–311.

36. Ekbloom B, Berglund B. Effect of erythropoietin administration on maximal aerobic power. Scand J Med Sci Sports 1991;1:88–93.

37. Roberts D, Shuh D, Smith DJ. Application of a modified INCSTAR Epo-trac 125/RIA for measurement of serum erythropoietin concentration in elite athletes. Clin Biochem 1995;28:573–580.

38. Souillard A, Audran M, Bressolle F, et al. Pharmacokinetics and pharmacodynamics of recombinant erythropoietin in athletes. Br J Clin Pharmacol 1996;42:355–364.

39. American College of Sports Medicine. Position stand on blood doping as an ergogenic aid. Med Sci Sports Exerc 1987;19:540–543.

40. Dyment PG. Steroids: breakfast of champions. Pediatr Rev 1990;12:103–105.

41. Goldberg L, Elliot D, Clarke G, et. al. Effects of a multidimensional anabolic steroid prevention intervention. JAMA 1996;276:1555–1558.

30

Special Considerations for the Female Athlete

JOHN W. CASSELS, JR., AND DAVID J. MAGELSSEN

Women who are participating in regular, vigorous exercise present the health care practitioner with several unique concerns. Increasing numbers of women participate in competitive athletics and recreational fitness programs. In fact, exercise for health benefit has become the mainstay of preventive medical care. Improved cardiovascular function, weight control, skeletal maintenance, and stress reduction are benefits gained by the active woman. The impact of exercise on her reproductive health can be divided into two broad categories: (1) exercise in the nonpregnant female and its influence on menstrual physiology, reproductive potential, and lower urinary tract dynamics; and (2) exercise in the pregnant athlete, with its impact on maternal and fetal well-being. This chapter reviews these areas of health care concern and provides guidelines for the health care practitioner in treating the female athlete.

GYNECOLOGIC REPRODUCTIVE PHYSIOLOGY

The outward manifestation of normal reproductive function in the female is menstruation, ultimately culminating in pregnancy and childbirth. At menarche, the prepubertal girl begins to experience regular hormonal variation. A finely tuned orchestration of physical, psychosocial, and hormonal events regulates cyclic ovulation and menses.

Normal menstrual function results from a coordinated hypothalamic-pituitary-ovarian axis. Details of this system are available in standard textbooks and have been reviewed by Yen.[1] The gonadotropin-releasing hormone (GnRH) pulse generator is located in the medial basal hypothalamus. It is affected by stimulatory and inhibitory control of hormones and neurotransmitters. Maturation of the hypothalamus appears to be a requirement for normal pubertal events; alteration in its function before or after menarche can affect timing of GnRH secretion. Alterations in GnRH cycles have a detrimental impact on gonadotropin (follicle-stimulating hormone [FSH]–luteinizing hormone [LH]) release.

Pituitary release of FSH and LH in both tonic and cyclic fashion is required for selection, growth, rupture, and maintenance of the follicle as it generates the monthly oocyte and transforms to the corpus luteum during the latter half of the cycle. During growth, the granulosa cell layer of the follicle produces estrogen. A surge of LH, initiated under the influence of adequate exposure of the hypothalamus and pituitary to estrogen, triggers ovum release from the follicle. Subsequently, FSH and LH stimulate further production of estrogen and progesterone from the corpus luteum. In the absence of pregnancy, the corpus luteum undergoes regression and menses occurs.

Alterations in gonadotropin release can occur normally by varying the hormonal environment in which the pituitary is bathed or by pathologic changes (tumors of the pituitary, aplasias of gonadotropin-producing cells, or extragonadal hormonal production). This dysfunction of pituitary release will lead to breakdown of the regular cyclic production of steroid hormones expected in normal reproductive function and required for maintenance of normal physiology.

EXERCISE EFFECTS

Unlike the injuries discussed elsewhere in this text, gynecologic aspects of sports medicine typically do not limit or prevent participation in any activity. Moreover, dysfunction is frequently seen in athletes performing at their personal best. It is the effects of exercise on normal function that leads to concern for the female athlete.

Menstruation

Many studies have investigated the effect of exercise on menstrual function. Reviews should be consulted for details.[2-4] In summary, studies have attempted to determine the links between the degree and type of exercise and regularity of menstrual function; to show relationships between body weight or morphology (low percentage of body fat) attained in or for a particular activity and menstrual function; or to relate the occurrence of abnormal menstrual function (amenorrhea) to detrimental effects (osteoporosis).

There appears to be some agreement that low body fat may adversely affect some athletes; however, the degree of effect may relate as much to diet as to the weight itself. Athletes who consume adequate calories with sufficient protein for energy needs maintain a greater degree of normal menstrual function compared with similar–body-weight athletes who consciously restrict dietary intake.

Similarly, psychological and physical stress may play a role in some individuals independent of body weight. When injuries occur to amenorrheic dancers and limit their practice and performance, menstrual function may return in the absence of body-weight changes. Several studies have suggested an increasing frequency of menstrual dysfunction at increasing levels of participation. This is not directly related to energy expenditure, as different sports with similar physical demands have a differing prevalence of oligo- and amenorrhea.

The synthesis of data available regarding emotional stress, body morphology, and physical activity suggests the conclusions illustrated in Figure 30-1.[5] Any single alteration may be tolerated and menstrual function maintained. Excessive alteration of one factor (exercise to the point of exceeding energy supplies from a nutritional standpoint, altering body weight or percentage of body fat, dieting in an obsessive fashion to the point of physical stress or emotional lability) or combinations of two or more factors will increase the likelihood of menstrual abnormalities.

A normally menstruating woman experiences menses every 21–35 days with a luteal phase of 12–16 days dominated by progestational effects on the endometrium. Increasing degrees of dysfunction will lead to alteration in luteal phase length and progesterone secretion followed by anovulation. Subsequently, the anovulatory woman may develop hypoestrogenism in the face of decreased gonadal activity. Attempts to treat the oligomenorrheic and amenorrheic woman are directed at restoring this cyclic hormonal balance.

Finally, the control of menstruation by use of oral contraceptives may have positive or negative effects on per-

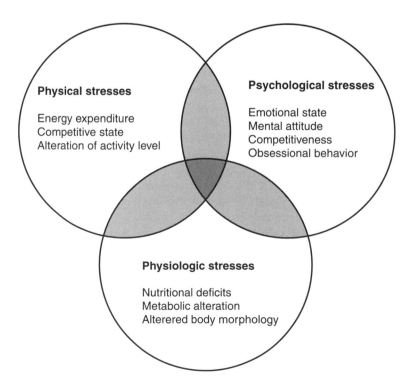

FIGURE 30-1

Normal reproductive health is maintained by interaction of physical, psychological, and physiologic well-being. As stresses occur, there is increased dysfunction. Extreme stress or interaction of stress between health issues may lead to complete cessation of function (anovulation and amenorrhea).

Physical stresses

Energy expenditure
Competitive state
Alteration of activity level

Psychological stresses

Emotional state
Mental attitude
Competitiveness
Obsessional behavior

Physiologic stresses

Nutritional deficits
Metabolic alteration
Alterered body morphology

formance. The "pill" blunts the hormonal swings that occur in the naturally menstruating woman and therefore may alleviate symptoms due to periodic waxing and waning of steroid hormone levels. On the other hand, use of oral contraceptives may have adverse effects on aerobic capacity, muscle strength, and endurance. Many studies of oral contraceptives were performed before the development of current progestin agents used in the pill. Dosage of both estrogen and progestin components of the pill have been drastically altered in current formulations. Details of contraceptive studies have been thoroughly reviewed by Lebrun.[6] The decision to use oral contraceptives should be individualized based on indications and personal effects.

Osteoporosis

A major concern for women who are amenorrheic is the risk of decreased calcium deposition in bone.[7] Bone density increases in both sexes until 25–35 years of age. The controls affecting maximum bone density have not been defined. Periods of hypoestrogenism during lactational amenorrhea result in loss of bone mass, which recovers after the resumption of normal ovarian function. It is unclear whether amenorrheic athletes are invariably at risk of permanent bone mass depletion, although it seems clear that risks are greater in a hypoestrogenic state.

With the onset of amenorrhea, one may expect to see development of osteopenia with long-term progression to osteoporosis. This is manifested in women undergoing surgical castration, natural menopause, or lactational amenorrhea. The effects of athletic amenorrhea are somewhat less clear. Euestrogenic athletes may maintain normal bone architecture, whereas those who progress to hypoestrogenism may experience calcium depletion. Additionally, the dynamic stress placed on bone by weight-bearing exercise may be protective to the structural integrity of the stressed site.

When women develop osteopenia, they increase their risk of traumatic and stress fractures. These occurrences must be considered in the athlete presenting with new-onset pain or limitation.

EVALUATION OF THE AMENORRHEIC ATHLETE

Athletic amenorrhea remains a diagnosis of exclusion. Initial evaluation should screen for genetic, hormonal, or anatomic abnormalities. If these are absent in the athlete/patient, then education and counseling should be used to address the problem. Athletes with intercurrent problems should be referred for further evaluation.

Adolescent

When the adolescent girl presents for consultation, she frequently manifests fear of being different from her peers, oblivious to the long-term health effects of altered puberty.[8] The physician who is aware of the needs of the physically active adolescent is proactive in counseling. While recommending adequate nutrition and rest, the physician should help the patient develop an appreciation for the impact of physical activity on development. Meticulous records of growth, weight, and pubertal changes should be maintained as these will be invaluable if further evaluation is required.

The young girl may present initially with symptoms of amenorrhea or delayed puberty. In the absence of menses at age 16, the absence of secondary sex characteristics by age 13, or a delay in menses of more than 5 years from onset of thelarche or pubarche, a full evaluation should be carried out.

Family history, general medical health, and nutrition should be evaluated. Average heights and age of puberty for parents and siblings should be recorded. A complete physical examination will ascertain secondary sexual characteristics and presence of a vaginal opening. A perineal vaginal opening does not necessarily imply an intact outflow tract. Laboratory testing should initially include prolactin, thyroid-stimulating hormone, free thyroxine, LH, and FSH. A karyotype should be obtained in those with elevated FSH. A bone-age radiograph of the nondominant hand and wrist may be helpful.

In the absence of obvious abnormality, close observation for 6–12 months with alterations of activity level, attention to energy-rich nutrition, and measurement of body growth may be allowed. If abnormalities of initial screening are noted or no change occurs under observation, referral to a pediatric or endocrinologic specialist for complete workup is appropriate.

Reproductive-Age Woman

Secondary amenorrhea is the absence of menses for 6 months or three times the longest prior interval, whichever is shorter. When the athlete presents with this symptom, a detailed history should evaluate recent increase in activity level, competition, nutritional or weight changes, and general health. Pregnancy should always be considered and ruled out in the sexually active patient.

Serum prolactin and thyroid function studies should be performed to rule out endocrinopathy. In the patient with increased body weight, hirsutism, and history suggestive of chronic anovulation since puberty (irregular episodes of bleeding characterized by prolonged spotting or heavy bleeding), serum LH, FSH, dehydroepiandros-terone-sulfate, and testosterone should be evaluated for possible polycystic ovarian syndrome (PCOS). The LH-to-FSH ratio usually exceeds 2.5 to 1.0 in the PCOS patient. Androgens are in the upper normal range or slightly elevated. The athlete with PCOS may benefit from weight reduction associated with increased activity and should otherwise be managed as the usual chronic anovu-latory patient.

In the absence of hormonal abnormalities, a progestin withdrawal test (medroxyprogesterone acetate [MPA], 10 mg by mouth each day for 7 days) should establish estrogen status: those withdrawing within 10 days of com-pletion of the MPA course are euestrogenic; those fail-ing to withdraw are hypoestrogenic or may have developed an anatomic outflow obstruction, although this should be suggested by prior history.

If the patient has abnormalities of prolactin secretion, thyroid axis, or progestin withdrawal, she should be fur-ther evaluated by an appropriate specialist.

Fertility

The amenorrheic athlete occasionally seeks advice regard-ing fertility potential. If she is anovulatory with a history of normal function in the past, then appropriate modifi-cations of exercise, diet, and lifestyle should reestablish normal function. In the absence of normal physiologic ovulation, induction of ovulation with clomiphene cit-rate, human menopausal gonadotropins, or GnRH is fea-sible. These therapies are expensive, time-consuming, not guaranteed, and fraught with potential complication. Every effort should be made to regain normal function through counseling and activity modification.

Menopause

The hallmark of the menopause is cessation of follicular function and development of a hypoestrogenic state. Diag-nosis may be established by persistent elevation of serum FSH. In the menopausal woman younger than 40 years of age, evaluation for premature ovarian failure by an appropriate specialist is recommended. The menopausal-aged woman with symptoms, including vasomotor changes, vaginal dryness, and sleep disturbance, will ben-efit from counseling and direction in hormonal replace-ment and exercise modification.

THERAPY

Athletic amenorrhea is diagnosed by exclusion of other specific conditions. The first step in therapy for all patients

is education regarding the proposed diagnosis and mech-anism of occurrence. All patients, both premenarchal and adult, may be observed for a period while training regi-mens and dietary habits are altered. If no improvement in function is noted, appropriate pharmacologic treat-ment should be offered.

Delayed Puberty

When delay of onset of puberty or menarche is of suffi-cient concern to the athlete or her family, the patient should be referred to a pediatric or endocrinologic specialist. Hor-monal therapies to stimulate or simulate puberty are avail-able, but they should be undertaken only in the most strictly supervised setting. Routine use of oral contraceptives as hormone replacement should be discouraged in these ath-letes, except when required for birth control.

Estrogen Replacement: Adult

The estrogen status of amenorrheic adult athletes should always be determined. An athlete who withdraws to MPA (see section on the reproductive-age woman) requires only cyclic withdrawal stimulation. When not at risk of preg-nancy or if using adequate barrier contraception, the patient may receive a course of 10 days of MPA (10 mg per day for 10 days) every 1–2 months.

The athlete who does not withdraw requires cyclic estro-gen replacement. A regimen of conjugated estrogen, 0.625 mg on days 1 to 25 of each month, combined with MPA, 10 mg on days 16 to 25, provides adequate stimulation. In postmenopausal women, a regimen of 0.625 mg conjugated estrogen with 2.5 mg MPA daily on a continuous basis has been gaining popularity. This regimen might be useful in athletes who do not want to experience cyclic withdrawal bleeding. There is currently no report available on use of a continuous regimen in reproductive-age athletes.

Neither of the preceding regimens provides contra-ception, and patients should be warned to use adequate barrier contraceptive methods or abstain from intercourse. Sexually active athletes may use low-dose oral contra-ceptives and will receive adequate estrogen replacement; in fact, all medically eligible athletes may use oral con-traceptives for replacement therapy. All patients should be aware that if normal function returns, the first spon-taneous ovulation may occur before menses is seen, and pregnancy is possible.

Fertility

When the amenorrheic athlete desires conception, she should be extensively counseled regarding nutritional demands of pregnancy and alterations of activity level, as discussed under Physiologic and Nutritional Changes of Pregnancy. Whether these patients should be offered ovulation induction if they fail to alter their training pattern has been discussed.[9] Preconceptional modification of activity most successfully prepares the patient for pregnancy and may lead to return of normal reproductive function.

Ovulation induction with clomiphene citrate may be attempted; however, this drug is less useful in the hypoestrogenic amenorrheic population. If the patient desires further attempts at ovulation induction, referral to a specialist in reproductive endocrinology is appropriate.

Calcium

Adequate levels of calcium intake should be encouraged for all patients, especially those at risk of osteopenia. A daily intake of 1,000–1,500 mg of elemental calcium provides maximal benefit. In the absence of adequate estrogen production or replacement, however, decrements in bone mineral content will continue.

FEMALE ATHLETE TRIAD

When the physician encounters a female athlete reporting menstrual dysfunction, it is imperative that he or she be sensitive to the potentially dire health consequences that may be hidden in the athlete's history. Although the patient may readily present reporting her recognized symptom of amenorrhea, she may neither recognize nor report the frequently associated problems—eating disorders (anorexia nervosa, bulimia) and osteoporosis. This triad of eating disorders, amenorrhea, and osteoporosis has been reviewed in detail.[10] It is the role of the primary care physician to recognize the individual at risk, gain the confidence and trust of the athlete, and provide direction for counseling and treatment.

Many sports and athletic endeavors appear to benefit from low body weight. Elite gymnasts, long-distance runners, pairs skaters, and ballerinas all tend toward low body weight and reduced percent body fat. The body image that society has encouraged through recognition of fashion models and cover girls also influences the goals of many young women. Whether reduction in weight to achieve elite levels in athletics or pursuit of exercise to maintain low body weight is the primary goal, the female triad leads to markedly disordered nutritional status and will have far-reaching effects on menstruation and reproductive function and bone health.

On investigation, it is found that young women with anorexia nervosa refuse to maintain normal body weight; they have unrealistic perceptions of body image, confounded by fear of becoming fat; they have no demon-

TABLE 30-1
Behavior Indicating Possible Eating Disorder

Dieting to excess
Poor weight gain in view of diet and energy expenditure
Unnecessary exercise outside of training program
Guilt about eating
Perceived fatness at normal weight
Hoarding of food
Unnecessary attention to details of diet such as calorie content, portion size, frequency of meals
Frequent "weigh-ins"
Evidence of self-induced vomiting
Use of laxatives, diet pills, and diuretics to attempt weight control

Source: Adapted from M Putukian. The female triad: eating disorders, amenorrhea, and osteoporosis. Med Clin North Am 1994;78: 345–356.

strable endocrine or medical illness accounting for their body weight; and they will experience varying degrees of oligomenorrhea or amenorrhea. Bulimia is characterized by episodes of binge eating with intake of high-calorie, easily digested foods; surreptitious intake of food; abdominal pain, excessive sleep, or vomiting (frequently self-induced) at the conclusion of a binge; and frequent efforts to lose weight with swings in weight of more than 4.5 kg. Bulimic patients are frequently depressed after a binge, appearing aware of their abnormal eating pattern but fearing they have no control over their ability to stop the behavior.

Patients at risk for eating disorders may be recognized by many characteristic behaviors as outlined in Table 30-1. Physical findings will confirm these suspicions in many cases. Rapid weight loss and extreme fluctuations in weight, unnecessary for athletic participation, may occur; a yellowish cast to the skin, thinning hair, and presence of lanugo (childlike) hair may be recognized; and laboratory examinations may demonstrate hypoglycemia, renal dysfunction, and electrolyte disorders. The athlete may report generalized swelling, swollen salivary glands, muscle cramps, gastrointestinal distress, headaches, dizziness, or weakness. She may experience numbness or tingling in limbs that is due to metabolic disturbance. Cardiac examination may demonstrate bradycardia or arrhythmias. Accompanying osteoporosis and reduced weightbearing stress to the bones may lead to more frequent stress fractures.

When recognized, these athletes should be approached in private and encouraged to seek professional help from a specialist in eating disorders. The athlete should feel confidence that her athletic role will not be threatened by this health problem. Cooperation with parents and other support persons may be important in providing the appropriate environment for successful treatment. Appropri-

TABLE 30-2
Assessment and Treatment of Urinary Stress Incontinence in the Female

Urogynecologic evaluation
    Genitourinary history and physical examination
    Urinalysis and urine culture
    Urodynamic testing as indicated
Treatment modalities for stress incontinence
    Timed voiding and Kegel exercises
    Estrogen replacement in postmenopausal women
    Surgical pelvic relaxation repair

ate follow-up is necessary to ensure continuing therapy. It is imperative that warning signs of the female triad not be ignored.

BREAST CONDITIONS

Runner's nipple has been popularized in the literature of recreational and elite runners. Although more commonly experienced by women and during exercise that rhythmically rubs the breast and nipple against the outer garment, men may experience this condition, and it can occur in many sport activities. Many small-breasted women may elect to compete braless; in these cases, protection of the elevated nipple may become necessary. Effective measures to reduce discomfort include lubrication or covering with an adherent bandage. A well-fitted sports bra that does not give against or chafe the skin protects the nipple from abrasion in most women.

Large-breasted women who participate in sports should be encouraged to wear good support to maintain center of gravity and prevent breast trauma. Many variations of sports bras are available. These should provide excellent nonslip support. When made of synthetic materials without fasteners or seams, these bras provide comfort for most activities.

As women become more active in contact sports (soccer, rugby, field hockey, and even football), attention should be given to appropriate padding and protective garments to avoid blunt trauma to the breast.

URINARY INCONTINENCE IN THE ACTIVE FEMALE

Urinary incontinence is uncommon in the young nulliparous female athlete, but it occurs more frequently in parous and older women. It is a frequent symptom of women presenting to gynecologic clinics. Surveys have shown that as many as 10–25% of women experience some

degree of clinically significant urinary incontinence.[11] Incontinence increases in incidence with age and is associated with menopause, childbearing, and obstetric injury to the pelvic floor. As the demographics of society change, with relatively larger numbers of the female population reaching menopause, urinary incontinence is anticipated to increase as a health concern among women. This problem is compounded by the increasingly active lifestyle of women, even in older age groups. Exercise, such as running, golf, tennis, aerobics, and even walking, may exacerbate urinary incontinence during physical activity to such a degree that a woman is unable to participate.

In the premenopausal woman who experiences urinary incontinence during physical exercise, a gynecologic consultation is recommended. This consultation should include a complete gynecologic examination of the lower genitourinary tract, possibly including urodynamic testing. Incontinence secondary to pelvic floor relaxation may be treated satisfactorily in some cases with timed voiding and Kegel exercises.[12] Kegel described in 1956 that by daily exercising of the pubococcygeal muscles, stress urinary incontinence may be eliminated or minimized in some women.

Postmenopausal women may experience urinary incontinence associated with decreasing serum estrogen levels. Adequate estrogen replacement is recommended and may be adjunctive for treating incontinence in this age group. Urinary incontinence in many women cannot be adequately treated, however, short of surgical pelvic repair for incontinence caused by anatomic stress. Surgery should be considered only after evaluation of the incontinence has been completed and other nonsurgical approaches have been deemed inappropriate (Table 30-2). Successful medical or surgical treatment for urinary incontinence allows women to return to physical activity without fear of significant urinary incontinence during exercise.

PHYSIOLOGIC AND NUTRITIONAL CHANGES OF PREGNANCY

Not infrequently, an athletically active woman who finds herself pregnant turns to her physician for guidance regarding the level of intensity and type of physical activities advisable during pregnancy. It has been well demonstrated that pregnancy alters the basic physiologic functioning of a woman in a number of significant ways. Increased nutritional requirements and changes in cardiopulmonary function are of particular concern. In establishing a physical training schedule, the health care practitioner must consider baseline changes in maternal physiologic functioning to avoid potential deleterious effects on her and the fetus.

Resting heart rate, blood volume, and cardiac output during pregnancy all significantly exceed nonpregnant values.[13] Pritchard,[14] in a study of 50 normal pregnant women, found that total blood volumes near term gestation averaged approximately 45% above their nonpregnant levels. The amount of change varied considerably, with some women demonstrating little change and others almost doubling their blood volumes. Artal and colleagues[15] reported that even at rest, pregnancy increased tidal volume, oxygen consumption, carbon dioxide production, and the respiratory exchange ratio. These basic maternal metabolic function increases coupled with nutritional requirements for appropriate maternal weight gain and fetal growth have led the Food and Nutrition Board to recommend a daily dietary caloric increase of 300 kcal throughout pregnancy.[16] In addition to a baseline daily calorie increase, most authorities recommend a multivitamin and mineral supplement during pregnancy and lactation. Iron supplementation is particularly needed in the last half of gestation (after week 20) to provide for increasing pregnancy and fetal demands on maternal iron stores. Thus, it is particularly important that pregnant athletes who already have increased dietary requirements to support their physical training regimen ensure that they increase their caloric, mineral, and vitamin intake appropriately for promoting maternal and fetal well-being. Table 30-3 lists special nutritional needs of pregnant women.[17] The pregnant woman should avoid any activities that require weight reduction or fluid restriction during competition, training, or recreational exercise.

A gradual average weight gain of 9–13 kg is recommended during pregnancy. Women who are 15% or more below their ideal body weight before pregnancy are at greater risk of preterm labor. Adequate dietary intake and weight gain are especially important during the gestational course to optimize the pregnancy outcome.

EXERCISE GUIDELINES DURING PREGNANCY

Regular exercise is to be encouraged in healthy women with uncomplicated pregnancies. In some cases, highly trained, competitive athletes will experience pregnancy during periods of rigorous training or competition. Management of the elite athlete has been reviewed.[18] Certain precautions should be followed to ensure continued fetal and maternal well-being.

Before instituting any regular exercise program during pregnancy, a full physical examination and a medical history should be obtained early in gestation and regular prenatal care instituted. Specific medical conditions are problematic for exercise in pregnancy (Table 30-4). Avoidance of high-impact exercise programs or sports is necessary during pregnancy. Low-impact aerobic exercise is generally well tolerated by healthy pregnant women and their fetuses. No prospective evidence demonstrates a need to reduce exercise intensity during pregnancy. Women should guide the intensity of exercise by their prior level of training and symptoms of fatigue. Because of reduced aerobic capacity in pregnancy, the gravida should guard against exercising to a state of exhaustion. Guidelines for exercise in pregnancy, adapted from the current Technical Bulletin of the American College of Obstetricians and Gynecologists, are found in Table 30-5.[19]

During pregnancy, the workload placed on articulating surfaces and ligamentous attachments increases with

TABLE 30-3
Special Nutritional Needs of Pregnant Women

Nutritional Need	Average Daily Required Increases
Kilocalories	Nonpregnant baseline plus 300 calories
Protein	12% of daily total calories
Elemental iron	>30 mg
Calcium	>400 mg
Folic acid	>0.4 mg
Prenatal multivitamin supplement with 100% RDA	1 tablet daily
Alcohol	Absolutely contraindicated

RDA = recommended dietary allowance, established in 1989.[17]

TABLE 30-4
Contraindications to Exercise in Pregnancy

Absolute
    Incompetent cervix or cerclage
    Ruptured amniotic membrane
    Risk of preterm labor
    Treatment of preterm labor
    Hypertensive disease of pregnancy
    Fetal growth retardation
Relative*
    Essential hypertension
    Thyroid disease
    Pulmonary disease
    Vascular disease (e.g., thrombophlebitis, recent pulmonary embolism)

*May engage in medically supervised program.
Source: Adapted from American College of Obstetricians and Gynecologists. Exercise during Pregnancy and the Postpartum Period. Technical Bulletin No. 189. Washington, DC: American College of Obstetricians and Gynecologists, 1994.

TABLE 30-5
Guidelines for Exercise in Pregnancy

Mild to moderate exercise may be continued. Regular exercise (three or more periods per week) is preferable to intermittent training.

Intensity of exercise should be modified based on maternal symptoms.

No exercise should be performed in the supine position after the fourth month of gestation is completed. Prolonged motionless standing should be avoided.

Exercise requiring balance should be limited as body changes of pregnancy alter the center of gravity in the woman. Activities that increase the risk of falls or abdominal trauma should be avoided.

Exercises that use the Valsalva maneuver are discouraged.

Caloric intake should be adequate to meet the extra energy needs of pregnancy and the requirements for the exercise.

Maternal core temperature should not exceed 38°C (100.4°F). Clothing and environments should be considered in allowing dissipation of heat. Saunas and hot tubs should be avoided.

Postpartum return to the nonpregnant physiologic state may require 4–6 weeks. Prepregnancy regimes should be resumed gradually as these changes occur.

Source: Adapted from American College of Obstetricians and Gynecologists. Exercise during Pregnancy and the Postpartum Period. Technical Bulletin No. 189. Washington, DC: American College of Obstetricians and Gynecologists, 1994.

advancing gestation and maternal weight gain. Special precautions should be taken by the exercising gravida. Each exercise activity should begin with a 10- to 15-minute warm-up period and conclude with a similar cool-down period. Some authorities believe excessive stretching should be avoided in pregnancy.[20] Relative ligamentous relaxation of joints in advancing pregnancy makes it unwise to pursue excessive weightbearing activities, such as weight training. Active training programs should be reduced in intensity or eliminated at any time they result in joint, muscular, visceral, or soft tissue pain during pregnancy. A sound, commonsense approach under proper medical supervision is needed to avoid maternal or fetal harm. Periodic assessment of fetal growth by regular prenatal care and appropriate antenatal fetal testing is recommended in all women who are regularly exercising during pregnancy.

Postpartum exercise programs should be initiated under medical supervision and begun slowly. After uncomplicated vaginal delivery, modest exercising can usually begin safely after the first postpartum week. Exercise after cesarean birth should begin only after appropriate medical consultation and generally no earlier than 4–6 weeks after delivery.

REFERENCES

1. Yen SSC. Female hypogonadotropic hypogonadism: hypothalamic amenorrhea syndrome. Endocrinol Metab Clin North Am 1993;22:29–58.
2. Elias AN, Wilson AF. Exercise and gonadal function. Hum Reprod 1993;8:1747–1761.
3. Bonen A. Exercise-induced menstrual cycle changes: a functional, temporary adaptation to metabolic stress. Sports Med 1994;17:373–392.
4. DiFiori JP. Menstrual dysfunction in athletes: how to identify and treat patients at risk for skeletal injury. Postgrad Med 1995;97:143–156.
5. Red RL (ed). Interactions between lifestyles, environment, and the reproductive system. Semin Reprod Endocrinol 1990;8:1–96.
6. Lebrun CM. Effect of the different phases of the menstrual cycle and oral contraceptives on athletic performance. Sports Med 1993;16:400–430.
7. Drinkwater BL, Nilson K, Chestnut CH III, et al. Bone mineral content of amenorrheic and eumenorrheic athletes. N Engl J Med 1984;311:277–281.
8. White CM, Hergenroeder AC. Amenorrhea, osteopenia and the female athlete. Pediatr Clin North Am 1990;37:1125–1141.
9. Abraham S, Mira M, Llewellyn-Jones D. Should ovulation be induced in women recovering from an eating disorder or who are compulsive exercisers? Fertil Steril 1990;53:566–568.
10. Putukian M. The female triad: eating disorders, amenorrhea, and osteoporosis. Med Clin North Am 1994;78:345–356.
11. NIH Consensus Conference. Urinary incontinence in adults. JAMA 1989;261:2685–2690.
12. Kegel AH. Stress incontinence of urine in women: physiologic treatment. J Int Coll Surg 1956;25:487–499.
13. Porter M, Nobel HB, Gerbie AB. Exercise in Pregnancy. In JJ Sciarra (ed), Gynecology and Obstetrics (Vol 2). Philadelphia: Lippincott, 1990.
14. Pritchard JA. Changes in the blood volume during pregnancy and delivery. Anesthesiology 1965;26:393–399.
15. Artal R, Wiswell R, Romem Y, Dorey F. Pulmonary responses to exercise in pregnancy. Am J Obstet Gynecol 1986;154:378–383.
16. National Research Council. Recommended Daily Allowances (10th ed). Washington, DC: National Academy Press, 1989.
17. Commission on Life Sciences, National Research Council. Diet and Health. Washington, DC: National Academy Press, 1989:64–73.
18. Hale RW, Milne L. The elite athlete and exercise in pregnancy. Semin Perinat 1996;20:277–284.
19. American College of Obstetricians and Gynecologists. Exercise During Pregnancy and the Postpartum Period. Technical Bulletin No. 189. Washington, DC: American College of Obstetricians and Gynecologists, 1994.
20. Artal (Mittelmark) R, Wiswell RA, Drinkwater BL. Exercise in Pregnancy (2nd ed). Baltimore: Williams & Wilkins, 1991:306.

31

Sports Oncology: Tumors in the Athlete

J. DAVID PITCHER, JR.

The last thing on the athlete's mind is the thought of being slowed down by a benign or malignant neoplasm. Likewise, the health care provider who treats musculoskeletal disorders should be acutely aware of the signs and symptoms of these disorders to facilitate early diagnosis, treatment,[1] and return to full activities if possible. When the athlete is diagnosed with a neoplasm, the publicity and the questions asked are often overwhelming.

Errors in diagnosis of malignancies can be devastating.[2] Common mistakes fall into two categories: (1) information-gathering errors, which include failure to recognize pain referred from a more proximal location, failure to adequately expose a patient to allow thorough observation and palpation, failure to obtain or review studies that will lead to the proper diagnosis, and failure to recognize a sports-related injury bringing attention to an underlying neoplasm's existence[1]; and (2) patient management errors, which include failure to refer or obtain consultation early and a misplaced biopsy (usually done outside the referral center).

The plain radiograph is the most useful study to obtain when bone is involved, and it can be diagnostic in some soft tissue lesions. Normal variations should not be confused with tumors, and many benign lesions need only periodic clinical and radiologic follow-up. Four initial questions should be answered when evaluating these lesions:[3]

1. Is the lesion large and what is its location? Generally, anything larger than 5 cm has a higher chance of being in an aggressive or malignant stage (Table 31-1).[4] Various lesions have characteristic locations within the bone.
2. What is the lesion doing to the host bone or soft tissues? Permeative or infiltrating patterns are indicative of high-grade neoplasms.

3. What is the host tissue doing to the lesion? If the lesion is slow growing, it will be walled off. Quick-growing lesions will not be contained by the host's response.
4. Is there a soft tissue mass or matrix being produced in the lesion?

The answers to these questions are further refined with other studies, such as the bone scan, computed tomography (CT), and magnetic resonance imaging (MRI), but the plain radiograph guides the workup and determines its expediency (Figures 31-1 and 31-2).

Primary musculoskeletal malignancies are termed *sarcomas*. These are distinguished from *carcinomas*, which arise from glandular or epithelial tissues. Both benign and malignant musculoskeletal tumors can be classified according to histologic type. An exhaustive review of all these lesions is beyond the scope of this chapter, but most common lesions are briefly described here, along with general principles to follow.

THE YOUNG ATHLETE

Nonossifying Fibroma and Fibrous Cortical Defect

Nonossifying fibroma and fibrous cortical defect is usually an incidental finding on radiographs taken for minor trauma. These lesions may occur in as many as 30% of patients, and knowledge of the radiographic early bubbly and later sclerosing patterns will alleviate anxiety on the part of the athlete's parents. Formal reading of the radiographs and consultation with the radiologist is always advisable.[5] The eccentric, metaphyseal, lucent nonossifying fibroma and smaller cortical equivalent

TABLE 31-1
Staging of Musculoskeletal Neoplasms

Benign	Malignant
Stage 1: Benign latent	IA: Low-grade, intracompartmental
	IB: Low-grade, extracompartmental
Stage 2: Benign active	IIA: High-grade, intracompartmental
	IIB: High-grade, extracompartmental
Stage 3: Benign aggressive	IIIA: Low-/high-grade, intracompartmental with metastases
	IIIB: Low-/high-grade, extracompartmental with metastases

(fibrous cortical defect) need only plain radiographic monitoring every 3–4 months until proved stable, then at increasing intervals thereafter. Typical locations include the distal femur, proximal or distal tibia, or proximal fibula. The large lesion may present with a pathologic fracture or impending fracture that may need curettage and bone grafting.

Simple Bone Cyst

The young athlete involved in upper-body activities may present with a pathologic fracture through a proximal humeral-metaphyseal, expansile, lucent, simple bone cyst. Lesions occurring in the proximal femur pose an extremely difficult problem for the treating physician. Often, the lesion is of extreme enough size to warrant curtailment of athletic activities to prevent a devastating femoral neck or subtrochanteric fracture. Bone scanning and often MRI are warranted to determine biologic activity and to differentiate from the rare telangiectatic variant of osteosarcoma. Aspiration and steroid injection are often successful, although curettage and grafting may be needed in the larger at-risk (for fracture)

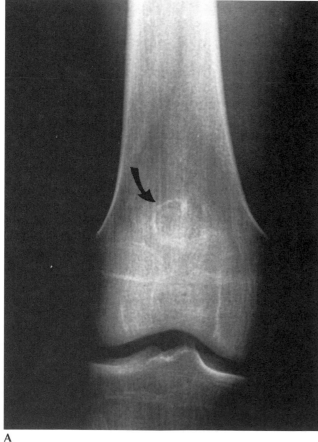

A

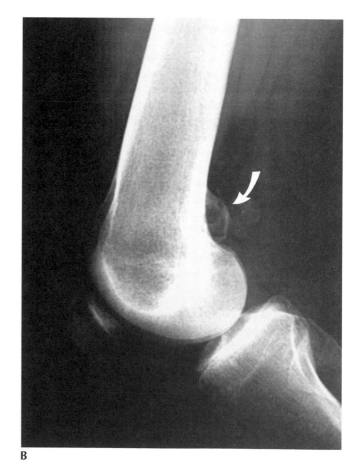

B

FIGURE 31-1

Plain radiographs (anteroposterior [A] and lateral [B]) of a distal femur in a U.S. Marine reveals the popliteal mass (arrows). From the x-ray alone, intramedullary and extraosseous involvement can be determined, a cartilage matrix can be determined, and the diagnosis of chondrosarcoma can be tentatively made. With this probable diagnosis, the expediency of further staging studies can be related to the patient, insurance companies, and radiologists involved in the case.

femoral lesions. Lesions rarely heal after fracture without surgical treatment.[6-8]

Osteochondroma

The athlete reports a painful distal femoral or subdeltoid mass exacerbated by running or overhead activities. Plain radiographs define the protruding metaphyseal to diaphyseal bony lesion, which can be sessile or pedunculated. Lesions may develop bursae beneath the adjacent structures, such as the iliotibial band, and become symptomatic. Bone scans should be obtained to determine the activity of the lesion and to identify multiple lesions so that monitoring can be planned.[5] If necessary, the pathognomonic intramedullary connection of the lesion to the host bone can be demonstrated with CT. Other, less common locations include the proximal tibia and scapula. Large lesions (cartilage cap more than 2 cm in thickness) or axial lesions (including scapular and pelvic lesions) should be removed because of the potential for low-grade malignancy.

Osteoid Osteoma

Because the osteoid osteoma often occurs in the lower extremities, its misdiagnosis as a stress fracture or shin

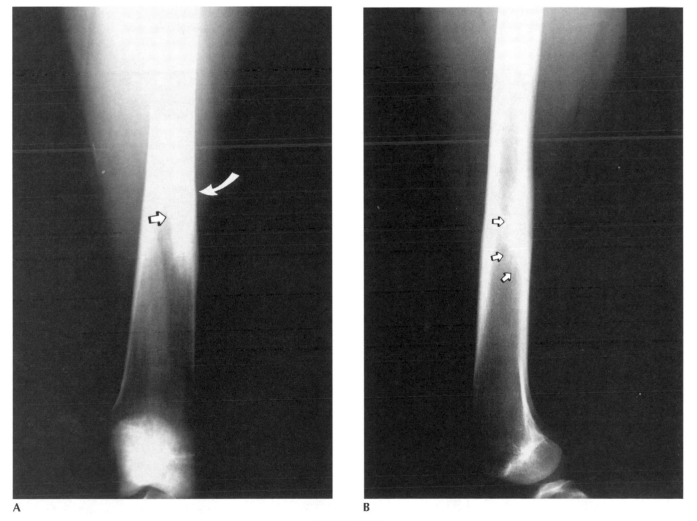

A   **B**

FIGURE 31-2

Plain radiographs (anteroposterior [A] and lateral [B]) of a distal femur in a runner reveals a blastic intramedullary lesion in a diaphyseal location (arrows). The differential diagnosis includes osteosarcoma, lymphoma, and infection. A lesion such as this should not be confused with that of a stress fracture. A magnetic resonance imaging and bone scan were promptly obtained, and a biopsy confirmed the unusual diagnosis of primary lymphoma of bone. A high index of suspicion is required to avoid costly delays in diagnosis and treatment.

splint delays definitive treatment. The characteristic night pain or pain relieved with aspirin can often be elicited with a careful history. Lesions occurring in the spine can be associated with scoliosis. Because of the vascularity of the lucent nidus (surrounded by reactive sclerotic bone), increased uptake on bone scan and increased density measurements of the nidus on CT with contrast, compared with noncontrast CT, can secure the diagnosis. Interest in the medical management of osteoid osteoma, particularly in difficult-to-excise locations, has shown promise.[5, 6]

Ewing's Sarcoma

Characteristically diaphyseal to metadiaphyseal in long bones, particularly the femur, Ewing's sarcoma usually presents with a soft tissue mass and often a destructive, permeative to moth-eaten radiographic picture (Figure 31-3). A layered periosteal reaction is often a late finding and is termed "onion skinning." An expeditious workup that includes a bone scan to rule out bony metastases, a chest x-ray film, chest CT, and MRI or CT of the lesion should be obtained. It is wise to consult an orthopedic oncologic surgeon as soon as the diagnosis is suspected to avoid repeating a study because of variations in methods of performing the sequences. The patient can be systemically ill, particularly in advanced stages, mimicking infection.[3, 5, 9]

THE SKELETALLY MATURE ATHLETE

Enchondroma

Typically, enchondroma is an incidental finding. If painful, the lesion is termed *atypical*. There are usually intra-

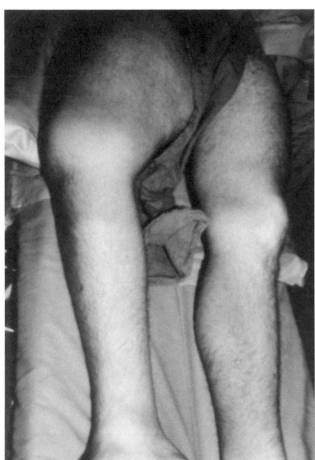

A

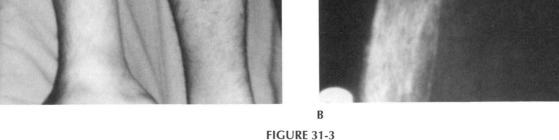

B

FIGURE 31-3

A. Clinical photograph at the time of biopsy in an adolescent athlete. More than 1 year of knee pain referred from the proximal femur had allowed the overlooked bone to weaken sufficiently to fracture. Alarmingly, a diagnostic knee arthroscopy had been performed. B. Pathologic fracture of the proximal femur with characteristic aggressive destructive pattern of Ewing's sarcoma.

FIGURE 31-4

Algorithm for evaluation of suspected bone and soft tissue tumors after a thorough history and physical examination. (CXR = chest x-ray; CT = computed tomography; MRI = magnetic resonance imaging.)

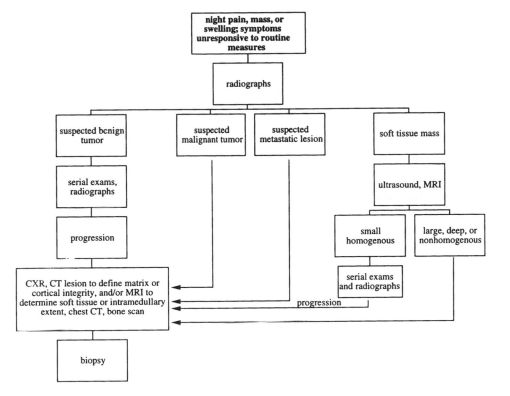

medullary nodules of calcification within a diaphyseal or metadiaphyseal lesion, which may be predominantly lucent with cortical scalloping or expansion. The athlete may present with a pathologic fracture of the phalanx or metacarpus from a blow or jamming injury. These fractures usually heal, and curettage and grafting can later be curative. A bone scan should be obtained to rule out multiple lesions and CT or MRI used in the case of large or atypical lesions. Lesions larger than 5 cm should be treated, but smaller asymptomatic lesions need only monitoring for radiographic or symptomatic change. Differentiation of an atypical enchondroma from a low-grade chondrosarcoma can be difficult even in the most capable of hands.[3, 5]

Giant Cell Tumor

Pain without fracture is the presenting symptom among the vast majority of patients with giant cell tumor. The distal femur and proximal tibia are characteristically involved. The remarkably lucent and expansile epimetaphyseal lesions can become quite large and extend to the articular cartilage. Rarely, the lesions metastasize to the lungs or other bones, so chest x-ray films and bone scans are always indicated. MRI demonstrates intramedullary extent and presence of any soft tissue mass before curettage. Various treatment options are available, including cryotherapy or phenolization in lesions in which the bony

architecture is maintained. Reconstructive measures with allografts or megaprostheses may be needed in advanced lesions or recurrent disease. Long-term surveillance is warranted to detect late recurrences.[4, 5, 10, 11]

Osteosarcoma

Advances in imaging techniques and adjuvant and neoadjuvant chemotherapy have made limb-salvage techniques possible in the second most common and most varied primary bone tumor, osteosarcoma. Occurring in low- and high-grade variants, from intramedullary to juxtacortical locations, any lesion with bone formed as a matrix must include this lesion in the differential. Most lesions occur in the femur and around the knee in the young adult, but a wide age group can be affected and all locations are possible. The bone scan shows uptake and rules out metastases, and both MRI and CT provide useful information. The MRI must also include the entire bone to rule out skip metastases, best seen in short tau inversion recovery and gadolinium-enhanced images. Chest x-ray films and CT should be obtained before biopsy, because chest CT after anesthesia shows atelectasis, which is difficult to differentiate from small metastatic foci. The biopsy should be done by the surgeon performing the resection to avoid a high rate of complications.[12, 13] An algorithmic approach can be helpful in avoiding pitfalls (Figure 31-4).

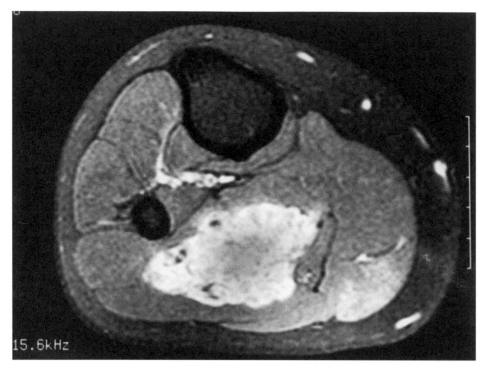

FIGURE 31-5
T2-weighted magnetic resonance image in a young female swimmer. A blow to the calf caused intralesional hemorrhage of a large hemangioma of the soleus. A biopsy was required and an eventual excision because of continued symptoms.

Lipoma and Hemangioma

Soft tissue tumors must never be taken for granted unless they are biopsy proved. Pain is not indicative of malignancy but is more likely a result of pressure on an adjacent nerve, inflammation in the reactive zone of a tumor, necrosis, or invasion of the adjacent periosteum. A lipoma characteristically has a lucent soft tissue shadow on plain radiographs. Hemangiomas may have soft tissue phlebolith calcifications. Both may occur in the thigh or shoulder regions, interfering with vigorous athletic endeavors. MRI defines the lipoma on T1-weighted images, and T2-weighted images reveal the vascularity of the hemangioma (Figure 31-5). Vascular channels and an infiltrative pattern may be difficult to differentiate from a soft tissue sarcoma in the hemangioma. Large lipomas should be excised, and hemangiomas should be biopsied or excised when the diagnosis is in doubt or symptoms are present. More than 270 types of benign and malignant soft tissue lesions have been classified.[14] It behooves the health care provider to be cognizant of and ready to present to the athlete a logical plan when confronted with the common question, "What's this?"

THE SENIOR ATHLETE

Metastatic Carcinoma

No older athlete is without concern about the abrupt end of activities by cancer. Lung, breast, and prostate carcinomas present in so many ways that they must be considered with any atypical pain. Warning signs should be kept in mind: (1) a previous history of cancer, family history of cancer, or history of smoking; (2) pain unresponsive to a short period of rest; or (3) night pain. The spine is often affected because of vascular drainage. The workup should include examination of the most likely sites for a primary lesion, such as the breast or prostate. Prophylactic fixation of an impending fracture may allow the previously active individual to avoid a completely sedentary lifestyle. The prognosis after metastasis to bone has occurred remains poor, except in breast and prostate carcinomas, which may respond to chemotherapy.[3, 5]

The most difficult diagnoses to differentiate are vertebral compression fractures that are due to metastatic cancer to bone and those that are due to osteoporosis. Because of marrow edema in both instances, MRI is not always able to definitively exclude malignancy. Nuclear bone scanning can be helpful if widespread bony disease is already present, but this is not common in the senior athlete, and a biopsy will often be requested by the orthopedic consultant after all other studies.

Multiple Myeloma

The most common primary bone tumor is multiple myeloma and its less common solitary lesion, the plasmacytoma. Characteristically lucent on plain radiographs, the lesion may present as an impending or pathologic fracture (Figure

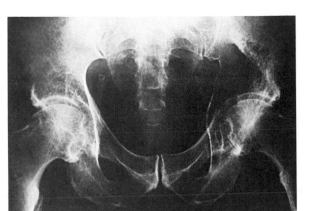

FIGURE 31-6

Hip pain was the presenting symptom in an elderly avid walker. The lucency in the ilium is typical for a plasmacytoma. When multiple lesions are present, multiple myelomas or metastatic lung or breast carcinomas are prime differentials.

31-6). Bone scans are frequently negative, because this process primarily involves osteoclastic activities, and the technician labels osteoblasts. Hypercalcemia should be ruled out as a life-threatening complication. Serum and urine protein electrophoresis should be obtained in addition to the standard laboratory tests (Table 31-2). Painful lesions, particularly in the spine, respond to radiation therapy. Impending fractures can be prophylactically fixed with intramedullary rods, either before or after radiation.[3, 5, 15]

Malignant Fibrous Histiocytoma and Liposarcoma

These two most common soft tissue sarcomas occur most commonly in the thigh. For the runner, skier, or other athlete, it is difficult to imagine how some of these lesions become as large as they do and remain undetected by the patient. It must be remembered that the doubling time for sarcomas is approximately 30 days, however, and as soon as suspected, the soft tissue sarcoma should be expeditiously evaluated. Because metastases occur in the lung and skeleton, chest x-ray films, chest CT, and bone scan, as well as MRI of the lesion, are indicated. If other symptoms are present, they should not be dismissed until metastases are ruled out. The long-term survival depends on the grade and size of the lesion.[14, 16, 17]

SUMMARY

The health care provider will only rarely encounter an athlete with a malignant lesion. However, night pain, a mass

TABLE 31-2

Laboratory Tests Recommended as Part of the Evaluation of Most Musculoskeletal Tumors

Study	Usefulness
Complete blood count	Elevated in leukemia, infection, malignancies associated with anemia
Erythrocyte sedimentation rate	Screening for myeloma, infection
Blood urea nitrogen	Elevated in renal osteodystrophy
Calcium	Elevated in metastatic disease and metabolic bone disease
Creatinine	Elevated in renal osteodystrophy
Urinalysis	Evaluation of myeloma and renal adenocarcinoma
Phosphorus	Elevated in metabolic bone disease
Alkaline phosphatase	Elevated in Paget's disease, metastatic disease, osteosarcoma
Lactate dehydrogenase	Elevated in osteosarcoma
Serum protein electrophoresis and immunoprotein electrophoresis	Elevated in multiple myeloma

or swelling with or without tenderness, or symptoms unresponsive to conservative modalities may be "red flags." Appropriate early studies and subsequent consultation are paramount to successful treatment of these disorders. Awareness of the basic principles and more common tumors can expedite return to athletic endeavors, if a return is possible.

REFERENCES

1. Damron TA, Sim FH. Soft-tissue tumors about the knee. J Am Acad Orthop Surg 1997;5:141–152.
2. Lewis MM, Reilly JF. Sports tumors. Am J Sports Med 1987;15:362–365.
3. Enneking WF. Clinical Musculoskeletal Pathology. Gainesville, FL: Storter Printing, 1986.
4. Enneking WF. A system of staging musculoskeletal neoplasms. Clin Orthop 1986;204:9–24.
5. Mirra JM, Picci P, Gold RH. Bone Tumors: Clinical, Radiologic, and Pathologic Correlations. Philadelphia: Lea & Febiger, 1989.
6. Healey JH, Ghelman B. Osteoid osteoma and osteoblastoma: current concepts and recent advances. Clin Orthop 1986;204:76–85.
7. Campanacci M, Capanna R, Picci P. Unicameral and aneurysmal bone cysts. Clin Orthop 1986;204:25–36.
8. Kaelin AJ, MacEwen GD. Unicameral bone cysts: natural history and the risk of fracture. Int Orthop 1989;13:275–282.
9. Neff JR. Nonmetastatic Ewing's sarcoma of the bone: the role of surgical therapy. Clin Orthop 1986;204:111–118.
10. Eckardt JJ, Grogan TJ. Giant cell tumor of bone. Clin Orthop 1986:204:45–58.

11. Campanacci M, Baldini N, Boriani S, Sudanese A. Giant-cell tumor of bone. J Bone Joint Surg Am 1987;69:106–114.
12. Simon MA. Current concepts review: limb salvage for osteosarcoma. J Bone Joint Surg Am 1988:70:307–310.
13. Yasko AW, Lane JM. Current concepts review: chemotherapy for bone and soft-tissue sarcomas of the extremities. J Bone Joint Surg Am 1991;73:1263–1271.
14. Sim FH, Frassica FJ, Frassica DA. Soft-tissue tumors: diagnosis, evaluation, and management. J Am Acad Orthop Surg 1994;2:202–211.
15. Goodman MA. Plasma cell tumors. Clin Orthop 1986;204: 86–92.
16. Lang TA. The Evaluation of a Soft-Tissue Mass in the Extremities. In JS Barr Jr (ed), Instructional Course Lectures. Park Ridge, IL: American Academy of Orthopaedic Surgeons, 1989;38:391–398.
17. Makley JT. Preoperative Staging Techniques for Soft-Tissue Neoplasms. In JS Barr Jr (ed), Instructional Course Lectures. Park Ridge, IL: American Academy of Orthopaedic Surgeons, 1989;38:399–405.

Index